Delmar's Radiographic Positioning & Procedures

Volume II: Advanced Imaging Procedures

Cynthia Cowling, BSc, MEd, MRT(R), ACR

Director of Program Development
The Michener Institute for Applied Health Sciences
Toronto, Ontario Canada

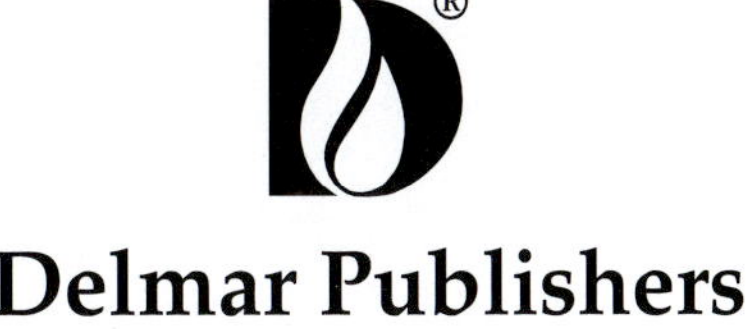

Delmar Publishers

an International Thomson Publishing company 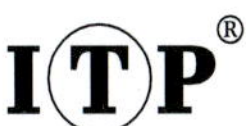

Albany • Bonn • Boston • Cincinnati • Detroit • London • Madrid
Melbourne • Mexico City • New York • Pacific Grove • Paris • San Francisco
Singapore • Tokyo • Toronto • Washington

Notice to the Reader

Cover Design: Bill Finnerty

Delmar Staff

Publisher: Susan Simpfenderfer
Acquisitions Editor: Marlene McHugh Pratt
Developmental Editor: Melissa Riveglia
Project Editor: William Trudell
Art and Design Coordinator: Rich Killar
Production Coordinator: Cathleen Berry
Marketing Manager: Darryl L. Caron
Editorial Assistant: Maria Perretta

Printed in the United States of America

For more information, contact:

Delmar Publishers
3 Columbia Circle, Box 15015
Albany, New York 12212-5015

International Thomson Publishing Europe
Berkshire House 168-173
High Holborn
London WC1V 7AA
England

Thomas Nelson Australia
102 Dodds Street
South Melbourne, 3205
Victoria, Australia

Nelson Canada
1120 Birchmount Road
Scarborough, Ontario
Canada, M1K 5G4

International Thompson EditoresCampos
Eliseos 385, Piso 7
Col Polanco
11560 Mexico D F Mexico

International Thomson Publishing GmbH
Konigswinterer Strasse 418
53227 Bonn
Germany

International Thomson Publishing Asia
221 Henderson Road
#05-10 Henderson Building
Singapore 0315

International Thomson Publishing—Japan
Hirakawacho Kyowa Building, 3F
2-2-1 Hirakawacho
Chiyoda-ku, Tokyo 102
Japan

1 2 3 4 5 6 7 8 9 10 XXX 03 02 01 00 99 98 97

Library of Congress Cataloging-in-Publication Data

Delmar's radiographic positioning and procedures.
p. cm.
Contents: v. 1. Basic positioning and procedures / [edited] by Joanne S. Greathouse—v. 2. Advanced imaging procedures / [edited] by Cynthia Cowling.
ISBN 0-8273-6782-1 (v. 1. : alk. paper).—ISBN 0-8273-6317-6 (v. 2. : alk. paper)
1. Radiography, Medical—Positioning. I. Greathouse, Joanne S. II. Cowling, Cynthia. III. Title: Radiographic positioning and procedures.
[DNLM: 1. Technology, Radiologic. 2. Posture. WN 160 D359 1997]
RC78.4.D44 1997
616.07'572—DC21
DNLM/DLC
for Library of Congress

97-43449
CIP

Contents in Brief

Contents in Detail

Preface

When I trained many years ago, I learned the art and science of radiography, reasonably confident that my knowledge would help keep me employed for the next 30 years or so. The graduate of today is exposed to a bewildering array of imaging modalities in existence and changes so rapid it is impossible to write a text that can guarantee to be on the cutting edge of all of them. It is becoming increasingly important, however, that radiography graduates be prepared for the variety of imaging in the field.

This volume is designed to provide the depth needed to learn about advanced imaging procedures and the breadth required to function within the concept of the diagnostic imaging environment.

It quickly became evident that the specialized nature of these procedures required the expertise of many individuals. We also realized that radiography knows no geographic boundaries and so we were able to work with contributors from three major countries: the United States, Canada, and Australia. As author and contributors worked through the chapters, other experts in such areas as anatomy, computers, computed tomography, ultrasound, magnetic resonance imaging, and radionuclide imaging were consulted to ensure relevance, currency, and accuracy until the numbers involved with the content of the book more than tripled. A 1-year project blossomed into a 3-year project, with the author and contributors always aware of the passage of time where future trends become everyday realities and routine procedures become rarities. All valued the importance of sufficient information to make this entire subject understandable. We believe that a good balance has been achieved and that graduates who wish to pursue additional studies as well as those wishing to remain within the confines of radiography will be well served by this text.

The text begins with an overview of those areas associated with advanced imaging procedures such as equipment, the use of computers in imaging, contrast media, the responsibilities of the technologist, and the care of the patient.

The design of the remainder of the chapters reflects the changing focus in health care and uses a body systems-based approach. Each chapter outlines the relevant anatomy, provides a brief historical overview of the special studies performed in the area, and then lists some of the more common reasons and pathologies for performing these studies. The description of the procedures themselves is written in a clear and concise manner, allowing the student to translate that information into the clinical environment. It assumes that the student and imager are concerned for the ongoing well-being of the patient and outlines any specific postprocedure care. Please also note that all elements are not applicable for each procedure. Review questions and case studies provide an opportunity for students to confirm that they have understood the information given. To assist students with visualization of the described content, over 500 illustrations (line drawings, photographs, and images) are provided in the text.

In addition to the text, an ancillary slide series has been developed to meet educators' needs for quality visual aids. A student workbook, which correlates closely with the text, assists students in organizing their study of the topic and provides additional opportunities for self-checks during the learning process.

The resultant text heralds the new multidisciplinary approach to imaging for the technologist and the hope is that students studying from this text will be challenged and prepared for their own future and the future of their chosen profession.

Acknowledgments

I would like to thank all the contributors who toiled long and hard to collect data and images for this text. I would also like to thank all those other colleagues, friends, and students who poured through film libraries and labored over computers creating all manner of images. In particular, I would like to mention Lorraine Ramsay, Tara Meneses, and St. Joseph's Hospital in Toronto; Rose Dileo and Toronto East General Hospital; Lilace Hudson and Mt. Sinai Hospital in Toronto; and Andrew Renner and The Royal Adelaide Hospital, South Australia.

The author and Delmar Publishers wish to express their appreciation to a dedicated group of professionals who reviewed and provided commentary at various stages. Their insights, suggestions, and attention to detail were very important in guiding the development of this textbook.

Paul Bober, EdD, RT(R)(ARRT)
Instructor, Radiology Department
Labette Community College
Parsons, Kansas

Jacklynn Darling, MS, RT(R)(M)(ARRT)
Associate Professor, Radiologic Technology Program
Morehead State University
Morehead, Kentucky

Mark Hagy, MS, RT(R)(ARRT)
Assistant Professor, Radiologic Technology Program
East Tennessee State University
Elizabethton, Tennessee

Emily Hernandez, MS, RT(R)(ARRT)
Director and Associate Professor of Radiologic Science
Indiana University
Indianapolis, Indiana

Christine Mehlbaum, BS, RT(R)(ARRT)
Instructor, Radiography Department
Penn State University
Schuylkill Campus
Schuylkill Haven, Pennsylvania

Michelle Miller, MEdRT(R)(M)(ARRT)
Program Coordinator, Radiography
Champlain College
Burlington, Vermont

Anita Phillips, BS, RT(R)(ARRT)
Program Director, Radiographic Technology
Wake Technical Community College
Raleigh, North Carolina

Barbara Smith, BS, RT(R)(ARRT)
Instructor, Radiologic Technology
Portland Community College
Portland, Oregon

Gary Watkins, PhD, RT(R)(ARRT)
Associate Professor, Department of Radiographic Sciences
Idaho State University
Pocatello, Idaho

An initiative of this nature has demonstrated again to me that the radiography profession is filled with caring, compassionate people and I am proud to be associated them all.

A special thank you must go to the project team at Delmar Publishers—Marlene Pratt, Melissa Riveglia, Rich Killar, Bill Trudell, Cathleen Berry, and Darryl Caron.

No text of this nature can be completed without the help and support of employers. The Michener Institute has supported my endeavors from the very start of this project.

And finally, but most importantly, a debt of thanks goes to my family, Ian and Andrew. None of us realized the time and effort this text would require and I thank them for their support, patience, and love throughout its development.

Cynthia Cowling, BSc, MEd, MRT(R), ACR

Contributors

Dennis Bair, AS, RT (R)(CV)(ARRT)
Supervisor of Angiography
Medical College of Wisconsin
Milwaukee, Wisconsin

Ron Bentley, BSc, MRT
Senior Anatomy Instructor
The Michener Institute for Applied Sciences
Toronto, Ontario Canada

Pamela Bonnert, BS, RDMS
Clinical Instructor
St. Luke's School of Diagnostic Sonography
St. Luke's Medical Center
Milwaukee, Wisconsin

Bronwyn Chapple, MIR
Chief Radiographer/Manger
South Australian Breast X-Ray Service
Wayville, South Australia

Susan Cleverly, MRT(R)
Senior Technologist, Angiography
The Toronto Hospital
Toronto, Ontario Canada

Cynthia Cowling, BSc, MEd, MRT(R), ACR
Director of Development
The Michener Institute for Applied Health Sciences
Toronto, Ontario Canada

Mary Susan Helene Crowley, MRT(R)(ARRT)
Instructor
The Michener Institute for Applied Health Sciences
Toronto, Ontario Canada

Holly Engle, RT(R)(CV)(ARRT), RCVT
Formerly at Bakersfield Memorial Hospital
Bakersfield, California

Michael Glisson, DipAppSci, RMelbIT, MAppSci, Monash
Head of School of Medial Radiation Science
Charles Sturt University
Wagga Wagga, NSW
Australia

Mary J. Hagler, MHA, BA, RT(R)(N)(M)(ARRT)
Clinical Coordinator
Cabrillo College
Aptos, California

Carolyn Kaut Roth, RT(R)(MR)(ARRT)
Director of MRI Technologist Program
University of Pennsylvannia Medical Center
Philadelphia, Pennsylvania

Evelyn Kelly, BSc, MA, RN, MRT(R)
Senior Instructor
The Michener Institute for Applied Health Sciences
Toronto, Ontario Canada

Peter Lloyd, DCR, ARMIT, Grad Dip, FEd
Former Lecturer at the University of South Australia
School of Medical Radiations
Adelaide, South Australia

Nancy Macklin, MRT(R)
Charge Technologist
The Wellesley Hospital
Toronto, Ontario Canada

Patricia McDonald, MRT(R)
Senior Technologist, GI Intervention
The Toronto Hospital
Toronto, Ontario Canada

Gail Rodrigues, MRT(R), RDMS
Senior Instructor
The Michener Institute for Applied Health Sciences
Toronto, Ontario Canada

Marsha Sorter, MHE, RT(R)(M)(N)(ARRT)
Assistant Professor of Radiology
Midwestern State University
Wichita Falls, Texas

HOW TO USE THIS TEXT

Delmar's Radiographic Positioning and Procedures, Volume II: Advanced Imaging Procedures is designed for and provides an opportunity for the learner to gain a better understanding of advanced procedures and comparative imaging. The text has many unique features which will make it easier for you to learn and integrate theory and practice, including:

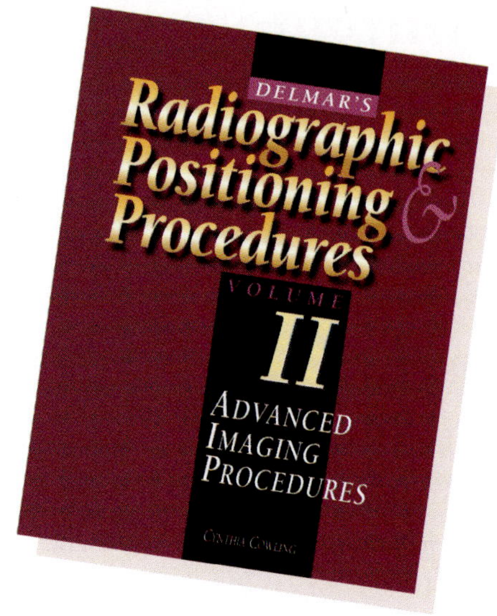

CHAPTER 3

Specialized Studies of the Skeletal System

CYNTHIA COWLING, BSc, MEd, MRT(R), ACR

INTRODUCTION AND HISTORICAL OVERVIEW
ANATOMY
Bone Formation and Composition
Articulations
The Vertebral Column
PROCEDURES
Arthrography
Arthrography of the Knee
Arthrography of the Hip
Arthrography of the Temporomandibular Joint
Arthrography of the Shoulder
Other Arthrographic Studies
OTHER IMAGING MODALITIES
Computed Tomography
Magnetic Resonance Imaging
Ultrasound
Radionuclide Imaging
OTHER SPECIALIZED SKELETAL STUDIES
Metastatic Survey
Long Bone Measurement
Scoliosis
Bone Density Measurement
Bone Age
INTERVENTIONAL PROCEDURES
Bone Biopsy

OBJECTIVES
At the completion of this chapter, the student should be able to:
1. Describe the procedures used in the diagnostic studies of the skeletal system as listed.
2. Describe the bony anatomy of all relevant areas of study.
3. List the major indications and reasons for performing the studies listed.
4. Compare the resultant images provided in the various imaging modalities used in each stu...
...ss safe practice procedures for each examina-
7. Identify common radiographic appearances of resultant images for each procedure.
8. List usual contrast media used, if any, for each procedure.
9. Identify appropriate patient care practice...

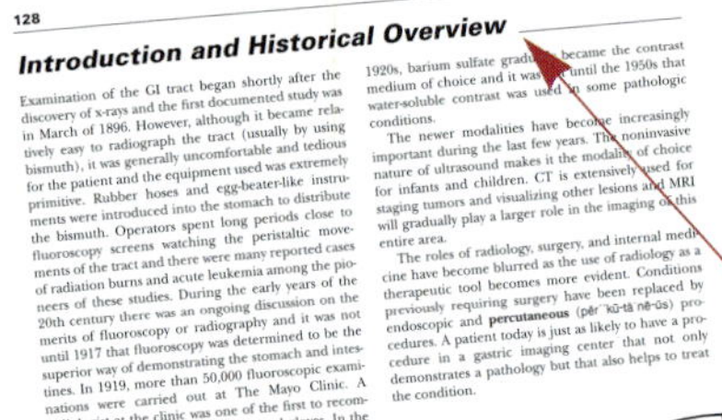

GASTROINTESTINAL SYSTEM 4

128

Introduction and Historical Overview

Examination of the GI tract began shortly after the discovery of x-rays and the first documented study was in March of 1896. However, although it became relatively easy to radiograph the tract (usually by using bismuth), it was generally uncomfortable and tedious for the patient and the equipment used was extremely primitive. Rubber hoses and egg-beater-like instruments were introduced into the stomach to distribute the bismuth. Operators spent long periods close to fluoroscopy screens watching the peristaltic movements of the tract and there were many reported cases of radiation burns and acute leukemia among the pioneers of these studies. During the early years of the 20th century there was an ongoing discussion on the merits of fluoroscopy or radiography and it was not until 1917 that fluoroscopy was determined to be the superior way of demonstrating the stomach and intestines. In 1919, more than 50,000 fluoroscopic examinations were carried out at The Mayo Clinic. A radiologist at the clinic was one of the first to recommend the use of protective aprons and gloves. In the 1920s, barium sulfate gradu... became the contrast medium of choice and it was ... until the 1950s that water-soluble contrast was used in some pathologic conditions.

The newer modalities have become increasingly important during the last few years. The noninvasive nature of ultrasound makes it the modality of choice for infants and children. CT is extensively used for staging tumors and visualizing other lesions and MRI will gradually play a larger role in the imaging of this entire area.

The roles of radiology, surgery, and internal medicine have become blurred as the use of radiology as a therapeutic tool becomes more evident. Conditions previously requiring surgery have been replaced by endoscopic and **percutaneous** (pĕr´kū-tā nē-ŭs) procedures. A patient today is just as likely to have a procedure in a gastric imaging center that not only demonstrates a pathology but that also helps to treat the condition.

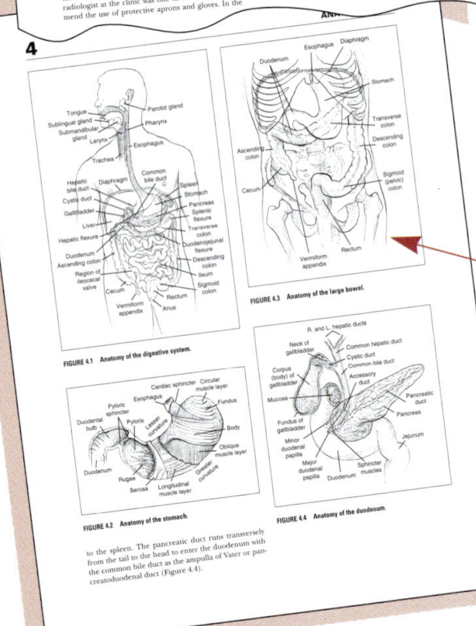

FIGURE 4.1 Anatomy of the digestive system.

FIGURE 4.2 Anatomy of the stomach.

FIGURE 4.3 Anatomy of the large bowel.

FIGURE 4.4 Anatomy of the duodenum.

Chapter Outline

1 At the beginning of each chapter is an outline listing the main headings covered within the chapter. Review these headings of topic areas before you study the chapter. They'll be a roadmap to the material in the chapter.

Objectives

2 Learning objectives identify the key information to be gained from the chapter. Use these objectives, together with the review questions, to test your understanding of the chapter's content.

Introduction and Historical Overview

3 This section provides a brief historical overview of the special studies performed for the particular body-system chapter.

Anatomy

4 Each body system chapter includes an overview of the structure and function of that particular system. Line drawings with labels help differentiate human structures and organs and explain physiological processes. The full-color anatomy and physiology figures, which can be found near the front of the text for easy reference, further assist you in visualizing and understanding anatomy and physiology concepts.

Key Terms

5 Important terms to know are presented in bold throughout the text. These terms are defined in the glossary at the end of the text. Phonetic spellings follow terms that may be difficult to pronounce the first time they appear in the text.

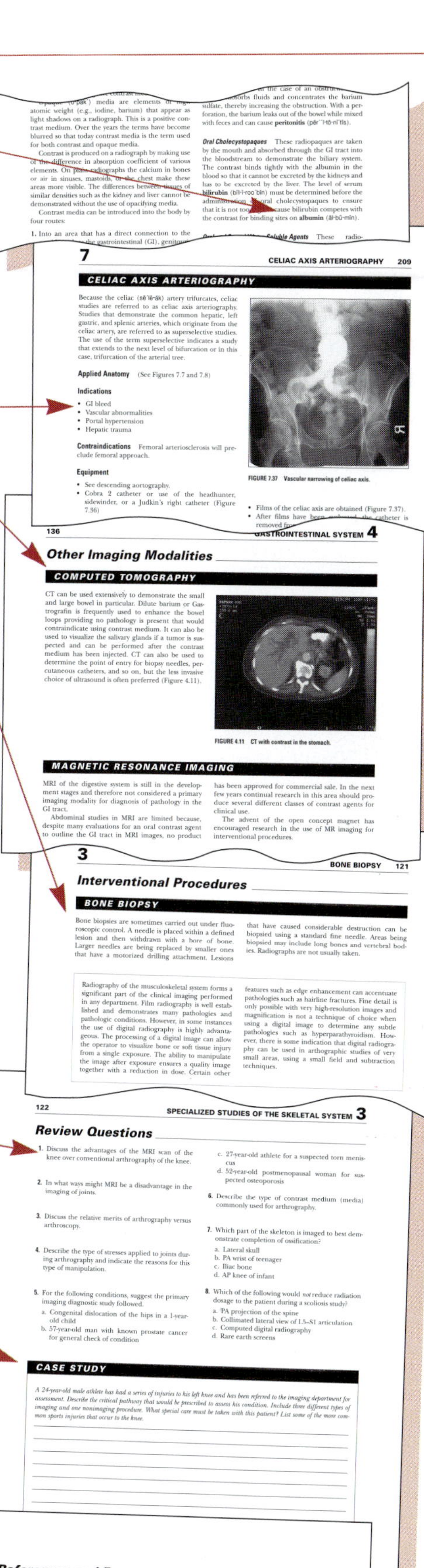

Procedures

6 The procedures are presented in an easy-to-follow bulleted format. Many photographs, images, and line art are included in the procedures section to help clarify the concepts presented.

**Preliminary Radiographs* and *Patient Preparation* describe how to prepare before the actual examination. *Indications* and *Contraindications* outline reasons for doing the procedure. *Equipment* and *Contrast Media* list exactly what is needed for the procedure, and *Radiation Protection* advises how to minimize the dose to the patient. The procedure itself is covered under *Procedure Sequence, Procedure Radiographs, Alternative Radiographs*, and *Post Procedure Care*. Some *Common Pathologies* visualized during a specific procedure are also listed.

*Modalities for each body system are presented within each body system chapter, allowing for comparison of the different imaging modalities.

* Interventional procedures are also indicated for each body system.

Review Questions

7 Various types of review questions are presented to test your knowledge of the chapter content.

Case Studies

8 The case studies provide a critical thinking scenario for you to put your knowledge of the chapter content into practice.

References and Recommended Reading

9 This listing includes both the references used in each chapter and additional sources for further study.

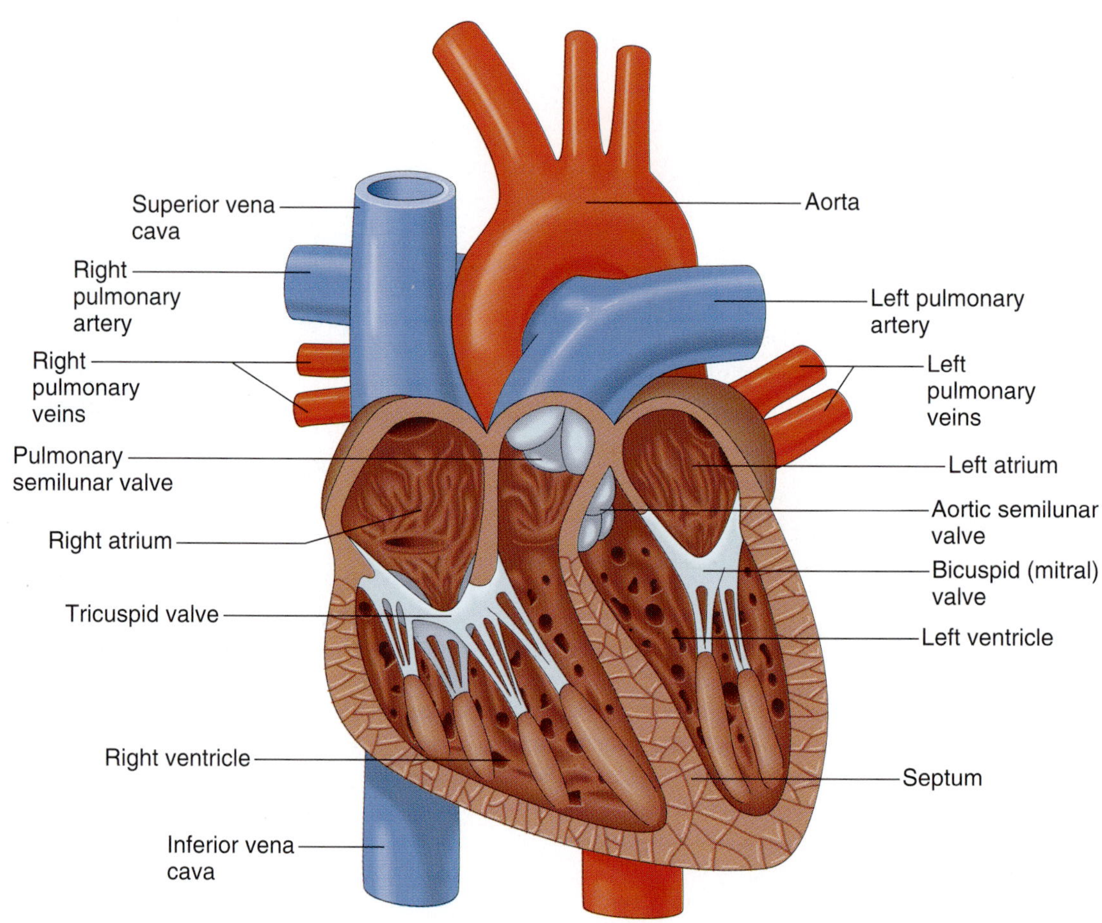

ILLUSTRATION 1 Anterior Internal View of Heart

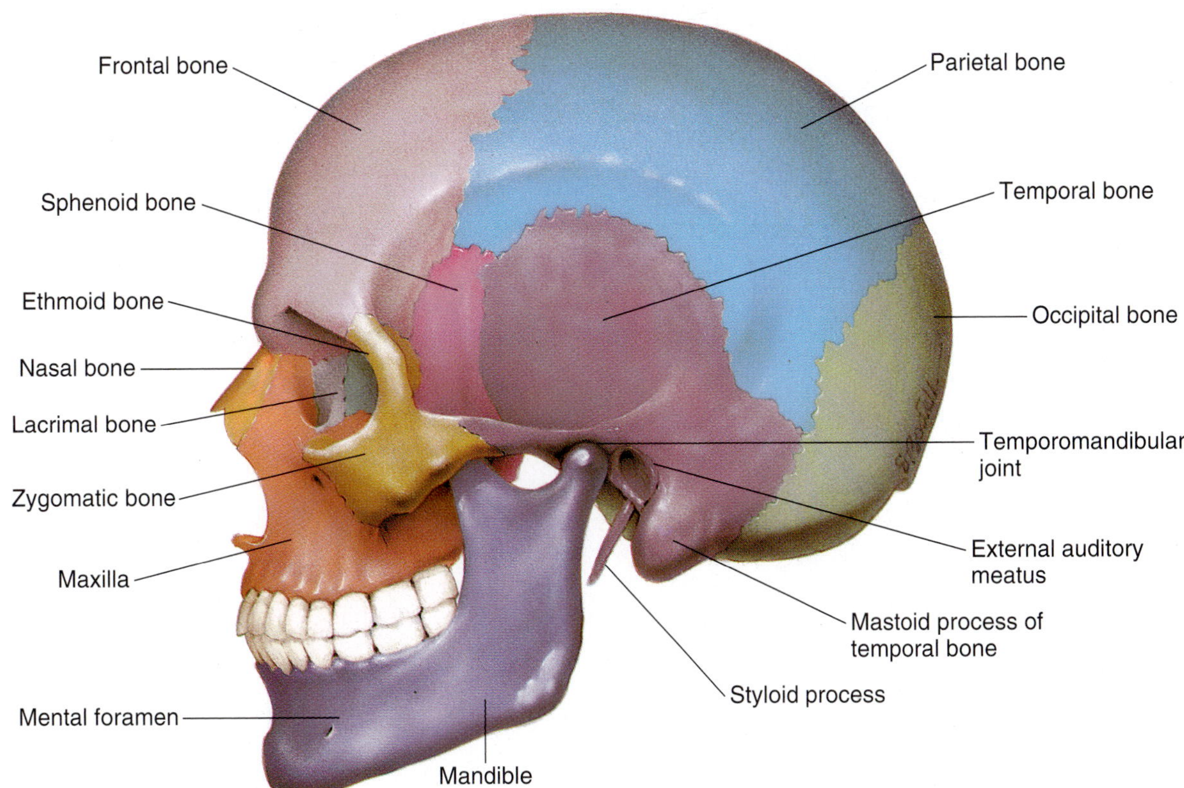

ILLUSTRATION 2 Lateral View of Skull

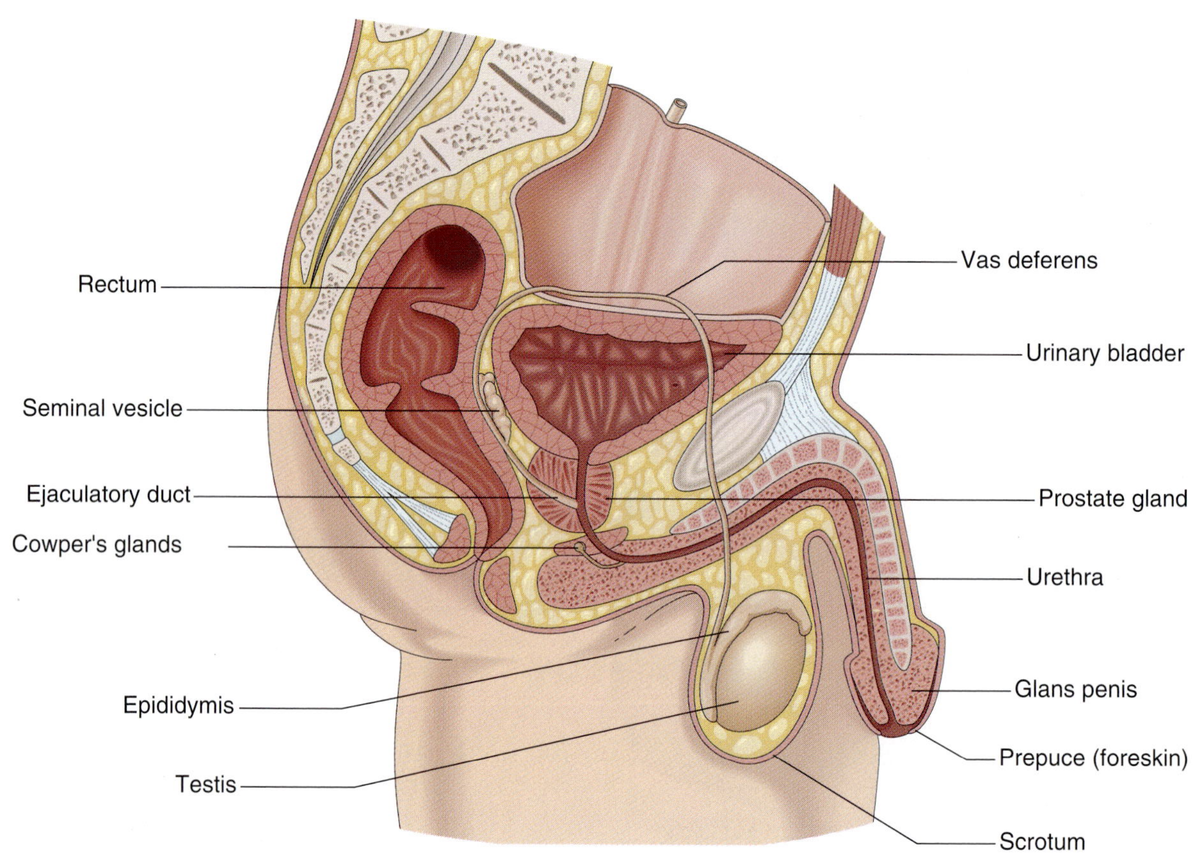

ILLUSTRATION 3 Male Reproductive System

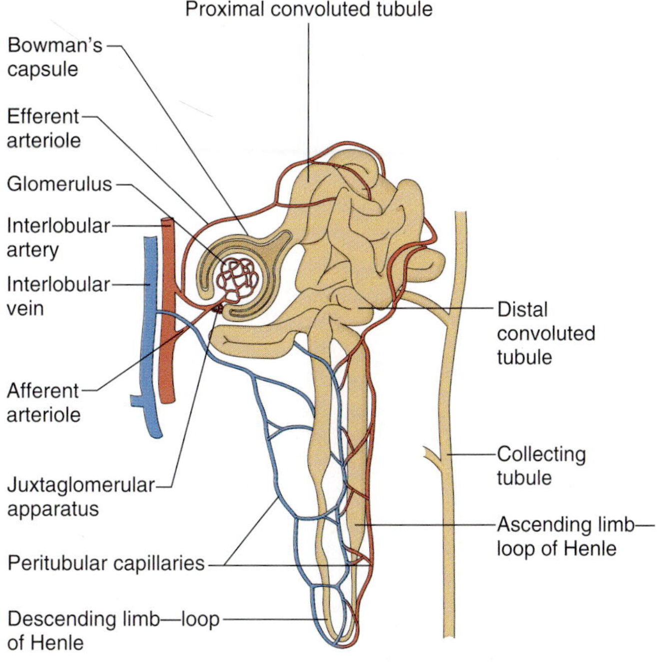

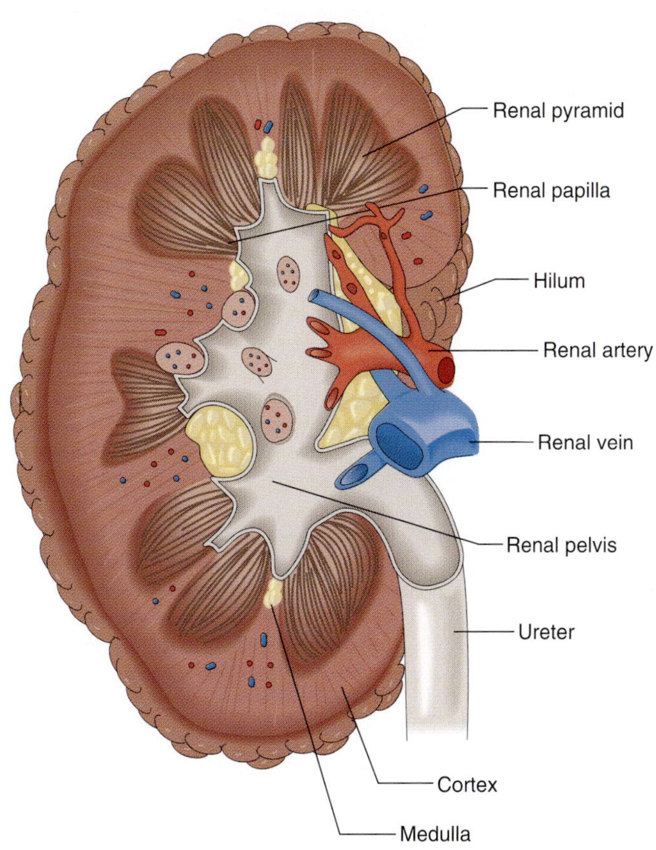

ILLUSTRATION 4 Nephron and Sagittal Section of Kidney

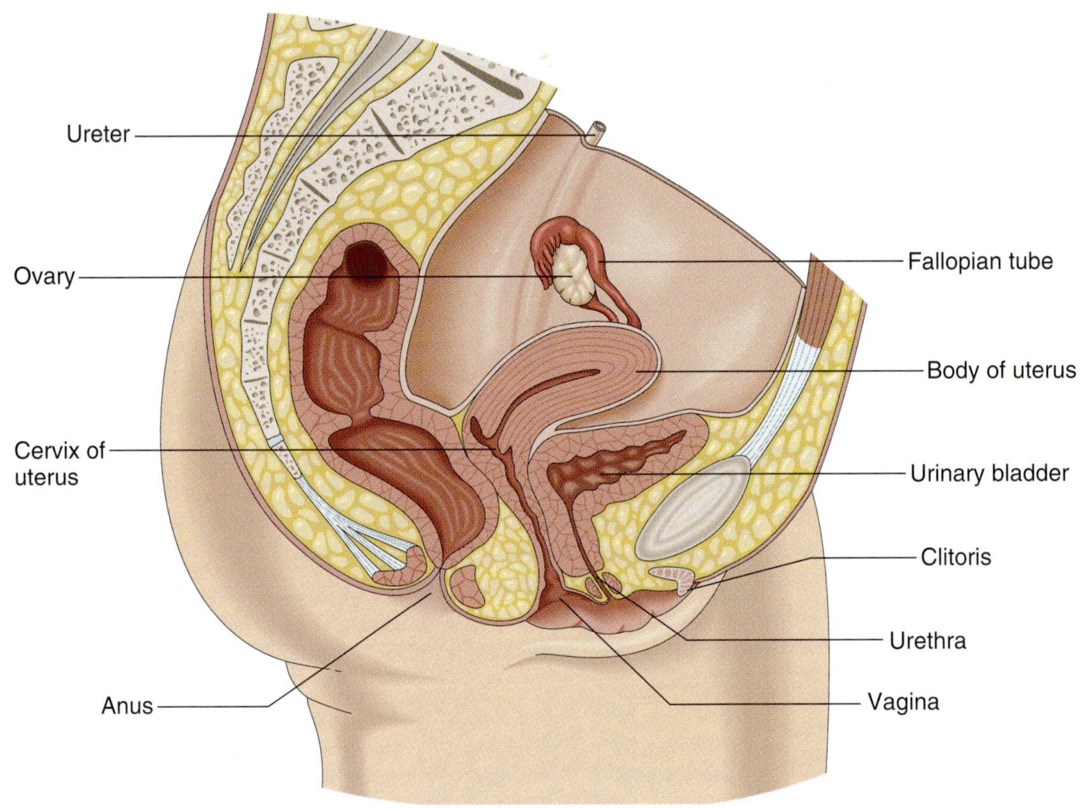

ILLUSTRATION 5 Female Reproductive System

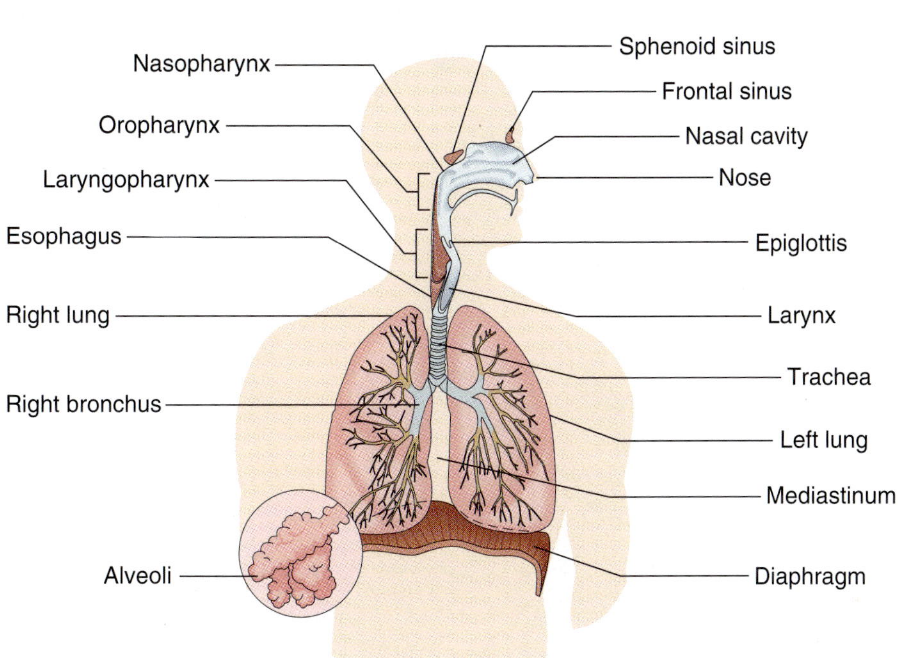

Respiratory System

ILLUSTRATION 6 Respiratory System

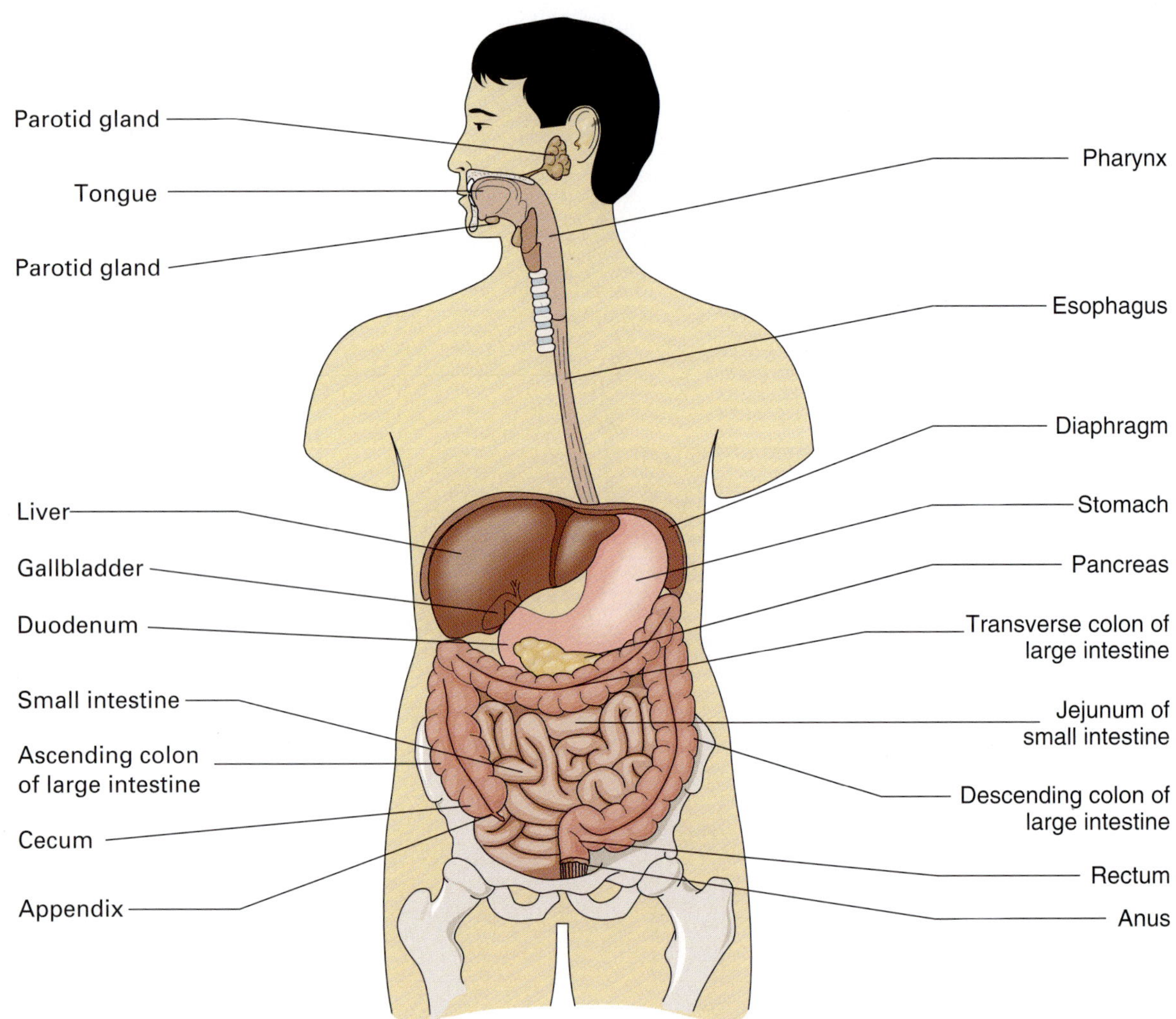

ILLUSTRATION 7 Digestive System

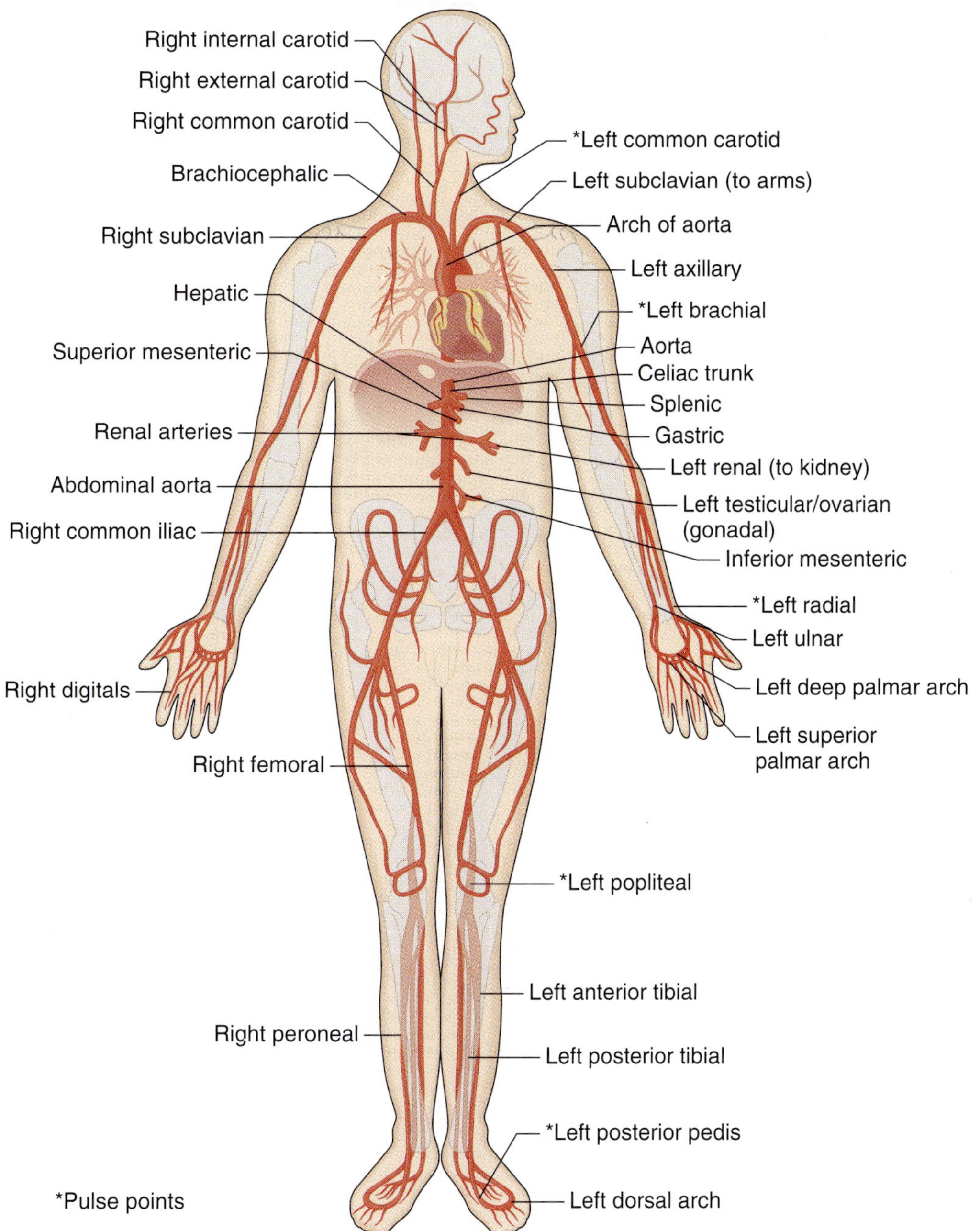

ILLUSTRATION 8 Arterial Distribution

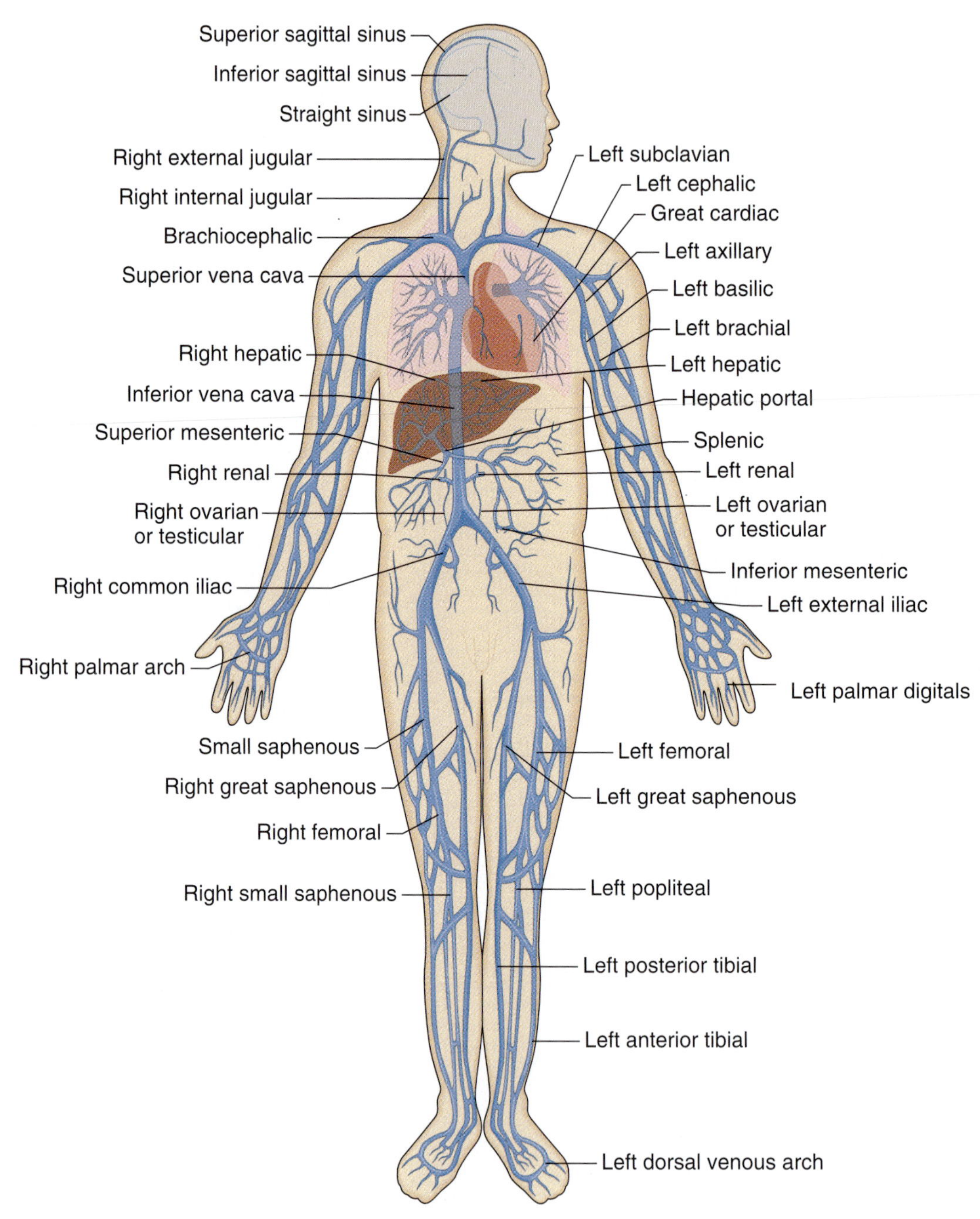

ILLUSTRATION 9 Venous Distribution

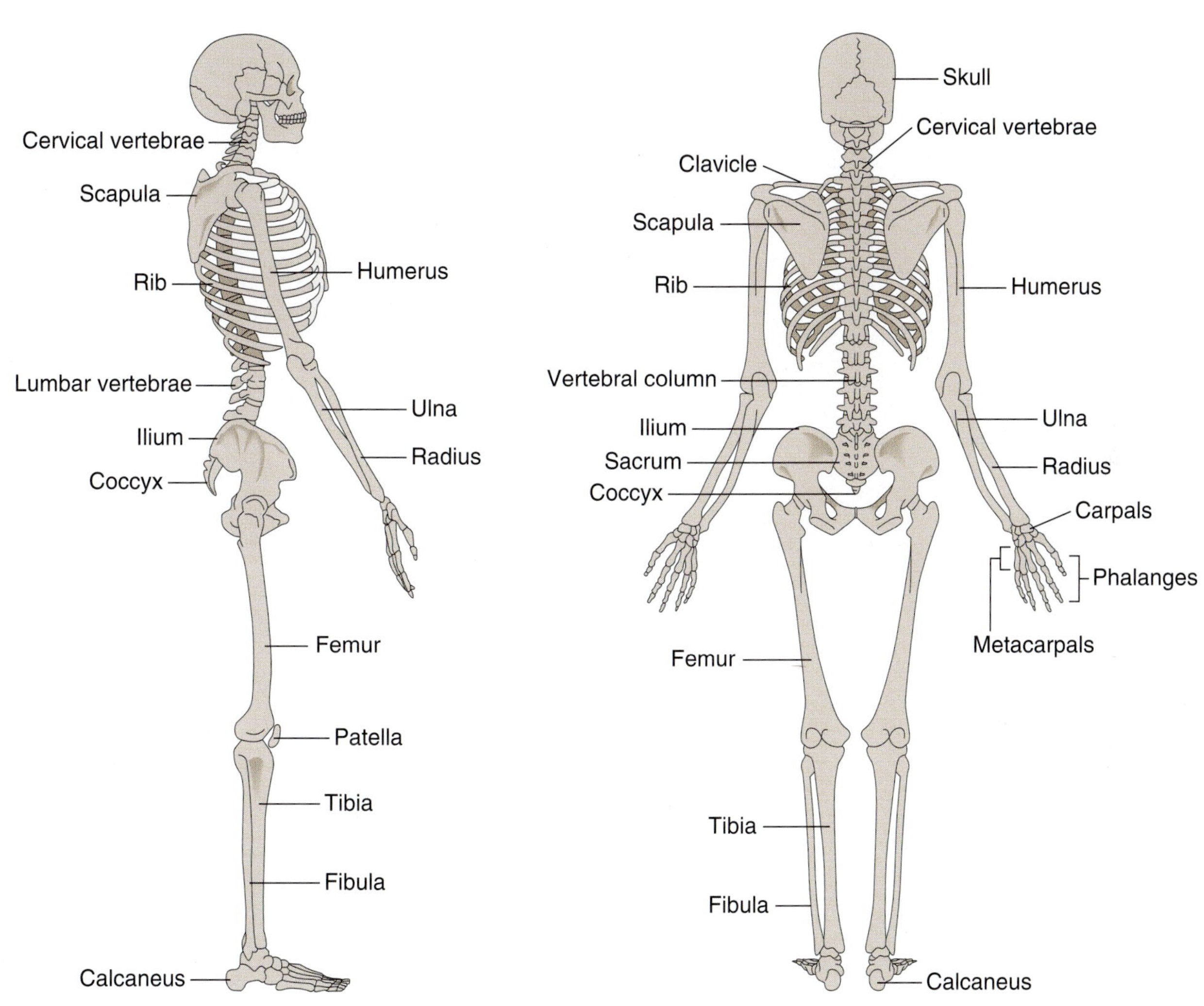

ILLUSTRATION 10 Skeletal System

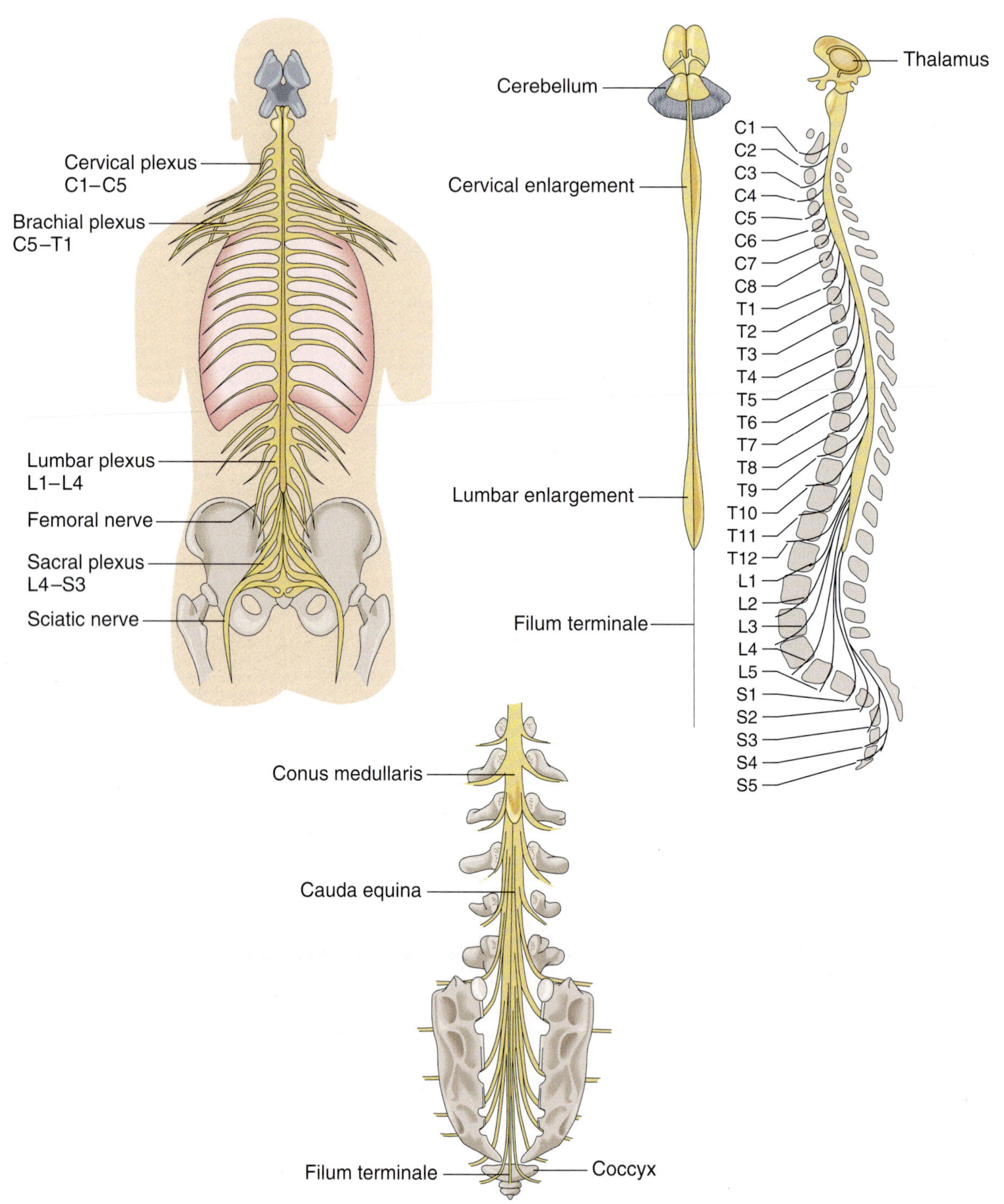

ILLUSTRATION 11 Spinal Cord and Nerves

SECTION I

INTRODUCTION to RADIOGRAPHIC and IMAGING PROCEDURES

CHAPTER 1

Introduction to Diagnostic and Interventional Procedures

SUSAN CLEVERLY, MRT(R)
NANCY MACKLIN, MRT(R)
EVELYN KELLY, BSc, MA, RN, MRT(R)
CYNTHIA COWLING, BSc, MEd, MRT(R), ACR

OBJECTIVES

At the completion of this chapter, the student should be able to:

1. List the main tasks of the technologist during any procedure.
2. Define contrast media.
3. List the different types of contrast media.
4. Compare nonionic with ionic water-soluble agents.
5. List the secondary effects of contrast media.
6. List other drugs used in an imaging department.
7. Describe the different methods of administration.
8. List precautions required when administering contrast media.
9. Describe the role of the technologist involved with the use and administration of medication.
10. Describe the historical development of interventional radiology.
11. List the main types of interventional techniques used.
12. Describe the uses of embolization.

Introduction

This is a text for and about radiologic technologists and deals with the special procedures frequently performed for diagnosis and sometimes for treatment. It describes the role and function of technologists working in the special suites, describes the type of care each patient should receive, and provides an overview of equipment and drugs used. This text, however, goes one step further and describes the other imaging modalities, demonstrating how they so frequently interrelate. The primary focus is radiography but each section also includes some of the studies performed using other modes of imaging. It provides an introduction to the increasingly complex era of sophisticated and highly technical equipment and procedures.

Historically, each imaging modality has been considered a separate entity, particularly for technologists. Radiographers studied angiography, nuclear medicine technologists studied gamma camera scans, and even within imaging departments, although these areas might be immediately adjacent to each other, the procedures carried out within these rooms were often unknown to technologists working elsewhere.

Each area is complex and does require a special focus. However, it is becoming increasingly important that technologists working in imaging departments become more familiar with their colleagues' procedures down the hall. They are, after all, working with and caring for the same patients! This book has been written for students technologists who need to know a good deal about the special procedures involving x-radiation and something about the other modalities that often form a complement to the studies they perform.

The second unique feature of this book is that the studies are grouped under anatomic and functional systems. In an effort to eliminate technologic barriers, each system has a listing of many of the imaging procedures performed, with an emphasis on x-radiation. This means that students learning about the biliary system will discover that although stones can be visualized in the operating room under fluoroscopic control using x-radiation, these same stones may already have been demonstrated using ultrasound or nuclear medicine. Furthermore, they will learn that certain radiologic procedures currently performed can resolve signs and symptoms without the need for extensive surgery.

Each chapter highlights the history, anatomy, equipment, patient care, and procedures undertaken. The first two chapters provide a background for imaging modalities and technologic advancements that have made special procedures possible. Although the text does not attempt to be comprehensive by including *everything* the student needs to know to perform special procedures, it does give an understanding of this growing area and provides the interested student with the knowledge to pursue each section further.

The care of the patient is fundamental to the role of the technologist, and nowhere is this more important than during special procedures. These examinations involve complex equipment, often large and intimidating. Studies frequently involve lengthy stays in the imaging room; invasive procedures often carry a higher risk and usually require an explanation to the patient and a signed consent form. This chapter examines the role of the technologist in special procedures, extremely important medicolegal issues, the pharmacology of contrast media and its effects and uses, and an overview of interventional procedures, a relatively new area that requires the highest level of patient care.

Role of the Technologist in Specialized Imaging and Procedures

Susan Cleverley, MRT(R) and Nancy Macklin, MRT(R)

The technologist working in special imaging and procedures is an integral part of a highly qualified team. Working with the radiologist and nurse, these technologists provide imaging to aid in the patient's diagnosis or treatment, and they offer visual assistance during interventional procedures.

The scope of the technologist's practice will vary from institution to institution, but expertise is essential to ensure that procedures are carried out efficiently and safely. Like radiologic technologists in any environment, they are expected to maintain a professional and ethical manner and to respect patient confidentiality.

EDUCATIONAL BACKGROUND

This text is not intended to provide the student with all the knowledge, skills, and attitudes needed to work at an experienced level in a special department or computed tomography (CT) or magnetic resonance imaging (MRI) equipment. It will highlight what these areas do. In most cases, technologists working in any of these areas will have gained certification in specialized areas such as MRI, CT, and angiographic procedures. It is important to note, however, that the education of the undergraduate technologist will provide the foundation needed to function successfully in this environment. A firm knowledge of anatomy, physiology, and pathology is needed as is an understanding of equipment, particularly the role of computers in imaging. Trouble-shooting and adherence to quality assurance principles are critical to the effective management of these areas. Patients are often more ill when these procedures are necessary. The technologist must use exemplary patient care skills and be aware of medicolegal issues. This is a rapidly growing and expanding part of medical imaging. Technologists have an obligation to pursue lifelong learning, ensuring that they remain cognizant of changes in their field.

TECHNICAL RESPONSIBILITIES

As technology advances, the roles of the various imaging modalities change with it. At one time angiography was primarily used as a diagnostic form of imaging, but technologic advances have allowed CT, MRI, and ultrasound to overtake, and in some cases, replace angiography as a diagnostic tool. Intervention and therapeutic techniques are now becoming the major procedures done in angiography. The technologist is responsible for preparing the room (Figure 1.1) and providing appropriate radiographic positioning specific to each examination whether the patient is on the fluoroscopic table, the angiographic table, or the CT or MRI table. Knowledge and understanding of the imaging modality being used together with knowledge of anatomy and the suspected pathology being examined or treated are critical to ensure that necessary information is obtained during preliminary imaging and the procedure itself.

Duties may include preparing sterile trays, preparing the patient, gowning and gloving to assist the radiologist, or circulating throughout the procedure. A knowledge of appropriate catheters, guidewires, pharmaceuticals, and other materials used for each particular examination ensures an active participation by the technologist.

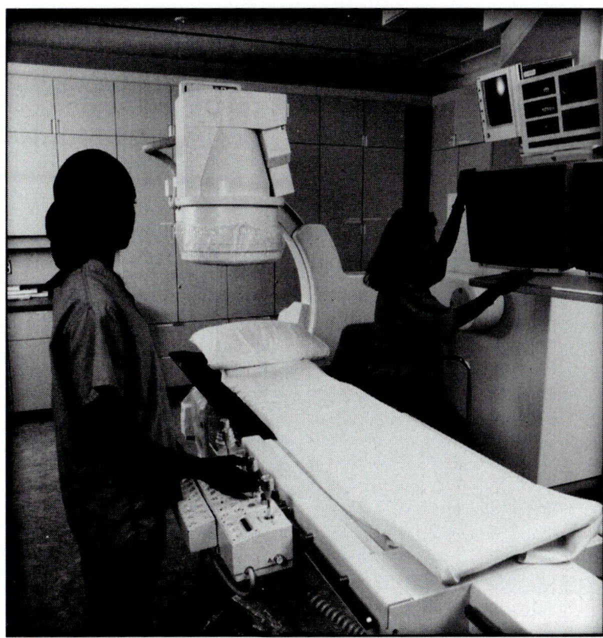

FIGURE 1.1 Technologists prepare the special procedures suite.

Awareness of standard precautions and infectious diseases is critical. Sterile technique may be required during some procedures. Safe work habits must be maintained throughout, such as when cleaning instruments, during the dismantling of trays, and during the manipulation of the equipment.

The technologist may be responsible for the correct use of the **electrocardiograph (ECG),** pressure monitoring devices, or other specific equipment used for therapeutic procedures. This equipment can be used to either diagnose or treat the patient's condition or may be an intricate part of the imaging equipment as in ECG **gating.**

Contrast media are used during angiography, CT, and MRI, and this may involve the use of a contrast media injector. An understanding of the reactions to contrast media is essential. An understanding of how the injector is integrated with the x-ray generator will assist the technologist in providing excellent images. It will also ensure that volumes and rates of injection are appropriate for each individual vessel examined (see Chapter 6, Angiographic Procedures and Equipment). The evolution of computers has added to the technologist's responsibilities. The manipulation of digital data during processing in digital subtraction angiography (DSA), CT, and MRI has given technologists the opportunity to participate in final image formation and to use the knowledge of anatomy and pathology to its fullest (Figure 1.2).

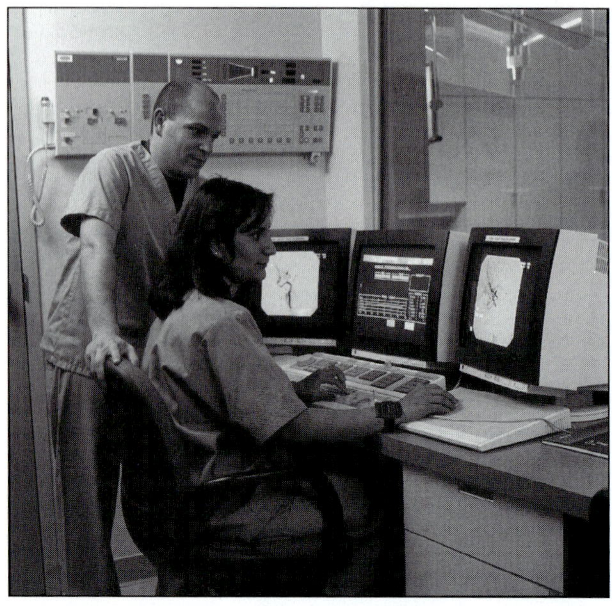

FIGURE 1.2 Technologists manipulate the digital image.

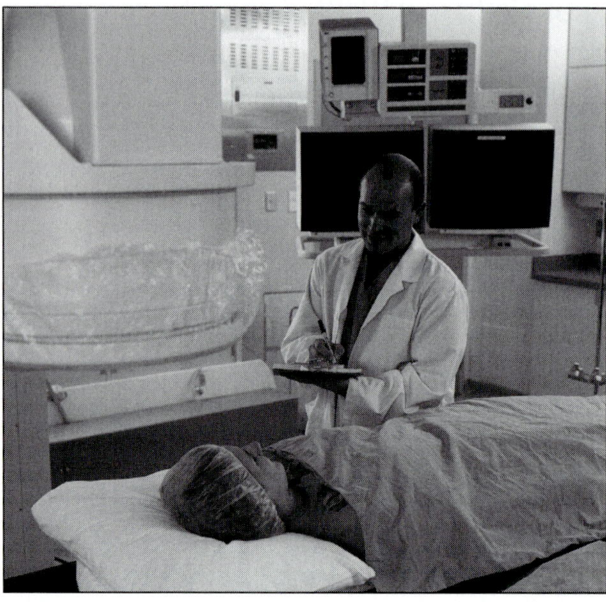

FIGURE 1.3 Technologist provides reassurance to the patient.

PATIENT CARE

In many of the procedures discussed in this text, the technologist will often see critically ill patients with special needs for long periods of time. Good communication skills among team members help create an optimal patient care environment. The technologist must develop a sensitive rapport with the patient at the start of the examination and maintain this rapport by offering constant reassurance throughout (Figure 1.3). Consent forms such as the one illustrated in Figure 1.4 will need to be completed and the explanation of its contents often becomes the technologist's responsibility. This relationship will help in the assessment of the patient's condition during the procedure and will aid in gaining the patient's cooperation during imaging.

The patient is always at risk with the injection of contrast agents. The technologist should be aware of any potential harm to the patient, allergies, previous contrast reactions, and appropriate measures to take to prevent and treat these reactions. Certification in basic cardiac life support/cardiopulmonary resuscitation is clearly an asset in dealing with arrest situations and in some institutions it is mandatory. In many facilities, a technologist may also be certified to administer intravenous (IV) contrast media. The technologist should fully understand the drugs used before and during the procedure and should always be aware of the adverse reactions these may incur.

Many advanced diagnostic and interventional procedures have their own inherent risks and these should be previously discussed between the referring physician and the radiologist. These potential problems should be explained to the patient or the power of attorney or equivalent before the examination. The technologist should have an acute awareness of these risks and complications and the appropriate actions to take should they occur.

There is also an obligation to adhere to the safe use of ionizing radiation to limit the dose to the patient and staff. Fluoroscopy times should be kept to a minimum and gonadal and thyroid shielding should be used whenever it is not in the way of anatomy being imaged. State, federal, and international regulations regarding the use of ionizing radiation must be rigorously adhered to, including the use of the **ALARA principle.** Knowledge of the science of radiation and instrumentation will always result in a better understanding and use of radiation. All technologists have a responsibility to the patient to keep radiation to the minimum and to ensure minimal dosage to themselves and other staff members.

RESEARCH

Imaging modalities are continuously evolving. An enthusiastic and interested technologist has endless opportunities to contribute to the development and eventual publication of these advancements. Keeping

Consent for treatment

Date ____________ Time ____________

I authorize the performance of the following procedure(s)

____

on ________ (name of patient) ____________ to be performed by ________ (name of physician) ________ ,MD.

The following have been explained to ____________ by Dr. ____________ (name physician) ____________.

Nature of the procedure (describe procedure)

____.

For the purpose of ________________________________

____.

The possible alternative methods of treatment are ________

____.

The possible consequences of the procedure are________

____.

The risks involve the possibility of ____________________

____.

The possible complications of this procedure are ________

____.

I have been advised of the serious nature of this procedure and have been further advised that if I desire a more detailed explanation of any of the foregoing or further information about the possible risks or complications, it will be given to me.

I do not request a more detailed listing and explanation of the above information.

Signed ________________________
(Patient/Parent/Guardian)

Witnessed by: ____________________

FIGURE 1.4 Typical consent form.

statistical records, writing papers, or presenting material at technical meetings are but a few possibilities for those willing to participate in professional growth. It can be rewarding and enjoyable to share new knowledge with peers.

Another growing area for technologic input is in the development and assessment of new materials and equipment used in undertaking these procedures. New designs in catheters, guidewires, and tools for intervention are continuously being evaluated. Technologists are often asked to participate in the selection of new x-ray equipment and to assist in the design of the imaging suite. The opportunities are limited only by the desire of technologists to become involved. As technologists acquire new knowledge and skills, it becomes more important that they be willing to share their information with other staff or technologists entering the field. Student technologists pass through many special imaging suites during their clinical semesters and technologists are primarily responsible for their training. Nurses, medical students, residents, and even radiologists may ask for technical advice. The knowledgeable technologist is invaluable.

As new procedures are undertaken, the technologist is responsible for assisting in the development of protocols and procedural manuals and keeping them current. Opportunities may also arise for technologists to present new procedures at departmental inservice lectures or during a more formal postgraduate course offered through the technical institution.

Newly qualified technologists would not be expected to fulfill all the tasks and responsibilities mentioned above. However, it is important to know that this area of specialized imaging holds opportunity and promise for well-educated and enthusiastic technologists. As barriers between professionals break down, the technologists with their wealth of knowledge and expertise will become the foundation of many of these departments.

Contrast Media

Evelyn Kelly, BSc, MA, RN, MRT(R)

Without contrast media, diagnostic radiology would be a limited investigative technique. The successful introduction and development of contrast media has been one of the foundations on which the practice of diagnostic radiology has been built. Within a month of the discovery of x-rays in 1895, it was realized that if roentgenography was to be useful for the study of anything other than bones, some type of chemical product that would enable the soft tissue vessels and organs to be seen with the rays would have to be used. The first contrast agent was a mixture of cinnabar, Vaseline, and gypsum and the first angiogram was done a month later on an amputated hand. The procedure took 57 minutes, but the images were very good for the standards of the time. Cadavers were found to be best suited for angiography because they did not move and could not be adversely affected by the chemical agent! A successful contrast agent for use on living humans would not be discovered for another 30 years.

Iodine was used in 1923 to make urine radiopaque and although it provided the basis for further advancement toward the development of an effective and yet safe contrast agent, at this time it could not be used in its inorganic form (sodium iodide) because of its high toxicity. It was not until 1950 that a safe intravascular water-soluble contrast agent was first tried with any success. Research continues to search for a contrast agent with negligible undesirable side effects.

Contrast media is a term used to describe substances of low atomic weight (e.g., hydrogen, nitrogen, oxygen) that appear as dark shadows on a radiograph. This is known as a negative contrast medium.

Opaque (ō-pāk′) media are elements of high atomic weight (e.g., iodine, barium) that appear as light shadows on a radiograph. This is a positive contrast medium. Over the years the terms have become blurred so that today contrast media is the term used for both contrast and opaque media.

Contrast is produced on a radiograph by making use of the difference in absorption coefficient of various elements. On plain radiographs the calcium in bones or air in sinuses, mastoids, or the chest make these areas more visible. The differences between tissues of similar densities such as the kidney and liver cannot be demonstrated without the use of opacifying media.

Contrast media can be introduced into the body by four routes:

1. Into an area that has a direct connection to the outside such as the gastrointestinal (GI), genitourinary (GU), or respiratory tract
2. Via injection into the bloodstream to demonstrate excretory organs such as the kidney or liver
3. By direct injection into the blood vessel to demonstrate the circulatory system
4. Via cavities that do not connect with the outside such as joint spaces or bile ducts

TYPES OF CONTRAST OR OPACIFYING AGENTS

Negative Contrast

Negative contrast such as oxygen, hydrogen, or helium can be used to demonstrate joint spaces or as a double contrast in the GI examinations. As long as the medium has a low atomic weight, it will produce a negative shadow.

Positive Contrast

Gastrointestinal Radiopaque Contrast Agents A radiopaque medium of high atomic weight and the undisputed leader of contrast in this area is barium sulfate. It has many advantages.

- It is not absorbed.
- It does not cause increased intestinal secretions.
- It is not toxic if aspirated.
- A flavoring agent can be added without deterioration in effect.
- An antiflocculation and antiprecipitation agent can be added without detriment.
- It maintains excellent opacity even in small amounts.

Although it has few disadvantages, it is not recommended if a large bowel obstruction or bowel perforation is suspected. In the case of an obstruction, the colon reabsorbs fluids and concentrates the barium sulfate, thereby increasing the obstruction. With a perforation, the barium leaks out of the bowel while mixed with feces and can cause **peritonitis** (pĕr′′ĭ-tō-nī′tĭs).

Oral Cholecystopaques These radiopaques are taken by the mouth and absorbed through the GI tract into the bloodstream to demonstrate the biliary system. The contrast binds tightly with the albumin in the blood so that it cannot be excreted by the kidneys and has to be excreted by the liver. The level of serum **bilirubin** (bĭl-ĭ-roo′bĭn) must be determined before the administration of oral cholecystopaques to ensure that it is not too high because bilirubin competes with the contrast for binding sites on **albumin** (ăl-bū-mĭn).

Oral and Rectal Water-Soluble Agents These radiopaques are used for studies of the gastrointestinal system when barium sulfate is considered dangerous (e.g., bowel perforation or obstruction). More precautions need to be exercised while using these agents because aspiration can cause pulmonary **edema** and they may cause electrolyte changes in infants and dehydrated patients. These agents must never be injected IV and are introduced in liquid form into the body in the same manner as barium sulfate.

Oily and Fat-Soluble Contrast Agents Iodized oils were developed for use in studies where absorption of contrast into the surrounding tissues or mixing with body fluids was not desired. They have been replaced by low osmolar aqueous contrast agents for many examinations and are therefore seen only rarely. They can be used to enhance many procedures, such as:

- Iodized oils for lymphangiography and sialography (e.g., Ethiodal)
- Iopanoic acid (e.g., Telepaque), the water-insoluble contrast agent for oral cholecystograms
- Iophendylate (e.g., Pantopaque) for myelography, now replaced with water-soluble low osmolarity agents
- Propyliodoine for bronchography (e.g., Dionisil)

Magnetic Resonance Imaging Agents

Gadolinium diethylenetriaminepenta-acetic acid (Gd DPTA), under the trade name of Magnevist, is used for central nervous system studies. This metal **chelate** (kē´lāt) is injected IV, is excreted by the kidneys, and has low toxicity. It accumulates in brain tumors because of extravascular leakage from tumor breakdown of the blood–brain barrier.

Inorganic Iodides

Inorganic iodides, potassium iodide and sodium iodide, were originally used for retrograde pyelography but because of their very toxic nature, they were quickly replaced by water-soluble contrast media.

Ionic Water-Soluble Organic Iodide

The water soluble Organic Iodides, both ionic and nonionic, are by far the most frequently used contrast agents, other than barium sulfate. Some of the examinations for which they are used are very sophisticated while others are so common to the day to day routine of a radiographer as to be considered a basic skill. See Table 1.1.

Monoacidic Monomer These compounds are called ionic because of the **anion** (ăn´ī-ŏn) and **cation** (kăt´ī-ŏn) that make up the compound. The basic structure of this compound is the benzene ring. The benzene ring with three iodine atoms attached comprises the anion, while the cation is either sodium, meglumine (mĕg´lū-mēn), or a combination of the two (Figure 1.5).

Three anions are:

- Diatrizoate—with the trade name of Hypaque Sodium
- Iothalamate—with the trade name Conray
- Metrizoate—with the trade name Isopaque

Monoacidic Dimer This compound has a similar composition to the iodide monomer, with a cation of sodium or meglumine. However, the anion is made up of two benzene rings. This allows for a lower osmolarity or the ability to deliver higher concentrations of iodine with fewer particles in solution, for example, six iodine atoms versus three atoms per anion in monomer (Figure 1.6).

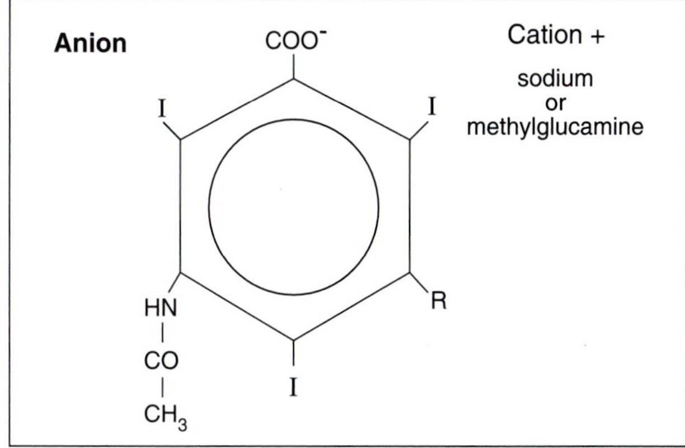

FIGURE 1.5 Schematic of basic structure of the ionic monomers.

Nonionic Water-Soluble Organic Iodide

Nonionic Monomer These agents are called nonionic because they do not dissociate into two charged particles in solution. A markedly lower osmolarity is a characteristic they share. Examples are Amipaque, Isovue, Omnipaque, and Optiray (Figure 1.7).

Nonionic contrast agents have many advantages over other agents:

- Less toxic to the patient
- Less likely to cause anaphylactic shock reaction
- Cause less heat and discomfort during injection
- Less neurotoxic due to the absence of carboxyl groups

Nonionic Dimer This contrast agent has six iodine atoms for each molecule in solution. This allows for a satisfying iodine concentration at isotonic strength. Manufacturers are still perfecting the development of this agent.

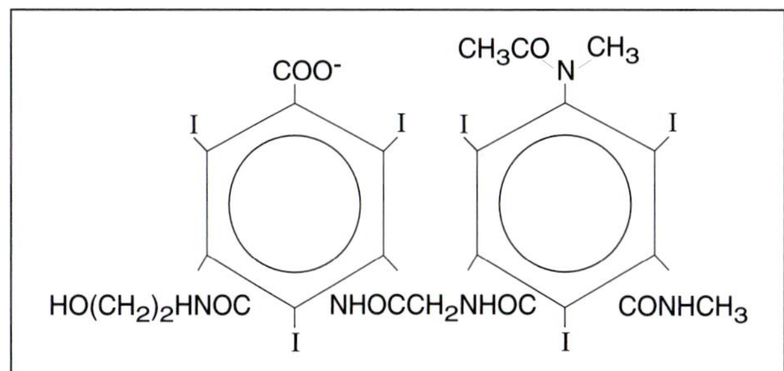

FIGURE 1.6 Schematic of ionic monacidic dimers.

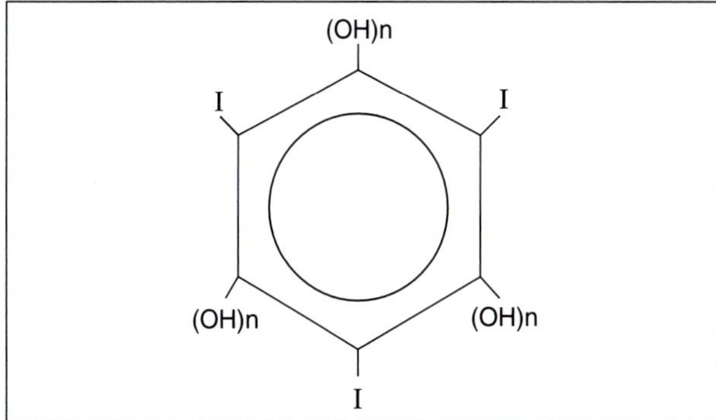

FIGURE 1.7 Schematic of examples of nonionic water-soluble organic iodide monomers.

SECONDARY EFFECTS OF CONTRAST MEDIA

Although the primary effect of a contrast agent is attenuation or absorption of radiation on its way from the source to the image detector, many secondary effects can be expected, which can render a compound unsuitable for use as a contrast. They have increased chemotoxicity due to binding proteins as well as osmotic effects or osmotoxicity, which can induce water movement across membranes of the body.

Ion toxicity, too high or too low in ion concentration, can interfere with cellular function or block enzymes or vasoconstrictor substances from the cell. Although it is impossible to make a contrast agent free from any secondary effects, an ideal injectable contrast agent should be water soluble, biologically inert, and chemically and heat stable with low viscosity and nonthreshold properties. It should be safe, low cost, easily stored and transported, and have the same or lower **osmolarity** as human serum. No contrast material has all of these properties, but the day might be close at hand as manufacturers strive to make the ideal agent, producing the best possible results.

OTHER DRUGS IN THE IMAGING DEPARTMENT

Over the years many drugs have come in and out of use as techniques change. The following is a list of some of the noncontrast drugs that may be used in the radiographic diagnosis or treatment of disease.

1. Astringents (e.g., tannic acid)
    - Helps to dry the mucous membranes so that polyps may be clearly visualized during a barium enema
    - Due to its damaging effects on the liver, rarely used today
2. Bicarbonate compound (e.g., UnikZoru, Varos)
    - Tablet or granular form used during a GI study as a gas-producing agent
    - Has the effect of giving a double-contrast GI series
3. Antispasmodic agents (hyosine butylbromide, e.g., Buscopan)
    - Control gastric hypersecretion and spasm of the bowel
4. Antidiuretic agents (e.g., vasopressin)
    - Dispel gas shadows on abdominal images
    - Control postoperative abdominal distention
5. Chymopapain (kī-mō-pă´pā-ĭn) (e.g., Discase)
    - Proteolytic enzyme that can be injected into the intervertebral disk during discography for relief of back pain due to ruptured disks (very rarely used; see Chapter 15)
6. Cathartics or laxatives (e.g., X-prep, Citromag)
    - Taken to cleanse the bowel of fecal material before investigation
7. Hypotonic agents
    - Produce a hypotonic state to relax the stomach, duodenum, and bowel
    - Makes it easier to outline with barium sulfate
8. Anticoagulant (e.g., heparin, Coumadin)
    - Prevent coagulation during vascular studies
9. Local anesthetic
    - Reduce sensation to an area during procedures requiring percutaneous injection
10. Allergy-reducing agents
    - Antihistamines—counter the effects of histamine release. Histamine causes urticaria or rhinitis, which is seen during a reaction.
    - Adrenalin or epinephrine—restores cardiac rhythm, raises blood pressure, and prolongs the effect of local anesthetic agents
    - Hydrocortisone for the relief of allergy symptoms
11. Patient preparation
    - Analgesics to reduce pain
    - Antiemetics to suppress nausea
    - Antianxiety sedatives or hypnotic to induce relaxation and sleep
    - Muscle relaxants

ADMINISTRATION OF MEDICATION

The reason for medication usually denotes the method of administration. The route of administration is determined by the desired effect—either local to the site of application or systemic intended for a more generalized effect.

For local effect, the drug may be applied to the skin (e.g., antiseptics, emollients) or to the mucous membrane (e.g., nasal spray, suppository).

For systemic effect, a drug may be given in several ways:

- Oral—in tablet, capsule, or liquid form. The effect is slower in onset but more prolonged.
- Sublingual (e.g., nitroglycerin)—absorbed through the membrane under the tongue, but has effects in other body parts
- Rectal—suppositories
- Inhalation—administered by aerosol and absorbed from the respiratory tract and alveolar surfaces
- Parenteral—injected into the body tissue or fluid
  —Intradermal—into upper layers of skin (e.g., allergy testing)
  —Subcutaneous—just under the skin
  —Intramuscular—into the muscle for large volumes and an immediate effect, or when the drug cannot be injected into the tissue

—Intra-arterially—into an artery
—Intrathecally—into a structure within a sheath (e.g., the spinal cord)

Whenever a medication is administered, safety is a priority. *Following the rights of drug administration ensures that safety for the patient:*

- Right drug
- Right patient
- Right route of administration
- Right dosage
- Right time of administration

Precautions for Administering Contrast Media

- Give simple and honest information to the patient regarding the drug and its procedure.
- Read the label.
- Do not prepare or administer a drug from a container that is not properly labeled or from a container where the label is not legible.
- Do not return an unused dose to the medication stock bottle.
- Never leave a medication unattended after it has been drawn up or poured.
- Never reuse disposable syringes and needles.
- Be sure the drug is compatible with the patient's age and size.
- Do not inject a cloudy or crystallized contrast media.
- Give only those drugs for which you have a physician's order.

Role of the Technologist with Regard to Medication

- Prepare medication properly according to instructions.
- Check patient identification and allergy history.
- Reassure the patient and explain the procedure.
- Assist with administration of the contrast media.
- Monitor the patient after the medication is given and report any unusual circumstances.
- Record dosage given, name of the drug, and any reactions.

Laws and regulations govern whether technologists are allowed to start IV lines and perform IV injections of contrast media. It is important to know the standards that prevail in your institution and area of the country. Maintaining the appropriate qualifications and training in all aspects of pharmacology, as it relates to contrast media, is essential. Knowledge of the drugs being administered increases your ability to cope with any adverse situation (Table 1.1).

TABLE 1.1 COMMONLY USED CONTRAST MEDIA

Trade Name	Generic Name	Approved Uses
Amipaque	Metrizamide	Myelography, CT
Angio Conray	iothalomate meglumine	Angiography
Cysto Conray	iothalomate meglumine	Retrograde pyelography
Cystografin	diatrizoate meglumine	Cystourethrography
Conray	iothalomate meglumine	IV pyelography (IVP), digital subtraction angiography (DSA)
Conray 30	iothalomate meglumine	Venograms
Conray 43	iothalomate meglumine	CT
Conray 325	iothalomate sodium	IV urography
Conray 400	iothalomate sodium	Angiography
Hypaque Sodium 20%	diatrizoate sodium	Retrograde pyelography
Hypaque Sodium 25%	diatrizoate sodium	IVP, CT
Hypaque Sodium 50%	diatrizoate sodium	Multipurpose
Hypaque M 30	diatrizoate meglumine	IVP, CT

continued

TABLE 1.1 CONTINUED

Trade Name	Generic Name	Approved Uses
Hypaque M 60	diatrizoate meglumine	Multipurpose vascular
Hypaque M 75	diatrizoate meglumine and sodium	Multipurpose vascular
Hypaque M 76	diatrizoate meglumine and sodium	Multipurpose vascular
Hypaque M 90	diatrizoate meglumine and sodium	Vascular studies
Hexabrix	sodium and meglumine ioxaglate	Multipurpose
Gastrografin	diatrizoate meglumine and sodium	GI studies, CT
Isopaque 280	meglumine metrizoate	Vascular studies
Isopaque	meglumine metrizoate	Angiography
Isovue 128	iopamidol	Arterial DSA
Isovue 200	iopamidol	Peripheral venograph
Isovue 300	iopamidol	Peripheral arteriography
Isovue 370	iopamidol	Selective visceral arteriography
Isovue M200	iopamidol	Myelography
Isovue M300	iopamidol	Myelography
Omnipaque 140	iohexal	Arterial DSA
Omnipaque 180	iohexal	Myelography
Omnipaque 240	iohexal	Multipurpose
Omnipaque 300	iohexal	IV, intrathecal, intra-arterial
Omnipaque 350	iohexal	IV, CT, DSA, Angiocardiography
Optiray 320	ioversal	IV urography, CT
Optiray 350	ioversal	IV urography, CT
Renografin 60	diatrizoate meglumine and sodium	Multipurpose
Renografin 76	diatrizoate meglumine and sodium	Multipurpose
Reno M 30	diatrizoate meglumine	Retrograde pyelography
Reno M 60	diatrizoate meglumine	Multipurpose
Reno M Dip	diatrizoate meglumine	Infusion urography
Renovist	diatrizoate meglumine and sodium	Multipurpose
Renovue	iodamide meglumine	IV urography
Renovue Dip	iodamide meglumine	Infusion urography
Sinografin	diatrizoate meglumine, iodipamide meglumine	Hysterosalpingography
Salpix	acetrizoate providone and sodium	Hysterosalpingography
Vascoray	iothalamate meglumine and sodium	Angiography and excretory urography
Bilopaque	tyrpanoate sodium	Oral cholecystography
Cholebrine	iocetamic acid	Oral cholecystography
Cholografin Meglumine	iodopamide meglumine	IV cholangiography
Cholografin Meglumine	iodopamide meglumine	Drip infusion IV for infusion cholangiography
Orografin Calcium	ipodate calcium	Cholecystography

TABLE 1.1 CONTINUED

Trade Name	Generic Name	Approved Uses
Orografin Sodium	ipodate sodium	Cholecystography
Telepaque	iopanoic acid	Oral cholecystography
Dionosil	propyliodone	Bronchography
Ethiodal	ethiodized oil	Lymhangiography
Pantopaque	iophendylate	Myelography
Lipiodil Ultra Fluid, Barium Sulfate for suspension	iodized poppyseed oil	Myelography, GI studies, oral and rectal
Vispaque	iodixanol injection	CT of the body and vascular studies
Ultravist	iopromide injection	Urography, tomography, vascular studies, hysterosalpingography
Magnevist	gadopentetate dimeglumine injection	MRI

Interventional Radiography

Cynthia Cowling, BSc, MEd, MRT(R), ACR

Interventions began in 1964 as a result of an incidental observation by Dotter, who noticed that an occluded iliac artery became patent after the insertion of an angiographic catheter. Trials were performed to determine the success of dilating a vessel and having it remain open. Initially, catheters were introduced over each other in a telescoping effect, widening the passage through the vessel, and pushing the plaque toward the side of the vessel. The size of the catheter limited the diameter (usually no more than 4 mm) and in 1974, Gruntzig devised the balloon catheter, which allowed for greater diameters, without compromising the initial puncture site. None of these procedures would have been possible without the introduction of the Seldinger technique, a mechanism for introducing catheters into the circulatory system (see Chapter 6). This technique became known as transluminal angioplasty. Since that time, numerous percutaneous procedures have enabled many patients to be treated in a less invasive and safer manner.

Interventional radiography is a relatively new technology, but it is expanding to become a significant part of an imaging department, changing the department from one functioning exclusively as a diagnostic unit to one of a therapeutic nature. Interventional radiography requires the cooperation of all sections of the imaging spectrum as well as medical and surgical staff. It is an area where the lines separating divisions in hospitals become fuzzy and is a good example of the reason technologists must be cognizant of all aspects of imaging and health.

Strictly defined, interventional radiography is an action taken to modify an effect. It is a procedure that aims to improve the condition of the patient, and although originally restricted to vascular work and considered part of angiography, it has expanded into all the body systems. Interventions as they relate to various systems are described in each appropriate chapter. The following list provides an overview of the types of interventional activities currently being practiced. Considerable experimentation with new techniques is being done.

Interventional radiography is performed in angiographic suites, GI suites, conventional radiographic rooms, and CT, MRI, and ultrasound facilities. It is carried out by radiologists, surgeons, and physicians, with the technologist having a vital role by assisting in these procedures. Often, radiographs or hard images are not required for the actual procedure, but they are often needed as a preliminary or follow-up to the procedure. Fluoroscopy is often used to determine placement and position, and technologies such as ultrasound are becoming more commonly used, as the technology seeks to find less invasive techniques.

TYPES OF INTERVENTIONAL TECHNIQUES

Each procedure is described in greater detail in its corresponding chapter.

Vascular Procedures

Percutaneous Transluminal Angioplasty (PTA) Angioplasty is a procedure that seeks to improve blood flow and supply by widening a vessel. The most common vessels involved are the iliac, femoral, renal, and coronary arteries. The original procedure used a telescoping device that gradually enlarged the lumen, but the width attainable was restricted by the size of the puncture through which these dilators had to pass. The advent of Gruntzig's balloon catheter resolved this problem. (See Chapter 6.)

Laser Angioplasty There has been significant interest in the development of a laser angioplasty catheter as a means to clear an occlusion. However, at this point no definitive study has demonstrated that the vessels remain patent any longer than after conventional balloon angioplasty.

Atherectomy It has been felt that the success rate and length of patency time could be improved if, as well as breaking up the plaque, it could somehow be removed nonsurgically. Several catheters have been designed to attempt this—pulsating, rotating, and ultrasonic—but at this time this has not replaced surgery, if the vessel does not or cannot respond to angioplasty.

Thrombolysis In some situations, occlusions are caused by a thrombus (usually in a vein). These can sometimes be treated by positioning a catheter at the occlusion and administering a thrombolytic agent. The use of streptokinase (strĕp´´tō-kī´nās) fell out of favor because of complications and studies are being done to find agents that will dissolve the thrombus without jeopardizing the condition of the patient.

Thrombus Filters The main pathway for a clot to follow is from the leg via the inferior vena cava to the pulmonary artery where its effects can be devastating. Filters can be placed within the inferior vena cava to catch the clots. This procedure would only be performed on individuals with a history of recurring clot development.

Embolization It is sometimes desirous to produce an occlusion rather than reduce one and this procedure introduces a substance, either a mechanical device or chemical material, to produce a temporary or permanent occlusion. Although this procedure has only been used regularly within the last 20 years, the first embolization occurred in 1904 when melted paraffin was injected into the external carotid arteries of patients suffering from tumors. However, it was not until the 1970s that embolytic agents were described and put to general use, Gelfoam and detachable balloons both in 1974. Since that time there has been a proliferation of devices (see Chapter 6, Angiographic Procedures and Equipment).

The three main reasons to perform this procedure are:

1. To control bleeding, usually from the GI tract or GU tract, or as a result of trauma
2. To reduce blood supply to tumors or organs or circulatory malformations
3. As a preoperative procedure to stem blood flow to a particular site

Interventions have now incorporated many body systems apart from the vascular system. Listed below are some of the procedures in general use. They will be covered in more detail under the specific systems.

Biopsies

The method of obtaining cell and tissue samples percutaneously by means of special needles and under imaging control has become a routine procedure. Fluoroscopy, CT, and ultrasound are all used to guide needles to the correct position.

Stents

The word stent originated from Charles Stent, a British dentist who made dental molds. The compound he used to make these molds was called a stent. It has since come to mean any material that gives support to or holds tissue in place. They are also termed endoprosthesis (ĕn´´dō-prŏs´thē-sĭs). Stents today are generally a catheter-like tube that provides drainage or an **anastomossis** (ă-năs´´tō-mōs´sĭs) during the healing process. They can be temporary or permanent and can be designed in many ways depending on their use.The role of imaging is to assist in their accurate placement and periodically check their patency. Stents are used in the treatment of the biliary, urinary, and GI systems, and new techniques are being developed using stents in vascular conditions.

Percutaneous Drainage

This procedure provides a tubal pathway from the outside to or from an organ or structure. Now that the site and size of abscesses, particularly in the abdomen, can be accurately determined by CT or ultrasound, percutaneous drainage can be put in place, with less trauma to the patient than a surgical procedure.

Percutaneous Nephrostomy The ability to create a pathway to the kidney percutaneously has allowed a number of interventions, such as dilatation of strictures, placement of stents, and retrieval of stones.

Prostrate and Urethral Intervention Procedures have been developed to open urethral strictures by means of balloon dilatation.

Biliary Intervention A number of procedures enable the biliary tree to be examined and treated percutaneously, without requiring surgical trauma. The efficacy of these procedures depends to an extent on the condition of the patient and the pathology under examination. Percutaneous decompression of the obstructed biliary system has become fairly routine. Percutaneous biliary cholangiography and drainage can be carried out in the imaging department, usually in a suite that offers an aseptic environment with which to perform these procedures as well as fluoroscopy control.

Stone Extraction

Certain conditions will allow renal and biliary stones to be removed percutaneously by means of a special extraction basket catheter. These procedures are performed under fluoroscopic control and aseptic conditions.

Lithotripsy is a mechanism for shattering kidney stones using an ultrasonic technique and allowing the patient to pass the stone fragments through the ureter and bladder.

Review Questions

1. Describe the main skills, knowledge, and attitudes needed to function successfully as a technologist in a special procedures environment.

2. Describe the four main methods of delivering contrast media.

3. Compare the chemical composition of ionic and nonionic compounds found in contrast media.

4. A positive contrast agent:
   a. can be helium or hydrogen
   b. is used in conjunction with barium sulfate
   c. is another term for any contrast medium
   d. is a contrast medium with a high atomic weight

5. An agent that relaxes the stomach is known as a/an:
   a. cathartic
   b. hypotonic agent
   c. astringent
   d. antidiuretic

6. A tube that provides drainage and gives support to a vessel is known as a:
   a. percutaneous drainage catheter
   b. filter
   c. stent
   d. balloon catheter

7. Embolization is used in:
   a. the control of internal bleeding
   b. the reduction of blood supply to tumors
   c. angioplastic procedures
   d. as a preoperative procedure to prevent excessive bleeding

CASE STUDY

Describe, from the point of view of the patient undergoing a special procedure, how you would like to be treated, from the time you enter the department until you leave the procedure room.

____

____

____

____

____

____

____

____

____

____

____

____

____

References and Recommended Reading

Ballinger, P. W. (1995). *Merrill's atlas of radiographic positions and radiological procedures* (8th ed., Vols. 1, 2, and 3). St. Louis: Mosby-Year Book.

Casteneda-Zuniga, W. R. (1988). *Interventional radiology.* Baltimore: Williams & Wilkins.

Chapman, S., & Nakielny, R. (1993). *A guide to radiological procedures.* London: Bailliere Tindall.

Clayton, B. D., & Stock, Y. N. (1993). *Basic pharmacology for nurses* (10th ed.). Toronto: Mosby-Year Book.

Cope, C., Burke, D., & Meranze, S. (1989). *Interventional radiology.* Gower Medical Publishing.

Eisenberg, R. L. (1992). *Radiology, an illustrated history.* St. Louis: Mosby-Year Book.

Ferrucci, J. T., et al. (1985). *Interventional radiology of the abdomen* (2nd ed.). Baltimore: Williams & Wilkins.

Kandarpa, K., & Aruny, J. E. (1996). *Handbook of interventional radiologic procedures* (2nd ed.). Boston: Little, Brown.

Rose, J. S. (1983). *Invasive radiology, risks and patient care.* Chicago: Year Book Medical.

Scherer, J. C., & Roach, S. S. (1996). *Introductory clinical pharmacology* (5th ed.). Philadelphia: Lippincott-Raven.

Snopek, A. M. (1992). *Fundamentals of special radiographic procedures* (3rd ed.). Philadelphia: Saunders.

Stolberg, H. (1988, Hong Kong; 1989, Montreal). *Proceedings of the Radiology Speakers Program.* Montreal: Medicopea International.

Sutton, D. A. (1993). *Textbook of radiology and imaging.* Edinburgh: Churchill Livingstone.

Torres, L. S. (1993). *Basic medical techniques and patient care for radiologic technologists.* Philadelphia: Lippincott.

Tortorici, M. R., & Apfel, P. J. (1995). *Advanced radiographic and angiographic procedures.* Philadelphia: Davis.

Wojtowycz, M. (1993). *Interventional radiology and angiography, handbooks in radiology.* St. Louis: Mosby-Year Book.

CHAPTER 2

Introduction to Specialized Imaging

MICHAEL GLISSON, DipAppSci (Med Rad) RMelbIT, MAAppSci, Monash
MARY SUSAN HELENE CROWLEY, MRT(R)(ARRT)
CAROLYN KAUT ROTH, RT(R)(MR)(ARRT)
GAIL RODRIGUES, MRT(R), RDMS
MARSHA SORTER, MHE, RT(R)(M)(N)(ARRT)

MAGNETIC RESONANCE IMAGING

INTRODUCTION AND HISTORICAL OVERVIEW

PRINCIPLES

Magnets
Nuclear Magnetic Fields
Polarization
Equilibrium
Net Magnetization
Precessional Frequency
Radiofrequency Pulse
Radiofrequency Coils
Excitation
Signal Detection
Relaxation
T1 Recovery
T2 Decay
Spin Echo

IMAGE PRODUCTION

Image Contrast Parameters
Time to Echo (TE)
Time to Repetition (TR)
T1-Weighted Image
T2-Weighted Image
PD-Weighted Image
Spatial Encoding
Slice Selection
Image Formation
View Options
Pulse Sequences

APPLICATIONS

Protocol Selections (Pulse Sequence and Parameter Choices)
Artifact Compensation (Image Optimization)
Coil Selection and Patient Positioning
Image Recording Systems and Photography for MRI
Safety and Patient Care for MRI

ULTRASOUND

INTRODUCTION AND HISTORICAL OVERVIEW

PRINCIPLES

What Is Sound?

IMAGE PRODUCTION

Doppler
Intercavity Ultrasound
Biologic Effects
Image Recording Systems

APPLICATIONS

Indications for Use
Clinical Applications
Patient Care Considerations

RADIONUCLIDE IMAGING

INTRODUCTION AND HISTORICAL OVERVIEW

PRINCIPLES

Physics of Nuclear Medicine
Choice of Radiopharmaceutical

IMAGE PRODUCTION

Gas Detectors
Scintillation Detectors
Gamma Camera
SPECT
Positron Emission Tomography (PET)
Computers in Nuclear Medicine

APPLICATIONS

OBJECTIVES

At the completion of this chapter, the student should be able to:

1. Describe the historical developments in conventional angiographic instruments.
2. Understand the basic principles and functions used in conventional angiography.
3. Appreciate the general developments in specialized imaging instruments.
4. Describe the basic functions of the digital computer in any imaging system.
5. Understand the concepts of analog and digital and the conversion of data.
6. Understand the construction of a basic digital image.
7. Appreciate basic image processing concepts.
8. Compare the relative advantages of the digital computer within an imaging system.
9. Describe the development of CT as an imaging modality.
10. Understand the basic principles underlying the evolution of CT scanners.
11. Describe the functioning elements of a typical CT scanner.
12. List some clinical applications for CT.
13. Describe the development of MRI as an imaging modality.
14. Describe the basic principles of MRI.
15. List some clinical applications for MRI.
16. Describe imaging systems used in MRI.
17. Discuss patient and operator safety issues when using MRI.
18. Describe the development of ultrasound as an imaging modality.
19. Describe the basic principles of ultrasound.
20. Understand the basic principles of image production in ultrasound.
21. Describe the basic principles of Doppler.
22. List some clinical applications for ultrasound.
23. Discuss patient care considerations when performing ultrasound examinations.
24. Describe the development of radionuclide imaging (nuclear medicine) as an imaging modality.
25. Understand the basic principles of physics in nuclear medicine.
26. List the uses and applications of radiopharmaceuticals.
27. Describe the image recording systems used in radionuclide imaging.
28. Define and briefly describe single proton emission computed tomography (SPECT).
29. Define and briefly describe positron emission tomography (PET).

Equipment in Specialized Procedures

Micheal Glisson, DipAppSci (Med Rad) RMelbIT, MAppSci. Monash

Introduction and Historical Overview

The equipment used in specialized radiographic and imaging procedures encompasses several **imaging modes,** each having its own particular historical development. Subsequent sections of this chapter will provide a generalized appreciation and a brief historical insight into the evolution of each mode.

Over the past 25 years, specialized equipment and techniques have made significant advances. These have resulted in great changes to the equipment and the methods of diagnostic investigation. Because this trend will no doubt continue, a sound understanding of the underlying equipment and related **protocols** is essential in preparation for future advances.

A key event that has facilitated and contributed to the rapid and continuing advances in all modes of medical imaging is the integration of the **digital computer** into imaging systems. This landmark occurrence is often cited as the major influence in the development of current specialized instruments. It is difficult to perceive a large imaging department today without a CT scanner. Without its inherent digital computer this technology could not exist. As important as the computer may be to all the specialized imaging modes, it is important to recognize that ongoing complementary developments have also occurred. These developments are often overlooked, such as major advances in improving the ratings and specifications of key imaging components (x-ray tubes, high-tension generators, image intensifiers, television cameras, CT detectors, ultrasound transducers, magnetic field production, radiofrequency coils, etc.). Furthermore, unique solutions to mechanical, electrical, imaging, or environmental difficulties have also allowed advances to be achieved (slip ring technology, ultrasound sector scanners, specialized instrument shielding, etc.). The evolution of the modern CT scanner is an excellent example of ongoing complementary advancements being incorporated into imaging technology. A similar trend is also evident in the development of the other specialized imaging modes.

Angiographic Equipment

Conventional radiographic imaging equipment has continued to develop in response to a basic requirement to produce time sequences of radiographic images of rapid vascular physiologic events. The configuration and complexity of this equipment is in part related to the duration of the vascular event and the imaging requirements of the desired vascular anatomy. Cardiac angiography requires rapid image acquisition to ensure that abnormalities that can last for less than a second are accurately imaged. Typically, in conventional equipment, a cine camera is chosen. In neurologic examinations the duration of the vascular event is longer, allowing relatively slower imaging rates to achieve acceptable image quality. Here a conventional cut film changer is suitable. Further, the manner in which the imaging equipment is configured is also influenced by the target vascular region. In coronary artery studies, high **resolution** and precise angular relationships of the imaging system are required to accurately visualize the vascular anatomy. These systems typically use a matched imaging chain to optimize the images produced and a **C- or U-arm system** to mount the imaging equipment and to provide the positioning precision required. Such high precision is not necessarily required in other vascular areas, such as abdominal and peripheral angiography, and the imaging components are matched and mounted in a manner to optimize the acquisition of these images. It is possible to broadly categorize angiographic instruments into specializing in four areas, neurologic, cardiac, abdominal/thoracic/general, and peripheral.

Principles

ANGIOGRAPHIC IMAGING SYSTEMS

All categories of angiographic instruments share common components. In relation to the x-ray beam and the final image, three subsections can be identified. These can be considered as primary, secondary, or tertiary image production systems. A primary imaging system uses the x-ray beam directly to produce the final image. In conventional imaging this is achieved by the use of a film/screen system. A secondary imaging system does not directly image from the x-ray beam but involves the use of a further intermediate imaging system before final image production. A photofluorographic imaging system, which involves the use of an image intensifier, is an example. A tertiary imaging system involves two intermediate imaging systems. Video imaging techniques are an example, where the image intensifier and video camera represent the two intermediate imaging stages. In all imaging systems, it is critical that all imaging components be matched to produce the highest quality images. Figure 2.1 divides a conventional angiographic system into the three image production subsections.

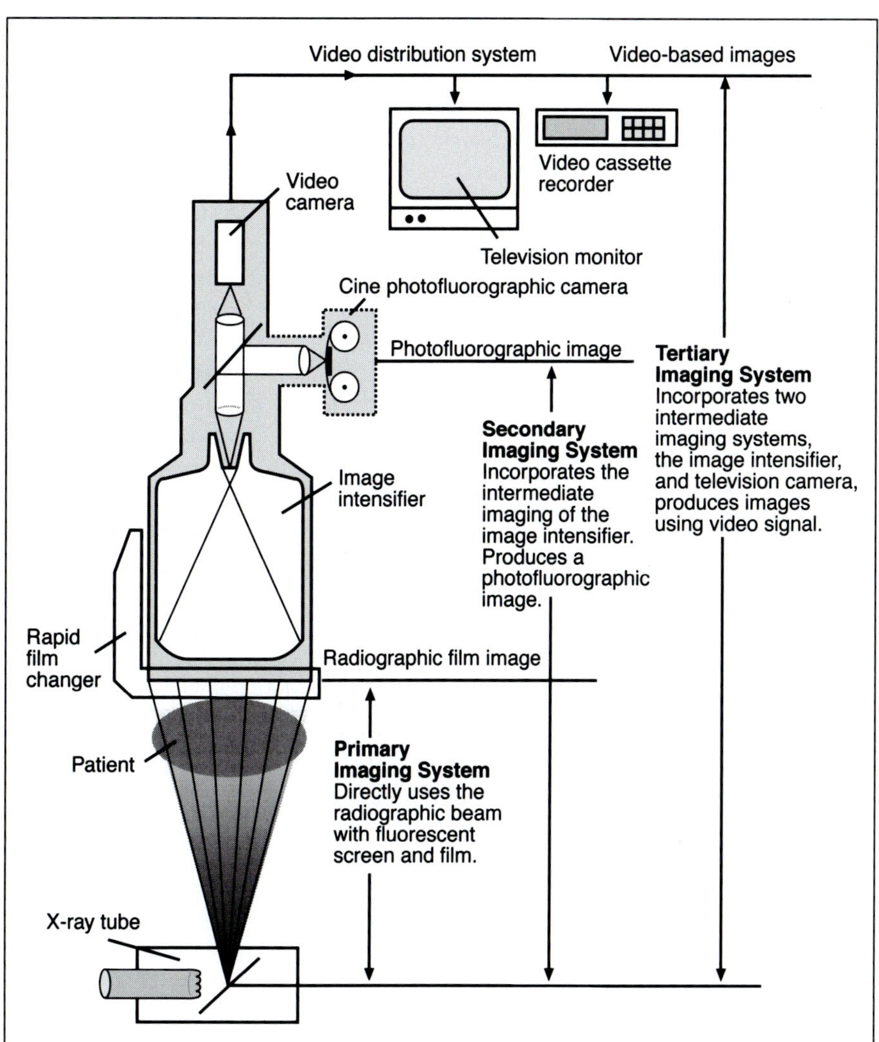

FIGURE 2.1
Imaging subsections of a conventionial angiographic imaging system. The relevant components of each of the primary, secondary, and tertiary subsystems are shown in relation to the primary x-ray beam.

Image Production

PRIMARY IMAGING SYSTEMS

Primary imaging systems directly use the radiographic beam to produce images. In angiography, a precision mechanical instrument involving radiographic film and screens is used to produce the rapid sequence of images. Early angiographic systems tried to use full-size film/screen cassettes, often stacked. As each radiographic exposure was completed, the exposed cassette would be manually removed from the exposure field and the next unexposed cassette would take its place. The timing of the exposure and precision and reproducibility of the imaging rate was operator dependent. Consequently, these early systems were unsuitable for extremely fast sequences, difficult to reproduce accurately, and limited to the number of cassettes in the changer. Compared to modern systems, this equipment appears to be inadequate. However, at the time, it reasonably matched the specifications of the film/screens and the capabilities of the x-ray generation system. The x-ray generation systems could not produce long sequences of short-time, high-intensity radiographic exposures; film/screens were not as sensitive as today, and x-ray tube ratings were significantly lower. Within these constraints, however, the manual system involved several inaccuracies in timing. To overcome these, automated cassette changing systems were introduced. These rather large instruments improved both the accuracy of timing and the changing rate but were limited in the number of cassettes they could hold and were cumbersome and prone to mechanical problems.

Film Changers

An improved solution to the problems already encountered was to discard the cassette itself and then precisely move each radiographic film through a fixed set of screens. Film is light and flexible and can be moved quickly and accurately. Two variations of rapid film changer evolved based on this principle. These are the roll film changer and the cut film changer. Roll film changers are similar in principle to a cinematic film camera with the shutter device removed. In radiographic applications, a large roll of unexposed film (typically 30 m of 35-cm wide film) is transported across an exposure area incorporating two fluorescent screens and a radiographic grid. Just before radiographic exposure, an unexposed portion of film is held stationary and pressured between the screens, ensuring film/screen contact. A coordinated radiographic exposure is made, thus avoiding the need for a shutter device. At the conclusion of the exposure, the now-exposed portion of film is released and transported forward onto a receiving drum. These changers could easily achieve filming rates of 1 to 12 exposures per second; however, they were physically large and bulky. Loading and unloading these systems involved specialist film rolls and darkroom facilities. It is now uncommon to see this system in use. Systems that transported single (cut) films provided a better solution.

The cut film or rapid serial film changers became the conventional rapid image acquisition device of choice in angiography. Many different manufacturers have produced essentially similar systems, all of which transport a single size of radiographic film. Two sizes are common (35 × 35 cm or 14 × 14 inches and 24 × 30 cm or 10 × 12 inches). These changers are typically capable of film rates up to six exposures per second and are operator controlled via an electronic interface and a program controller. Unlike the roll film changers, individual sheets of radiographic (cut) films are loaded into a loading magazine and then internally transported via a roller system. The film path passes across an exposure area that incorporates two fluorescent screens and a radiographic grid. A compression table containing the two screens holds the unexposed film stationary for exposure ensuring screen film contact. When exposure is completed the pressure is released and the exposed film is transported onto a receiving magazine. Simultaneously the next unexposed film is transported into the exposure area and held stationary. The changer is now ready for the next radiographic exposure. This is shown in Figure 2.2. This cycle is repeated until the loading magazine is emptied or the external program controller ends the sequence. The program controller is the electronic control system that basically allows the operator to set the film rate. Initially these devices were simple and could only control film rates for selected short periods of time. They have evolved to complex electronic systems capable of coordinating all activities within an angiographic examination such as injector initiation, radiographic exposure initiation, variable film rates for select periods of an examination, and coordination of table movements in particular examinations. Subsequently manufacturers introduced a computer punch card system to allow pre-programming of these complex sequences.

The most common cut film changer in general use today is the PUCK system (see Figure 2.2). This instrument is relatively compact, versatile in its mounting options, and available in biplane models. It can be purchased to mount on C- or U-arm systems. Some

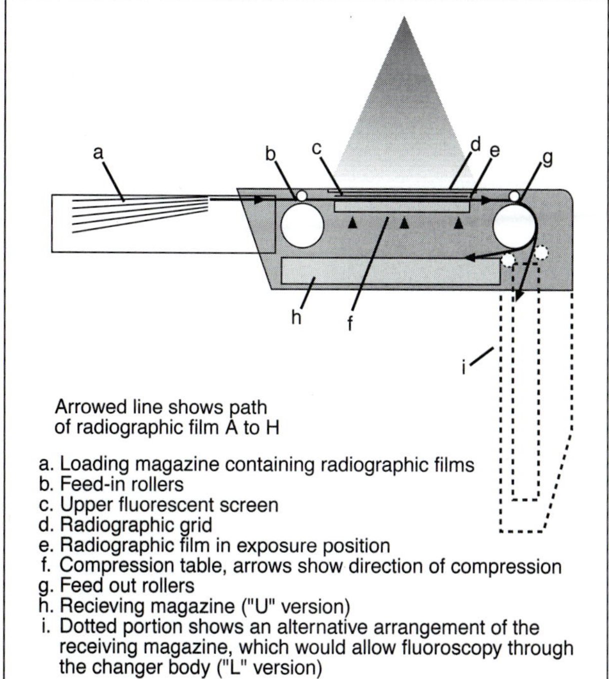

FIGURE 2.2 Schematic diagram of a Siemens PUCK rapid film changer, "U" and "L" model. The models are named in relation to the path taken by the film during transport. The film turns under in the "U" model into a shielded receiving magazine below the exposure area. In the "L" the film passes into a receiving magazine at right angles (*dotted outline*) to the exposure area.

models allow direct fluorographic screening through the changer, before rapid filming to ensure accurate patient position; in others the changer can be rotated away from the face of the image intensifier to allow accurate patient positioning and can then be rotated back into its position for the angiographic run.

The rapid film changer has improved its efficiency as an imaging system over time. The fast fluorescent screens have been replaced with rare earth phosphors and the radiographic film appropriately matched. This has allowed the actual film/screen combination to be effectively optimized for the angiographic procedure. The radiographic grid has seen improvement in both scatter removal and radiation transmission. Aluminum components, also used in the exposure area, generally to support the front screen and protect the grid, have been replaced with carbon fiber. This improvement has reduced beam attenuation and hardening. Overall, these improvements have allowed the changer to achieve a constant standard of image quality with less radiographic exposure. Practically, exposure times have been lowered allowing the system to decrease contrast media motion blur and capture improved stop motion images for analysis. The program controller has likewise developed into a sophisticated electronic control and coordination unit. As the changer has improved so have the controlling units. Modern controllers typically control two rapid film changers, the initiation of radiographic exposures, the injector, and other critical functions of other instruments in the angiographic suite (such as a moving table).

Complementary to the particular developments in film changers has been the rapid improvements in x-ray generation systems and tube technology in the past 20 years. These improvements alone have allowed angiographic imaging systems to acquire at higher repetition rates over longer times. High-power **three-phase** and constant potential high-tension generators have been developed for specialized applications in angiography and other imaging modes. To match the generator, the x-ray tube has likewise developed matching specifications for use in specialized imaging applications. A modern x-ray tube system for angiographic applications is air cooled, has a high-speed rotor, high rating dual foci capabilities, and a high thermal capacity.

Also influential in the development of primary image acquisition systems, and generally on all angiographic systems, has been the characteristics and delivery of vascular contrast media. In the past the relative chemotoxicity and risks associated with unfavorable patient reactions led to developments to limit its volume to achieve a diagnostic imaging sequence. It was rapidly realized that for certain procedures the use of biplane imaging systems could acquire two angiographic images for one volume of contrast media. The total volume of contrast media used per examination and the examination times could be theoretically halved. This concept, although theoretically sound, introduced a new series of related complexities to be overcome. Radiation scatter cross-talk between the image receptors was a problem, the use of crossed grids placing limitations on tube angularity. High-tension generators were devised to switch the exposure factors alternatively between two tubes or controls developed for two generation systems. Depending on the manufacturer, simultaneous or sequential exposures are used to acquire biplane images. The delivery of the contrast media also was an important influence in the development of angiographic imaging systems. Developments in catheter and catheterization techniques combined with the use of image intensifiers as a positioning aid allowed the accurate catheterization of select vascular structures. This directly resulted in a reduction in the volumes of contrast media required to produce quality radiologic images. For other angiographic studies involving large vascular beds, it was found that the use of large-volume hand injections of contrast media did not always provide adequate visualization of the anatomy desired. Contrast media delivered was rapidly distributed in the vascular structure without forming an adequate bolus for visualization. To overcome this, contrast media required introduction at a rate much greater than could be reliably delivered by hand. Pressure injectors were introduced. Initially gas injectors were used but precision electromechanical devices are now used extensively. These contrast media injection devices are able to deliver precise volumes and rates of contrast media at body temperature. These units provide accurate reproducible injections and readily interface into a coordinated sequence of events in an angiography room.

Photographic subtraction methods were developed in angiographic imaging procedures to simplify the resultant radiologic images for analysis (Figure 2.3). Angiography strives to provide concise information concerning the vascular anatomy; the bone detail in an angiographic sequence is therefore redundant. Subtraction techniques in use provide a photographic elimination of common bone detail between a noncontrast and contrast media-filled image in an angiographic sequence. The next major development in angiography was to improve the visualization of the minute subject contrasts. Digital imaging systems are inherently sensitive to the changes required. Most angiographic suites still incorporate a rapid film changer and even with the advent of extensive digital instruments, this primary imaging device often can be found firmly attached to the tube mount, just in case it is required.

Primary imaging devices are not the only method of acquiring angiographic images because for certain vascular examinations they are incapable of film rates quick enough to ensure quality diagnostic image production. The image intensifier becomes a vital link in a secondary imaging system.

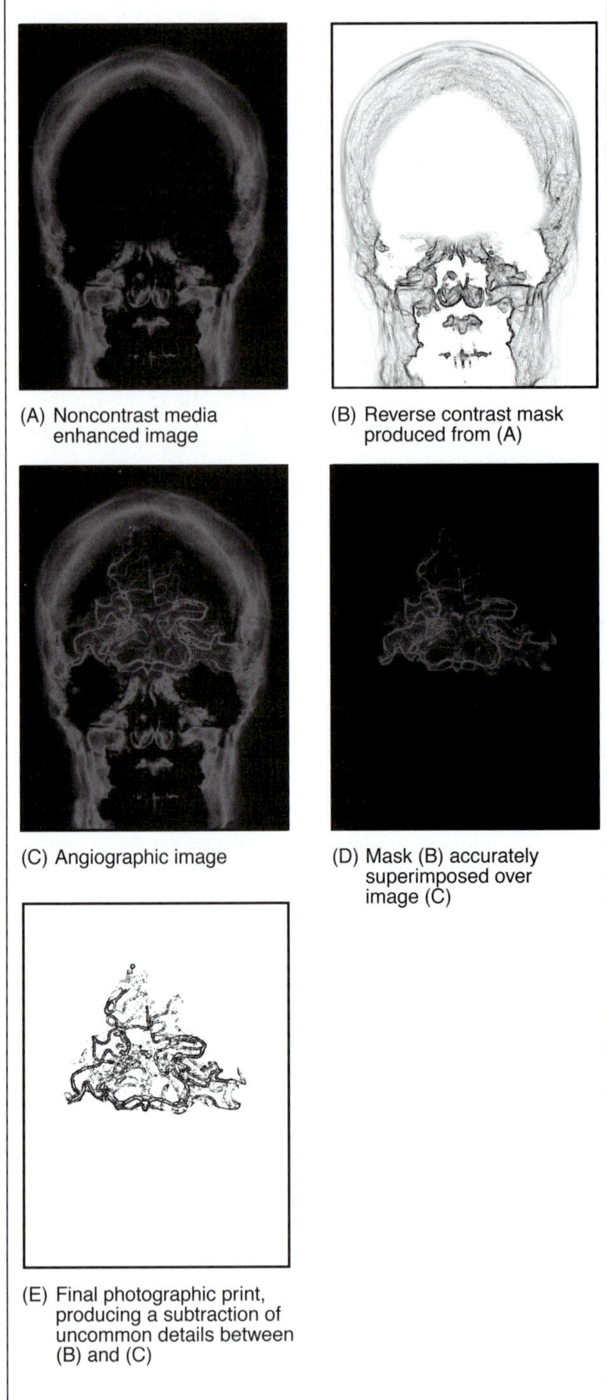

(A) Noncontrast media enhanced image

(B) Reverse contrast mask produced from (A)

(C) Angiographic image

(D) Mask (B) accurately superimposed over image (C)

(E) Final photographic print, producing a subtraction of uncommon details between (B) and (C)

FIGURE 2.3 Photographic mask subtraction method (analog equivalent of digital mask mode subtraction). A reversed contrast polarity mask image (B) is prepared from the nonenhanced image (A). This mask (B) is now accurately superimposed over a contrast media-enhanced angiographic image from later in the same series (D). A photographic subtractive print is then produced (E).

SECONDARY IMAGING SYSTEMS

All secondary and tertiary imaging systems incorporate the use of an intermediate imaging component known as the image intensifier. An image intensifier is a photoelectric system that increases the original relative brightness of a radiographic image produced by a fluorescent screen. The system uses a large input phosphor screen of a fixed diameter (typically 35, 30, 24, 18 cm in diameter) that converts the radiographic latent image to a proportional light representation. This light image is then converted to a proportional electronic representation via an interaction with a photocathode. The electrons comprising this image are both accelerated and focused on a small diameter output phosphor screen (typically 2.5 cm) by an applied electric field. The kinetic energy gained by the electrons is converted into light via collision with the output phosphor and produces an image. The whole system is enclosed in an evacuated glass envelope and apart from the input surface and the output screen, the entire assembly including its power supply, is encased in an electromagnetic shield. The basic design of the unit has not changed since its introduction into imaging applications 30 to 40 years ago. Major improvements have, however, been made in its efficiency and imaging capabilities. A major advance was the introduction of cesium iodide (CsI) as the input phosphor 20 years ago. This new phosphor made significant improvements in both resolution and radiation conversion efficiency. Further improvements have resulted in the introduction of dual field systems. Such systems are able to select a smaller input diameter thus matching the anatomy being examined.

Typically, secondary imaging devices use the bright minified light output of the image intensifier to produce diagnostic images. These recording systems are all inherently photographic and are generally termed photofluorographic systems. All these devices rely on a complex optical coupling lens distribution system to receive the image produced for recording. To allow the distribution of the image from the image intensifier to more than one secondary or tertiary imaging device at a time, use is made of a semitransparent reflective mirror. Mounted typically within the optical coupling unit, this mirror is inclined at 45°. It reflects a large proportion of the light output into a selected photofluorographic camera while a minor percentage is transmitted to a television camera (which is a tertiary imaging device). The system described allows the operator to view an image run on the television camera as it is acquired. Other systems preferentially rotate the mirror to direct all the light output into a selected photofluorographic camera when acquiring the image. This configuration improves the radiation and imaging efficiency of the system, but leaves the operator unsighted via the television camera during the actual image acquisition.

Photofluorographic cameras include serial spot cameras. These can use either roll or cut film and are available in several film widths. Typically 70-, 100-, 110-mm spot film cameras are found in departments, and although these cameras are capable of up to 12 frames a second they are not generally used for angiographic image acquisition procedures. Cine film cameras, similar in principle to a cine movie camera are the conventional choice in very fast image acquisition procedures. Typical film sizes encountered are 35 mm or 16 mm width. A typical roll of film is 50 m long. The camera itself is a precision unit with modern systems capable of up to 200 frames a second but used at much slower rates typically 75 to 100 or slower depending on the vascular anatomy and abnormality sought. The film sensitivity of the cine film has been matched spectrally to the light output of the image intensifier for maximum efficiency. The intensity of the light needs to be maintained to avoid both image over- or underexposure. Automatic exposure systems were developed to ensure the latter requirement because it is not possible to manually compensate radiographic exposure factors for the rapidly changing subject contrasts encountered in these angiographic procedures. These automatic exposure devices function on maintaining a set level of light intensity from the center of the image intensifier output and they generally sample the light via a shadow-free system. This is rather like the light meter system in a single lens reflex camera. The sampled light is then converted to an electronic representation via a photosensitive device. This proportional electronic signal is used to alter the radiographic exposure factors dynamically during a procedure. A simple system manipulates the x-ray tubes milliamperage within a set range to maintain image brightness at a fixed beam quality. The same principle is generally used for automatic screening control or exposure control of a photofluorographic camera (Figure 2.4).

Another improvement in rapid cine camera image acquisition was the development of pulsed radiation acquisition of cine images. As the camera shutter is closed, it is not efficient to continue to irradiate the patient when there is no image being recorded. Pulsed synchronized radiation systems certainly increased the switching complexity of the generator used for image acquisition but potentially reduced radiation dose to the patient. The cine camera remains the fastest image acquisition device in use for high-speed imaging of select vascular events in angiography.

TERTIARY IMAGING SYSTEMS

In common with secondary imaging systems, tertiary imaging systems also use the minified output of an image intensifier to produce an image for display, but incorporate a further conversion of the light image before final image display. A television camera and associated control circuitry is a typical tertiary imaging device, converting the secondary image of the

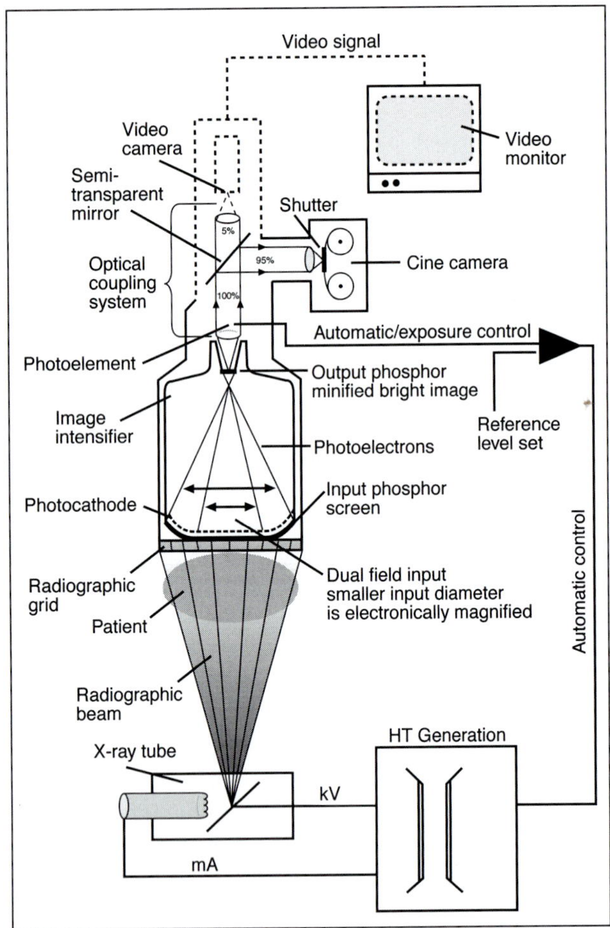

FIGURE 2.4 **A secondary conventional angiographic imaging system incorporating cine radiography.**

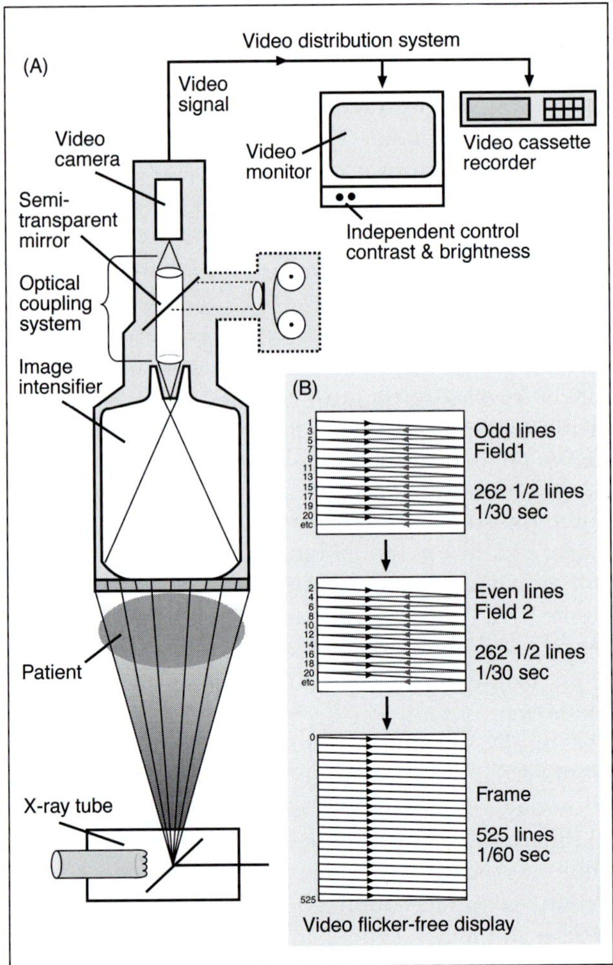

FIGURE 2.5 **A tertiary angiographic imaging system. (A) Illustrates the basic components and relationships in a tertiary imaging system in angiographic application. (B) Schematic shows how flicker free video display is achieved using interlaced scanning.**

image intensifier into an electronic representation. This **video signal** can then be distributed via a video distribution system. It may be simultaneously displayed on several video monitors, recorded on magnetic tape or video disk, or stored in an intermediate electronic digital memory (freeze-frame). Figure 2.5 demonstrates the relationships between the imaging components in an angiographic video display and recording system.

Conventional modern television cameras used in medical imaging have improved over time to become both smaller in physical size and more sensitive to low light conditions. It is a combination of the television camera and its control unit that produces the video signal. A video signal represents an array of horizontal scan lines made within the camera of the light image of the image intensifier. Typically 525 lines are present, scanned at a maximum of 30 times a second and the camera control unit coordinates the scanning sequence and adds appropriate synchronization pulses to allow display devices to decode and display the signal. Each complete set of lines is termed a frame. A frame rate of 30 times a second causes display flicker. To overcome this a rate of at least 50 frames a second is required, but not possible. To solve this dilemma, the even-numbered scan lines in a frame are scanned first and then the odd-numbered lines second. Each half-frame is a field and is scanned in one-sixtieth of a second. When displayed these 60 half-frames overcome the flicker problem without loss of image information. This process is known as interlaced raster scanning. The **spatial resolution** of the television image has two elements, each related to the number and bandwidth of the scan lines on the image. It is possible to increase the scanning rate, which in turn improves resolution, but this involves the use of specialized cameras and video distribution, recording, and display systems. These high-resolution television systems are generally encountered in highly specialized angiographic installations where instant high-quality video replay is required.

The video recorder produces a dynamic recording of the video signal on a moving magnetic tape. Video recordings are especially useful in cases such as cine studies where long times are involved in the immediate processing or display of the angiographic images. Cine studies often incorporate the use of video replay to provide an instant playback of the cine run recorded. The actual spatial and contrast resolution of a video tape is inferior to the actual film but is adequate to allow a decision regarding the relative adequacy of a filming sequence.

Video disk systems are similar to magnetic tape in that they record the video signal on a high-speed rotating disk coated with magnetically sensitive material. An advantage of this system is that it can be accessed randomly, so that it is possible to access any image stored directly without having to fast forward or reverse a tape to find the desired sequence. In some systems, images can be stored in an intermediate electronic memory. These systems generally leave the last frame of the television signal displayed on the monitor for inspection. This can result in a saving of fluoroscopic radiation dose if the stored image can convey enough information to the primary operator, avoiding continuous screening.

Applications

Conventional angiographic equipment has developed to improve the visualization of select vascular structures. Several different forms of angiographic instrument can be identified. However, all use imaging subsystems that can be considered either primary, secondary, or tertiary image production sequences. Overall conventional rapid film angiographic recording systems have developed to become reliable and important investigative instruments in diagnostic imaging.

The primary and secondary imaging systems of conventional angiography all incorporate the use of photographic film. Photographic film provides outstanding spatial resolution but is relatively insensitive in discriminating small changes in subject contrast. Angiographic procedures inherently involve the artificial manipulation of subject contrast via the introduction of contrast media. Photographic subtraction methods were developed to allow a better visualization of the vascular anatomy unencumbered by other anatomy. These techniques were undoubtedly an improvement but still did not improve the inherent sensitivity of the system. This is where conventional imaging systems have reached their limit and unless a major breakthrough can be made, it appears the development of these systems has been exhausted.

Digital imaging systems, however, are inherently sensitive to small changes in subject contrast and are readily suited for this application. The current problem with digital angiographic systems is that their spatial resolution does not equal that of conventional film/screen. With the advent of digital video processing and the incorporation of the digital computer into a fluoroscopic unit, the digital vascular unit was introduced. Initially it was hoped that these units would enable angiography to be performed by IV injection alone, based on their improved sensitivity to low subject contrasts. Experience demonstrated that the selective intra-arterial procedures provided superior diagnostic outcomes. Digital subtraction techniques, which are relatively simple to effect by digital **postprocessing,** rapidly developed to enhance the diagnostic capabilities of these units. A digital vascular unit also has added advantages. In addition to being able to subtract images, it can display an examination in realtime. It allows the operator a series of postprocessing options (such as a mask selection, image smoothness and sharpness, image **contrast manipulation** including polarity inversion, analysis and measurement), not possible with conventional radiographs. The digital computer has now been incorporated into angiography, with specialized digital units available for both general angiography and specialized cardiac studies.

Computing in Special Instruments

Principles

BASIC FUNCTIONS OF A COMPUTER-BASED IMAGING SYSTEM

All modern specialist imaging instruments, irrespective of mode, have incorporated a digital computer into their imaging chain. In certain modes (CT, MRI, SPECT, DSA) the digital computer is an essential component in the production of the image; in others (such as sonography, conventional nuclear medicine) it enhances the collection and subsequent production of images and data for analysis. Irrespective of the application, several important functions of the computer can be identified, as summarized in Figure 2.6.

Image Acquisition

Image acquisition involves the coordinated collection of the image **data.** A digital computer is ideally suited to accurately control and coordinate the image acquisition components of an imaging instrument. This may involve coordinating the magnitude and motion of the imaging energy(s) while accurately locating the detector(s) in space. The computer must then receive output data from the detector(s) and convert these signals ready for digital processing. This conversion process is called an **analog to digital conversion (ADC).**

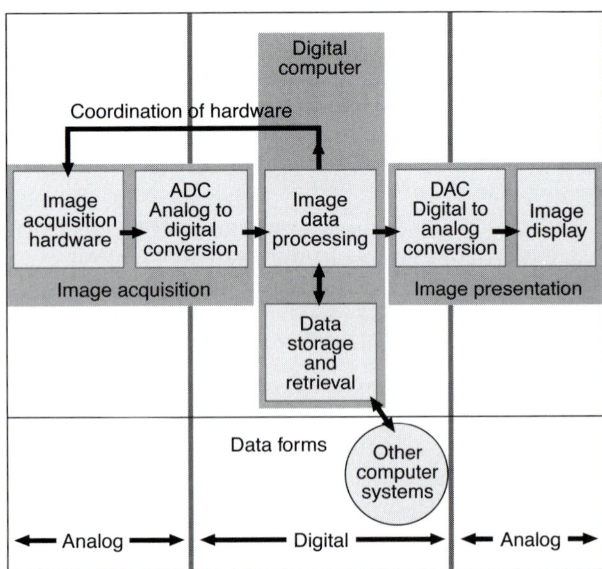

FIGURE 2.6 Basic function areas and data forms in a digital imaging system. Four basic functions can be identified in a digital imaging system. These are image acquisition, image data processing, data storage and retrieval, and image presentation. Only two data forms can be identified—analog and digital.

Image Data Processing

All computers follow set instructions in manipulating digital data. These instructions are coded via a computer language into a program of activities. These programs represent algorithmic solutions to select imaging problems. A computer program is collectively known as software. An advantage of software is that it can be readily rewritten. Computer-based imaging systems characteristically have regular updates of their imaging software. Each new update generally provides improved capabilities and an increase in options. The physical and electrical components of imaging system are by definition known as hardware.

An imaging computer receives data from the ADC to perform its specific tasks. In many systems an initial task is to correct for problems in the input data and then proceed to process the image data. An example of a processing routine is a reconstruction algorithm such as that found in CT or MRI. Once the **digital image** is created the system is then required to provide processes to allow the operator to manipulate the image produced. All these tasks together can be considered image processing. This is now a familiar term in specialized imaging techniques. For this discussion, image processing will be broadly divided into three basic areas of operation. These are **preprocessing,** image data processing, and **post-processing** routines. These are somewhat arbitrary, and as already noted, the processes are interconnected. The output of the processing routines is passed on for conversion to an analog response for image presentation.

Data Storage and Retrieval

The computer is also required to coordinate the format, exchange, and retrieval of digital data from both within itself and with external storage devices. Internal storage devices can be temporary holders of information such as the **random access memory (RAM)** or permanent media for storage such as a hard drive or a floppy diskette. The computer must also format data for exchange or receipt from outside storage devices such as tape drives or optical disk systems. In a similar manner a computer is able to exchange data with other compatible computer systems using common communication protocols. The protocols are important in establishing networks of computers and in the exchange of imaging data between computer systems from different manufacturers. A joint committee of the **ACR (American College of Radiologists) and NEMA (National Electrical Manufacturers Association)** in the United States has already proposed an industry-wide protocol for the interchange of imaging information in medical imaging. To achieve this aim, several versions have been developed, the current protocol being known as **DICOM 3.**

Image Presentation

Data presentation is essentially the reverse of image acquisition. The computer organizes and then converts the discrete digital data representations into the format of an analog signal. Such analog signals can be displayed by a variety of display devices thereby producing images for qualitative analysis or numerical representations for quantitative analysis. An essential conversion is required to allow data presentation and it is termed a **digital to analog conversion (DAC).**

INTRODUCTION TO DIGITAL IMAGING IN SPECIALIZED MEDICAL IMAGING INSTRUMENTS

Although four major functions can be identified in a basic computer-based imaging system, another important observation can be made. Two of the four functions primarily handle analog data in conversion processes and the remaining two are entirely digital in nature. Irrespective of the complexity of a computer-based imaging system, it is always possible to identify only two forms of data being manipulated, one that is **analog** and the other that is **digital.**

Analog and Digital

All medical imaging modes use the interactions of an imaging energy or source with the human body as the method of creating an image. For example, CT involves the transmission and attenuation of a continuous imaging energy waveform. This process is considered to be analog, the tissue attenuation process not breaking the continuous flow of the x-ray energy. The detection device (a CT detector), correctly termed a **transducer,** is also an analog device. It now converts the continuous waveform of attenuated x-ray energy into a similar continuous and smooth electrical representation. Further, the actual production of the x-ray beam is an analog process. The kinetic energy of the projectile electrons within the x-ray tube is smoothly and continuously converted into the x-ray photons of the beam by interaction with the tube anode material (Figure 2.7).

Although these analog transitions and processes retain their continuous nature, they do have inherent problems. Analog transition processes are capable of distorting signals, so that the shape of the output signal may not be a faithful reproduction of the input.

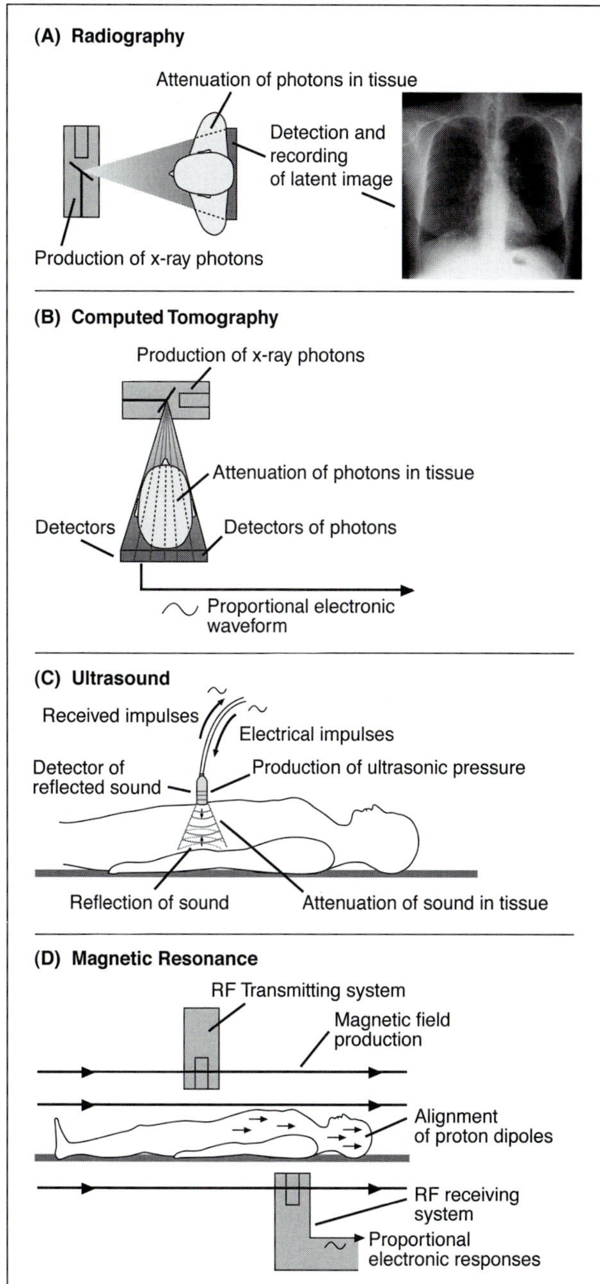

FIGURE 2.7 Examples of analog signal transitions in medical imaging. The processes labeled in each mode represent either an analog signal production or transition.

Analog signal production processes also involve inherent uncertainties in the accuracy of the signals being produced. These are known as **noise products.** It is important to limit both of these problems because they will directly influence the capabilities of an imaging system to accurately discriminate properties of the image signals produced.

The analog output of an imaging transducer is unsuitable for direct use in a digital computer. Analog representations are fundamentally opposite in nature to digital data. Digital data are composed of discrete precise components called **bits.** A single bit is capable of describing only two states, that of on or off or 1 or 0. This simple digital expression can only allow the temporal presence of a varying analog signal to be described but no detail of its magnitude. To improve the precision of this digital description, a sequence of bits is used. Eight bits sequenced together is termed a **byte.** Using the binary counting system a single byte can describe numerical values between 0 and 255. Now in relation to our original analog signal, some 256 temporal measurements of its magnitude can be made.

A byte is also a basic measurement of digital data. It is used to describe the capacity of computer storage devices, such as the internal memory (RAM) and the internal and external storage devices such as floppy diskettes, hard drives, tape drives, and optical storage media. In describing these capacities, the terms kilobyte, megabyte, and gigabyte are commonly encountered. Although each uses a metric prefix, the actual number of bits in each is slightly larger, being related to the power of two closest to the specification. For example, 1 kilobyte is 1024 (2^{10}) bits.

Digital computers are not restricted to processing or describing data as single bytes. Modern systems now group a sequence of bytes into what is termed a word. A word length is specified by each particular computing system but is typically, 16 bits (2 bytes), 32 bits (4 bytes), or 64 bits (8 bytes) long. The word length is influential in the precision of the digital data and the speed (in conjunction with the **system clock**) of data transfer within any computer system.

Analog to Digital Conversion

To overcome the inherent incompatibility between the analog signal output of the imaging transducer(s) and digital representations required by the computer, a device known as an analog to digital converter (ADC) is used. This process is also known as **digitization.** An ADC is an essential component of a computer imaging system and its specifications are highly influential in the final quality of the images produced or data to be analyzed. The output of an imaging transducer is a continuous electrical representation of the incident imaging energy. The amplitude of this waveform is related to the attenuation, transmission, reflection of the imaging energy, or the magnitude of its presence depending on the imaging mode. The function of the ADC is to create a representative discrete digital signal that will accurately characterize the continuous analog waveform. To achieve this the ADC must accurately perform two basic processes: **sampling** and **quantization.** It must also complete these processes quickly, accurately, and be reproducible. The speed of the process will directly influence the number of images the system can acquire per unit time.

Sampling involves the division of the continuous waveform into discrete parts. This is achieved by selecting discrete points on the continuous signal. This process is generally time based. Sampling rate is the number of times a second an analog waveform is sampled and then subsequently converted to a digital number by the second process of quantization (Figure 2.8A). The quantization process converts the magnitude of the analog signal at each sample point into a digital number, selected from a predetermined range.

The transfer of analog data to a digital representation involves certain unavoidable errors and a consequential loss of image data (Figure 2.8B). Because it is impossible to infinitely sample an analog waveform, minute amounts of information will always be lost. This is called sampling error. The higher the sampling rate the smaller will be the sampling error and associated loss of image information. In a computer imaging system the sampling rate influences the physical size of a single sampling point in relation to the volume within the object being imaged. Because a digital image is a two-dimensional rendering of the object, the sampling rate is directly related to the number of pixels (generally expressed as a row by column number) that will be displayed to produce the digital image. Depending on the medical imaging mode, 320 × 320, 512 × 512, 1024 × 1024, and 2048 × 2048 are typical image display matrix specifications. As the size of the matrix is increased, the spatial resolution or spatial frequency response of the image is also increased. Practically, this results in an increased ability to accurately resolve smaller features within the image. However, because of the discrete nature of the samples producing the pixels on the display, a limit will be eventually reached, where features will not be resolved. This is known as the **Nyquist limit.**

Quantization also potentially involves loss of image data. In the process of awarding a digital value to an analog sampled value, the ADC can only draw on a fixed and predetermined range of digital numbers (see Figure 2.8A).The range of these numbers is expressed in terms of bits and is referred to as the **bit depth** or depth of digitization. Typically, medical imaging systems use expansive **quantization ranges** and 10 to 12 bit (2^{10-12}) ranges are common. Irrespective of these magnitudes, it is not possible to precisely quantify each sample magnitude, requiring the system to either round up or down. This uncertainty, termed a **quantization error,** will cause a loss of image information (see Figure 2.8B). Practically, in an imaging system, the smaller the quantization uncertainties the more accurate will be the discrimination of differing tissue types within the patient. When quantization values are translated to a proportional **gray scale** on a video monitor, the observer will then be able to accurately discriminate individual **pixels** based on their relative luminance. The quantization range is therefore directly influential in the **contrast resolution** of the final image.

The ADC process is highly influential in the characteristics and quality of the final digital image. It is important to note that in certain imaging modes, this digital image cannot be directly gained from the coordinated raw digital responses collected at the ADC. To construct the final image, a further intermediate process is used that initially orders and then calculates the digital data to form the final image. The use of a digital computer is vital in this reconstruction process. Irrespective of the manner the final digital image is constructed, it retains the following properties. A digital image is composed of a square or rectangular matrix of discrete sampling points, the digital matrix. Each point represents a finite volume (voxel) within the object examined and has a discrete digital value, which is a correlated representation of the imaging energy (such as attenuation, reflectivity, intensity, etc.). When passed through a DAC process, each discrete sampling point is awarded a proportional gray scale value for display. When displayed, each sampling point is now known as a pixel (or pel). The spatial resolution of the image is related in turn to the number of sampling points in an image and the sampling rate of the ADC. The contrast resolution of the image is directly related to the range of discrete values awarded to each point during the quantization process in the ADC. The construction of a digital image is shown in Figure 2.9.

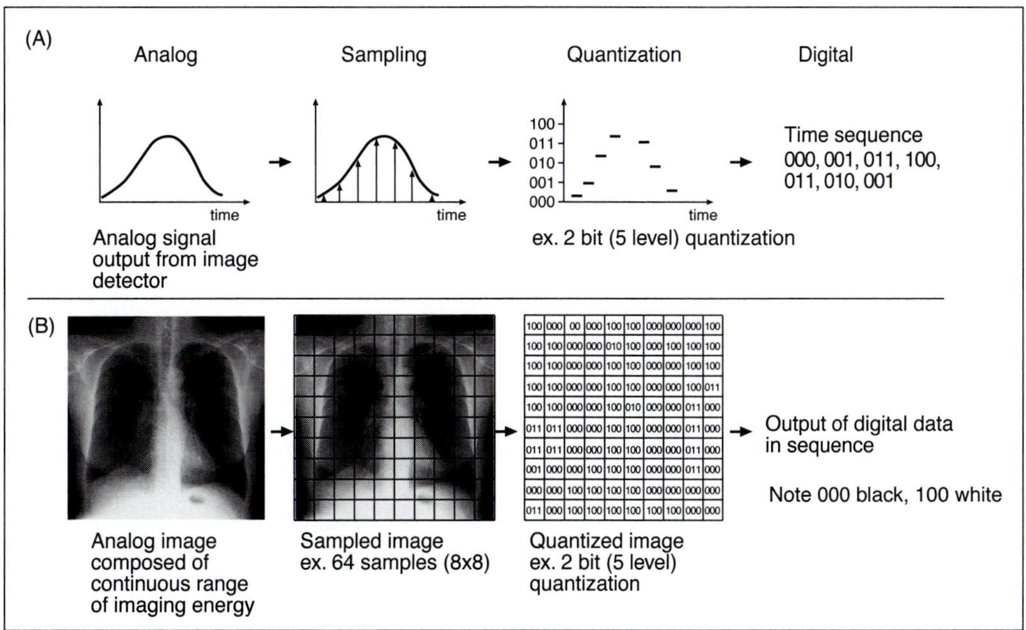

FIGURE 2.8 Analog to digital conversion (ADC) process. (A) An analog signal waveform is sampled a finite number of times and quantized using a 2 bit (5 level) process. Note the errors in sampling and those in quantizing, which introduces errors (uncertainties) in the accuracy of the digital data representation. (B) An analog image is digitized to show the influence that finite sampling has on spatial details and limited quantization range on the accuracy of the digital image data. To diminish these errors in the digital data (image), both sampling and quantization magnitudes need to be increased.

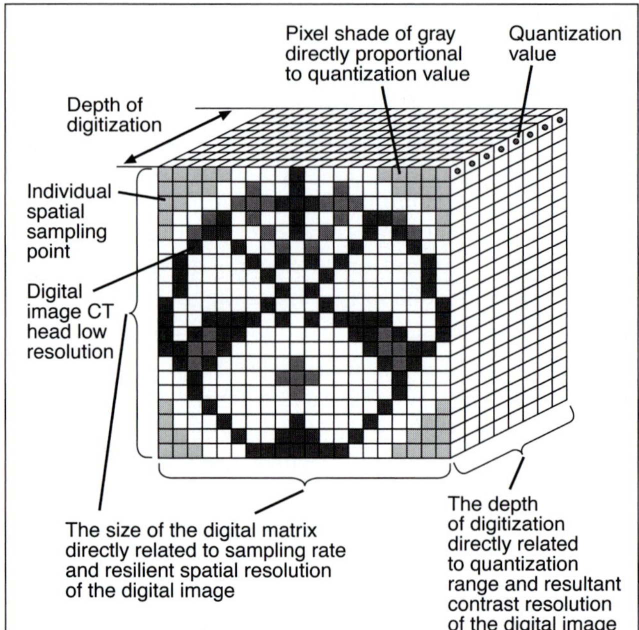

FIGURE 2.9
A digital image can be pictorially shown as a three-dimensional solid composed of many smaller cubes. Each of these cubes can contain only one bit of information. If we increase the depth of the solid (the depth of the digitization), it is possible to describe smaller changes in the imaging energy between each cube (spatial point). The depth of digitization (quantization range) directly influences the contrast properties of the final image. To display a digital image, the value at each cube is translated to a proportional gray scale and displayed as a pixel (picture element) on a display monitor.

Image Production

IMAGE DATA PROCESSING

Image data processing relates to the manipulation and analysis of digital image data and can be broadly divided into three basic areas of operation. These are preprocessing routines, image data processing, and postprocessing routines. Individually and collectively each area of operation strives to improve the quality of the final digital image (Figure 2.10).

Preprocessing Routines

Preprocessing routines are used to reformat the digital data produced by the ADC. The reformatting of the data is used to overcome some of the known inherent problems of analog image acquisition devices. If a detector produces a nonlinear response to the image energy, this can be rectified by a preprocessing routine. In these routines, at each sample point, the quantization value is modified according to a mathematic statement to yield a new value. Once the data has been corrected, if required, they are then passed on for further image data manipulation. Generally, medical imaging systems do not allow the operator to manipulate these preprocessing routines.

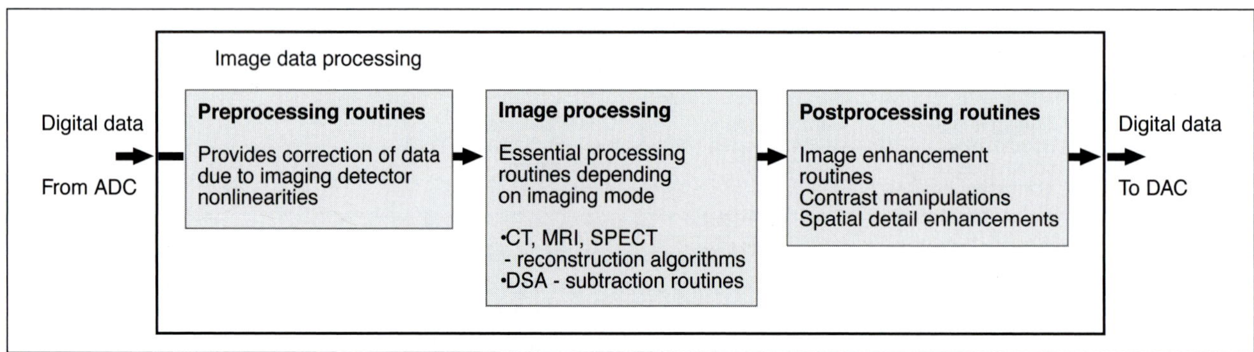

FIGURE 2.10 Three basic operations of digital image processing. (A) Preprocessing routines, (B) image processing, and (C) postprocessing routines.

Image Processing

Once the corrected digital data are received from the preprocessing routine, the actual processing routine can then occur. An image processing routine is no more than an **algorithm,** in the form of a program, which directs the computer to perform mathematic and organization processes on the raw digital data. In certain modes such as CT, MRI, and SPECT, this image processing routine is essential. This routine is responsible for the reconstructed digital image. Image processing routines in these modes also may contain options that allow raw data to be reconstructed in other than planar responses (three-dimensional reconstruction, coronal and sagittal reconstructions, operator-directed line of reconstruction). In other imaging modes, reconstruction may not be necessary, but other processing routines are applied to the raw digital data. In DSA, rapid sequences of digital image data are processed. Each digital image in the rapid sequence is digitally subtracted from generally the first in the series. This results in images with **contrast media enhancement** of the vascular anatomy being subtracted from a noncontrast mask. Additionally, image data processing routines may also allow quantitative data to be extracted in any mode of imaging. In summary, image data processing takes the raw preprocessing digital data and manipulates it into a form suitable for later postprocessing manipulation and digital storage.

Postprocessing Routines

Postprocessing manipulation of digital images has no equivalent in conventional analog imaging, in its ability to selectively enhance **features** or alter the contrast ranges within the image. It is these routines that have generically become known as digital image processing. Postprocessing routines have essentially two related parts. The first allows an operator the ability to selectively manipulate the digital data forming the image to enhance select target features. The second is largely automated, in that the routine automatically prepares and matches the manipulated image data for conversion in the DAC process.

Most operator-directed postprocessing routines seek to enhance the inherent contrast range of the digital image or its select spatial features. Contrast modifications have become an essential postprocessing routine in specialized instruments such as CT and MRI. Both these imaging modes are capable of producing digital images whose quantization ranges (2^{12}) far exceed the gray scale display capabilities of monitors (2^8) and the contrast discrimination of the human eye (2^{4-5}). Contrast postprocessing routines such as **windowing** have overcome this obvious mismatching problem. An operator is able to choose a quantization level within a digital image and then a corresponding width of quantization values to display. An automated postprocessing routine then maps the selected values via a **look up table (LUT)** to match these values to the gray scale available on the monitor. In this manner, it is possible for the operator to view all the digital image data via a series of selected levels and **window widths.** At no time is the display range of the display device exceeded.

Postprocessing routines can also seek to enhance specific structures within the digital image. These spatial **enhancements** include routines that sharpen edges, others that smooth features, and others that seek to remove noise artifacts.

In spatial domain image processing, the computer mathematically manipulates the quantization values within the digital image to produce the output enhanced digital image. It is this form of processing that is extensively used to provide the majority of postprocessing routines in use. There are only three mathematic operations in spatial domain image processing (Figure 2.11A). They are termed **point, local** or neighborhood, and **global operations.** Point operations manipulate the digital value at each sampling point, one by one, according to a mathematic function and place the new value in the same corresponding spatial position in the enhanced output image. Local operators mathematically calculate each new digital value in the output image by the weighted contributions of its surrounding neighbors in the original image. Variations in the weighting factors will produce edge sharpening, edge detection, or edge smoothing. A global operation mathematically treats the digital image as a large set of digital values. Rotation and magnification (zoom) are examples of this operator. Spatial domain image processing is robust and versatile; however, not all postprocessing imaging problems can be readily solved by this method. Frequency domain methods provide other options in seeking solutions to difficult problems.

Frequency domain imaging processing must initially reformat the digital data before the application of the actual processing routine. Digital images have clear relationships between the position and quantization values of each sampling point. It is possible using mathematics to also describe these relationships in terms of the frequency spectrum. Using mathematics known as a **Fourier transform,** an entire digital image can be re-expressed as a function of spatial frequency. The new image is now said to be in Fourier or Frequency space. In specialized imaging systems, both forms of image postprocessing are used to achieve select image outcomes.

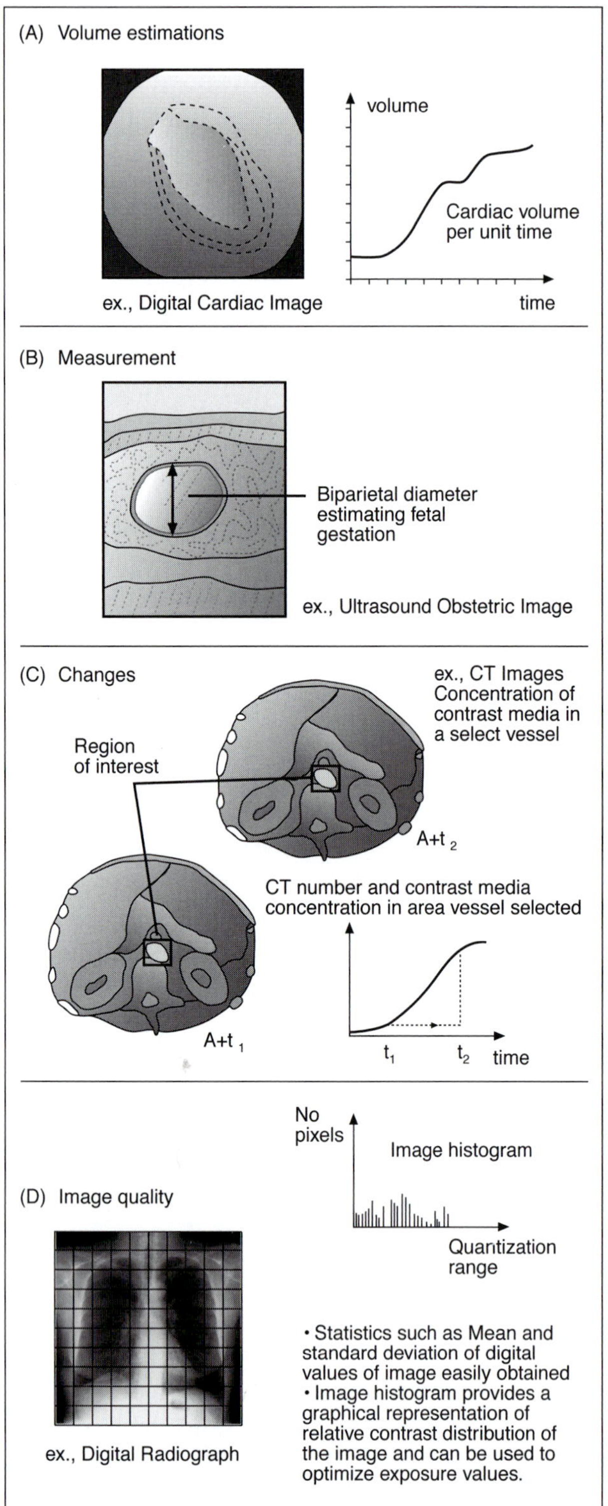

FIGURE 2.11 Quantitative data extraction. Four examples are provided of quantitative data extraction from digital medical images.

Postprocessing can be used in addition to the manipulation of images for analysis, to extract and prepare quantitative data for analysis. In many imaging modes, additional statistical data concerning an image are readily available due to the inherent numerical nature. Histograms can be constructed of the whole image or of selected subregions. The latter, referred to as regions of interest, can be useful in analyzing dynamic sequences, where particular statistics can be displayed as a function of time. These new curves can yield quantitative information of physiologic function, such as the buildup and elimination of contrast medium or a radiopharamacetical, within a specific body region or target organ. Other quantitative postprocessing routines involve measurement. It is relatively simple to provide digital calipers to gain accurate measurements within a digital image. In obstetric ultrasound, such measurements are often directly referred to a postprocessing algorithm that provides a direct estimate of fetal age. Using measurement tools, areas and volumes can be determined. The latter postprocessing routines are used to determine cardiac or other volumes in various phases from the images produced. A selection of four examples of quantitative data extraction is shown in Figure 2.11.

Digital to Analog Conversion

Digital to analog conversion is required to allow the production of the final image form for analysis. To display the digital information a reverse conversion process is required. The digital data now needs to be converted back into analog format. Most display and review instruments are typically analog devices. The output digital data from the operator-directed and automatic postprocessing are passed onto a DAC. DAC is essentially the reverse of an ADC. The DAC organizes the data and then converts these digital values into corresponding analog values. Typically DAC systems produce video outputs or drive computer video monitors directly to produce the output image.

Applications

The incorporation of the digital computer into imaging systems has brought great benefit to medical science and its diagnostic accuracy. Now a variety of modern imaging modes cannot function without the vital assistance of the integrated computer system.

Digital computers are characterized by their ability to manipulate digital responses and digital data. All medical imaging procedures involve the use of analog processes. As a direct consequence, essential ADC and DAC processes are an important and influential function of digital computer imaging systems. ADC of analog data, also known as digitization, is an important part of the image acquisition process. DAC, which is essentially the reverse of ADC, is vital to prepare images for display. Both these conversion processes are highly influential in the quality of the digital image produced.

The major advantage of the digital computer is that once the data have been transformed to digital format, they can be manipulated easily and efficiently. This allows these systems to rapidly organize and manipulate the imaging data to identify complex relationships. Such flexibility has facilitated planar image reconstruction methods, helical scanning techniques of data acquisition, three-dimensional visualization, virtual reconstruction of internal structures, and real-time image procedures such as subtraction. A range of options is now available that would be impossible with conventional analog (film/screen) imaging systems. Further, because the computer is directed by a software program, any subsequent improvement in a particular algorithm in terms of increased processing speed, accuracy, or improved options can be readily incorporated through a software upgrade. An existing system can more readily take advantage of improving computer technology to enhance image quality. In a conventional imaging system most advances have been made by replacing hardware items.

Another major benefit of the digital computer in imaging is the comparative ease of image data storage, retrieval, and distribution. Digital data being inherently numerical are readily and efficiently stored on a range of permanent and nonpermanent media. Unlike its analog film counterpart, mass storage takes up little physical space and also unlike photographic copy techniques, digital images do not degrade. Being inherently discrete numerical representatives, a copy is an exact copy of these representations. Retrieval methods have developed to provide fast, efficient access to large data sets of images by many operators at once. Such solutions have seen the introduction of radiologic image information systems and the distribution of images and associated information throughout the imaging department. In the wider clinical environment efficient distribution of digital data has been made possible by the efficient linking or networking of computers. Although a **network** may consist of a few computers linked together locally, the modern trend has been to link many computers over a wide area and to share and exchange image and other information. This can assist in the management of a patient transferred from a regional to metropolitan clinical center or between centers in a city, or even within the one hospital. A networked system can make a patient's images obtained during an imaging scan available to other sections of the hospital. This can allow simultaneous image analysis to be performed by an imaging specialist or presurgical image evaluation carried out by a surgeon, thus saving valuable time. In these systems, the individual computers can be linked together by direct wires, telephone lines, optical cables, radiofrequency devices, or a combination of these telecommunications methods. However, to communicate with each other, they must share compatible formats of the data and use common communication protocols.

Image preparation and manipulation techniques are a major beneficiary of the use of the digital computer in medical imaging systems. The use of pre- and postprocessing image manipulation routines has markedly influenced the accuracy and ease of image data presentation. Essential postprocessing routines have enabled exceedingly large data sets to be accurately displayed without loss of important detail. An ability to manipulate the digital image to readily enhance contrast ranges within an image or to enhance spatial details, has no equivalent in analog imaging.

As technology advances it is highly probable that all medical imaging modes will incorporate a computer to enable diagnostic image production. Already, much change has occurred and many clinical and technologic advances have been made through the judicious incorporation of a digital computer in medical imaging science. What will the next 25 years bring?

Review Questions

1. In relation to a typical conventional angiographic installation, explain the primary, secondary, and tertiary imaging subsystems and the relationships that exist between them.

2. Name and discuss the four basic functions and two basic data states found in a computer-based imaging system.

3. Describe the basic "construction" of a digital image. What relationships exist between the sampling rate, size of the digital matrix, and spatial resolution of the final displayed image; and the depth of digitization, quantization range, and contrast resolution of the final displayed image?

4. Which of the following conventional angiographic imaging instruments produces the fastest filming rate?
   a. cut film changer
   b. cassette changer
   c. photospot camera
   d. 35-mm cine camera
   e. 35-cm wide roll film changer

5. The spatial resolution of a digital image is increased by which of the following?
   a. increasing the depth of digitization
   b. acquiring the images at a faster rate
   c. increasing the sampling rate
   d. decreasing the size of the digital matrix
   e. using larger pixels on the screen

CASE STUDY

You have completed an examination using a computer-based imaging system (say a CT or MRI or SPECT); you note a subtle abnormal appearance in a sequence of the images acquired. Discuss what options you have available to you to render this appearance more visible for medical analysis and what other options you may use to gather quantitative information to further aid medical analysis.

References and Recommended Reading

Awcock, G. J., & Thomas, R. (1995). *Applied image processing.* London: Macmillan.

Baxes, G. A. (1994). *Digital image processing.* New York: Wiley.

Bushberg, J. T., Siebert, J. A., Leidholdt, E. M., & Boone, J. M. (1994). *The essential physics of medical imaging.* Baltimore: Williams & Wilkins.

Curry, T. S., Dowdey, J. E., & Murry, R. C. (1990). *Christensen's physics of diagnostic radiology* (4th ed.). Philadelphia: Lea & Febiger.

Dendy, P. P., & Heaton, P. (1987). *Physics for radiologists.* Cambridge, MA: Blackwell Scientific.

Hendy, W. R., & Reitenour, R. (1992). *Medical imaging physics* (3rd ed.). St. Louis: Mosby-Year Book.

Romans, L. E. (1995). *Introduction to computer tomography.* Baltimore: Williams & Wilkins.

Russ, J. (1994). *The image processing handbook* (2nd ed.). Boca Raton, FL: CRC Press.

Snopek, A. M. (1992). *Fundamentals of special radiographic procedures* (3rd ed.). Philadelphia: Saunders.

Woodward, P., & Freimarck, R. (Eds.). (1995). *MRI for technologists.* New York: McGraw-Hill.

Computed Tomography

Mary Susan Helene Crowley, MRT(R)(ARRT)

Introduction and Historical Overview

The discovery of x-rays allowed the transmission of human body images that yielded an immense amount of interesting and often useful diagnostic information. However, because a three-dimensional structure was being projected onto a two-dimensional display, much of the information about a specific internal structure was masked by shadows of overlying structures. Radiographs at various angles helped to separate the planes but at a greatly increased radiation dose to the patient. This method however, did not overcome the basic problem of the overshadowing of the denser materials. To eliminate the unwanted structure detail, various "tomographic" techniques were developed.

A complete history of tomography in radiology includes the development of a variety of techniques during the several decades preceding the first implementation of CT.

These developments included mathematic techniques for reconstruction contributed by Radon and others, the development of medical x-ray technology, and the introduction of inexpensive mini- and microcomputers and array processors. All these necessary technical elements were in place by the late 1960s.

CONVENTIONAL TOMOGRAPHY

Before the advent of CT, conventional tomography used the basic principle of blurring out unwanted structures. With conventional linear tomography the plane of interest was held in focus while the overlying and underlying anatomic structures were blurred. The overhead x-ray tube and the film under the patient were linked by a pivoted rod and the plane of focus occurred along the horizontal plane. A sharp image of the object plane was obtained by moving the film and moving the x-ray tube above the patient at the same time, but in opposite directions (Figure 2.12). The resultant image enhanced radiographic contrast in the area of interest while blurring the adjacent unwanted structural information. By moving the pivot point up and down, the plane of interest was adjusted. By changing the tomographic angle the thickness of the cut could be controlled.

Increased patient dose is one of the principal disadvantages of of conventional tomography. For a complete conventional tomographic examination the focal plane as well as the planes above and below are exposed to the full beam for each exposure. The resulting dose received by the patient can be as high as several grays (abbreviated Gy).

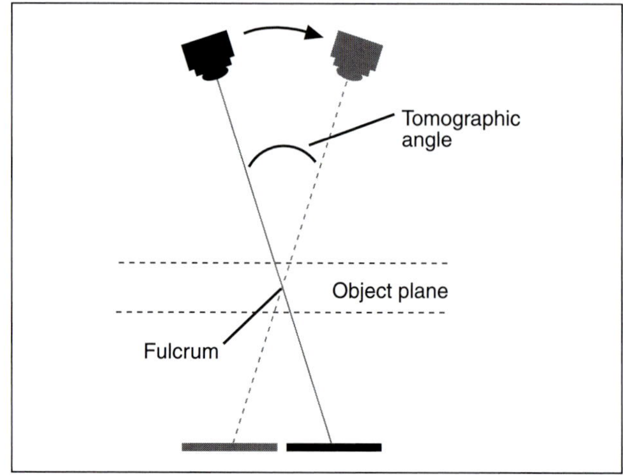

FIGURE 2.12 In the simplest form of tomography, linear, the cassette and tube simultaneously move in opposite directions. Only objects lying in the object plane will be imaged in focus.

The next development was transversal planograph. The patient either sat or stood on a rotating disk that was coupled to a turntable holding the film (Figure 2.13). As the exposure was made with an angled overhead stationary x-ray tube, the film and patient rotated synchronously in the same direction. The final image was an approximate representation of density distributions of the scanned area but contained considerable blurring, limiting the use of this method. Further attempts to develop this method with electronic means in 1960s ended when it became clear that the resolution was less than with the normal planographic views.

A solution to this problem of blurring required a specifically programmed computer. That technique became known as computed **axial tomography.**

COMPUTED AXIAL TOMOGRAPHY

Cormack was the first to apply the techniques of image reconstruction from projections to radiogra-

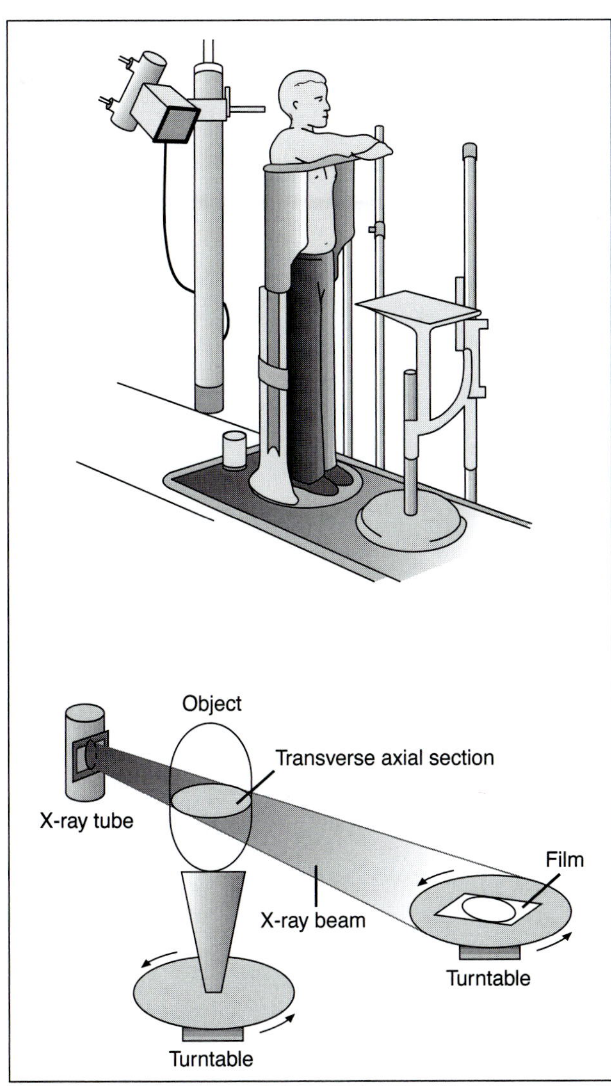

FIGURE 2.13 Transverse axial tomography (TAT) produced transverse cross sections of selected anatomy. The patient (either standing or sitting on a pedestal) and the film simultaneously rotated in the same direction.

phy. Houndsfield, along with EMI, a records and electronic components company, launched the first clinically viable CT scanner. The EMI neuroscanner was an immediate success during the early 1970s. For their discovery Cormack and Houndsfield shared the Nobel Prize for medicine in 1980.

The commercial development of CT in the early 1970s introduced the possibility of excluding confusing superimposed structures. The ability to differentiate the various structures within the brain allowed for the display of tumors, hematomas, and infarcts according to their size and position without the use of contrast medium. The elimination of patient distressing diagnostic examinations such as pneumoencephology (nū´´mō-ĕn-sĕf´ă-lŏg´ră-fē) was truly the advent of a new era in imaging.

CT is a quantitative method of imaging. Accuracy when differentiating between **absorption values** in tissues is highly valued. After the tremendous diagnostic capabilities of CT were recognized, dozens of x-ray equipment manufacturers joined in the production of CT scanners. In this competitive atmosphere, the technical refinement of CT equipment evolved quickly. From 1973 to 1978, four **generations** or geometric configurations (types) of CT scanning systems emerged. The gradual reduction of scan times from 300 seconds to approximately 2 seconds was accomplished.

Principles

Although today's scanners have many technical advancements, the same basic principles of axial tomography are used. Instead of producing an image on radiographic film from a wide-angle beam of x-rays passing through the patient, readings are taken of the intensity of the x-rays emerging from the patient. Profiles of these readings are processed by a computer and then displayed on a television screen or cathode ray tube (CRT). The CT is displayed without any superimposition or blurring of the anatomy of interest. The ability to vary the contrast and brightness of the displayed image without rescanning the patient was also a great advancement in diagnostic imaging. The method of computing and reconstructing the image is addressed later in this chapter.

EQUIPMENT DESIGNS

A modern CT scanner consists of a **gantry,** a collimated x-ray source, a **detector array**, a computer data acquisition and reconstruction system, a motorized patient couch, and one or two CT display consoles. The major data acquisition geometry differences between the various commercial scanners lies in the computer capabilities and gantry design. The design of the CT gantry relates the number and type of **detectors** used as image receptors as well as the geometric configuration and scanning motion of tube and detectors.

Originally scanners were divided into "generations" for identification purposes but as the number of companies involved increased, scanners became identified by their geometric configuration. Manufacturers continuously strive to improve their data acquisition geometry and components to produce high-resolution artifact-free images and faster scan times.

Components of Typical CT Unit (Figure 2.14)

Patient Table The table is comprised of carbon fiber molded into a ridged, strong platform that supports the patient during the CT examination. Each manufacturer has a maximum allowable patient weight for their tables. For example,

Picker—450 lb distributed weight
Elscint—475 lb distributed weight

The table is mounted on a pedestal that houses the mechanical and electrical components to move the table vertically and horizontally. A few companies produce a table that swivels about 12° to the left or right of midline.

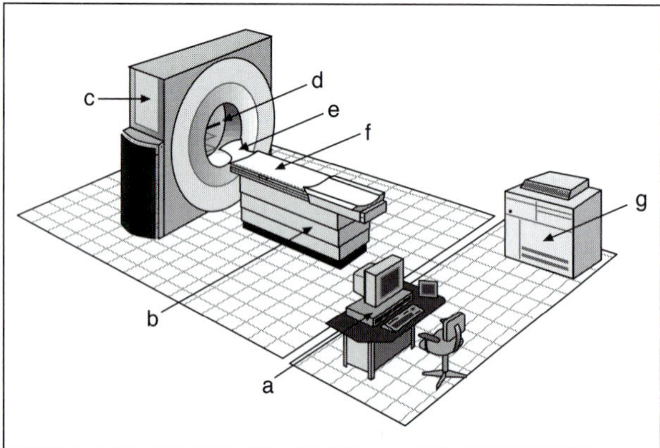

FIGURE 2.14 Main components of a typical modern CT imaging system; (a) operator's control console; (b) motor driven adjustable table support; (c) gantry, which houses the x-ray tube, generator, slip rings, collimators, detectors, and detector electronics; (d) aperture; (e) head holder; (f) patient couch; (g) laser imager.

Gantry The gantry houses the x-ray tube, slip rings, high-tension generator, collimators, detector array, and detector electronics. Several gantries have a cephalic and caudal tilt range of 12° to 30° to accommodate all types of patient conditions. For accurate patient positioning a laser beam is located at the top and side of the aperture of the gantry.

Aperture To accommodate the various patient types and scans performed, the circular opening in the gantry in which the patient is positioned for the CT scan is commonly 70 cm in diameter. For easy access to the patient, the aperture is approachable from the front and back of the gantry. A camera to constantly monitor the patient is usually mounted at the back of the gantry.

X-ray Tube Originally, the first and second generation scanners used stationary, oil-cooled x-ray tubes. As the demand for faster scan times and increased tube output escalated, the adoption of rotating anode x-ray tubes and eventually **slip ring technology** significantly increased the heat storage capacity of CT units (Figure 2.15).

Today's generators vary from 30 to 60 kW depending on the manufacturer. Modern x-ray tubes have large diameter anodes made of rhenium, tungsten, and molybdenum alloy (RTM) with a smaller target angle (~12°) and 3600 to 10,000 rotations per minute (rpm). Typically a small focal spot is 0.6 × 1.6 mm in size and 0.9 × 2.4 mm for a large focal spot, but this varies with each manufacturer.

SCANNERS

First Generation

The EMI Mark 1 was the only scanner of this type built. It was installed in the Atkinson Morley Hospital at Wimbledon under the supervision of Dr. Ambrose in 1971. The patient was placed horizontally on a couch with his head enclosed in a "waterbag" (Figure 2.16). The x-ray tube (emitting a pencil-shaped beam) and two side by side thallium-doped crystals of sodium iodide coupled to photomultipliers moved in a linear **translate** and circular rotation movement. Between each scan the couch moved in increments of 1 to 2 cm. The readings were then processed by a microcomputer and displayed. Scan time was approximately 5 minutes per slice for a total of 25 minutes per clinical examination.

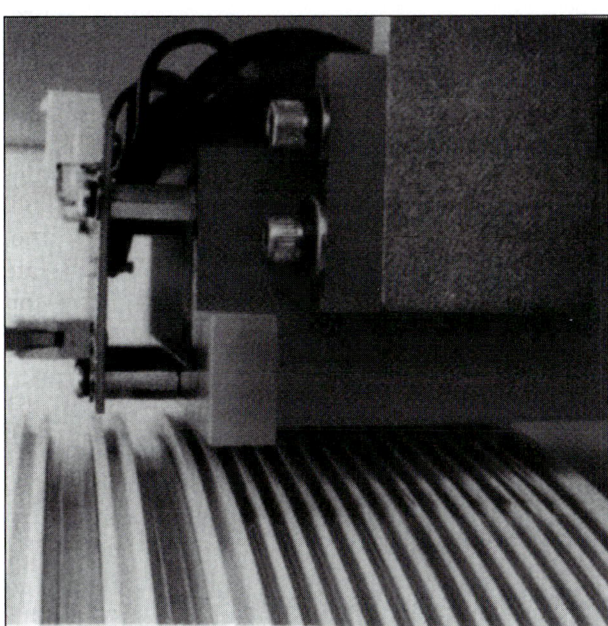

FIGURE 2.15 The cylindrical slip ring design scanners are intended to provide continuous rotation of the gantry components by eliminating the conventional high-tension cables from the generator to the x-ray tube. The electromechanical slip rings consist of circular electrical conductive rings and brushes. Modern on board generators provide power to the slip rings, which in turn supply power to the x-ray tube. (Courtesy of Picker International)

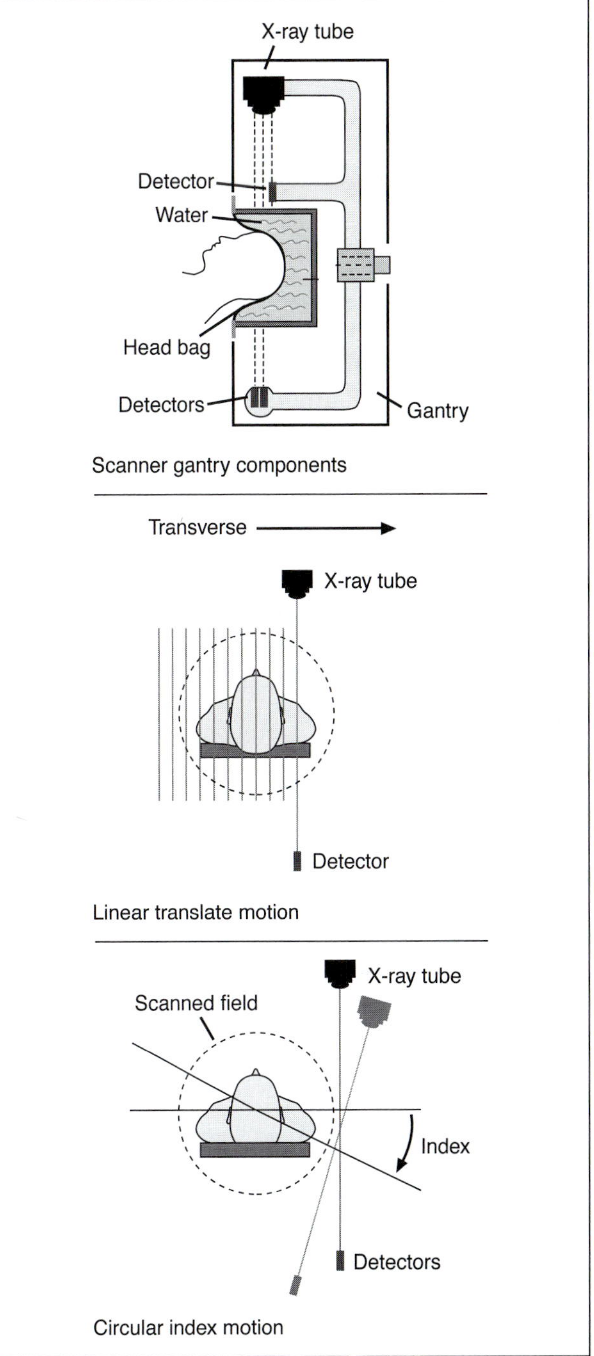

FIGURE 2.16 First generation CT scanner with a translate-rotate gantry motion. Note the paired detector and pencil shaped x-ray beam.

Second Generation

The second generation, similar in configuration to the first, used multiple solid state detectors and a diverging fan beam. The linear detector array varied from 10 to 100 detectors and were often made of cesium iodide. The scan motion was still one of transverse and rotate, but by increasing the number of detectors, the indexing steps were less, thus reducing the scan time. The fastest scan was approximately 6 seconds (Figure 2.17).

In 1973, Pfizer Corporation, in conjunction with Dr. Langley, produced a large aperture version of the EMI brain scanner enabling the scan of whole bodies. Because the scan time was still 5 minutes, inherent motion of the internal anatomy caused the resultant images to appear blurred. Other techniques for body imaging were at that time more diagnostic.

Third Generation

The third generation scanners are based on fan-beam geometry with a "rotate-rotate" motion. The x-ray tube and detectors are mounted on a circular track and rotate 360° in tandem around the patient. The detector array consisting of 700 to 1000 detectors is wide enough to cover the whole patient with a diverging

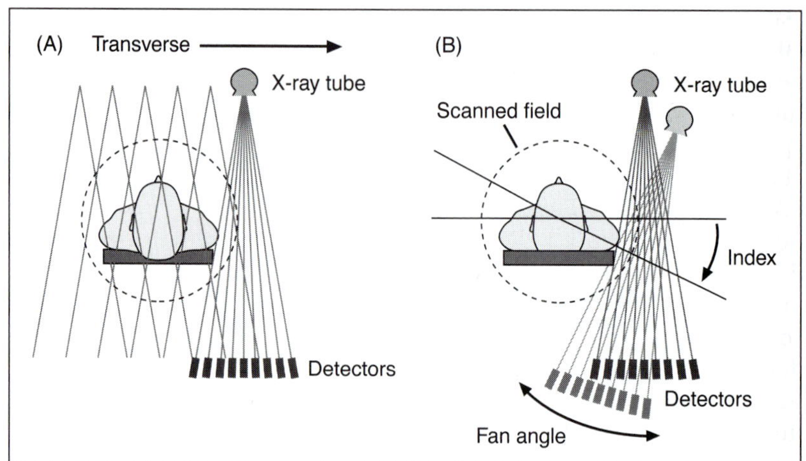

FIGURE 2.17
Basic second generation CT scanner. (A) Demonstrates the linear transverse motion of the x-ray tube and (B) the angular movement of the x-ray tube and detector assembly between each translation. Note the fan x-ray beam and multiple detectors.

fanned beam of x-rays. Rotate-rotate scanners generally collect data within a few seconds (the more detectors the shorter the scan time). Third generation geometry is used by most companies today (Figure 2.18).

Fourth Generation

The basic fourth generation consists of a stationary ring of 1200 to 2000 detectors that completely surround the patient. The x-ray tube, with a collimated fan-shaped x-ray, rotates inside the ring of detectors. Another fourth generation geometric configuration motion has the beam rotating outside the ring of detectors as the ring of detectors tilt. This tilting motion, referred to as nutation (nū-tā´shŭn), allows the fan beam to hit an array of detectors located on the opposite side of the detector ring. Since there is no lateral movement in both third and fourth generations, scan times as low as 0.7 seconds per 360° data acquisition are possible (Figure 2.19).

SPIRAL CT

With conventional CT scanners, the motion of the tube and detector array was limited to single 360° turns alternating clockwise and counterclockwise.

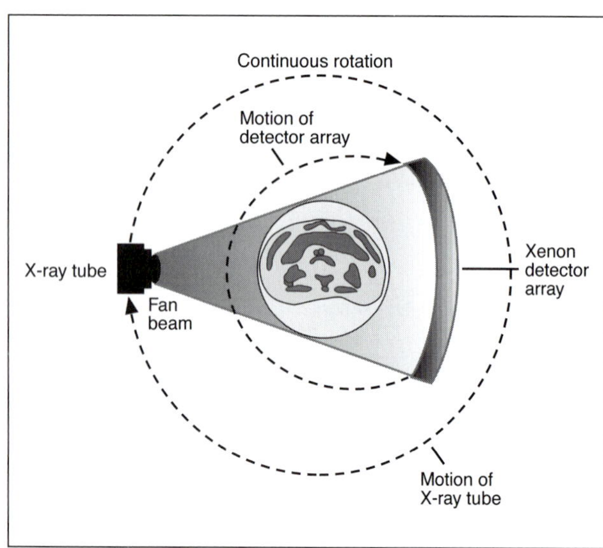

FIGURE 2.18 Third generation geometric configuration of x-ray tube and detectors (in conjunction with slip ring technology) is the most commonly used in modern CT scanners.

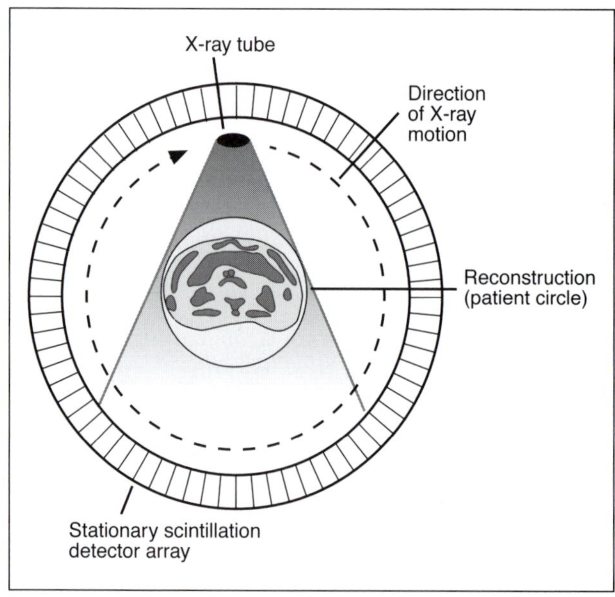

FIGURE 2.19 Fourth generation data acquisition geometry with stationary detectors and a rotating x-ray tube.

Data are acquired contiguously, slice by slice, at 2 to 10 seconds per slice. Included in scan time is a scan delay as the table moves to the next position and the tube is ready for the next exposure. This allows for approximately one to three scans per minute. A CT abdomen and pelvis with 10-mm slice thickness would take approximately 30 to 45 minutes. Slip ring technology has allowed for the continuous circular rotation of the x-ray tube and detector array. This mechanical movement permits a volume of data to be collected in 60 seconds or less. The x-ray tube and detector assembly continually rotate around the patient while the table top moves at a constant speed through the gantry (Figure 2.20). The patient table travels typically at a speed of one **slice thickness** per 360° rotation. **Pitch** is a term used in spiral CT to describe the distance between revolutions or turns of a **helix.** If the pitch is increased, the distance between the revolutions increases. Pitch can be expressed as table speed divided by the chosen slice thickness. If the table speed is the same as the slice thickness, it can also be expressed as 1:1 ratio or a pitch of 1; when the table speed is two times the slice thickness, pitch is expressed as a 2:1 ratio or a pitch of 2. Extending the helix provides greater z-axis coverage but may affect the ability to detect small pathologies due to the increased slice thickness.

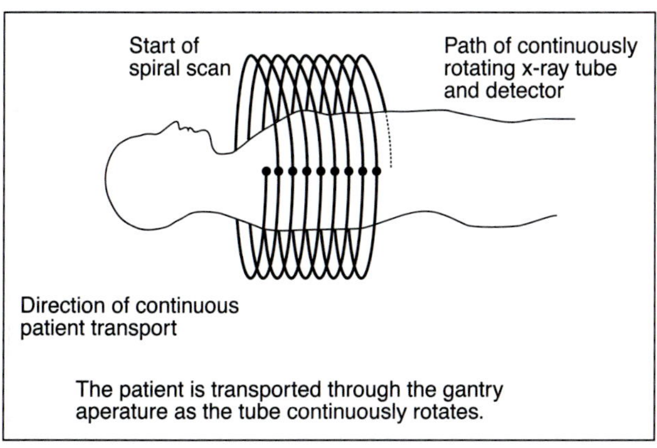

FIGURE 2.20 Spiral or volume data acquisition geometry.

Two of the biggest advantages associated with spiral CT are speed of data acquisition and minimal patient motion artifacts resulting from different levels of respiration. In conventional CT the patient is required to breathe in and out and hold for each slice scanned. Inevitably the breathing pattern varies with each breath hold. Spiral CT requires one breath hold to acquire a whole volume of tissue from the diaphragm to the symphysis. The data can be acquired in 60 seconds, with no shifting of anatomic structures. (If the patient is unable to breath hold for 60 seconds, the volume acquisition can be divided into two 30-second acquisitions.)

Advantages of Spiral CT

1. Scan times of less than 60 seconds are possible.
2. Interscan delays are minimized, which is important when investigating the dynamics of contrast media flow or the physiology of organs.
3. One single exposure and one breath hold allows complete coverage of the anatomic area.
4. Patient motion artifacts are reduced.
5. Shifting of anatomic structures position is reduced.

Limitations of Spiral CT

1. Because the x-ray tubes must be able to sustain high power levels for longer periods of time, tubes with improved cooling rates and higher capacity are required.
2. Reconstruction time for spiral CT is a little longer because it requires that an interpolational algorithm be applied to all the collected data. This algorithm removes streak artifacts.
3. Unshapen images may appear as a result of partial volume averaging.

Image Production

DATA ACQUISITION

Acquisition of CT data first requires an x-ray source to be aligned with a detector array. After the x-ray beam passes through the patient, the detector samples or reads the intensity of each ray of the fan beam and then measures the transmitted beam's intensity. The patient's internal anatomic structures attenuate the x-ray beam according to their mass, density, and effective atomic number. The transmitted beams from the many projection angles seen throughout the scan are absorbed by the detector. The attenuation of each ray sum is then calculated and correlated with the position of each ray.

Once the detector has received all the projection data, an electrical or analog signal is produced representing the **attenuation** profile of the view. The attenuation profile created for each view is projected back onto a matrix. The intensity of the analog signal produced is directly proportional to the intensity of the transmitted x-ray beam absorbed by the detector. The signal proceeds to the data acquisition system (DAS), located within the gantry, where the analog signal is amplified and then sent to an ADC. Because the computer cannot understand analog information, the analog signals are converted to digital form and transmitted to an array processor. By using algorithmic calculations the array processor solves the statistical information fundamental for the mathematic reconstruction of the CT image. A numerical value is assigned to each signal according to the intensity of signal emitted from the detector. These numerical values (raw data) are stored in the computer where reconstruction filters are applied to the raw data to optimize a balance between spatial resolution and contrast resolution to best represent clinically relevant detail.

DETECTOR ARRAY

The detector array is the image receptor for the CT scanner just as the x-ray film is for conventional radiography and the image intensifying screen is for the fluoroscopy. The number, size, and type of detector in the arrays used in today's CT scanners varies according to the manufacturer. Although scintillating crystal detectors are used in most CT scanners today, gas-filled detectors are also a viable choice as an image receptor.

Gas-filled detector arrays consist of a large metallic chamber with grid-like tungsten strips spaced at approximately 1-mm intervals. The strips divide the large chamber into many smaller chambers, about 15 detectors per centimeter, each functioning as a separate radiation detector. The entire array is hermetically sealed and filled under pressure with a high atomic number inert gas such as xenon or xenon-krypton mixture. All gas-filled detectors use the ionization of gas by the incoming radiation to produce an electrical signal. The ionization of the gas in the chamber is proportional to the radiation incident on the chamber (Figure 2.21).

Scintillation detectors have evolved from sodium iodide crystals-photomultiplier assemblies (Figure 2.22) with excessive afterglow and bulk to smaller more efficient cesium iodide or cadmium tungstate crystal-photodiode assemblies. A ceramic material used by one company has been pronounced as the superior scintillating material of the 1990s. The intensity of the light signal produced from the crystal as the attenuated x-ray interacts with the crystal is proportional to the beam incident on it.

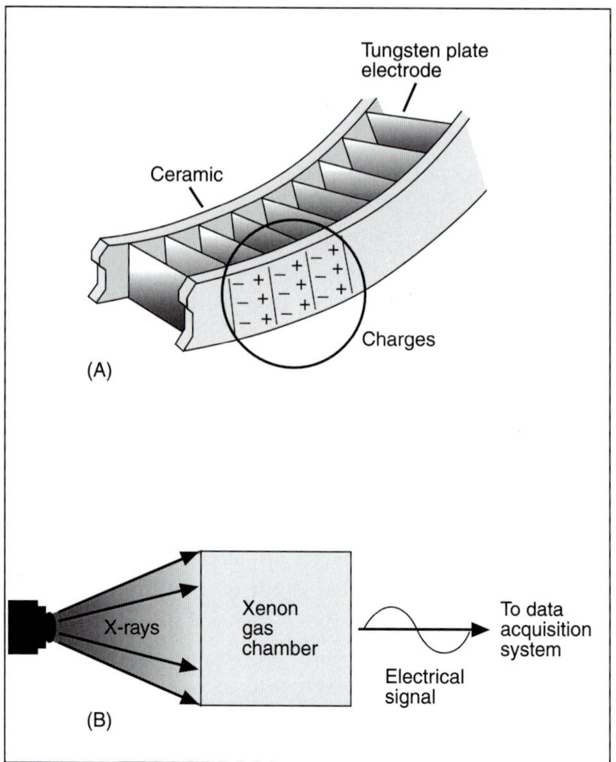

FIGURE 2.21 (A) Array of xenon gas-filled ionization CT detectors. (B) X-ray photons are captured by the gas ionizing chamber and converted to an electrical signal that is sent to the data acquisition system.

The spacing of these detectors varies from one to eight detectors per centimeter. Even with the differences in the design of each detector type the overall intrinsic detection efficiency of both types of detectors is 45%.

Image Displayed

The CT image is usually displayed on a black and white or color CRT. The CT images are displayed in gray scale and the text can be displayed in color (Figure 2.23). By using the touch screen or keyboard commands the choice of image display and manipulation techniques can be communicated to the computer.

The Displayed Image

The internal anatomic structures are reconstructed from a multitude of projections taken of the area. The scanned anatomy is projected back onto a **matrix display** of rows and columns with each tissue having its own location in the matrix. The matrix of a displayed image is comprised of a number of blocks called **pixels**

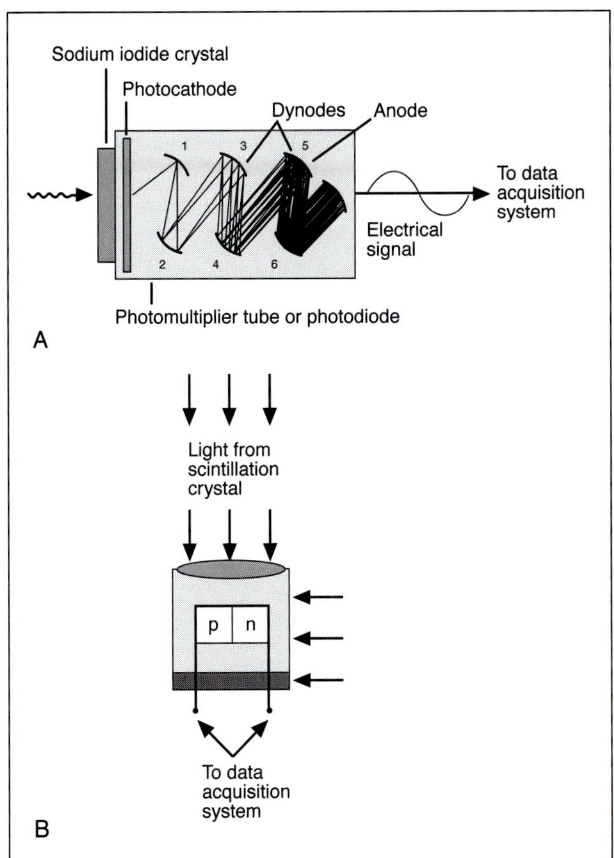

FIGURE 2.22 (A) X-ray photons are captured by the scintillation crystal detector assembly. The emitted light photons enter the photomultiplier tube at (B), are amplified and exit at the anode as an electrical signal that is sent on to the data acquisition system.

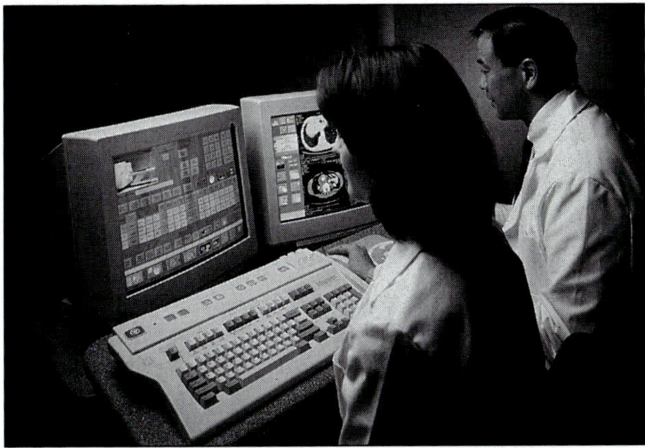

FIGURE 2.23 CT operator's console (Courtesy of GE Medical Systems, Milwaukee, WI).

or picture elements. The smaller the **pixel size** the better the spatial resolution because each pixel will contain a smaller amount of data. Each pixel in a CT image is a two-dimensional representation corresponding to a **voxel** or volume element in the body (Figure 2.24). The voxel depth equals the slice thickness chosen for the scan. Each cell is displayed as a density or brightness level on the CRT. Current CT scanners provide matrices of up to 512 × 512, resulting in 262,144 cells of information.

The size of the pixel is determined by the size of the scan circle chosen and the matrix size. To calculate the size of a pixel in the matrix chosen the scan field of view (FOV) is divided by the matrix size:

FOV of 240 mm, matrix of 512,
$240 \div 512 = 0.4$ mm

The smaller the scan circle the less area there is to display. The larger the matrix used the smaller the pixel.

Ideally the smallest pixel measurement will be obtained from using the largest matrix and the smallest scan circle (must include the desired anatomy).

Therefore:

- Longer reconstruction times are available with a large matrix.
- The smaller scan circle covers less anatomic area.
- The patient's dose is increased with a larger matrix.

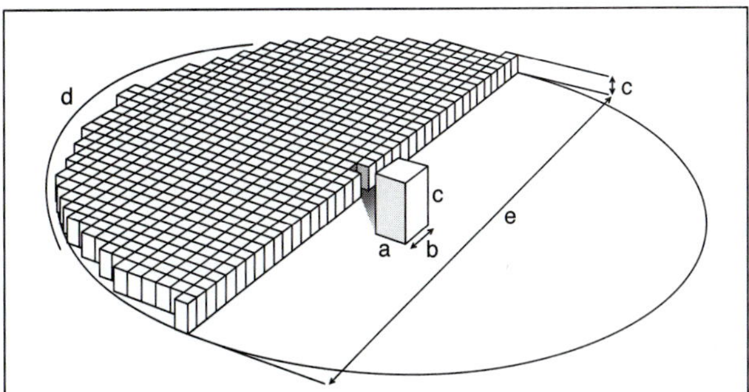

FIGURE 2.24 Schematic of a scanned CT slice. (A) Volume of tissue or 1 voxel; (B) length and width of pixel; (C) slice thickness; (D) entire matrix; (E) scanned field of view. A scanned slice has dimensions of depth, representing the slice thickness. The pixel is a representation of a volume element (voxel) within a patient. As x-rays pass through each voxel, the information is computed to generate a CT number for each pixel displayed. Voxel size depends on slice thickness, matrix size, and field of view.

Each pixel is assigned a numerical value or **Houndsfield unit,** which represents average attenuation of the tissue relative to water, which has a value of zero.

Although all the information is displayed in this array of numbers, it is difficult to interpret, so the numbers are translated into gray levels and the axial image is displayed on the screen of the CRT. Adjustments to the image contrast can be accomplished by controlling the **window width** and **window level.** Window level and window width controls are based on the CT attenuation number system. According to the Houndsfield scale, the range of attenuation numbers could be from –2000 (air) to +3000 (dense bone). (Houndsfield units and CT numbers are synonymous.)

Because the human visual range encompasses 32 or fewer shades of gray, and the photon beam exiting the patient encompasses more than 2000 subtle shades, only a portion of the total range of stored densities is displayed at one time. Once the axial image is displayed on the CRT, the window level and width are adjusted to display the diagnostically relevant information. Information outside these levels will be lost from diagnosis. Adjustments to the image can be accomplished by controlling the window width and level. Window width and level controls are based on the CT attenuation number system. Choosing the window width dictates the number of attenuation values each step on the gray scale will represent.

For example, on an 18-step gray scale, a window width is narrowed from 1600 to 100; each gray scale step now represents 10 Houndsfield units rather than 100. So 2 pixels differing by 20 Houndsfield units would be displayed as separate shades with the narrower window width and displayed as the same shade at a wider window width. Sometimes the acquired data need to be displayed and filmed as two separate images to discriminate the various densities (Figures 2.25 and 2.26).

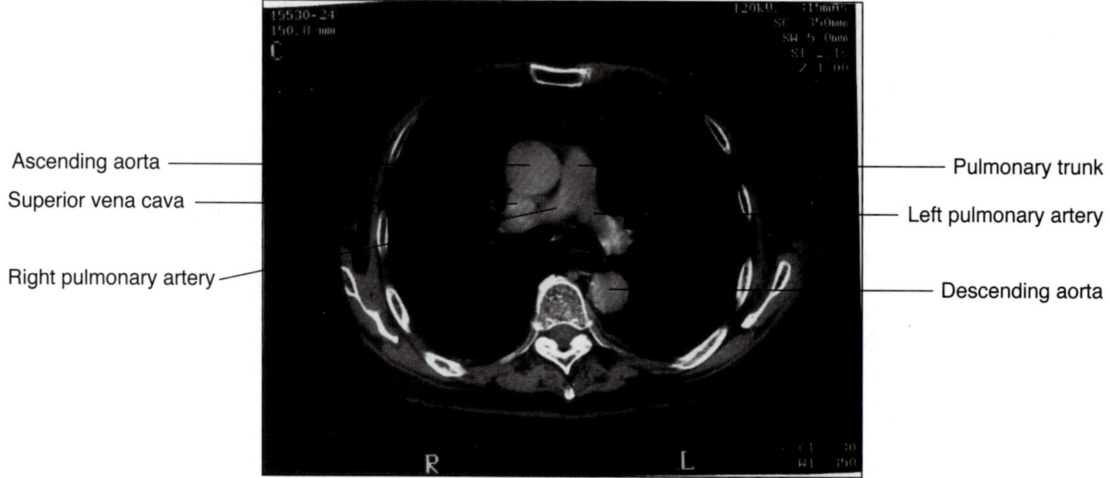

FIGURE 2.25 Axial CT scan of chest at the level of the pulmonary trunk. The window level is 30 and window width is 350.

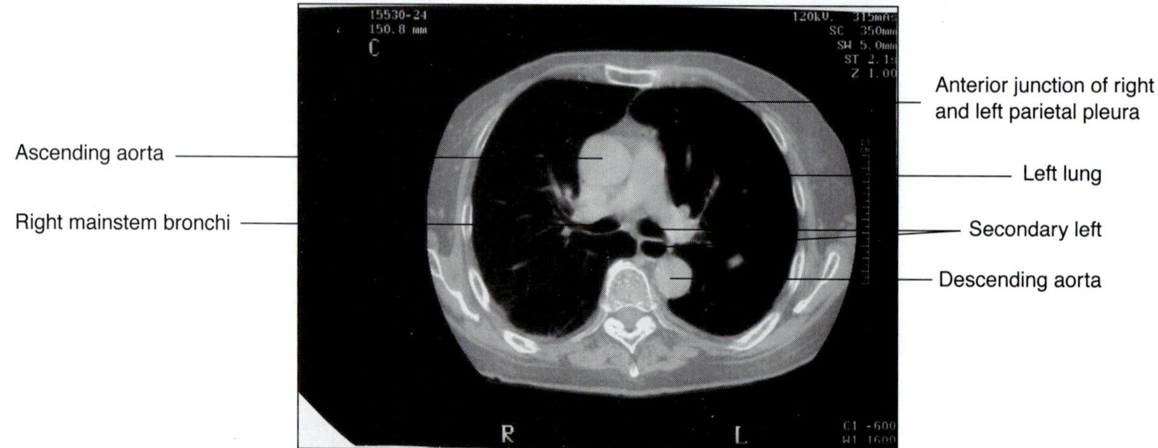

FIGURE 2.26 This scan is of the same patient and level as Figure 2.25. Note the window level of this image has been adjusted to –600 and the window width to 1600.

The primary area of interest is focused on since the full range of CT numbers cannot be displayed. In the abdomen, where there are many variations in tissue densities, a wide window width would be chosen (Figure 2.27A), whereas in the brain and liver, where there is less variation, a narrower window width would be chosen (Figure 2.27B). The window level is considered the center of the range. To visualize the type of tissue desired—bone, soft tissue, or lung parenchyma—select a window level that is the center of this range of CT numbers assigned to this tissue.

THREE-DIMENSIONAL RECONSTRUCTION IMAGING

Three-dimensional imaging was developed and refined throughout the 1980s. It is often used by surgeons and other physicians in planning surgery or therapy and evaluating the complex human anatomy because it offers a unique perspective for the review and diagnosis. Clinical application of three-dimensional CT scanning originally began with craniofacial surgery and orthopedics. Since that time many other applications have been developed (Figure 2.28).

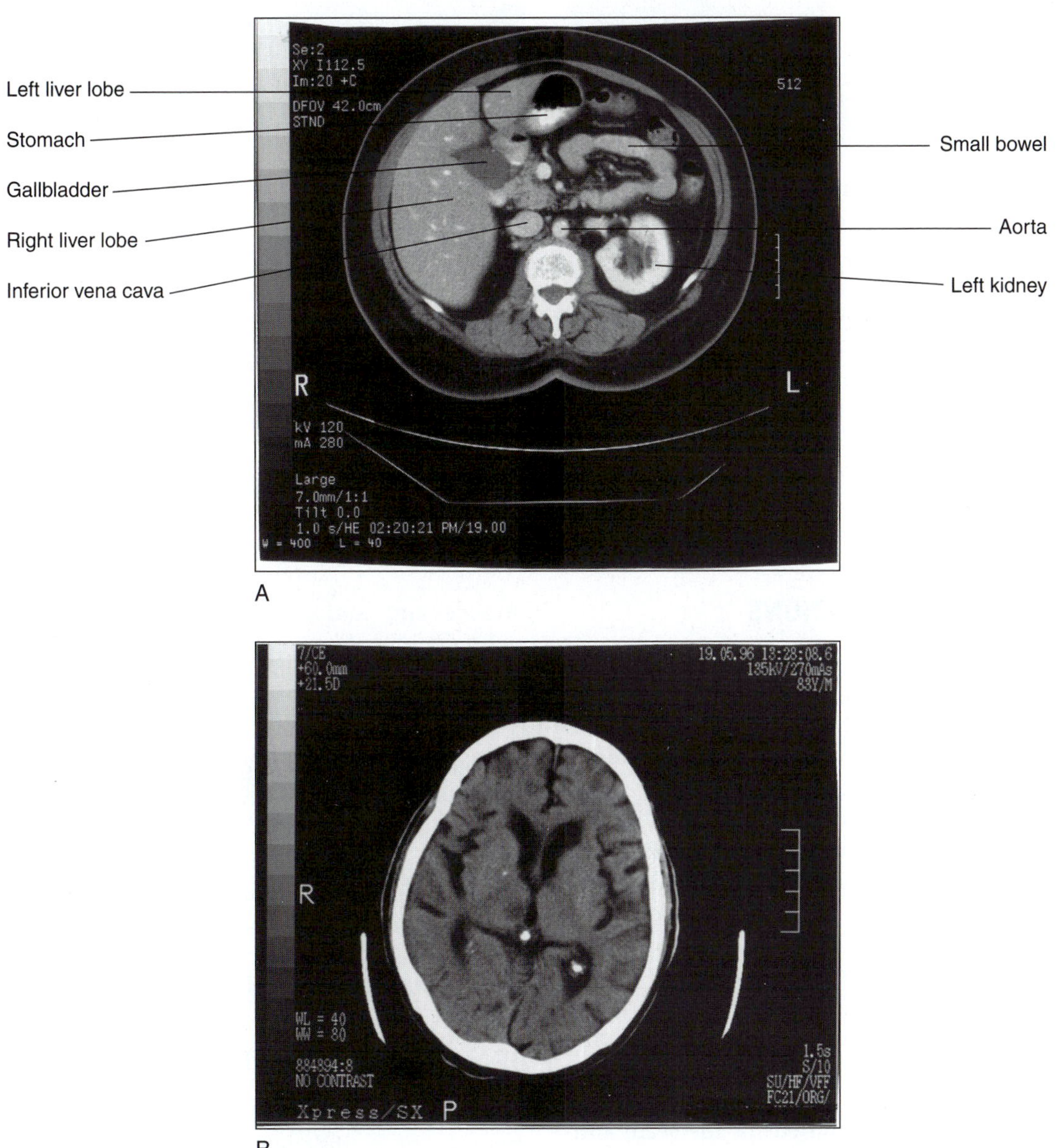

FIGURE 2.27 (A) Abdominal scan with a window level of 40 and window width of 400. (B) Axial CT through the ventricles with a narrow window width of 80 and a level of 40.

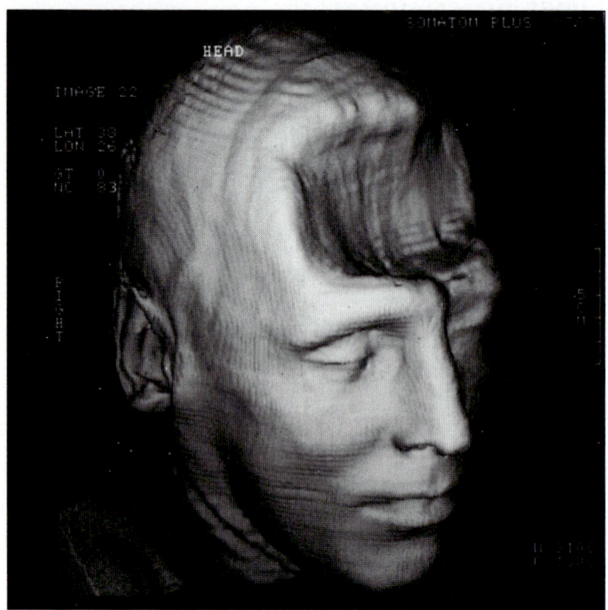

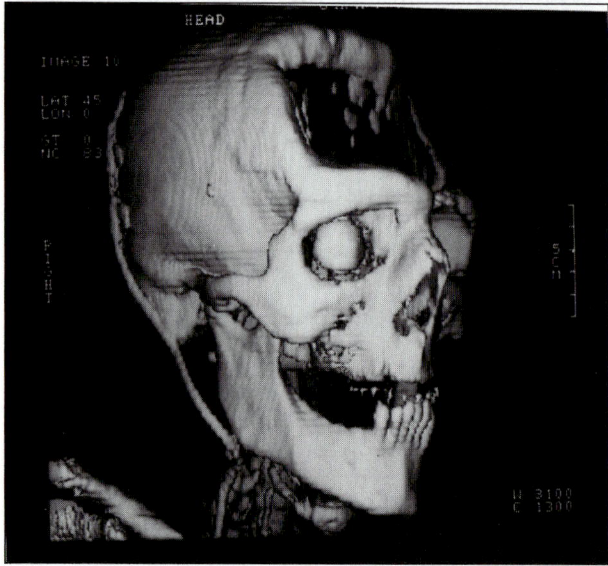

FIGURE 2.28 Three-dimensional reconstruction of skull.

IMAGE STORAGE

Storage devices for CT images include magnetic tape and disks, digital videotape, optical disks, and optical tape. Multiformat video camera and laser electronic image recording are the two hard copy recording methods of CT images. Generally, multiformat video cameras are no longer used and laser cameras are now used for hard copies of digital images. Long-term storage of the studies is done on optical disk or magnetic tape.

Applications

PATIENT CARE CONSIDERATIONS

The technologist positions the patient correctly while ensuring that the patient is as comfortable as possible. All artifact-causing objects should be removed. If the patient is having an abdomen or chest scan, the arms (if possible) should be placed out of the scan area above the head. The region of interest should be centered within the gantry aperture and the correct scan field of view selected to avoid out-of-field artifacts. The patient's history should be taken and the procedure fully explained.

Explanation should include all parts of the procedure starting from the scout, to localize and prescribe the scan parameters; the direction and speed of the table movement; the expected noises; contrast administration and any possible reactions that might occur; the respiratory technique required for the scan; and when to remain still and the expected length of the examination. The patient should be aware of the position of the technologist at all times. This provides reassurance and understanding, and ensures that the technologist is always aware of difficulties encountered during the scan. The technologist should communicate with and observe the patient throughout the scan to ensure the above instructions are being followed. Any movement will cause misrepresentation of the data. Communication with the patient also ensures the person's well-being. Many scanners are now equipped with programmed breathing instructions in a variety of languages. With the availability of technology for faster image acquisition we are able to acquire more accurate diagnostic CT scans with greater speed and with less discomfort to patients (Figure 2.29).

ORAL AND INJECTABLE CONTRAST MEDIA

Oral contrast media given to outline the bowel will increase the confidence and accuracy in the diagnosis. The amount and timing of the dose given depends on the area of bowel to be examined (Figure 2.30).

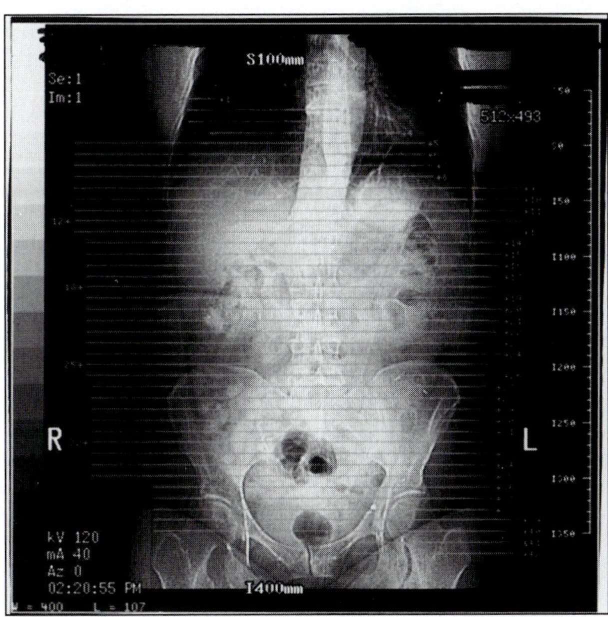

FIGURE 2.29 Scout view of the abdomen to localize the scan parameters. Each horizontal line indicates the level of one slice.

An injectable contrast medium opacifies the blood vessels, organs, and surrounding structures. It improves the definition of organ boundaries by increasing the contrast between normal parenchyma and intraparenchamal lesions. Some studies require pre- and postcontrast scans and some only one or the other (Figure 2.31).

CLINICAL APPLICATIONS

With all of the rapid advances in imaging, the radiologist acts as a consultant to the referring physician in choosing the most expeditious and cost-effective method for diagnosing and treating the patient. The following are indications for using diagnostic CT:

Head

- Contusions
- Hematomastomas
- Subdural or epidural hematomas
- Cerebral abscess
- Herpes simplex encephalitis
- Meningitis (to check for increase in cranial pressure before lumbar puncture)
- Congenital brain abnormalities
- Intracranial and extracranial tumors (Figure 2.32)

Spine

- Disk herniation
- Spinal stenosis
- Spinal infection of disk space or epidural area
- Trauma (Figure 2.33)
- Intraspinal tumor

Neck or Face

- Developmental anomalies
- Inflammation or infection
- Trauma (Figure 2.34)
- Tumors

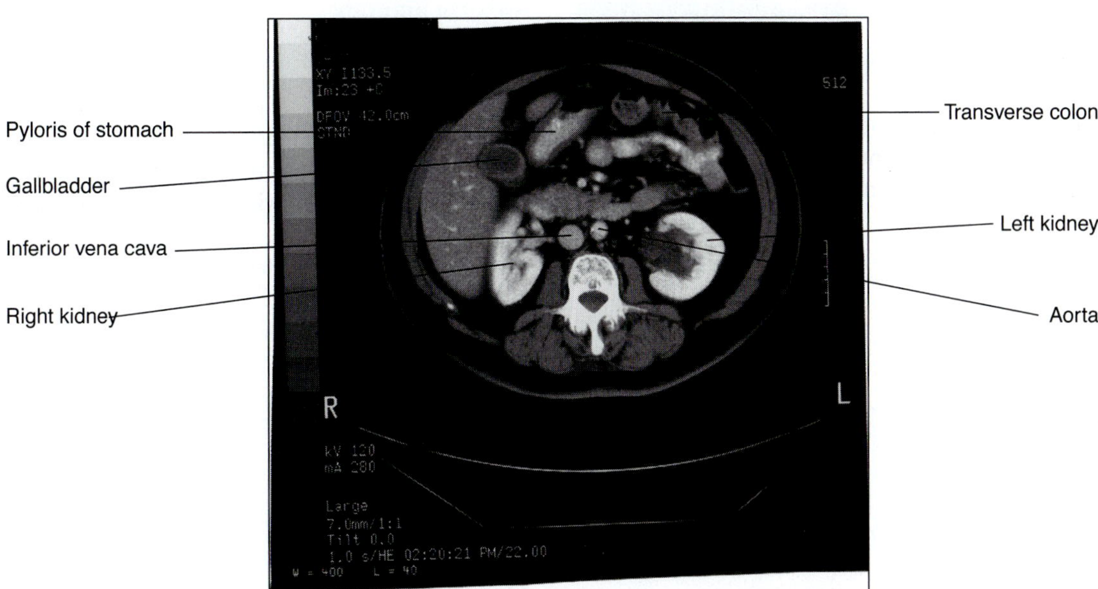

FIGURE 2.30 Oral contrast can be seen in the pyloric part of the stomach and the transverse colon.

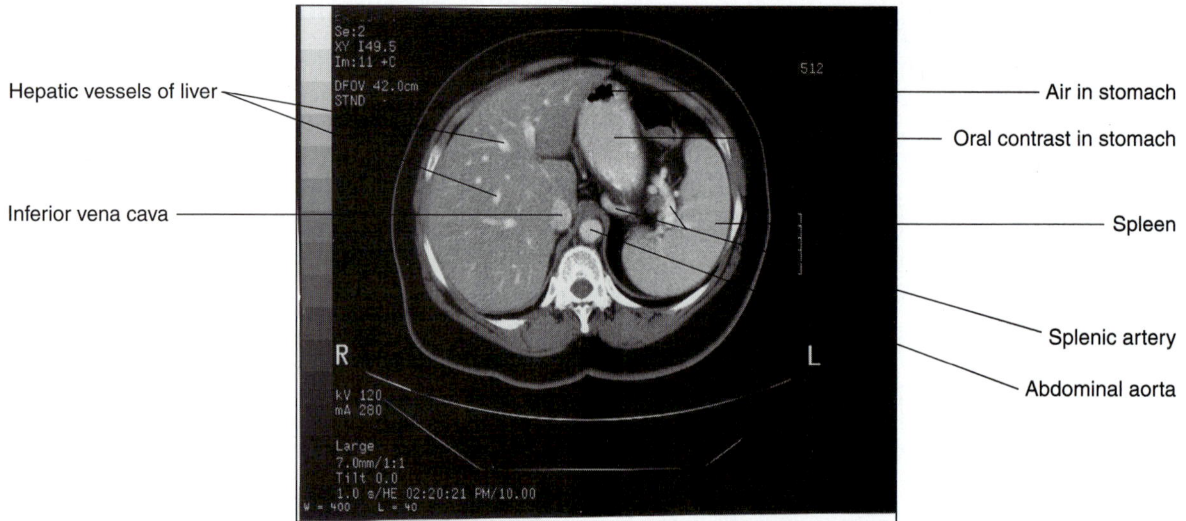

FIGURE 2.31 The positive contrast seen in the text and the highlighted hepatic vessels, inferior vena cava, aorta, and splenic artery denotes the administration of IV contrast media.

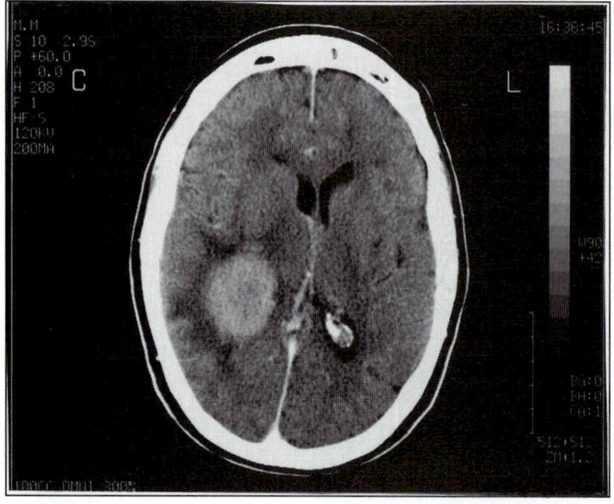

FIGURE 2.32 Axial CT scan demonstrates a meningioma surrounded by edema.

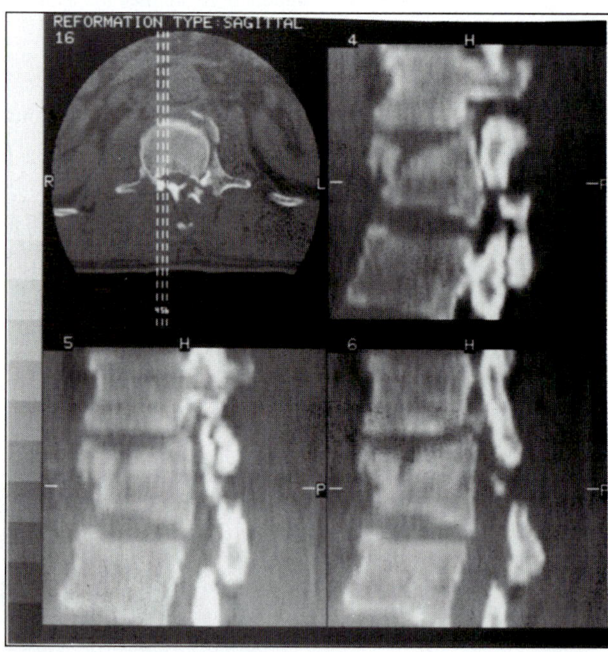

FIGURE 2.33 Axial scan showing a fractured thoracic vertebra. The three sagitally reconstructed images depict the area denoted by the dotted lines.

Chest and Mediastinum

- Lymphadenopathy
- Bronchogenic carcinoma (chest wall invasion)
- Lymphoma
- Other malignancies
- Mediastinal masses
- Presence or extent of aneurysms and aortic dissections (Figure 2.35)
- Pulmonary metastases
- Primary lung tumor

Abdomen

- Metastases in liver
- Metastases in adrenal glands
- Cysts
- Fatty deposits versus tumor
- Lymph node involvement
- Chronic pancreatitis (Figure 2.36)

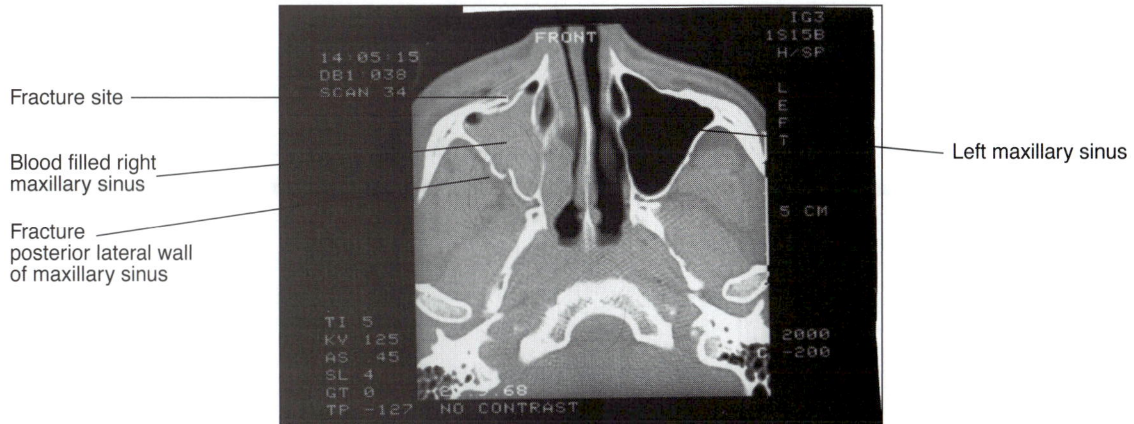

FIGURE 2.34 Axial CT scan of sinuses. Note the fracture of the anterior and lateral wall of the right maxillary sinus.

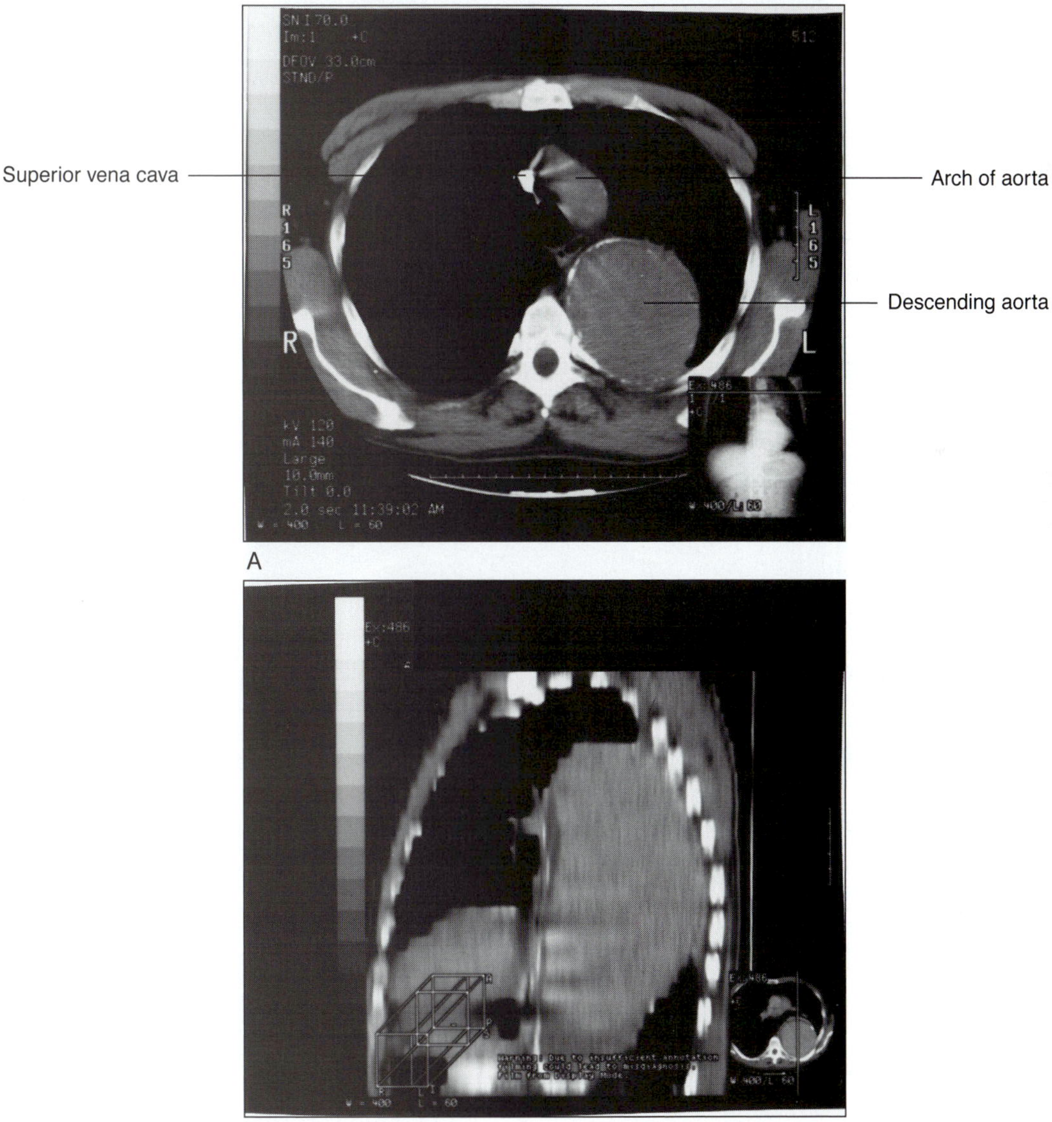

Superior vena cava

Arch of aorta

Descending aorta

A

B

FIGURE 2.35 (A) Axial scan through the arch of the aorta shows a large aortic aneurysm in the descending aorta. (B) Sagittal reformat of (A). Inset shows the level of the reformat.

- Solid pancreatic masses
- Hemangiomas
- Cirrhotic liver
- Focal masses in spleen

Kidney

- Cystic and solid masses (Figure 2.37)

Retroperitoneum

- Tumors
- Lymph node enlargement/metastases

Adrenal Glands

Pelvis

- Extent of tumor (Figure 2.38)
- Abscess

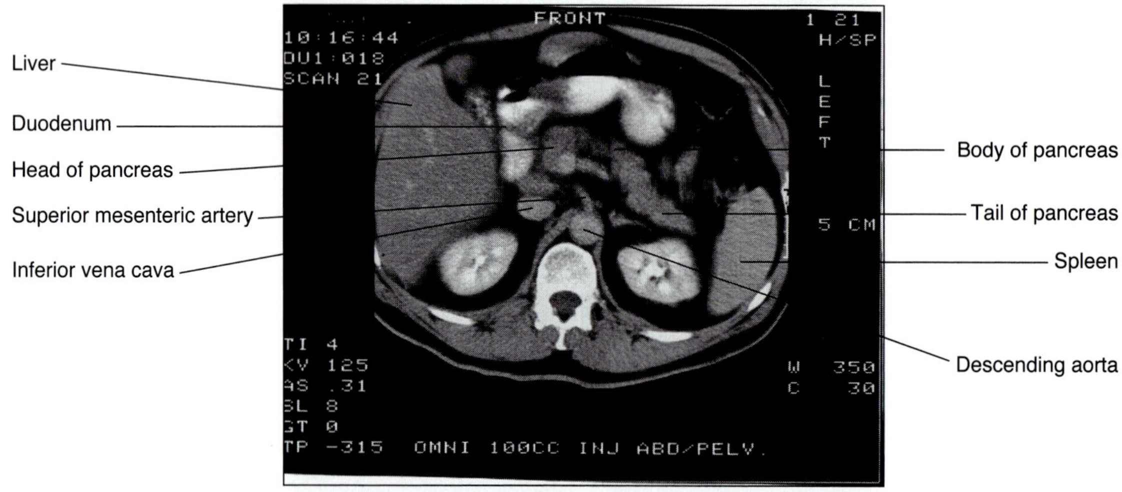

FIGURE 2.36 Axial CT scan through the pancreas with oral and IV contrast media administered.

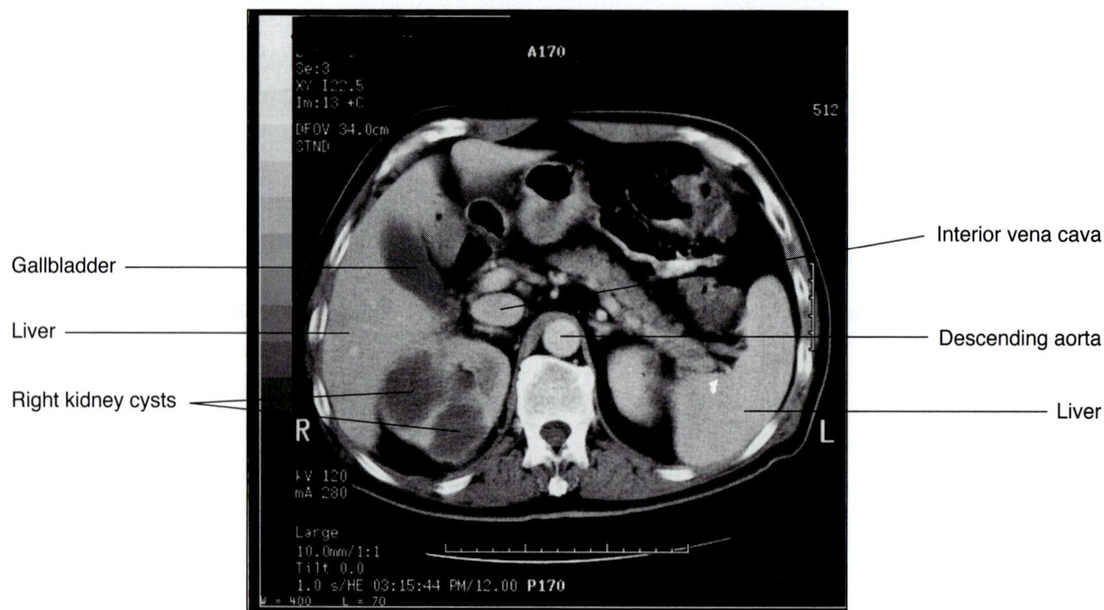

FIGURE 2.37 Noncontrast axial CT scan of abdomen showing cysts in right kidney.

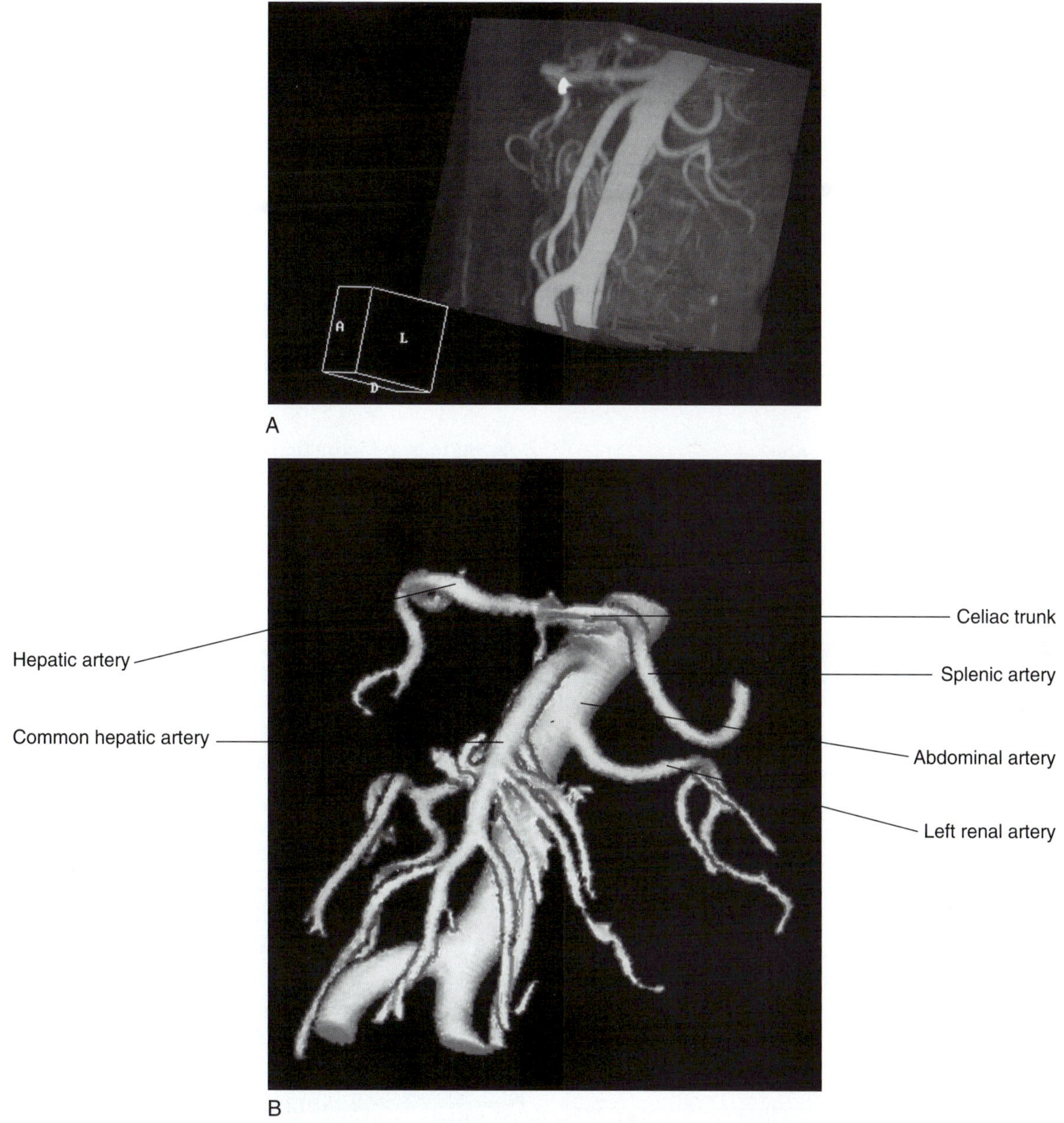

FIGURE 2.38 (A) Computed tomography angiography demonstrates the abdominal aorta with its main branches. (B) Three-dimensional reconstruction of (A).

Review Questions

1. Which term is used to define the table increment in distance per millimeter per 360° rotation of the tube and detector assembly in spiral computed tomography?
   a. helix
   b. pitch
   c. nutation
   d. scan arc

2. When changing the slice thickness from 10 mm to 5 mm for a CT scan, what happens to the number of photons detected?
   a. decrease in number by 50%
   b. increase in number by 50%
   c. increase in number by 100%
   d. decrease in number by 25%

3. The maximum number of shades of gray displayed on the CT monitor is determined by the:
   a. matrix size
   b. window width
   c. window level
   d. pixel size

4. Discuss the most important factor in obtaining artifact-free diagnostic CT study.

5. State one factor that contributes to an increase in patient dose and one factor that increases reconstruction time.

CASE STUDY

An artifact appeared on this CT scan of a spine (Figure 2.39). The original scout film had a stripe along its length. What do you think caused this problem and how can it be corrected?

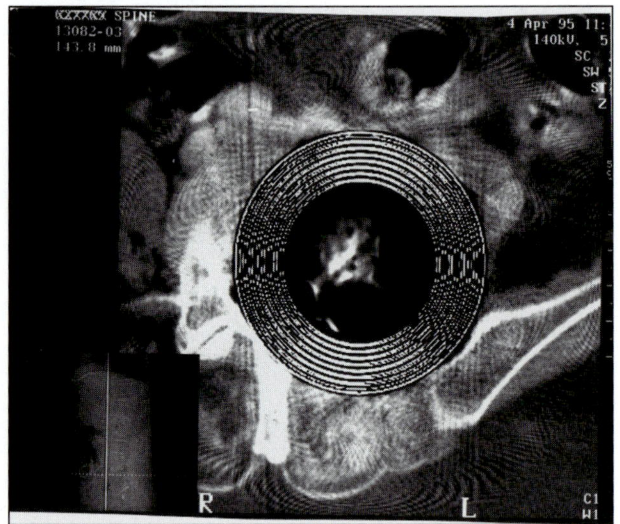

FIGURE 2.39

References and Recommended Reading

Berland, L. L. (1987). *Practical CT technology and techniques.* New York: Raven Press.

Bushong, S. C. (1993). *Radiologic science for technologists* (5th ed.). St. Louis: Mosby-Year Book.

Carlton, R., & McKenna Adler, A. (1992). *Principles of radiographic imaging: An art and a science.* Albany, NY: Delmar.

Curry, T., III, Dowdey, J., & Murray, R. (1990). *Christensen's physics of diagnostic radiology* (4th ed.). Philadelphia: Lea & Febiger.

Clark, S. (1995). *An introduction to CT scanning.* Elscint (Canada). (Unpublished notes).

Dummling, K. (1984). 10 years computed tomography—A retrospective view. Electromedia, 52. Siemens.

Haaga, J., Lanzieri, C., & Sartoris, D. J. (1994). *Computed tomography and magnetic resonance imaging of whole body* (3rd ed.). St. Louis: Mosby-Year Book.

Philips Medical Systems. (1992). *Computed tomography principles and practice.* Netherlands: Philips Medical Systems.

Scroggins, D., Reddinger, W., Carlton, R., & Shappell, A. (1995). *Computed tomography review.* Philadelphia: Lippincott.

Seeram, E. (1994). Computed tomography physical principles clinical applications & quality control. Toronto: Saunders.

Steenbeek, J.C.M. (1993). *Principles and applications of volumetric CT. MedicaMundi, 38,* 1.

Kalender, W. A. (1994). *Technical foundations of spiral CT. Seminars in ultrasound, CT, and MRI, 15* (2), 81–89.

Magnetic Resonance Imaging

Carolyn Kaut Roth, RT(R)(MR)(ARRT)

Introduction and Historical Overview

Before the development of MRI, several methods were used to evaluate the human body for anatomy and pathology. Methods such as plain film radiography were used to evaluate bone, CT to evaluate brain and intra-abdominal organs, ultrasound to evaluate abdominal viscera and the pelvic structures, pneumoencephalography to evaluate ventricular anatomy, and angiography to evaluate the vascular system. Exploratory surgery was performed to evaluate anything that could not be seen by these techniques, all of which were invasive procedures. Some used ionizing radiation or the introduction of iodinated contrast agents and some invaded the body surgically. Because of its high soft tissue contrast, multiplanar capabilities, and noninvasive technique, MRI has, in many cases, become the imaging modality of choice for the evaluation of the body.

Unfortunately, when technologists are introduced to MRI, they are faced with an imaging modality unlike those in radiography to which they are accustomed. For this reason, some are initially intimidated. There seems to be several reasons for this impression, including terminology that is unique to MRI, sophisticated hardware and software, and fundamental principles based on quantum mechanical physics. To fully understand the methodology of MRI, the technologist should combine small portions of the principle with the clinical application. This section presents an overview of the history of MRI, an introduction to the MRI principles, typical examples of clinical applications, the safety considerations of MRI, and frequently used MRI terminology.

Magnetic resonance imaging is the offspring of scientific experiments performed by physicists in the 1930s and 1940s, which blossomed in the 1960s and 1970s into what became known as **nuclear magnetic resonance** (NMR). NMR and MRI refer to experiments involving the interactions of nuclei with magnetic fields and radiowaves. It is a technique that is now commonly used for clinical imaging as well as a laboratory tool. Today scientists, physicians, radiographers, and lay persons have become familiar with applications and techniques for MRI.

Even though MRI units seemed to appear in radiology departments and imaging centers overnight, MRI is not the result of a single invention. Therefore, contrary to popular belief, MRI has a long history that dates back to the beginning of this century and beyond. Several landmark dates led to MRI as it is known today.

Static electricity was recognized early in Greece as the invisible attractive force that was produced as fur was rubbed over amber. Black rocks mystified the natives of ancient Magnesia because when they were spun, they returned to their original orientation. In the 1800s Oersted discovered that electricity produces magnetism by noticing that the needle of a compass would deflect in the presence of an electrical charge. Not long after, Faraday noticed that magnetic fields induce currents.

Although the concepts of spin angular momentum for atoms was accepted, the idea of the result (magnetic moment) was yet to be realized. In the early 1920s Pauli suggested hyperfine splittings in high-resolution optical spectra to arise from different spin angular momentum states. This was proven in the late 1920s by Stern and Gerlach who sent a collimated beam of silver ions through an inhomogeneous magnetic field in such a way that the beam was perpendicular to both the magnetic field and its gradient. A deflection of the beam was detected in two locations on the detector plate suggesting two discrete states, parallel and anti-parallel.

Rabi coined the term nuclear magnetic resonance in 1938. In the early 1930s and 1940s, Gortier attempted to prove thermal equilibrium and failed. It must not have been such a bad idea because in 1946, Purcell, Torrey, and Pound studied absorption of radiofrequency (RF) energy in paraffin wax by means of a resonant cavity. Bloch, Hanson, and Packard described "an electromotive force resulting from a force precession of the nuclear magnetization in the applied RF field."

In 1953, Varian and associates of Palo Alto, California first commercialized NMR and acquired patents from Bloch and Hansen, built research systems 7000 to 14,000 gauss (0.7–1.4 tesla [T]). By 1960, about 1000 spectrometers were operating worldwide in chemistry laboratories at universities and at pharmaceutical laboratories.

In 1971, Damadian published a controversial paper that claimed that NMR was capable of detecting cancer on the basis of increased T1 relaxation times. In 1973, Lauterbur tested an imaging technique known as "zeugmatography" that generated multiple projections of an object then reconstructed with the use of projection reconstruction algorithms. EMI Ltd. produced a 1500-gauss human body in 1978. In 1981, Dr. Ian Young, at Hammersmith Hospital in London, conceived imagers with clinically acceptable times. Today MRI systems range from 0.01 T to 2.0 T in field strength.

Although MRI techniques have taken approximately 70 years to evolve, the time from the first image to today is less than 20 years. At this time, technologists and physicians are learning principles and applications of MRI simultaneously and their responsibilities frequently overlap.

Principles

Magnetic resonance is the study of the interactions of magnetic fields and **radiowaves** with the **nuclei** of atoms. Quite simply, to perform MRI, a patient is placed into a scanner whose main component is a strong magnetic field. Once in the field, nuclei of some of the hydrogen atoms in the body align with the magnetic field. RF energy is then used to tip the hydrogen out of alignment. After the RF is removed, the nuclei realign with the magnetic field. As they realign they produce an MRI signal. This signal is translated into the images (Figures 2.40 and 2.41).

MAGNETS

To perform MRI the patient is placed into a powerful magnetic field. The magnetic field located within the imager is usually referred to as B or $\mathbf{B_0}$. The strength of the B_0 can be expressed in units of **tesla (T)** and **gauss (g)** whereby 1 T = 10,000 g. Magnetic fields can be created by either magnetizing materials that can maintain magnetization (iron or steel) or by passing current through a wire. The latter forms what is known as an **electromagnet** and the former a **permanent magnet** (Figures 2.42 and 2.43). Magnetic fields in MRI typically range from about 0.1 to 0.3 T in permanent magnet imagers and 0.5 to 2.0 T in superconductive electromagnets. Typically, permanent magnets have vertical fields and electromagnets have horizontal fields.

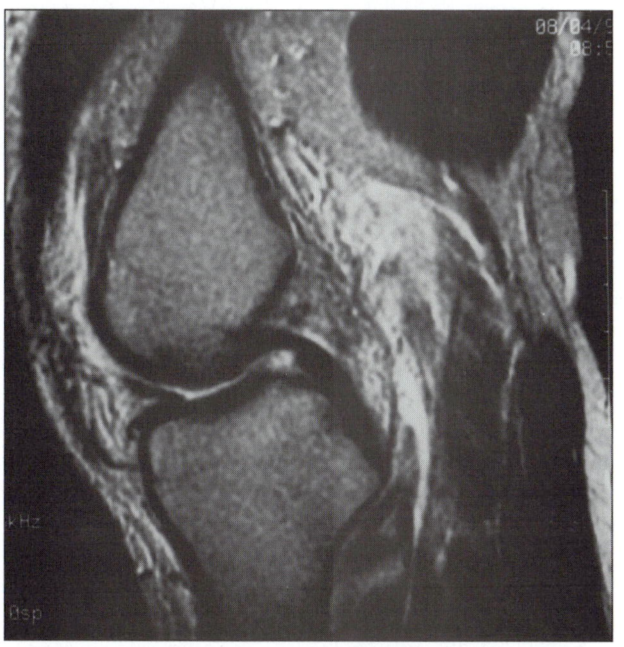

FIGURE 2.40 MRI of the knee acquired in the sagittal plane. Image was acquired with image parameters (PDWI) such that anatomy is well visualized.

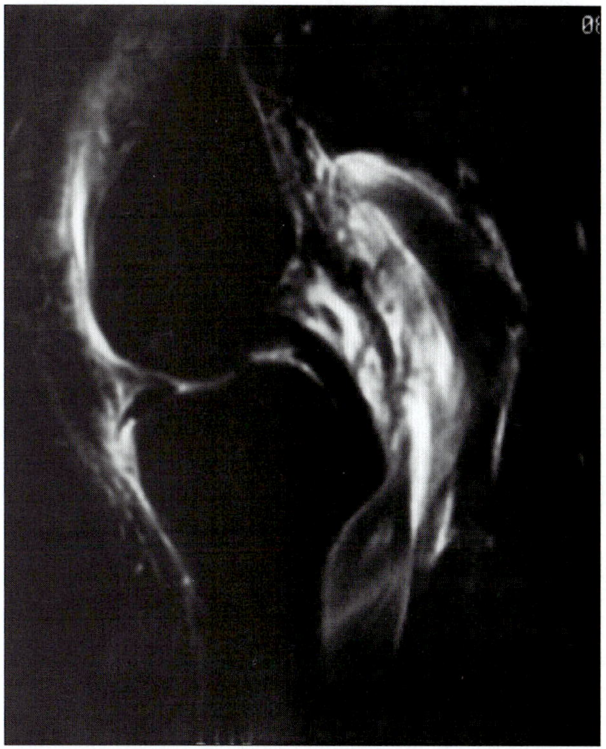

FIGURE 2.41 MRI of the knee acquired in the sagittal plane. Image was acquired with imaging parameters (STIR) such that pathology is well visualized.

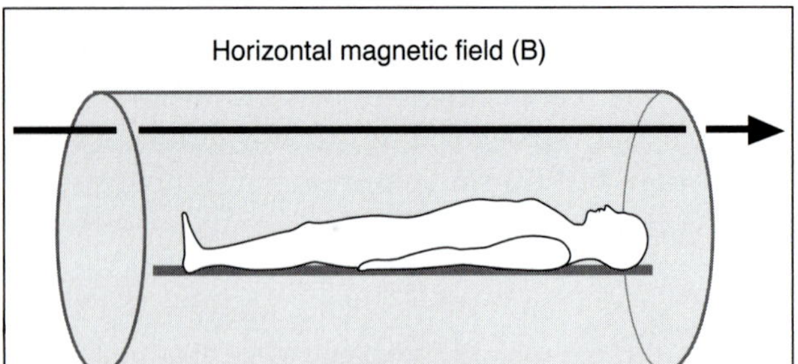

FIGURE 2.42 Typical configuration of electromagnets.

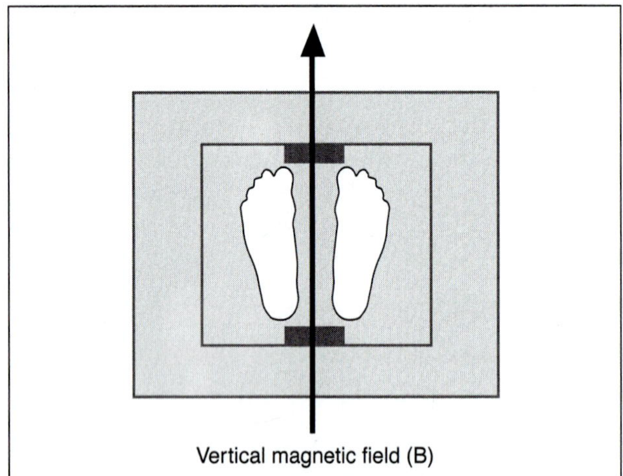

FIGURE 2.43 Typical configuration of permanent magnets.

NUCLEAR MAGNETIC FIELDS

Because of its sensitivity to detection and its abundance within the body, we observe the nucleus of the hydrogen atom, or the **proton,** for clinical MRI. In fact, the human body is made up of approximately 75% water with each water molecule containing two hydrogen atoms (H_20). Because water is the basis for MRI, the structures best visualized on MRI scans are soft tissues. On placing the subject into the MRI scanner the protons have a positive charge and are spinning. Because moving charged particles make magnetic fields, protons act like microscopic bar magnets. The microscopic magnetic field associated with each proton is known as its **magnetic moment**. The magnetic moment has magnitude and direction, and can be illustrated as a vector (Figure 2.44).

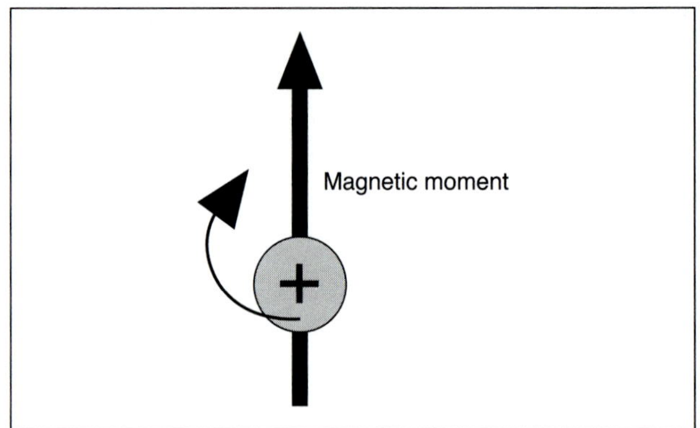

FIGURE 2.44 Spinning charge.

POLARIZATION

On exposure to an external magnetic field (B_0) these magnetic moments behave like bar magnets and either attract or repel B_0. Those magnetic moments that attract are said to **align** with the magnetic field and those that repel oppose the field. More magnetic moments align with the field than oppose it. Therefore, when the number of attracted and opposed moments are totaled, there is an excess of magnetic moments aligned with the field. This excess is known as the **spin excess** or the **proton density**. The proton density increases as the external magnetic field strength (B_0) increases because in higher fields, more protons align with the field (Figure 2.45).

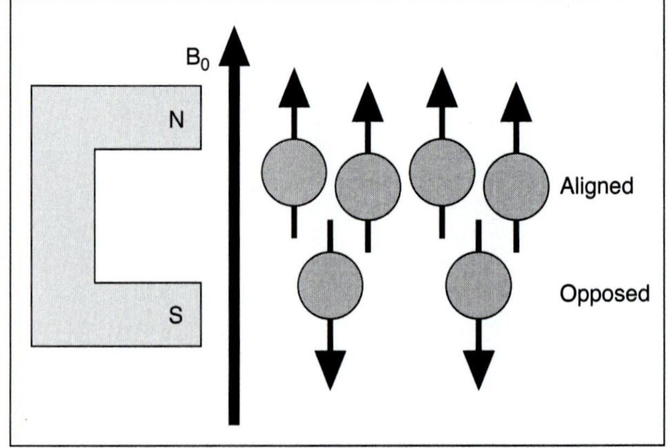

FIGURE 2.45 Nuclei in a magnetic field.

EQUILIBRIUM

Protons not only align but also spin in the presence of the strong magnetic field. For this reason they are called spins. For hydrogen there are two discrete **spin states** permitted. These are known as the low- and high-energy states. Spins that align with the field are in the **low-energy state** and those that oppose the field are in the **high-energy state**. It is the excess spins in the low-energy state that are the nuclei responsible for the images. This spin excess occurs in a condition known as **thermal equilibrium** (Figure 2.46). To visualize the net effect of thermal equilibrium, spins can be drawn on the Cartesian coordinate system.

NET MAGNETIZATION

Thermal equilibrium occurs seconds after interaction with the magnetic field. The sum of magnetic moments in the spin excess adds to form a macroscopic or measurable component known as the **net magnetization** (Figure 2.47). Because the net magnetization has direction and magnitude, it is often represented by a vector known as the **net magnetization vector.** When the net magnetization is along the Z axis, it is known as Mz and when it is in the XY plane, it is known as Mx,y.

PRECESSIONAL FREQUENCY

The nuclei do not align directly with but at an angle to the direction of the magnetic field. This, in combination with the spin of the nucleus, permits the

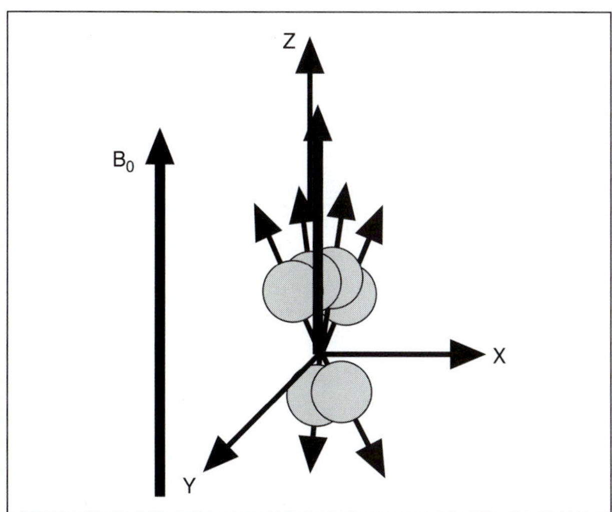

FIGURE 2.46 Thermal equilibrium.

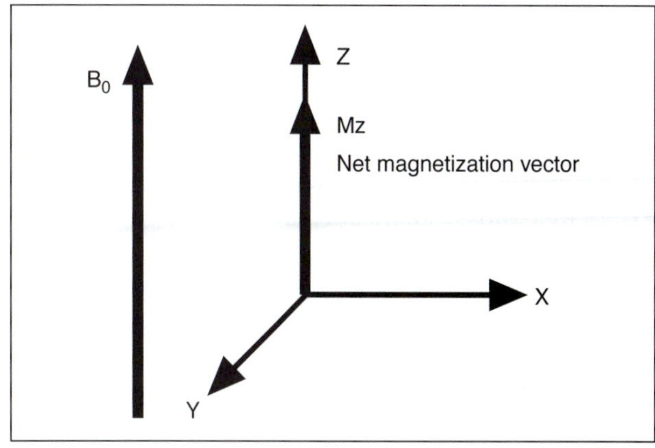

FIGURE 2.47 Net magnetization.

nucleus to wobble or **precess** in the presence of the applied field (B_0). The rate, or **frequency of precession** can be calculated by knowing the strength of the applied field and the spin angular momentum and the magnetic moment of each nucleus. The latter is known as the **gyromagnetic ratio** and is constant for each atom. We calculate the frequency of precession with the **Larmor equation**

$$w_0 = b_0 g$$

where w_0 expressed in **megahertz** (MHz) is the frequency, b_0 expressed in Tesla is the strength of the applied field, and g expressed in megahertz/tesla is the gyromagnetic ratio (Figure 2.48).

RADIOFREQUENCY PULSE

The net magnetization (the sum of the magnetic moments) is macroscopic and measurable, but minuscule compared to the strength of the applied field, which usually ranges from 0.03 to 2.0 T. Therefore, to

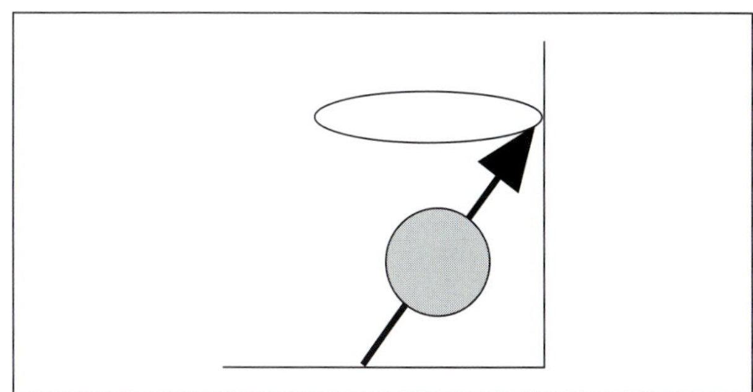

FIGURE 2.48 Precession.

get information from the tissues in which protons reside we add energy into the system in the form of an **RF pulse.** The frequency of the RF pulse must match the frequency at which the nuclei precess in the presence of the applied field to achieve a condition known as **resonance.** Because the energy needed to excite the spins depends on the strength of the magnetic field, a high magnetic field strength requires a higher frequency to accomplish **excitation**. Interestingly, the RF necessary to perturb the spins is approximately 63 MHz in a 1.5-T magnetic field. This incidentally is the same frequency at which channel 3 broadcasts in many metropolitan areas (Figure 2.49).

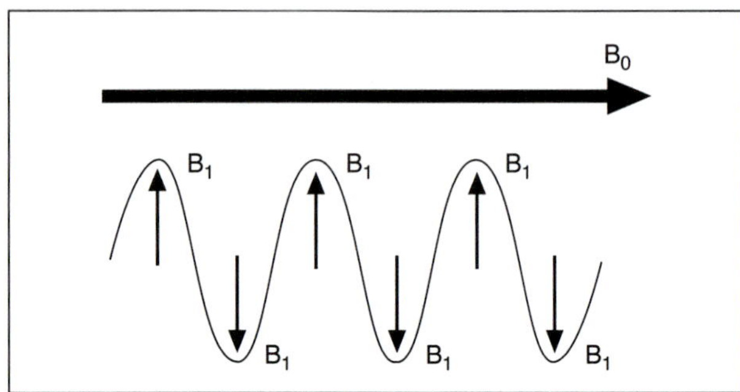

FIGURE 2.49 Electromagnetic radiowaves.

RADIOFREQUENCY COILS

The RF pulses are introduced by way of an RF transmitter known as an **RF coil.** RF transmitter coils produce an oscillating electromagnetic radiowave. The secondary magnetic field produced by the RF coil is known as B_1 and should be positioned at right angles to the main magnetic field B_0 (Figure 2.50).

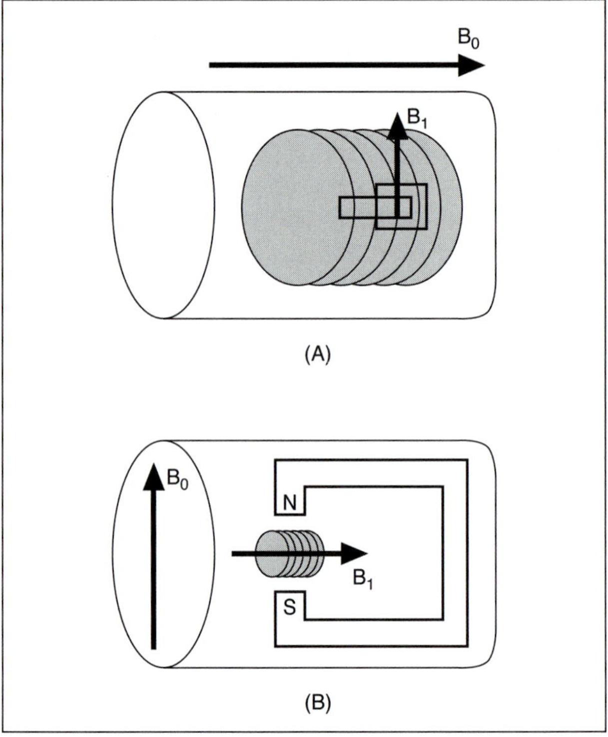

FIGURE 2.50 RF coil orientation in an (A) electromagnet and (B) permanent magnet.

EXCITATION

Energy is added to the system in the form of a short intense blast of RF energy known as an RF pulse. This is also known as an **excitation pulse** (Figure 2.51). Energy can be added such that the net magnetization vector is tipped 90° away from its original position in line with the magnetic field. Therefore this can also be referred to as a 90° RF pulse. On the Cartesian coordinate system, the original position of the net magnetization vector was along the longitudinal (Z) axis and the new position is in the transverse (X,Y) plane. Longitudinal net magnetization is expressed Mz, and transverse magnetization is expressed as Mx,y.

During the excitation process, two discrete processes occur with respect to the individual nuclei.

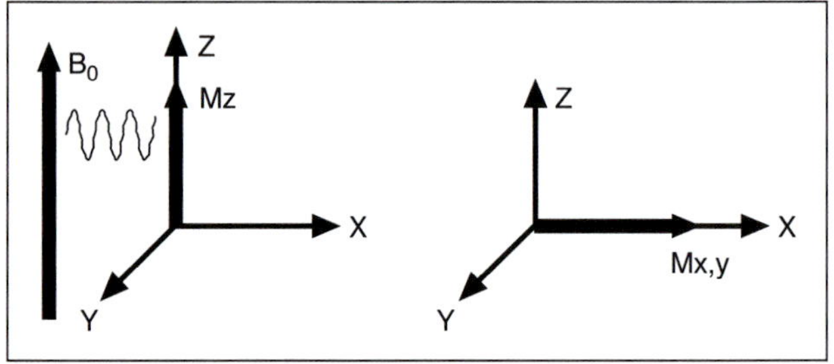

FIGURE 2.51 RF excitation.

First, the RF pulse forces the nuclei into **phase coherence,** whereby they begin to precess together or in phase. Secondly, some of the low-energy spins absorb energy from the RF pulse and enter the high-energy state.

SIGNAL DETECTION

The spins precess in the transverse plane as the result of the 90° pulse. This precession of spins in the transverse plane (transverse magnetization) induces a signal voltage within an RF receiver coil. The RF coil is selected on the basis of desired anatomy and pathology. *(The size of the anatomic structure and the nature of the pathology to be imaged determines the size and type of RF coil that is optimal for the examination.)* It is this induced signal that is known as the **free induction decay (FID)** and is responsible for the image (Figure 2.52).

RELAXATION

During the excitation process, two discrete processes occur with respect to the individual nuclei. The first process forces the nuclei into phase coherence, whereby they begin to precess together or in phase. The second process allows some of the low-energy spins to absorb energy from the RF pulse and enter the high-energy state. After the termination of the RF pulse, spins begin to relax back to thermal equilibrium. During this process the net magnetization grows back to its original position along the Z axis.

T1 RECOVERY

The time it takes for the spins to recover part of their original position along the longitudinal or Z axis (in line with B_0), is one T1 time. **T1 relaxation** recovers exponentially. Therefore, in one T1 time the spins have recovered 63% of their original magnetization. By knowing the T1 relaxation time of a given tissue type, extrinsic parameters can be selected that maximize the T1 effect on the image.

During excitation, the spins absorb some of the transmitted RF energy and enter the high-energy state and are said to be hot. At that time they are situated at right angles to the direction of the magnetic field. When the external RF energy has been removed, the spins release some of that energy (or heat) to their environment (**lattice**) and begin to realign themselves with B_0. Because the spins release some of their energy to the lattice, T1 relaxation can also be called spin-lattice relaxation. Since this recovery occurs along the Z or longitudinal axis, T1 relaxation is also called **longitudinal relaxation** (Figure 2.53).

T2 DECAY

The time constant by which spins lose phase coherence is known as the **T2 decay** time. T2 decays exponentially, in half-lives. Therefore, in one T2 time, 63% of the transverse magnetization is lost. By knowing the T2 decay time, extrinsic parameters can be selected that maximize the T2 effect on the image (Figure 2.54). T2 decay is also known as spin-spin relaxation.

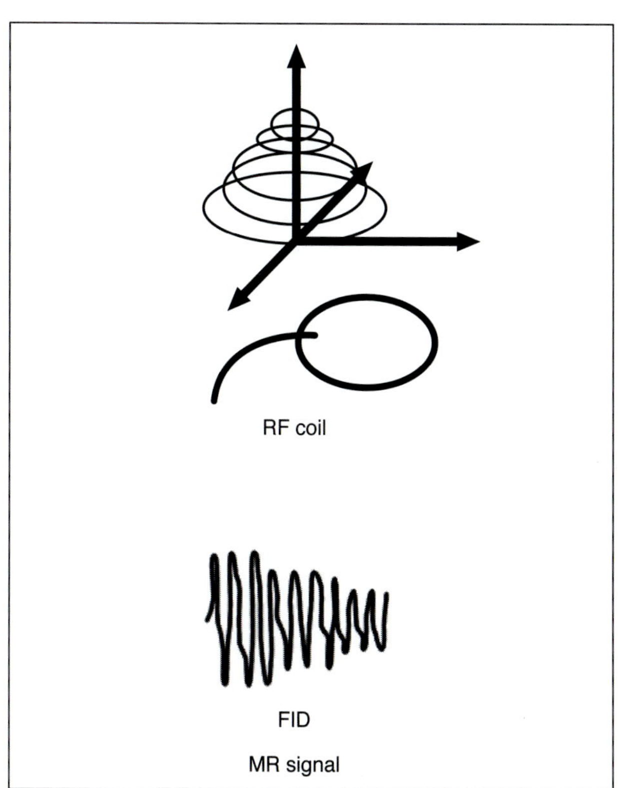

FIGURE 2.52 Signal detection during relaxation.

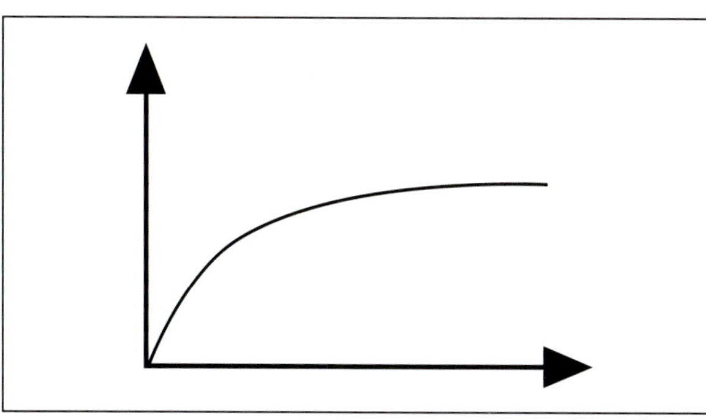

FIGURE 2.53 T1 recovery curve.

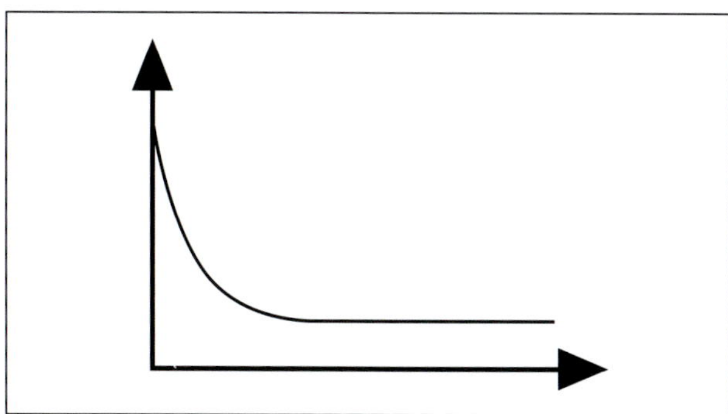

FIGURE 2.54 T2 decay curve.

SPIN ECHO

Signal that decays in the transverse plane is the result of T2 decay but is also influenced by imperfections known as inhomogeneities in the magnetic field and in the patient. The combination of T2 plus the inhomogeneity effect is known as T2* decay.

Following the RF pulse, a signal voltage is induced in a receiver coil. This voltage is displayed as an FID. The rate at which the transverse magnetization (shown on the FID) decays depends on the T2 relaxation times of the tissues. The 180° RF pulse refocuses the signal from the FID. This refocused signal is known as the **spin echo** (Figure 2.55).

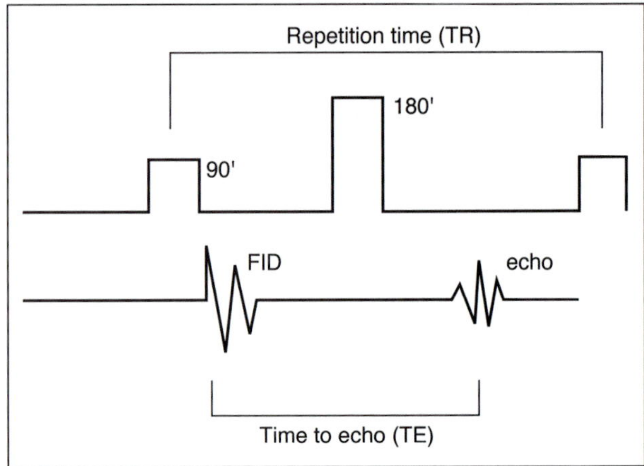

FIGURE 2.55 Spin echo pulse sequence.

Image Production

IMAGE CONTRAST PARAMETERS

Because water is the basis for MRI, water-laden soft tissue structures are best visualized. The beauty of MRI is that structures can be made to appear different with the simple adjustment of MRI parameters. With some parameter selections, fat can appear bright with water dark. With other selections water can appear bright with fat dark (Figure 2.56).

TIME TO ECHO (TE)

The **echo time (TE)** is the time between the 90° RF pulse and the echo signal (Figure 2.56).

TIME TO REPETITION (TR)

The **repetition time (TR)** is the time between consecutive 90° RF pulses in a pulse sequence. In spin echo pulse sequences the 90° pulse creates transverse magnetization. After the RF pulse is removed, longitudinal magnetization recovers at a rate dependent on the T1 relaxation time of the tissue (Figure 2.57).

T1-WEIGHTED IMAGE

To acquire image with different degrees of T1 information, the TR can be manipulated. In general, images acquired with short TR values produce images with high T1 contrast. TE is also selected for such images and is chosen to minimize the T2 effect on image contrast. Therefore to acquire images with a large T1 effect, short TR and short TE values should be used. These images are known as T1-weighted images because image contrast is weighted in the favor of T1. Contrast characteristics on T1 images demonstrate high signal from fat, intermediate signal from brain, viscera, and muscle, and low signal from water and water-filled structures. Because image quality is usually high, T1-weighted images are generally acquired for anatomic information (Figures 2.58 and 2.59).

T2-WEIGHTED IMAGE

To acquire images with different degrees of T2 information, the TE can be manipulated. In general images acquired with long TE values produce images with high T2 contrast. Because TR is also set on such images, it is selected to minimize the T1 effect on image contrast. Therefore to acquire images with a large T2 effect, long TR and long TE values are chosen. These images are known as T2-weighted images because contrast is weighted in the favor of T2. Contrast characteristics on T2 images demonstrate high signal from water, intermediate signal from brain, viscera and muscle and low signal from fat-filled structures. Because image contrast is usually high, T2-weighted images are generally acquired for pathologic information (Figure 2.60).

PD-WEIGHTED IMAGE

When images are acquired using short TE and long TR values, minimizing both the T1 and T2 effects, the resultant image is known as a proton density (PD)-weighted image. These images are also known as spin

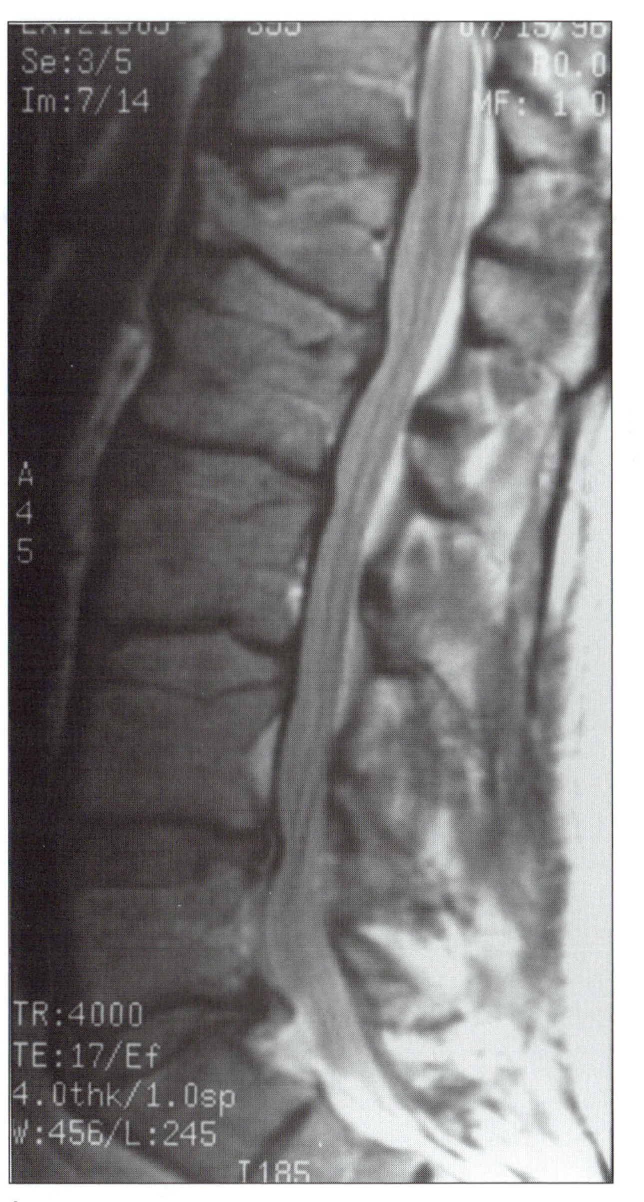

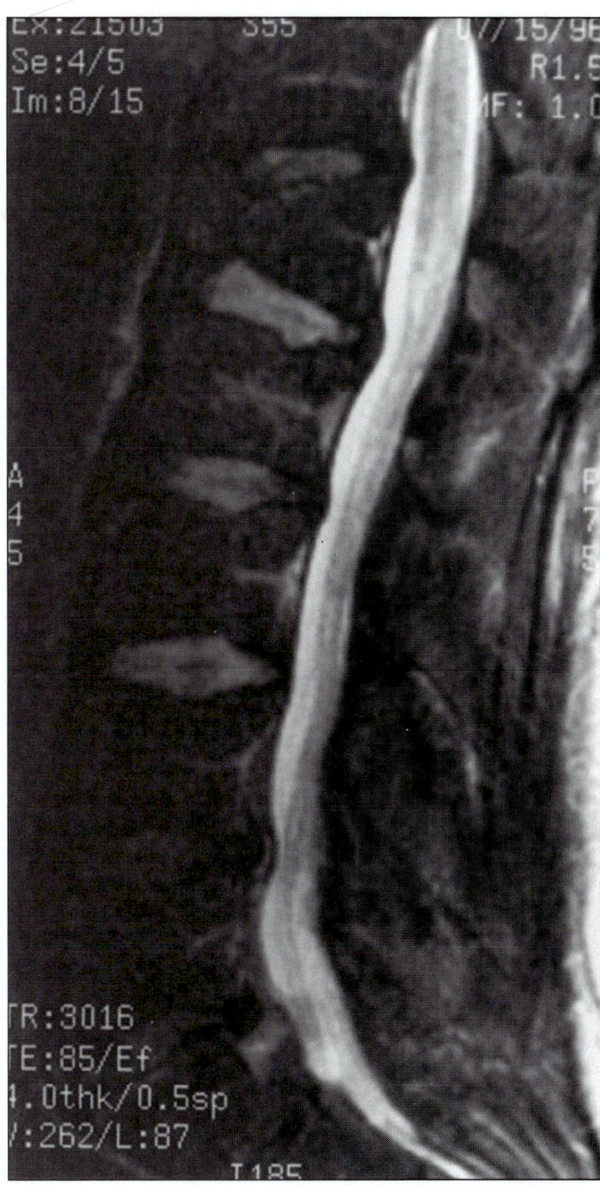

A B

FIGURE 2.56 Sagittal lumbar spine with (A) short TE time and (B) long TE time.

density, mixed mode, or first echo images. In this case with a long TR and a short TE selected, most structures demonstrate intermediate to high signal intensity (Figure 2.61).

SPATIAL ENCODING

The various views obtained in MRI are the product of a process known as spatial encoding accomplished with the use of **magnetic field gradients.** The gradients provide position-dependent variation of the magnetic field strength and signal frequency. Therefore, each RF signal represents a specific position within the magnet or a specific location within the body. Signals are encoded with information by using magnetic field gradients placed along the X (right to left), Y (front to back), and Z (head to feet) axis of the magnet.

Images can be reconstructed from these signals in a variety of scan planes using techniques analogous to those used in CT. However, unlike tomographic imaging, which enables visualization of the anatomy of interest by blurring out the structures above and below the fulcrum point, MRI scans are obtained by observing the MRI signals from the body in the presence of magnetic field gradients (Figure 2.62).

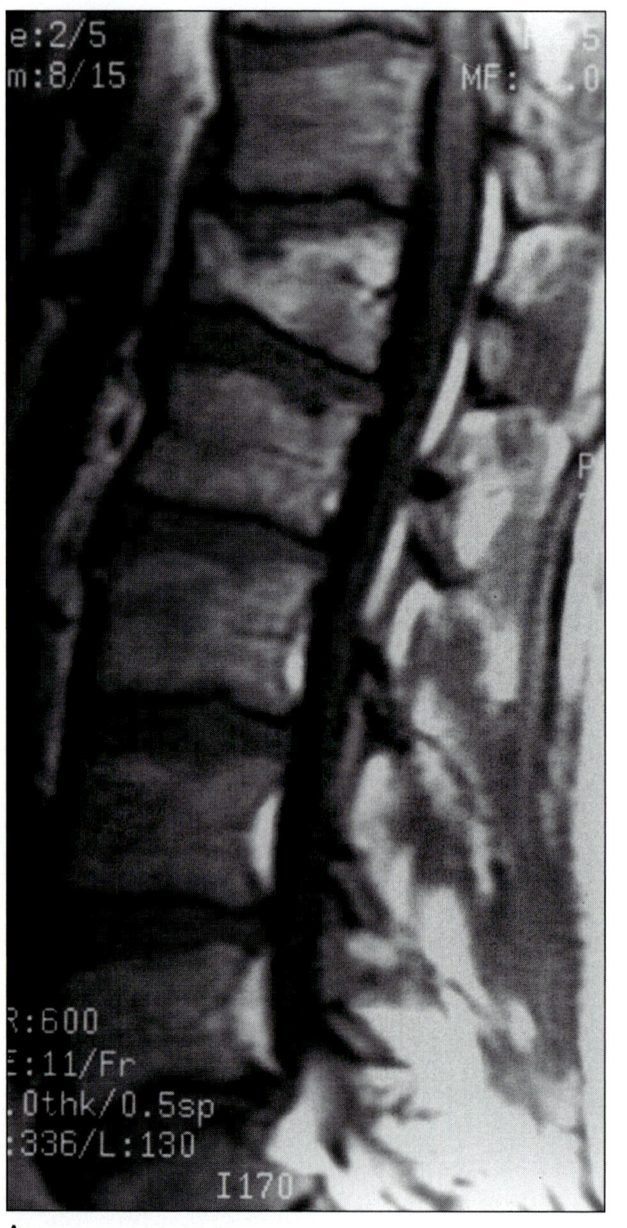

A

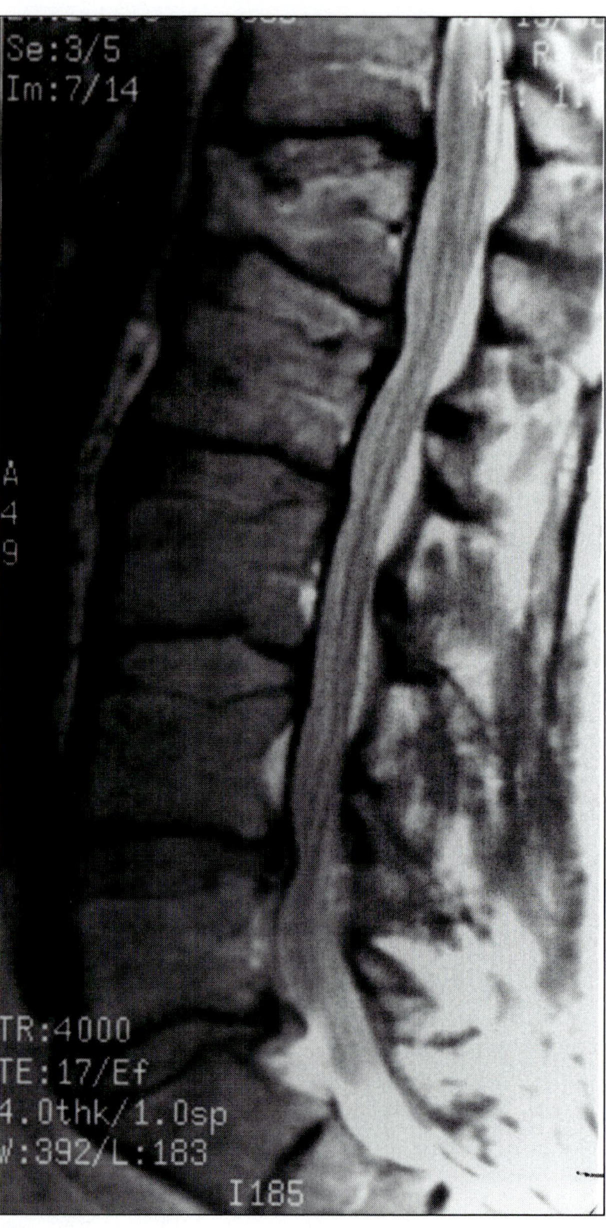

B

FIGURE 2.57 Sagittal lumbar spine with (A) short TR time and (B) long TR time.

SLICE SELECTION

The frequency required to excite the spins is directly proportional to the strength of the magnetic field in which the spins reside. Given that, if the magnetic field strength was changed, the frequency of the signal would change. This change is achieved by applying another magnetic field superimposed over the main magnetic field. The superimposed field is deliberately higher at one location in the magnet than in another. This is known as a magnetic field gradient. Magnetic field gradients provide position-dependent variation of magnetic field strength for the purpose of spatially encoding MRI signals. For example, a patient lying in the magnet with the gradient applied can have a low magnetic field located inferiorly (toward the feet) and the higher magnetic field located superiorly (toward the head). This scenario would produce signals with higher frequencies at the head than the feet.

To detect a particular signal, the imager must be tuned to the frequency of that signal. Setting this frequency is like dialing a radio. If a radio was to be tuned to a particular station (or frequency), the broadcast could be heard from only that station even

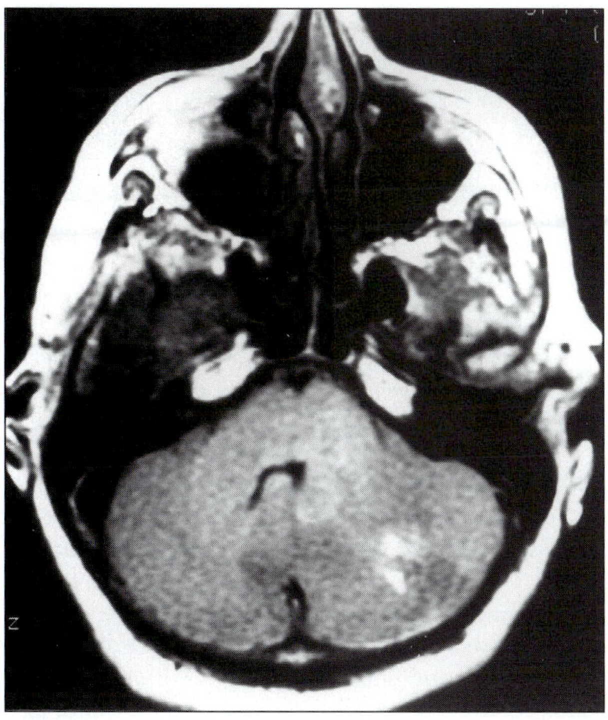

FIGURE 2.58 T1-weighted image of the brain.

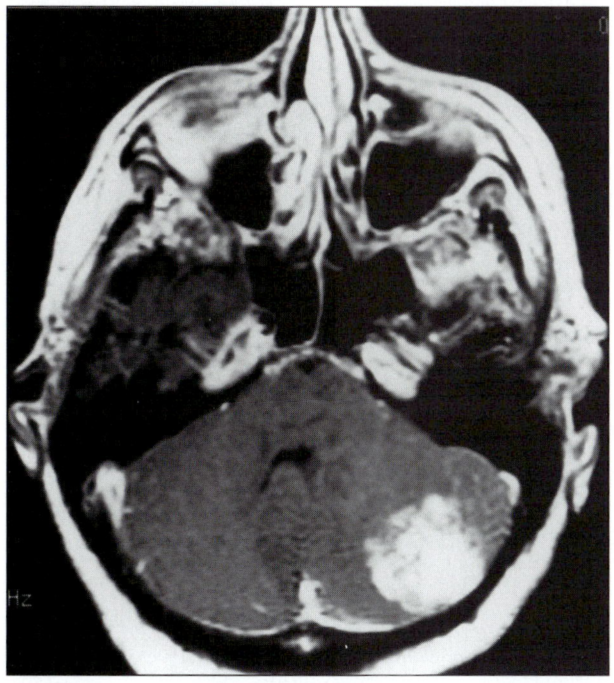

FIGURE 2.59 Brain demonstrating contrast enhancement.

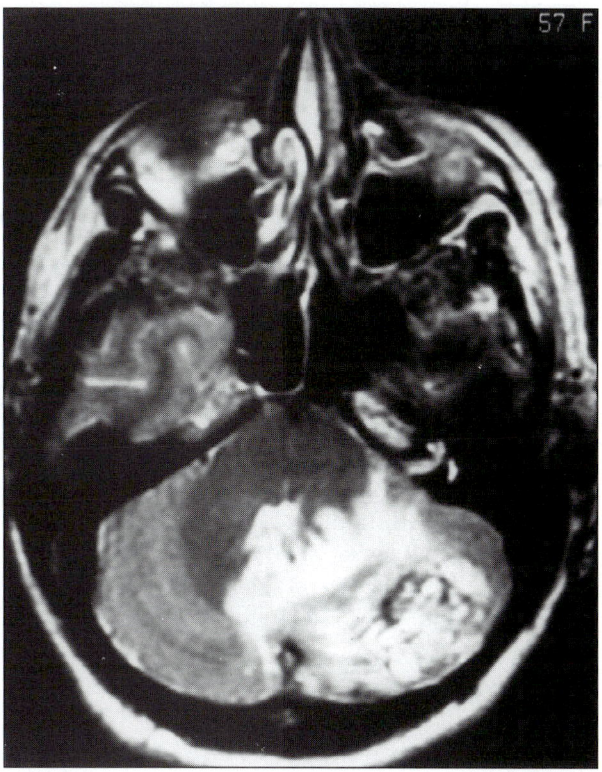

FIGURE 2.60 T2-weighted image of the brain.

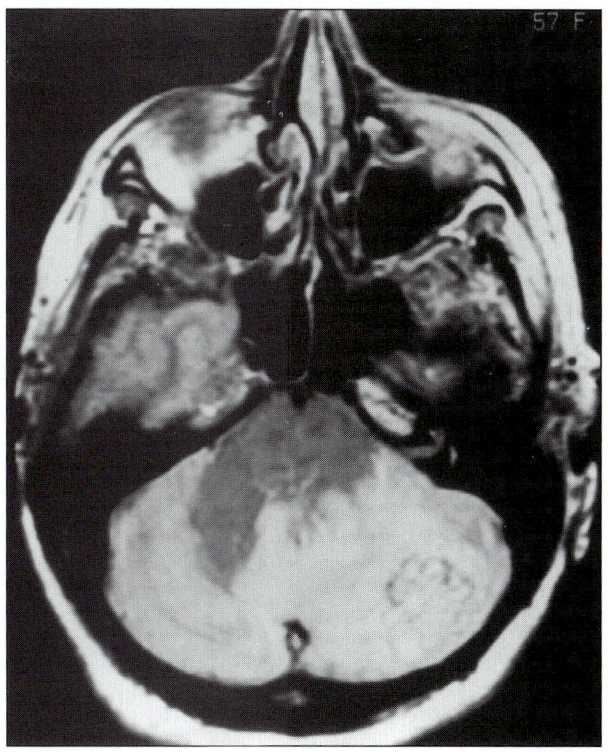

FIGURE 2.61 Proton density-weighted image.

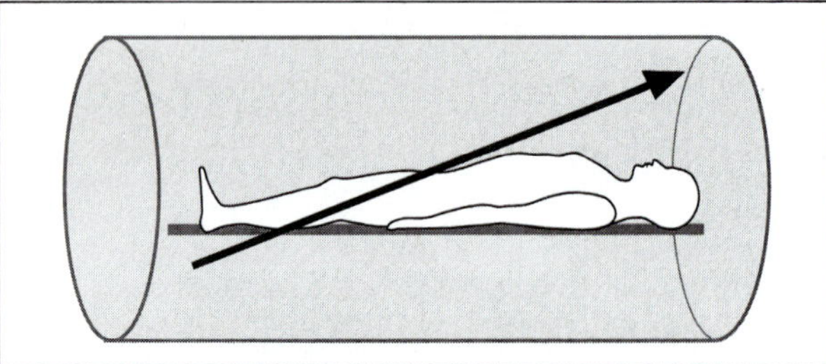

FIGURE 2.62 Magnetic field gradient applied along the Z axis.

though other radio stations may be transmitting at the same time. The same is true in MRI; with the gradient applied, setting the frequency ensures that only the signal emerging from a specific location within the magnet is detected. In the example mentioned above, by tuning in to the higher frequencies, signals only from the patient's head could be detected and therefore create an image of the brain.

IMAGE FORMATION

The signal is then translated by a series of mathematic processes into numbers and subsequently into shades of gray, which are assigned specific locations in the imaging matrix on the TV screen. This process produces the image. On the image, tissues with high signal intensities produce bright areas and those with low signal intensities produce dark areas. Manipulating the imaging parameters can alter the signal intensities obtained and drastically change the appearance of the images.

VIEW OPTIONS

In MRI, views are referred to as **imaging planes.** There are three straight plane options in MRI, including sagittal, axial, and coronal. In addition to the straight planes an unlimited number of oblique projections can be acquired. The sagittal imaging plane corresponds to a lateral radiograph by looking like a side view. A sagittal image is the product of slicing from head to feet, parallel with the midsagittal suture, dividing the body into right and left. The coronal plane would look like an anteroposterior (AP) view and is the product slicing from head to feet, parallel with the coronal suture, dividing the body into anterior and posterior. The axial plane divides the body into superior and inferior and produces images that look similar to CT images (Figure 2.63).

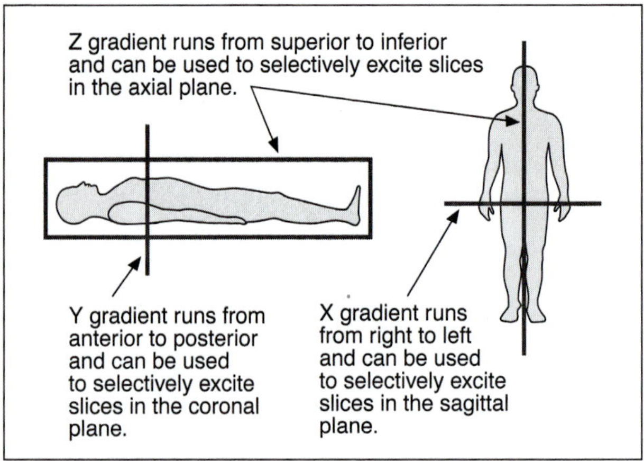

FIGURE 2.63 Orientation of physical gradients.

The imaging plane is selected on the basis of the anatomy to be examined. For example, in head imaging, a sagittal image is usually selected for **localization** as the best plane to demonstrate anatomy of the brain. If instead the abdomen is imaged, the coronal plane may be a better choice for localization. In the head and the abdomen axial images are almost always acquired after the localization images. All studies performed in MRI require more than one imaging plane, because like in other diagnostic imaging modalities, "one view is not enough" (Figure 2.64).

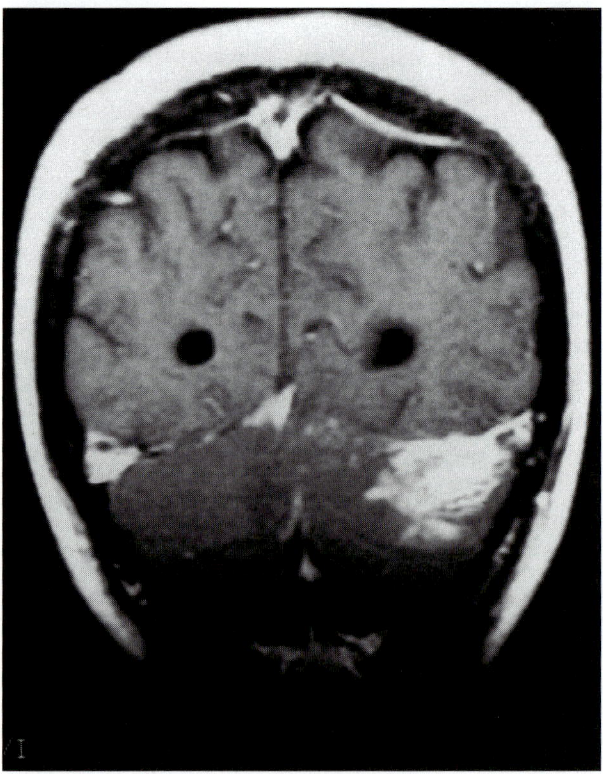

FIGURE 2.64 T1-weighted image of brain.

PULSE SEQUENCES

Finally, to create an MRI a series of RF and gradient pulses are applied. This series of pulses is known as a pulse sequence. A few pulse sequences that are fairly standard for MRI include spin echo, gradient echo, and inversion recovery. Each sequence has its unique characteristics; therefore, many imaging protocols usually include combinations of sequences to provide a variety of clinical information (Figure 2.65).

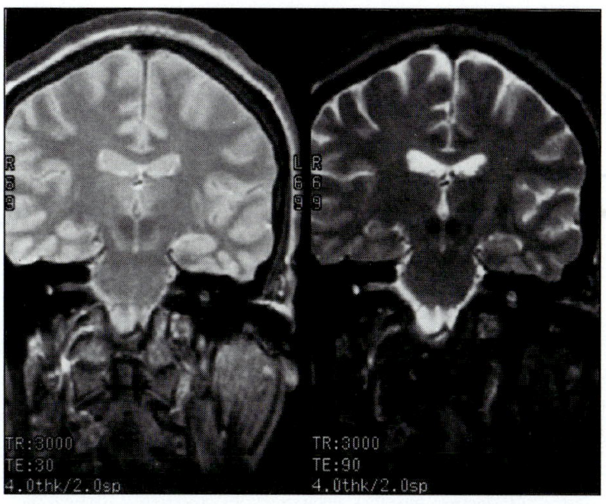

FIGURE 2.65 Coronal images acquired with a spin echo sequence.

Applications

MRI is probably the imaging modality of choice in situations in which soft tissues structures are of interest. In the early 1980s MRI was almost exclusively used for imaging of the central nervous system (brain and spine), in combination with or compared to CT. Later in the decade, MRI became proven for its usefulness in the musculoskeletal system. Musculoskeletal MRI scanning was compared with the gold standard, the arthrogram. Today MRI is used for almost any part of the body including the brain, spine, joints, abdomen, pelvis, and thorax.

PROTOCOL SELECTIONS (PULSE SEQUENCE AND PARAMETER CHOICES)

When an MRI is requested for a particular patient, imaging planes, pulse sequences, and imaging parameters are chosen to optimize the study. Such selections are incorporated into what is known as a **protocol.** Each protocol includes several imaging sequences per study such that the anatomy and pathology are appropriately imaged.

ARTIFACT COMPENSATION (IMAGE OPTIMIZATION)

The quality of the MRI can be degraded by a number of imaging **artifacts.** Artifacts can be caused by physical forces (**susceptibility** and chemical shift) and sampling artifacts (motion). This section describes these artifacts and some compensation techniques.

An MRI can be incredibly sensitive to motion because imaging times are long relative to physiologic motion. When considering effects detrimental to image quality, motion is probably first. For this reason, most system manufacturers have made an effort to develop imaging parameters and options to help compensate for motion (Figure 2.66).

COIL SELECTION AND PATIENT POSITIONING

Along with the protocol, imaging planes, parameters, and options, the RF coil is selected on the basis of the anatomy and pathology to be imaged. Some RF coils are designed to transmit and receive MRI signal, whereas others are designed only to receive signal. In general, the smaller the coil, the more coils and the closer the coil is placed to the anatomy of interest, the better the signal and the better the image (Figure 2.67).

IMAGE RECORDING SYSTEMS AND PHOTOGRAPHY FOR MRI

The images are digital images and can be stored by a number of mechanisms. These storage methods include transfer to hard copy, **magnetic tape, optical disk,** or **dat tape.** The former requires a lot of space and patience to keep track of bulky films without losing them. The latter requires sophisticated hardware and software. Many facilities use a combination of one or more methods for the storage of MRI data.

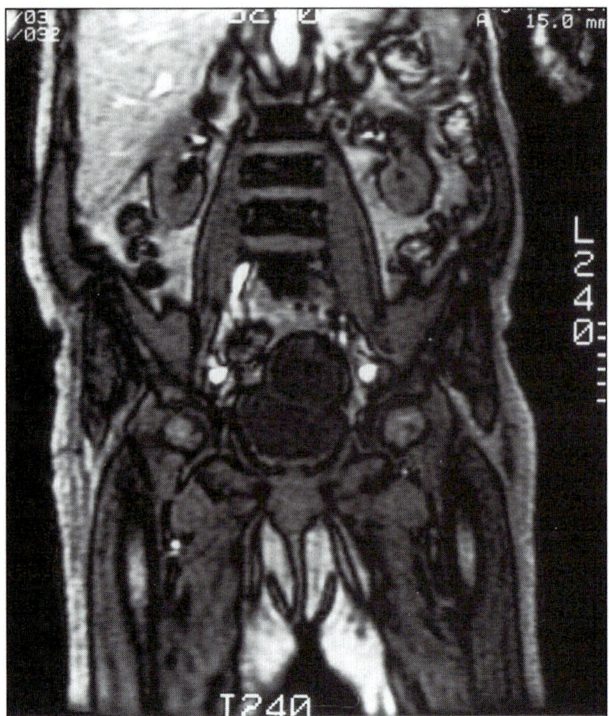

FIGURE 2.66 Coronal image of abdomen acquired during a breath hold.

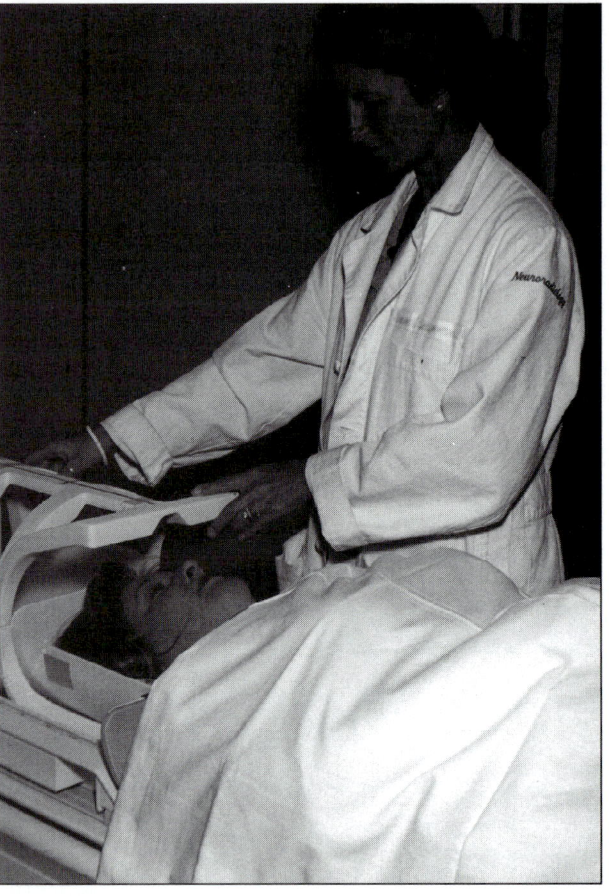

FIGURE 2.67 RF coil used for vascular system from aortic arch to circle of Willis.

The most commonly used, but nearly outdated, method is to transfer image data to hard copy. In this case images are filmed onto a piece of single emulsion film and stored with other film radiographs in the radiology film library. Because space is difficult to find and costly to maintain, the large radiology file rooms of the past are shrinking.

The next method to store MRI data is with magnetic tape. This method is also bulky because each tape only holds 211 images. Then tapes are stored in large storage racks outside of the magnetic field. One must be careful not to allow tapes to enter the magnetic field because the field will erase the image information from the tape. Newer methods to store digital information include optical disk and dat tape. Each holds 10,000 to 14,000 images and is small and easy to store. The dat tape is faster and easier to access than the optical disk, but it can be written over.

SAFETY AND PATIENT CARE FOR MRI

To date there have been virtually no long-term adverse biologic effects of extended exposure to MRI as a whole. However, if separate components of the MRI process are examined, several inconsequential and reversible effects of magnetic, gradient, and RF fields are observed.

Biologic Effects of the Static Magnetic Fields, Static Fields Below and Above 2 T

At this time there seems to be no long-term biologic effects to exposure to magnetic fields, at least in fields below 2 T. Above 2 T some biologic effects were noticed including fatigue, headaches, and irritability. Below 2 T the only effect reported was reversible.

Fringe Fields (Magnetically or Electrically Activated Devices and Projectiles)

In most cases the magnetic field is not confined to the bore of the magnet, but also extends outside of the bore and into the scan room, sometimes outside the scan room. This outside magnetic field is known as the fringe field. There are electrically, magnetically or mechanically activated or electrically conductive implanted devices that can be influenced by the fringe field. For this reason, all implanted devices (including cardiac pacemakers or pacer wires) or ancillary equipment must be tested before they enter the MRI scan area.

Implants and Prostheses in the Magnetic Field

The biggest concern for implants and prostheses in the magnetic field is the potential of **torque** and heating. Torque occurs as an implant moves across the magnetic field lines and twists or turns as the result of that motion. Heating occurs as the gradient and RF fields are turned on and off during the MRI sequence. All **implants** and prostheses should be evaluated before the patient enters the scan room for imaging. *Absolute contraindications* for MRI include patients with **cardiac pacemakers, intracranial vascular clips,** and **intraocular foreign bodies.** All other implants should be considered on a case by case basis.

Another concern for implants includes artifacts from metallic implants. Although this effect is not life-threatening, it may render the MRI poor quality and in some cases useless. For this reason, care should be taken to evaluate all implants within patients, including those safe for an MRI.

Gradient Magnetic Field and Time-Varying Field Effects

Faraday's law states if a magnetic field moves with respect to a conductor, a current can be induced within the conductor. Because the human body is a good conductor and because magnetic field gradients are switched on and off during MRI acquisition, the concern for time-varying fields is the possibility of peripheral nerve stimulation. This results in involuntary muscle contractions, mild cutaneous sensations, and visual disturbances, all of which are reversible effects.

The Food and Drug Administration (FDA) has regulations regarding the exposure of patients to loud acoustic noise. Switching gradients produces loud noise that depends on the pulse sequence. For these reasons, it recommended that all patients are provided with earplugs or headphones during MRI procedures.

RF Fields and RF Absorption

The predominant effect of RF exposure is the heating of tissue. The FDA limit for the heating of tissue is 1°C in the body's core.

Pregnancy

The FDA recommends that patients can be imaged with MRI if the information gained would have required more invasive testing. Such patients are evaluated on a case by case basis. For pregnant health care employees, the FDA leaves the decision to the discretion of the facility. The Society for Magnetic Resonance (SMR) safety committee recommends that pregnant associates may enter the magnetic field to position patients but must leave the scan room while the RF and gradient fields are on.

Patient Screening and Safety Education

Patient and personnel screening is, to date, the most effective way in which to avoid potential health hazards to patients in MRI. Patients and employees with questionable ferromagnetic foreign objects either in or on their bodies should be rigorously examined to avoid any serious health risks and accidents. Maintaining this controlled environment can be achieved by careful questioning and education of patients and all personnel. In addition, routine preventive maintenance checks by the service engineer and continuing education are also important. Careful planning and diligent upkeep of an MRI facility can provide a safe environment for both patients and employees.

Review Questions

1. Gradient coils provide a means for:
   a. magnetic field homogeneity
   b. position-dependent variation of magnetic field strength and signal frequency
   c. a strategic magnetic field
   d. an oscillating magnetic field

2. In MRI, after RF excitation:
   a. the receiver coil detects the emitted RF signal
   b. the RF signal is induced within the receiver coil
   c. the receiver coil transmits a 90° RF pulse
   d. the receiver coil is tackled in the end zone

3. An absolute contraindication for MRI would be:
   a. ferrous foreign body within the eye
   b. pregnancy
   c. cardiac pacemaker
   d. a and c

4. Describe the different imaging planes and how they are acquired using gradients.

5. Describe four major features that distinguish MRI acquisition from CT acquisition.

CASE STUDY

A man has been admitted with acute pain in his head. Because he is a recent immigrant with no language skills, it is impossible to take any history. The question becomes: Is this a trauma injury involving fracture or a pathology? Discuss how an MRI could be taken to provide maximum visualization for these two different scenarios.

References and Recommended Reading

Applegate, E. J. (1991). *The sectional anatomy learning system.* Philadelphia: Saunders.

Berkow, R. (Ed.). (1987). *The Merck manual.* Rahway, NJ: Merck Sharp & Dohme Research Laboratories.

Bontrager, K. (1997). *Textbook of radiographic positioning and related anatomy* (4th ed.). St. Louis: Mosby-Year Book.

Brasch, R. (Ed.). (1993). *MRI contrast enhancement in the central nervous system: A case study approach.* New York: Raven Press.

Bushong, S. (1988). *Magnetic resonance imaging: Physical and biological principles.* St. Louis: Mosby-Year Book.

Edelman, R. R., & Hesselink, J. R. (1990). *Clinical magnetic resonance imaging.* Philadelphia: Saunders.

El-Khoury, G. Y., & Bergman, R. A. (1990). *Sectional anatomy by MRI/CT.* New York: Churchill Livingstone.

Hayman, L. A., & Hink, V. C. (1992). *Clinical brain imaging normal structure and functional anatomy.* St. Louis: Mosby-Year Book.

Higgins, C. B., Hricak, H., & Helms, C. A. (1992). *Magnetic resonance imaging of the body.* (3rd ed.). New York: Raven Press.

Kaut, C. (1992). *MRI workbook for technologists.* New York: Raven Press.

Kaut, C., & Westbrook, C. (1993). *MRI in practice.* Oxford: Blackwell Scientific Publications.

Kaut, C., & Faulkner, W. (1994). *Review questions in MRI.* Oxford: Blackwell Scientific Publications.

Lane, A., & Sharfaei, H. (1992). *Modern sectional anatomy.* Philadelphia: Saunders.

The Lippincott Manual of Nursing Practice. (1991). (5th ed.). Philadelphia: Lippincott.

Lufkin, R. (1990). *MRI manual.* Chicago: Year Book Medical Publishers.

Lufkin, R. B., Bradley, W. G., Jr., & Brant-Zawadzki, M. (Eds). (1990). *The Raven MRI teaching file.* New York: Raven Press.

Middleton, W. D., & Lawson, T. L. (1989). *Anatomy and MRI of the joints: A multiplanar atlas.* New York: Raven Press.

Mills, C. M., DeGroot, J., & Posin, J. P. (1988). *Magnetic resonance imaging: Atlas of the head, neck, and spine.* Philadelphia: Lea & Febiger.

Pomeranz, S. (1991). *Orthopaedic MRI: A teaching file.* Philadelphia: Lippincott.

Schitzlein, H. N., & Murtagh, F. R. (1990). *Imaging antomy of the head and spine: A photographic color atlas of MRI, CT, gross, and microscopic anatomy in axial, coronal, and sagittal planes.* Baltimore: Urban and Schwarzenberg.

Shellock, F. G. (1994). *Pocket guide to MR procedures and metallic objects: Update 1994.* New York: Raven Press:

Snopek, A. (1992). *Fundamentals of special radiographic procedures* (3rd ed.). Philadelphia: Saunders.

Stark, D. D., & Bradley, W. G., Jr. (1988). *Magnetic resonance imaging.* St. Louis: Mosby-Year Book.

Westbrook, C. (1994). *Handbook of MRI technique.* Oxford: Blackwell Scientific Publications.

Ultrasound

Gail Rodrigues, MRT(R), RDMS

Introduction and Historical Overview

In 1881, Pierre and Jacques Curie using quartz and a battery discovered the piezoelectric effect, which produces ultrasound. Since that time ultrasound has been used to locate schools of fish (sonar) and catch speeding motorists (Doppler radar). It was also used in an attempt to locate the sunken Titanic off the shores of Nova Scotia, Canada in 1912.

World War I was the real starting point for research into the practical usage of ultrasound. The war departments were looking for a way to detect submarine activity using ultrasound. This led the way for further research, and the development of sonar (sound navigation and ranging) during World War II. During that war ultrasound was also being used to detect flaws in metals. In 1937, K. T. Dussik, an Austrian, designed the first ultrasound imaging device; he tried to image the ventricles of the brain, but the process proved impractical.

In 1949, Howry and Bliss from the United States using naval sonar equipment, constructed the first usable ultrasound imaging machine. It was able to produce an image of the anatomy in the form of dots. Both the patient and the transducer were immersed in water to obtain the images. A worker in the laboratory replaced the transducer crystal they were using with barium titanate and lead zirconate titanate, materials still being used in modern ultrasound practice. In 1954, Howry and Holmes built an ultrasound unit made from an old gun turret. Patients were submerged in water again, this time inside the gun turret with weights tied to them to keep them submerged.

The early 1960s brought the first commercially manufactured ultrasound scanner. The patient was out of water but now was covered with mineral oil, which was used as a coupling agent between the patient's skin and the transducer. The image was primitive; we would find it next to impossible to diagnose from it today. The mineral oil has been replaced with gel and the equipment is much more sophisticated, but the basic principles of ultrasound imaging carry on from the first research done for the war effort in the early 1900s. Modern diagnostic ultrasound equipment (Figure 2.68) uses high-frequency sound waves (higher than the audible range). These waves travel into and out of the body to create sectional images of soft tissue organs.

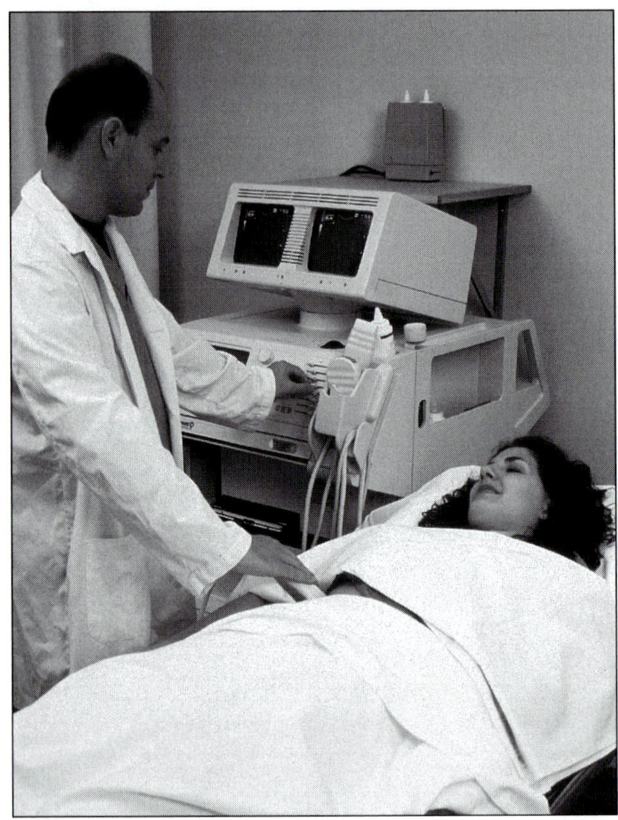

FIGURE 2.68 Modern ultrasonic equipment.

Principles

WHAT IS SOUND?

Sound is a form of mechanical energy or pressure waves. The mechanical energy creates molecular vibrations that move through a medium (the body). These molecular vibrations caused by pressure waves occur in a pattern, with the compressed portion of the wave known as a **compression** and the relaxed portion of the wave as a **rarefaction** (Figure 2.69). These two portions of the ultrasound wave occur over and over,

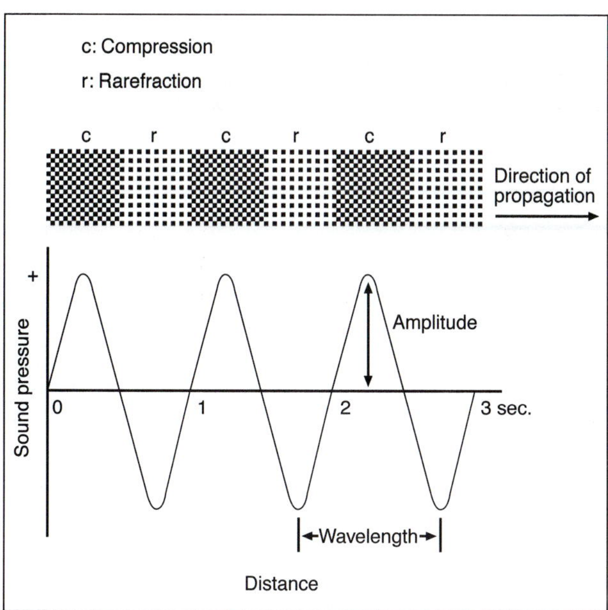

FIGURE 2.69 Longitudinal sound waves.

in a cyclic pattern, and therefore can be drawn as a sine wave and can use wave parameters. One of the wave parameters used is frequency.

Frequency is the number of cycles per second. The unit is the **hertz** (Hz), named for physicist Heinrick Hertz (1857–1894), who was the first to broadcast and receive radiowaves. Frequency can be expressed as:

1 cycle/sec = 1 Hz
1000 cycles/sec = 1 kHz (kilohertz)
1,000,000 cycles/sec =1 MHz (megahertz)
Audible sound range = 15–20 kHz
Ultrasound = > 20 kHz
Diagnostic ultrasound = 2.25–10 MHz

Sound waves travel in a line parallel to their origin (longitudinal wave travel), whereas x-rays are transverse waves. Sound needs a medium in which to travel; x-rays require a vacuum. As you speak, the molecules in the air are the medium in which the sound is traveling or propagating. With ultrasound the patient's body (soft tissue) is the medium.

An ultrasound beam is created by a vibrating crystal (piezoelectric crystal), which is housed in a **transducer**. With ultrasound, the pressure waves are produced in the transducer by the crystal when it is applied with electricity. The crystal has the ability to create electricity when hit by ultrasound (mechanical energy). Thus one form of energy is transformed into another, which is known as the **piezoelectric effect.** Piezoelectric (pī-ē´zō-ē-lĕk´trik) is Greek for "pressure electricity." The piezoelectric crystal is typically made from lead zirconate and lead titanate.

electrical energy + crystal →
ultrasound (mechanical energy)

mechanical energy (ultrasound) + crystal →
electrical energy

When the ultrasound pulse (mechanical energy) is emitted from the crystal, the pulse enters the patient's body, interacts with the tissues, and reflects back to the transducer. At the crystal, the ultrasound reflection (mechanical energy) is transformed to electrical energy, and this electricity is displayed as a brightness dot on the TV monitor, which is our image. The greater the percentage of reflection from the tissue, the more electricity will be produced at the crystal and the whiter the dot on the TV monitor. What controls the percentage of reflection from the tissues? The tissues themselves!

Not all tissues have the same characteristics, in particular elasticity (or stiffness) and density. It is the difference in stiffness and density of adjacent tissues that creates the percentage of reflection. The greater the difference in stiffness and density (known as **acoustic impedance mismatch**), the greater the percentage reflection, the more electricity produced, the whiter the dot on the final image on the monitor. A small acoustic impedance mismatch will produce a black dot on the monitor. A large range of grays can be produced from the tiny stiffness and density changes within the tissues, producing the ultrasound image as multiple shades of gray representing the anatomic structures. The radiographic image is produced by that portion of the x-ray beam that has *passed through* the body, whereas the ultrasound image is produced by the beam *reflecting back* to the transducer.

Image Production

An ultrasound pulse will interact with tissue and a percentage of the beam will be reflected. The remainder of the beam will continue to the next interface (point at which two tissues meet) and reflect; this process will continue until the beam is completely attenuated or used up. This creates one line of dots or information. Multiple lines together make up a **sector** or rectangular **field of view** or image. The general beam shape (sector or rectangular) is controlled by the manufacturer. Each section that is imaged is a few millimeters thick; therefore, a great number of sections are required to demonstrate an entire organ or structure. An organ is imaged by moving or angling the transducer across the patient's body. The images are created automatically and simultaneously once the operator has set up the controls and placed the transducer on the patient's skin. All organs or structures are examined in at least the sagittal and the transverse plane.

Ultrasound does not image well through bone or air because of the large differences in stiffness and density between bone (or air) and soft tissue. There will be a large acoustic impedance mismatch at the bone-soft tissue interface, a large percentage of reflection, and therefore little or no ultrasound left to transmit into the tissues. No image is seen beneath the bone or air and the area appears black on the screen. This is known as **acoustic shadowing,** which is a useful artefact in ultrasound. It helps identify strong attenuators like calcifications, bone, and gallstones and kidney stone (Figure 2.70). An ultrasonic gel is used between the skin and the transducer to eliminate air and facilitate transmission of ultrasound into the body.

Another type of useful artefact is **through transmission** or acoustic enhancement. Through transmission is a white area produced posterior to a cyst or fluid collection (Figure 2.71). If a fluid is compared to solid liver tissue, there is more attenuation of the ultrasound beam through the solid liver than through the fluid, due to the higher percentage of reflection at the solid interfaces. Therefore, if the same beam interacts with the fluid and the solid, more energy remains in the beam at the posterior aspect of the cyst or fluid as compared to the solid. Due to the increased energy, the area posterior to the cyst will be whiter on the monitor. The beam is more intense, will reflect more energy, and thus be whiter. Through transmission is useful in the identification of cysts or fluid collections.

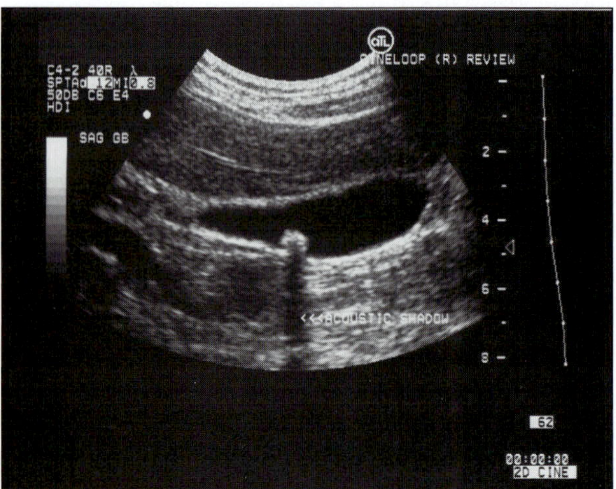

FIGURE 2.70 Acoustic shadow (gallstone).

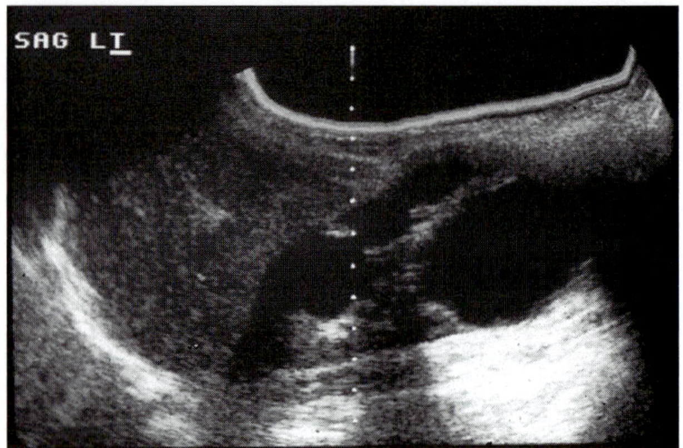

FIGURE 2.71 Through transmission.

As the ultrasound beam moves through the tissues it is attenuated. If there were two reflectors that were absolutely the same but one sat anteriorly in the body and the other posteriorly, then we would want them to appear the same on the TV monitor. However, due to attenuation they would not; the more anterior reflector would be displayed as whiter than the posterior one because there is more energy remaining in the beam more anteriorly. To compensate for this distance attenuation the time gain compensation (TGC) control is used. The TGC adds voltage to the returned echo according to depth to allow reflectors that are the same to be displayed the same. The greater the depth a reflector returns from, the more voltage applied. The TGC controls are set up by the equipment operator, an important factor for image quality. The TGC must be set for every patient and for the different organ depths within that patient. A poorly set TGC can make it difficult to properly identify structures (Figure 2.72A). Figure 2.72B represents a scan of the liver with the TGC set correctly.

DOPPLER

Christian Johann Doppler, an Austrian physicist, recorded the theory of **Doppler** in 1842 by watching the changing color of the stars. Doppler uses ultrasound waves to determine the velocity, direction, and

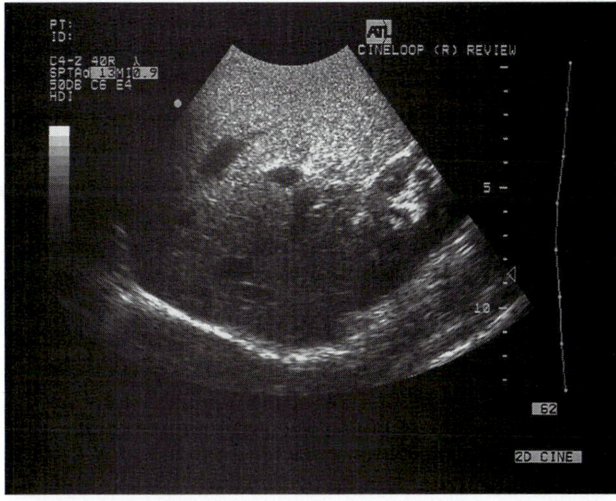

A

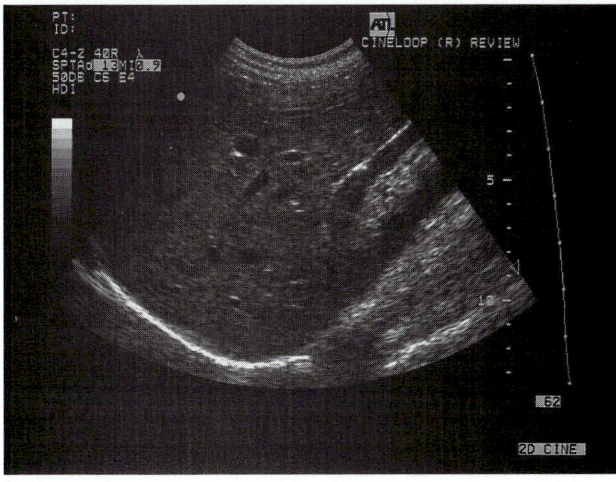

B

FIGURE 2.72 (A) TGC poorly set and (B) TGC accurately set.

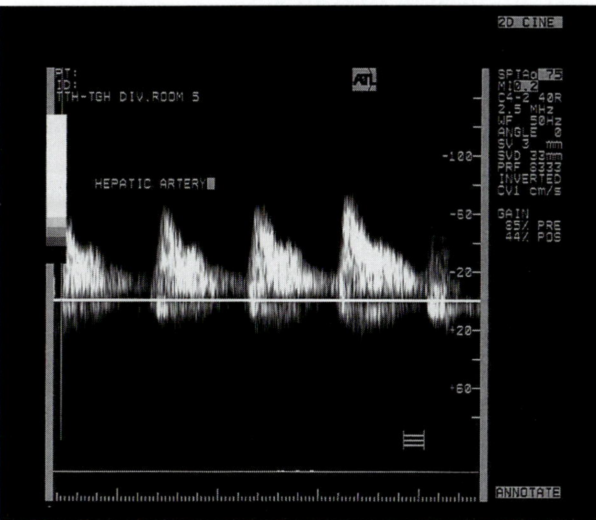

FIGURE 2.73 Spectral analysis display.

characteristics of the flow of red blood cells (RBC) in the body. Instead of determining the amplitude of the reflected ultrasound wave, Doppler determines the difference in frequencies. A known, fixed frequency is emitted from the transducer and when it interacts with a moving object (RBCs) a different frequency is reflected back to the transducer. This difference between the emitted and reflected frequencies is known as the Doppler shift. In diagnostic ultrasound the Doppler shift is proportional to RBC velocity. The Doppler shift is always in the audible range and will account for the funny sounds emanating from ultrasound departments. Doppler can be displayed graphically (spectral analysis display) and in color.

Spectral Analysis Display

This graphic display of Doppler signals does not look like any anatomic structure. It appears as a bunch of dots on a graph, which typifies a particular pattern of blood flow (Figure 2.73). For example, flow through a normal renal artery will have a specific expected graphic pattern.

With spectral display blood flow toward the transducer is displayed above the zero baseline and flow away from the transducer is below the zero baseline. Velocity is recorded on the Y axis. The maximum or peak blood flow velocity reading in numbers can be obtained from this graph. These readings are compared to the normal expected parameters to determine if the patient's flow is normal or not. The technologist must learn to recognize the appearance of the normal and abnormal blood flow patterns.

Color Flow Doppler

Color Doppler is achieved by coding blood flow toward the transducer in red and coding blood flow away from the transducer in blue. This color image is overlaid onto the normal two-dimensional image of the area being scanned. To remember these directions: BART = *B*lue *A*way *R*ed *T*oward

The color does *not* indicate arterial or venous flow. A vessel could be either color depending on whether the blood is moving toward or away from the transducer. The intensity of the color indicates the velocity of flow, but an actual number reading for peak velocity is not possible to obtain. This necessitates the combined use of spectral analysis display and color Doppler to get an accurate peak velocity reading. Color flow Doppler is used to quickly identify if there is flow, stenosis, occlusion of a vessel, or regurgitant flow.

INTERCAVITY ULTRASOUND

There are ultrasound transducers that are specifically made for intercavity scanning. These transducers have the crystal at the end of its length. This allows for the structure that is being imaged to lie closer to the crystal, achieving better detail. The two areas most commonly imaged in this way are the uterus and adnexa (**endovaginal**) and the prostate and seminal vesicles (**endorectal**).

BIOLOGIC EFFECTS

The unit of intensity for ultrasound is milliwatt per centimeter squared (mW/cm^2). There are no known biologic effects to ultrasound below an intensity exposure of 100 mW/cm^2. Intensity readings evaluate the power of the ultrasound beam and the area over which the power is applied. Scans should be performed considering the benefit to the patient.

IMAGE RECORDING SYSTEMS

Ultrasound images can be recorded by a multiformat camera (film), videotaping, or computerized images and storage.

Applications

INDICATIONS FOR USE

Ultrasound can image any soft tissue structure in the body that is not surrounded by either bone or air, for example, the liver, gallbladder, pancreas, uterus, the fetus, or the heart to name a few areas. Ultrasound is a detailed precise examination that compares to CT in its clarity and diagnostic value.

Ultrasound cannot assess the function of an organ as radiography or nuclear medicine can, for example with the kidneys, but it can assess dynamic structures like the heart without any radiation. It can also assess nonfunctioning organs for morphology, for example, a kidney in failure (Figure 2.74). The ultrasonic study of the abdomen is limited by the amount of bowel gas the patient has (going back to our high percentage of reflection); air and fat are limiting factors for imaging.

Some developing areas in ultrasound are the use of contrast agents to better visualize Doppler flow; three-dimensional imaging of fetuses, vessels, tumors, and cardiac chambers; and hysterosonography in which saline with microbubbles is injected into the uterus.

CLINICAL APPLICATIONS

Most soft tissue pathologies that are greater than 3 to 5 mm can be imaged using ultrasound. Some examples would include abscesses, tumors in a number of organs, abdominal aortic aneurysm, obstructions in the urinary system, and physical fetal abnormalities (Figures 2.75, 2.76, and 2.77).

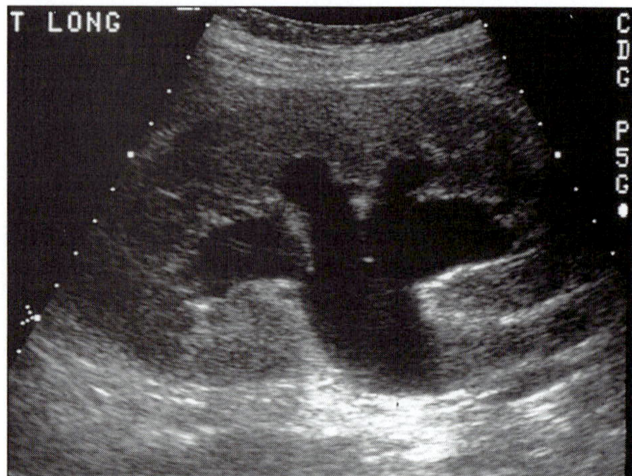

FIGURE 2.74 Hydronephrosis.

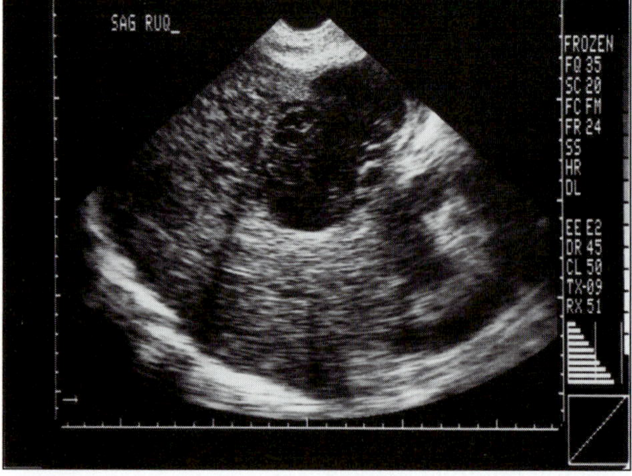

FIGURE 2.75 Abdominal aortic aneurysm.

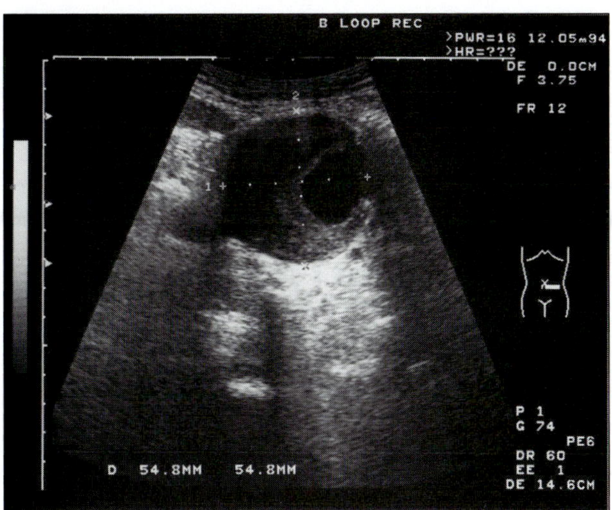

FIGURE 2.76 Hydrocephalus.

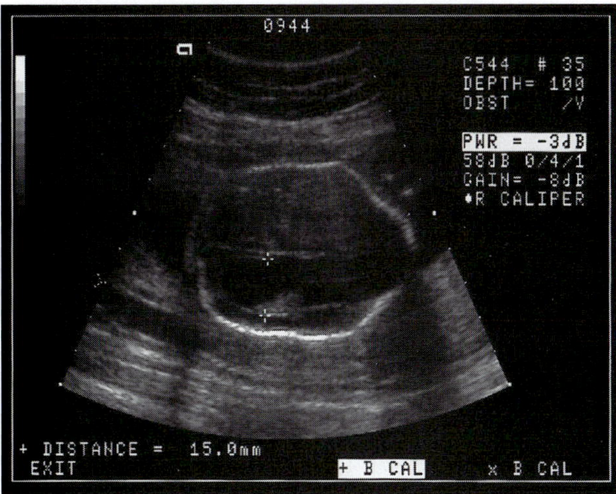

FIGURE 2.77 Liver abscess.

PATIENT CARE CONSIDERATIONS

For abdominal examinations the patient is asked to fast from the night before until the test. This is an attempt to minimize the amount of abdominal gas to allow for better visualization.

Pelvic ultrasounds require the patient to drink three to four 8-oz glasses of water. This will fill the bladder and push the small bowel up and out of the way of the transducer. The full bladder moves the uterus and unfolds it away from the vagina, and acts as a 'window' to better visualize the male and female pelvis. Ultrasound travels well and is less attenuated through a fluid, including urine.

Endovaginal scans require the patient to empty her bladder to allow the transducer to be closer to the pelvic organs. With the bladder empty the uterus can fall back into its normal position, in closer proximity to the vagina and therefore in closer proximity to the transducer.

For all ultrasound examinations it is important to properly inform the patient about what the examination entails and exactly what will be done. This is absolutely critical with endovaginal and endorectal scanning. Proper communication helps to keep the patient calm and allows the procedure to move along smoothly. With any type of invasive scanning the examination must be clearly explained to patients to allow them to choose to have it done or not and to make sure that they know exactly what will be done to them, how, and by whom.

Review Questions

1. In a diagnostic imaging department which study should be performed first, a barium enema or an ultrasound of the abdomen or pelvis? Why?

2. A sound wave is best described as a:

a. transverse wave
b. longitudinal wave
c. oblique wave
d. perpendicular wave

3. What is *not* true regarding ultrasound?

a. it cannot travel in a vacuum
b. it is a form of mechanical energy
c. it emanates from the piezoelectric crystal
d. it easily travels through air

4. Which of the following is true?

a. doppler assesses blood flow.
b. with color flow Doppler red flow indicates an artery
c. a great percentage of reflection at an interface will result in a black dot on the image
d. through transmission is caused by a strongly attenuating structure

CASE STUDY

A patient is admitted with abdominal pains. She is overweight and has recently eaten. How would you ensure maximum picture quality? What anatomic areas in the abdomen would best be seen by ultrasound?

References and Recommended Reading

Bushong, S., & Archer, B. (1991). *Diagnostic ultrasound physics, biology, and instrumentation.* St. Louis: Mosby-Year Book.

Goldberg, B., & Liu, J. B. (1993). *Textbook of abdominal ultrasound.* Baltimore: Williams & Wilkins.

Kremkau, F. W. (1993). *Diagnostic ultrasound principles and instruments* (4th ed.). Toronto: Saunders.

Rodrigues, G., & Daniel, G. (1991). *Medical diagnostic ultrasound.* Toronto: The Michener Institute for Applied Health Sciences.

Rumach, C. M., & Wilson, S. R., Charboneau, J. W. (1991). *Diagnostic Ultrasound.* Vol. I. Toronto: Mosby-Year Book.

Radionuclide Imaging

Marsha Sorter, MHE, RT(R)(M)(N)(ARRT)

Introduction and Historical Overview

In the early 1940s, reports of the use of **radioactive** iodine to treat thyroid diseases and radioactive phosphorus to treat leukemia and polycythemia vera were greeted with great enthusiasm. Many envisioned these achievements as forerunners of a whole series of similar radioactive "magic bullets" that would seek out and destroy diseased tissues within the human body. Indeed, radioiodine has helped many patients with overactive thyroid glands. Although similar types of **radionuclide** therapy have not developed as hoped, the medical imaging modality of nuclear medicine—defined as the application of radionuclides to help diagnose and treat a wide variety of diseases and disorders as a study of the functions of organ systems—has flourished. (In recent years the terms **isotope** and **radioisotope** have fallen into disfavor. These two terms had been used for many years to describe all forms of all elements. Because this is not entirely correct usage of the two terms, they have been replaced by the terms **nuclide** and **radionuclide**, respectively. The term nuclide was proposed as a more precise term than isotope because the meaning of nuclide is any nucleus plus its orbital electrons. The term isotope refers to two or more forms of the same element.)

As with x-rays, the great value of nuclear technology lies in its capability for nondestructive measurements, but there are important differences. Where radiographs provide information primarily about the body structures, radionuclide tracers make possible measurement of regional function. Although it is true that contrast angiography and other imaging techniques also provide functional information, the ability to use hundreds or even thousands of safe and potentially useful radioactive tracers makes it theoretically possible to study nearly every function of the body.

Nuclear medicine technology brings together structure and function, which in biologic systems can be thought of as two aspects of a unitary process. In biologic systems we deal with individual molecules, individual cells, and individual persons, with certain intrinsic qualities, including spatial location and changes in location and composition with time. We are taught to distinguish between structure and function, but in light of the concept of the dynamic state of body constituents, we realize that what we call functions are fast processes of short duration, and what we call structures are slow processes of long duration. For example, the beating of the heart is usually thought of as a function, while the skeleton is thought of as a structure, although it, too, changes constantly throughout life.

We have come a long way from the time when a small amount of cyclotron-produced radioactive iodine was administered and a Geiger-Mueller counter tube was held directly over the thyroid gland to measure its iodine uptake; yet the basic principles of nuclear medicine remain essentially the same.

Just two months after the discovery of x-rays by Roentgen in 1895, Henri Becquerel was credited with discovering radioactivity. Marie Curie, in her doctoral thesis, proving that these mysterious "rays" were different from those of Roentgen, almost immediately suggested the term "radioactivity." She actually identified three emissions from "pitchblende" (now known to be radium and its **daughters**). Marie Curie subsequently received the Nobel Prize for her work.

The first medical application of radium came only a few years later. It was thought that the penetrating gamma rays of radium, discovered by Villard in 1900, might, like x-rays, have a greater destructive effect on cancer than on normal tissues. It is not generally known that Alexander Graham Bell suggested in 1903 the possibility of placing sources containing radium in or near tumors, a technique that is used still in the treatment of some cancers.

The rapid advancements of nuclear medicine included many developments happening almost at the same time. The following highlights are some contributors to the science and imaging of nuclear medicine.

- Marshall Brucer, MD, was chairman of the medical division of the Oak Ridge Institute in Tennessee and was associated with the Manhattan Project. He developed many of the instruments of nuclear medicine and wrote the definitive chronicle of nuclear medicine. Brucer was instrumental in the development of radiopharmaceuticals and the transfer of radioactive materials for civilian use.
- John Lawrence is one of the early significant pioneers in nuclear medicine. In the 1930s Lawrence used radiophosphorus (^{32}P) to treat leukemia patients.
- Enrico Fermi, an Italian, successfully generated the first nuclear fission reaction and produced the first radioactive isotope of iodine.

- Sam Seidlin, from Montfiore Medical Center in New York, reported the complete disappearance of multiple functioning metastasis in a patient who had a tumor removed. This news spurred Congress to support further study of the use of radioisotopes for cancer treatments. Seidlin used radioiodine for the treatments.
- Benedict Cassen, PhD, in 1951, gave nuclear medicine a boost with his development of the first nuclear (**rectilinear**) scanner. The device moved back and forth across the organ generating a picture, by means of an activated moving pen, of the organ based on the amount of radioactivity in it.
- George Mueller further improved the scanner by replacing the pen with a metal stylus that contacted teledeltos paper grounded to a metal plate. More detailed images of the thyroid were possible with the improved scanner.
- David Kuhl, in 1956, with others from the University of Pennsylvania used a glow lamp aimed at x-ray film in a light-proof box to develop the first photoscanner. This group was also responsible for the early conceptual development of positron emission tomography (PET).
- Merrill Bender used a photoscanner to create the first photoscans of brain tumors. Later, in 1962, Bender developed a camera with a matrix of 293 sodium iodide crystals. This invention was called the autofluoroscope.
- Hal O. Anger, in 1958, developed the **scintillation** (sĭn´´tĭ-lā´shŭn) **camera**. This device allowed for the imaging of an entire organ at one time, creating the possibility of performing not only **static images** of organs but images of their dynamic functions as well. This discovery, timed with the discovery of technetium 99m (^{99m}Tc), allowed nuclear medicine to move into a position of prominence as a medical specialty in the early 1970s.
- R. Jaszcar, in 1979, introduced the single photon emission computed tomographic camera (SPECT). For the first time three-dimensional views could be acquired through the use of SPECT. This is perhaps one of the most significant developments in the history of nuclear medicine.

Nuclear medicine has made and continues to make vast leaps in instrumentation and application. The field of nuclear medicine has expanded with the advent of sophisticated measuring equipment and imaging devices that have been interfaced with computers. Clinical nuclear medicine studies have become a standard inclusion in the modern day medical diagnosis.

Principles

PHYSICS OF NUCLEAR MEDICINE

Physics is the study of both matter and energy and the properties, forces, and interactions that influence the behavior of matter. As applied to nuclear medicine, physics encompasses atomic structure, the properties of radiation, radioactive decay, and the interaction of radiation and matter. To understand nuclear medicine, it is essential to have a working knowledge of the constituent particles of the atom. A basic understanding of the principles that govern radioactivity, the use of radioactive materials, and radiation-detecting instrumentation is critical to the learning process.

Nuclear Reactions

A nuclear reaction involves changes in the structure of the nucleus of an atom. As a result of such changes, the **nucleus** gains or loses one or more **neutrons** or **protons**. Thus, it changes into the nucleus of a different nuclide or isotope. If the nucleus changes into the nucleus of a different **nuclide,** the change is called a transmutation.

Most of the naturally occurring radionuclides have long **half-lives** (500 years or more); because of this their use in nuclear medicine is not practical. Radionuclides used in nuclear medicine are man made. The three basic methods of radionuclide production are:

1. Irradiation of stable nuclides in a reactor (reactor produced)
2. Irradiation of stable nuclides in an accelerator or **cyclotron** (accelerator or cyclotron produced)
3. Fission of heavier nuclides (fission produced)

Radioactive Decay

Radioactive decay, or radioactivity, is the process by which a nucleus spontaneously (naturally) changes into the nucleus of another isotope or nuclide. The process releases energy chiefly in the form of particles and rays called nuclear radiation. Uranium, thorium, and several other natural elements decay spontaneously and so add to the natural, or background, radiation that is always present in the earth's atmosphere. **Nuclear reactors** produce radioactive decay artificially.

Nuclear radiation consists largely of alpha and beta particles and gamma rays. An **alpha particle,** which is made up of two protons and two neutrons, is identical with a helium nucleus. A **beta particle** consists of a negative electrical charge and so is identical with an electron. It results from the breakdown of a neutron in a radioactive nucleus. That breakdown also produces a proton, which remains in the nucleus. The beta particle is released as energy. Alpha and beta particles are sometimes known as alpha and beta rays. **Gamma rays** are electromagnetic waves similar to x-rays.

Radioactive decay is measured in units of time called half-lives. A half-life equals the time required for half the atoms of a particular radioactive nuclide or isotope to decay into another nuclide or isotope. Half-lives of radionuclides range from a fraction of a second to billions of years.

CHOICE OF RADIOPHARMACEUTICAL

Nuclear medicine embraces a wide range of both diagnostic and therapeutic procedures. All, except **in vitro** tests, require the administration of a radiopharmaceutical to the patient. The term radiopharmaceutical emphasizes the essential characteristics that it contains a radionuclide as an integral part and also that it is a medicinal product and therefore must be suitable for administration to humans. A wide selection of radiopharmaceuticals is available to meet the very different requirements of the various procedures. Radiopharmaceuticals differ both in their physical and chemical form as well as in the radionuclide involved.

In considering a radiopharmaceutical both its pharmacologic behavior and its nuclear properties must be understood. The radiopharmaceutical must distribute itself in such a manner that the aim of the test is fulfilled and an accurate understanding of its biologic behavior is essential. The properties required of the radionuclide will differ according to the procedure and correct selection of the radionuclide will, in the case of diagnostic procedures, minimize the radiation dose to the staff and patient and maximize the information gained.

Four basic factors are involved in choice of a radiopharmaceutical:

1. Biologic behavior—The radiopharmaceutical must achieve a satisfactory distribution in the body or trace a particular metabolic absorptive, excretory, or other pathway.
2. Radionuclide characteristics—The radionuclide must have suitable properties with regard to radiation emitted and half-life.
3. Availability—This will depend on the mode of production of the radionuclide. (^{99m}Tc is the most widely used radionuclide in nuclear medicine and is readily available.)
4. Pharmaceutical—Most agents are injected intravenously and must therefore be of high pharmaceutical quality.

A **generator** system for producing radionuclides is a system for the production of radionuclide pharmaceutical with short half-lives. The most widely used are ^{99m}Tc and iridium 113m (^{113m}In). The desired nuclide is continuously produced by the **decay** of its long-lived parent. When a dose is needed, it is separated from the parent by chromatography, solvent extraction, or other means, and is then used before most of it can decay. A generator system must meet six criteria to be useful in nuclear medicine:

1. Be sterile and pyrogen-free
2. Be capable of multiple separations
3. Have a daughter's half-life of less than 24 hours
4. Be safe and simple to operate
5. Be able to yield a daughter with high radiochemical and radionuclide purity
6. Be convenient for the preparation of radiopharmaceuticals

Nuclear medicine procedures requiring radiopharmaceuticals are illustrated in Table 2.1.

TABLE 2.1 NUCLEAR MEDICINE PROCEDURES REQUIRING RADIOPHARMACEUTICALS

Purpose	Organ/System	Radiopharmaceutical
Imaging Organ flow Organ localization Abnormal uptake Function	Bone	^{99m}Tc-labeled pyrophosphate, methylene diphonate (MDP), ethylene hydroxydiphosphonate (EHDP), and hydroxymethylene diphosphonate (HMDP)

continued

TABLE 2.1 CONTINUED

Purpose	Organ/System	Radiopharmaceutical
Imaging	Brain	*do not penetrate intact blood–brain barrier*
Organ flow		^{99m}Tc pertechnetate
Organ localization		^{99m}Tc diethylenetriamine-pertechnetate acid (DTPA)
Abnormal uptake		^{99m}Tc glucoheptonate (GHA)
Function studies		^{67}Ga citrate
		^{201}Tl chloride
		^{99m}Tc phosphonates (MDP, HDP)
		^{99m}Tc red cells (in vivo)
		penetrate intact blood–brain barrier
		^{133}Xe (xenon gas)
		^{123}I iodoamphetamine (IMP) or
		^{131} IHIPDM
		^{99m}Tc d, 1-hexamethylpropylene amine oxime (HMPAO)
Imaging	Cisternography (cerebrospinal fluid compartment)	^{169}Yb DTPA
Organ flow		^{111}In DTPA
Organ localization		
Function studies		
Imaging	Heart	^{201}Tl chloride
Organ flow		^{99m}Tc-labeled pyrophosphate
Organ localization		^{111}In antimyosin
Function studies		^{99m}Tc isonitriles
		^{99m}Tc dioximines BATO
		^{99m}Tc diphosphines
Imaging	Kidney	^{99m}Tc-Sn DTPA (aerosol)
Organ flow		^{99m}Tc macroaggregated albumin
Organ localization		^{133}Xe gas
Abnormal uptake		^{127}Xe gas
Function studies		^{81}Kr gas
		^{99m}Tc microspheres and human albumin microspheres
Imaging	Liver/gallbladder	^{99m}Tc sulfur colloid
Organ flow	Spleen, gastrointestinal	^{99m}Tc albumin colloid
Organ function	Blood volume	^{99m}Tc-labeled red blood cells
Abnormal uptake	Plasma volume	^{99m}Tc iminodiacetic (IDA derivatives: HIDA, DISIDA, mebrofenin)
Function studies	Malabsorption	^{123}I human serum albumin
Dilution and excretion	GI blood loss	^{51}Cr-labeled red blood cells
	Iron metabolism	^{58}Fe citrate
	Red metabolism	^{59}Fe chloride
	Red cell survival	^{57}Co and ^{58}Co
Imaging	Lung	^{99m}Tc-Sn DTPA (aerosol)
Organ flow		^{99m}Tc macroaggregated albumin
Organ localization		^{133}Xe gas
Abnormal uptake		^{127}Xe gas
Function studies		^{81}Kr gas
		^{99m}Tc microspheres and human albumin microspheres

continued

TABLE 2.1 CONTINUED

Purpose	Organ/System	Radiopharmaceutical
Imaging Abnormal uptake	Lymphatic	^{99m}Tc antimony sulfide
Imaging Abnormal uptake Function studies	Bone marrow	^{99m}Tc sulfur colloid
Imaging Organ localization Abnormal uptake Function studies	Pancreas	^{75}Se selenomethionine ^{67}Ga citrate
Imaging Organ flow Organ localization Abnormal uptake Function studies	Parathyroid	^{75}Se selenomethionine ^{99m}Tc sestamibi ^{201}Tl
Imaging Organ flow Organ localization Abnormal uptake Function studies	Thyroid	^{99m}Tc sodium pertechnetate ^{131}I sodium iodine ^{127}I sodium iodine

Image Production

Because humans cannot detect the presence of radiation, it makes sense to have a device that can detect the presence of radiation. This section reviews the various instruments used in nuclear medicine, their use, and some of the differences in the types of detectors.

GAS DETECTORS

The basic function of a **gas detector** depends on the collection of **electrons** produced in a gas volume by the passage of radiation through the detector. As the electrons are produced by the radiation passing through the gas, they migrate to the positive wall (anode) of the detector, when an exterior voltage is applied. The general concept of the gas detector is that the electrons are collected by the anode, flow through a very sensitive current meter, and collect at the negative electrode. The measurement of this current flow is a function of the amount of ionization that has occurred inside the enclosed gas volume, which is in turn a measure of the amount of radiation to which the meter has been exposed.

SCINTILLATION DETECTORS

Certain materials have the property of emitting a flash of light (**scintillation**) when struck by ionizing radiation. A scintillation detector is a sensitive device used to detect ionizing radiation by observing the scintillations induced in the material. This is accomplished by fixing a light-sensitive device to a special photosensitive material that changes the flash of light into small electrical impulses. The electrical impulses are then amplified so they may be sorted and counted to determine the amount and nature of radiation striking the scintillating materials. Scintillators are used for diagnostic purposes to determine the amount and distribution of radionuclides in one or more organs of a patient.

The procedure for recording a scintillation involves several systems: the detector, a photomultiplier, a high-voltage power supply, the pulse height analyzer, and display modes.

GAMMA CAMERA

The rectilinear scanners of yesterday have expanded into complex imaging systems called gamma cameras. The gamma camera is still a scintillation detector but it uses extremely large sodium iodide crystals to detect radioactive emissions and transform those emissions into light energy or photons. The light energy is amplified and electronically located to record and produce an image (Figure 2.78).

Basic Structure

Collimator The **collimator** is located at the face of the detector where the photons first enter the camera. The collimator is used to limit the field of view, to increase resolution of the image, and to vary the sensitivity by reducing the amount and the course of photons coming into the detector. The collimators can be interchanged. They are made of material with a high atomic number, such as lead. Different collimators are used for various types of examinations to provide the best combination of sensitivity and resolution.

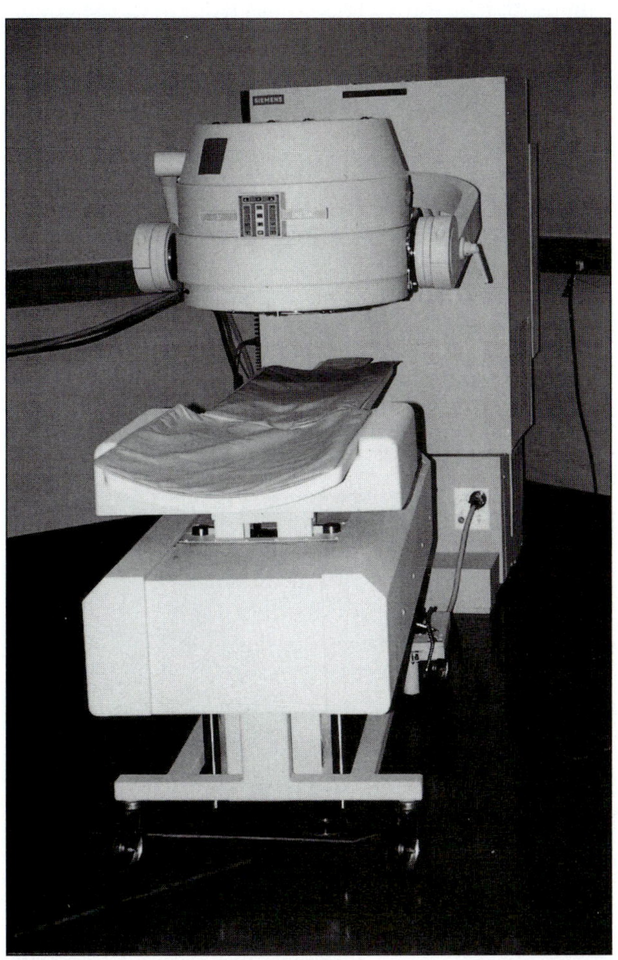

FIGURE 2.78 Typical gamma camera.

Crystal Sodium iodide crystals with a trace of thallium added are the scintillation crystals most widely used in gamma cameras. This crystal combination is effective in stopping most common gamma rays emitted from the radionuclides and radiopharmaceuticals used in nuclear medicine. Crystals may vary in thickness from one-fourth to one-half inch. The thicker the crystal the better it is for imaging radionuclides of energies over 180 KeV. The thicker crystal will also decrease resolution. The **photomultiplier tubes (PMTs)** or the light pipe may be attached to the crystal. The PMTs help direct the photons.

Detector Electronics

The PMTs are attached to the crystal inside the detector. These instruments convert and detect light photons emitted from the crystal. When the light from the crystal has been detected, it is then converted into an electronic signal and amplified by a factor of as much as 10^7. Usually a gamma camera detector head will contain 80 to 100 PMTs.

The detected signal is sent through a series of electronic processing steps. Some of the steps include determining location (x, y) and amplitude or energy (z). The values of x and y are determined by the location of the photon hitting the crystal. A pulse height analysis is used to discriminate those z signals that are not within a desired preset energy range for a particular radionuclide. The **pulse height analysis** eliminates scatter and other unwanted photons that would have a detrimental effect on resolution of the image.

After the information is processed, the signals are transmitted to the display system, which will include a film imaging system or a computer to record the image and display it on a **cathode ray tube (CRT)**.

Multihead Gamma Camera Systems

The most common gamma camera systems have a single detector that can be moved in various positions around the patient. There are systems that have dual heads to allow simultaneous imaging of anterior and posterior views. There are systems that have as many as three detectors (heads). These systems allow simultaneous imaging in three views (Figures 2.79 and 2.80).

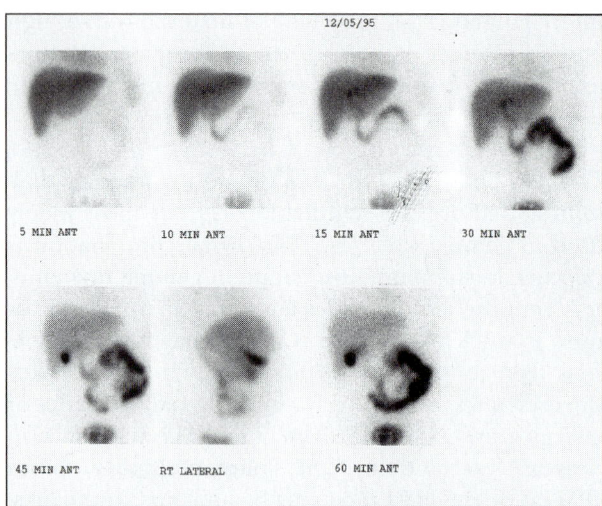

FIGURE 2.79 Series demonstrating function of the liver.

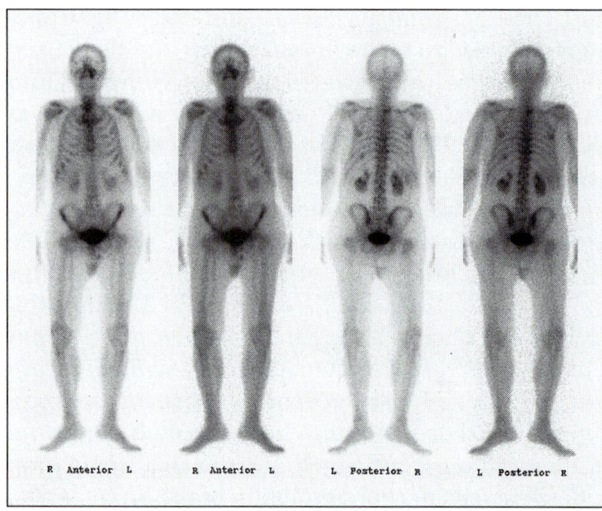

FIGURE 2.80 Complete bone scan.

SPECT

Single photon emission computed tomography (SPECT) can use from one to three gamma camera detectors to produce tomographic or sectional images of a structure. The detectors in SPECT rotate 360° around the patient's body while collecting data. The data collected are reconstructed in a computer in various formats including transaxial, sagittal, coronal, planar, or three-dimensional representation. Like CT and MRI these computer-generated images allow for the display of thin slices through various planes of an organ or structure in the body. Thus, the display will help in identifying small abnormalities in the various planes (Figure 2.81).

An excellent example of a SPECT study is the myocardial perfusion study used to detect perfusion defects in the left ventricular wall. While exercising, the patient is injected intravenously with ^{201}Tl, which is distrubuted in the heart muscle in the same manner as blood flow to the heart muscle. A set of images is taken after the initial injection of the ^{201}Tl. After several hours a second set of images is taken while the patient is at rest. The delayed images determine if any blood perfusion defects seen on the first images have resolved. The physician can determine if the patient has damaged heart tissue by comparing these images. Defects or damage are usually caused by a myocardial infarction or myocardial ischemia (Figure 2.82).

POSITRON EMISSION TOMOGRAPHY (PET)

An exciting tomographic technique in nuclear scanning is PET imaging. This comes from both the chemistry and physics inherent in **positron** tomography. The radionuclides used in PET imaging are carbon 11, nitrogen 13, oxygen 15, and fluorine 18; these isotopes of elements occur naturally in organic molecules.

Useful PET radiopharmaceuticals are now available to measure in vivo such important physiologic and biochemical processes as blood flow, oxygen, glucose and free fatty acid metabolism, amino acid transport, pH, and neuroreceptor densities. The physics of PET permits greater quantitative accuracy and preci-

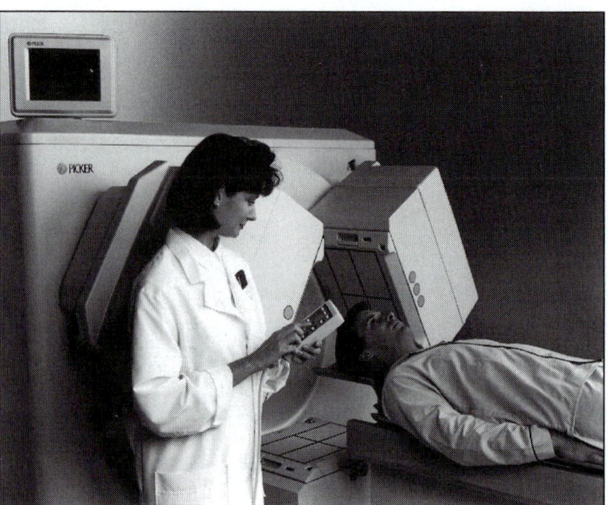

FIGURE 2.81 SPECT camera (Courtesy of Picker International Inc., Cleveland, OH).

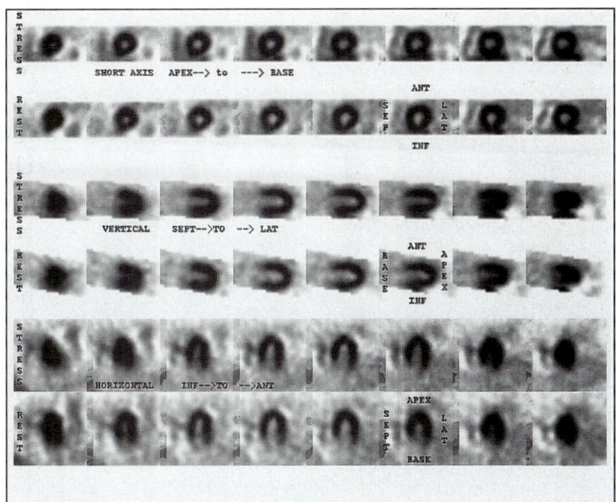

FIGURE 2.82 SPECT myocardial perfusion study.

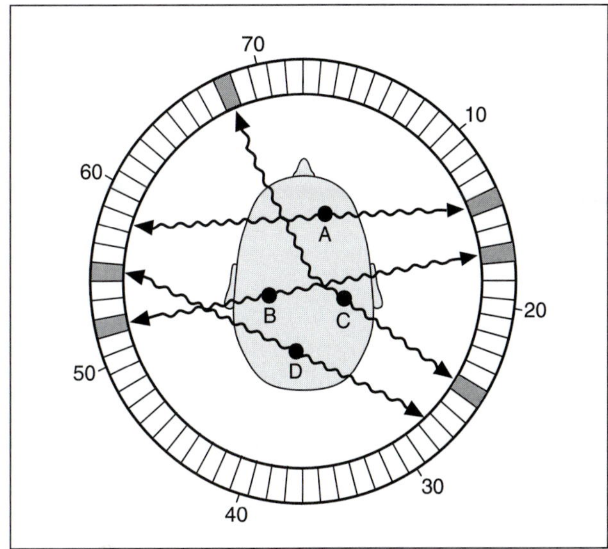

FIGURE 2.83 Geometry of PET detection system. Event *B* represents true coincidence detection, simultaneous detection of one gamma ray each from events *A* and *D* produces accidental coincidence detection, and event *C* represents scatter coincidence detection.

sion. The use of small, high-density crystal improves spatial resolution.

Recall that a positron is an antimatter electron, and consider a positron-emitting radiopharmaceutical distributed in a patient. As the positron is emitted, it travels several millimeters in tissue, depositing its kinetic energy. It then will meet a free electron in the tissue, and mutual annihilation occurs. Thinking back to conservation of energy, two 511 keV annihilation photons appear (511 keV is the energy equivalent to the rest mass of an electron or positron); from conservation of momentum, they are emitted 180° back to back. Therefore, it would make sense to use an Anger camera to individually detect these 511-keV gamma rays. However, it makes more sense to surround the patient with a ring of detectors and electronically couple opposing detectors to simultaneously identify the pair of gamma rays (Figure 2.83).

PET imaging differs from SPECT in that the "electronic collimation" of coincidence counting reduces the need for actual lead collimation, thus increasing sensitivity. Coincidence detection allows mathematically accurate attenuation correction.

PET scanners cost over $2 million. They require more space, more electricity, and more air conditioning than Anger cameras. Cyclotrons cost a minimum of $1 million as well, and are expensive to install and operate. Because of the short half-lives of the radionuclides used in PET imaging, the cyclotron is generally on site.

Human disease is biochemical in nature; therefore, the most effective treatment is a biochemical solution. It would then make sense that the most important method of diagnosis addresses the biochemical nature of the disease. For these reasons, laying the cost aside for the moment, the future of PET seems secure.

COMPUTERS IN NUCLEAR MEDICINE

One of the most vital parts of the nuclear medicine imaging system is the computer. The computer systems are used to acquire and process data from gamma cameras. They allow for the collection of data over a specific time frame; the data can then be analyzed to determine functional change over time. One such study that is an example of computer use is the renal function study. The radiopharmaceutical is administered and is cleared by normally functioning kidneys in usually 20 minutes. The computer has the capability to collect imaging data over a 40-minute period, then analyze the imaging data to determine how quickly the kidneys clear the radiopharmaceutical. The computer will allow manipulation of the image data to enhance a particular structure by adjusting the brightness and contrast of the imaging data collected. It is impossible to perform SPECT imaging without the computer. These studies are complex and require a great deal of computer processing to create images in the sagittal, coronal, and transaxial planes. Three-dimensional images can also be generated from computer acquisition of SPECT imaging data.

Applications

Although a variety of nuclear medicine studies are done in a nuclear medicine facility, radionuclide imaging of the cardiovascular system and radionuclide imaging of the skeletal system are the studies done most often.

Approximately 69 million Americans have one or more forms of acquired heart or blood vessel disease. Hypertension occurs in 63 million adults; coronary artery disease occurs in 6.1 million (3 million have angina); rheumatic heart disease occurs in 1.3 million; and stroke occurs in 2.9 million. Myocardial infarction causes over half a million deaths in the United States each year.

Cardiovascular studies would include SPECT imaging evaluation of ventricular function of the heart, gated blood pool studies of the heart, myocardial perfusion imaging of the heart with planar imaging and SPECT imaging, myocardial infarct imaging of the heart, and PET imaging of the heart.

The skeleton performs several functions for the body, including support, protection, movement, and blood formation. Bone, like other connective tissues, consists of living cells and a predominant amount of nonliving intercellular substance that is calcified. It is a metabolically active tissue with large amounts of nutrients being exchanged in the blood supplying the bone. Thus the skeleton and body fluids are in equilibrium. Tracer techniques have been used for many years to study the exchange between bone and blood. Radionuclides have played an important role in understanding normal bone metabolism, in addition to the metabolic effects of pathologic involvement of bone.

Radionuclide imaging of the skeleton includes whole body imaging of the skeleton, SPECT imaging of specific areas that are suspicious of disease, white blood cell imaging in bone and joint diseases, and flow imaging in bone and joint diseases (Figures 2.84 and 2.85).

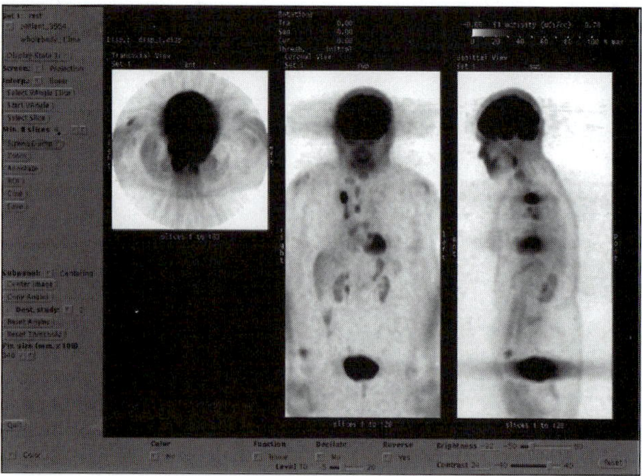

FIGURE 2.84 PET body scan demonstrates tumor in the right lung.

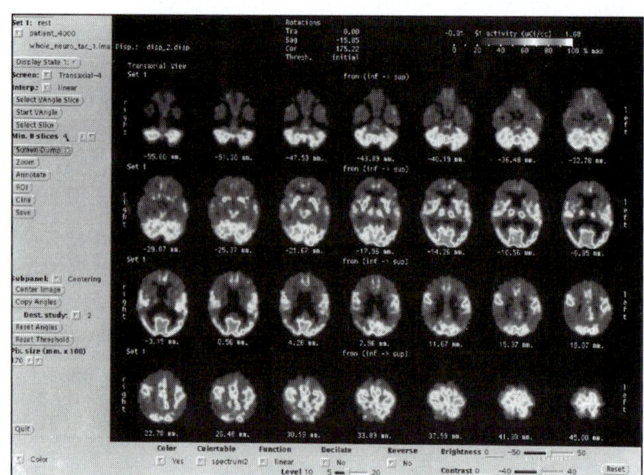

FIGURE 2.85 PET scan demonstrates Alzheimer's disease.

Review Questions

1. Which of the following scientists discovered radioactivity?
   a. Marie Curie
   b. John Dalton
   c. Amedeo Avogadro
   d. Henry Becquerel

2. Which of the following is *not* true of nuclear medicine studies?
   a. nuclear medicine studies provide high resolution images
   b. quantitative results provide physicians with detailed information regarding organ function
   c. nuclear medicine is used to identify a wide range of abnormalities
   d. nuclear medicine looks at anatomy based on physiology

3. Which of the following type of detector is used as the basis for obtaining images in nuclear medicine studies?
   a. geiger counter
   b. scintillation detector
   c. dose calibrator
   d. dosimeter

4. What are the basic components of the modern gamma camera?

5. How does SPECT imaging differ from static nuclear medicine?

6. Name five differences among PET imaging, static nuclear medicine imaging, and SPECT imaging.

CASE STUDY

A patient has a nonspecific heart condition. Describe the various radionuclide examinations that could be performed in the nuclear medicine departments.

References and Recommended Reading

Ballinger, P.W. (1995). *Radiographic positions and radiologic procedures* (8th ed.). St. Louis: Mosby-Year Book.

Bernier, D. R., Langan, J. K., & Christian, P. E. (1994). *Nuclear medicine technology and techniques* (3rd ed.). St. Louis: Mosby-Year Book.

Early, P. J., & Sodee, B. D. (1995). *Principles and practice of nuclear medicine* (2nd ed.). St. Louis: Mosby-Year Book.

Heart-facts—1995. (1995). Dallas: American Heart Association.

Hendee, W. R. (1979). *Medical radiation physics* (2nd ed.). St. Louis: Mosby-Year Book.

Krisnamurthy, G. T., Tubis, M., Hiss, J., et al. (1977). Distribution patterns of metastatic bone disease—a need for total skeletal image. *Journal of the American Medical Association, 237,* 2054.

SECTION II

SKELETAL SYSTEM

CHAPTER 3

Specialized Studies of the Skeletal System

CYNTHIA COWLING, BSc, MEd, MRT(R), ACR

OBJECTIVES

At the completion of this chapter, the student should be able to:

1. Describe the procedures used in the diagnostic studies of the skeletal system as listed.
2. Describe the bony anatomy of all relevant areas of study.
3. List the major indications and reasons for performing the studies listed.
4. Compare the resultant images provided in the various imaging modalities used in each study.
5. Identify radiographs indicated for each procedure.
6. Discuss safe practice procedures for each examination.
7. Identify common radiographic appearances of resultant images for each procedure.
8. List usual contrast media used, if any, for each procedure.
9. Identify appropriate patient care practices for each examination.

Introduction and Historical Overview

Radiography of the bony skeleton has been the mainstay of the radiology department since Roentgen first discovered x-rays. Until recently it was felt that x-radiation was the best and most accurate method of evaluating bones and their associated structures, such as joints. It still produces the gold standard of images when examining the fine structure of bone, but the newer modalities, particularly those that can be used without the risk of ionizing radiation, such as ultrasound and MRI, are rapidly expanding in the area of musculoskeletal imaging. Joints are still imaged radiographically, but the radiographer should be aware that the skeleton is no longer the unique domain of radiology.

Arthrography (ăr-thrŏg´ră-fē), the radiologic study of articulations, was first described in 1905 by Werndorff and Robinsohn who used air as the contrast medium, but the combination of a painful procedure and a possibility of an air embolus drastically reduced the frequency of this examination. The development of positive diodized contrast agents in the 1930s improved the quality of the image, but also caused irritation of the joint tissues. The first **double-contrast** arthrogram was performed by Bircher in 1933 but did not come into common use until the 1960s. In the 1990s, MRI is becoming the imaging modality of choice for soft tissue injury of the joints.

Anatomy

Special procedures of the skeletal area focus on the articulations, the vertebral column, and the early development of bone formation.

BONE FORMATION AND COMPOSITION

During the eighth week of embryonic development bone begins its formation in hyaline cartilage, a process known as endochondral ossification (ŏs´´ĭ-fĭ-kā´shun). (Certain bones develop within fibrous membrane.) In this ossification process, the future bone is represented by a cartilaginous model, surrounded by a membranous perichondrium. Blood vessels from the periosteum permeate the cartilage, carrying **osteoblasts,** which deposit a collar of bone around the middle of the long axis of the cartilaginous model, which then becomes the primary center of ossification (Figures 3.1 and 3.2).

Secondary centers of ossification appear at the proximal and distal ends of the bone and represent the secondary centers of ossification or the epiphyses (ĕ-pĭf´ĭ-sĭs). A plate of cartilage between the diaphysis (dī-ăf´ĭ-sĭs)and epiphysis remains for some time and represents the site of bone growth in length known as endochondral growth. The ossification produces living bone, which is comprised of approximately two-thirds inorganic salts and one-third organic material. The inorganic component is calcium phosphate and carbonate; the organic portion is composed of collagen fibers, cells, and a protein matrix, a mucopolysaccharide. The inorganic portion of the bone forms the hard bone matrix, which forms the framework and stores 90% of the body's calcium. It is this

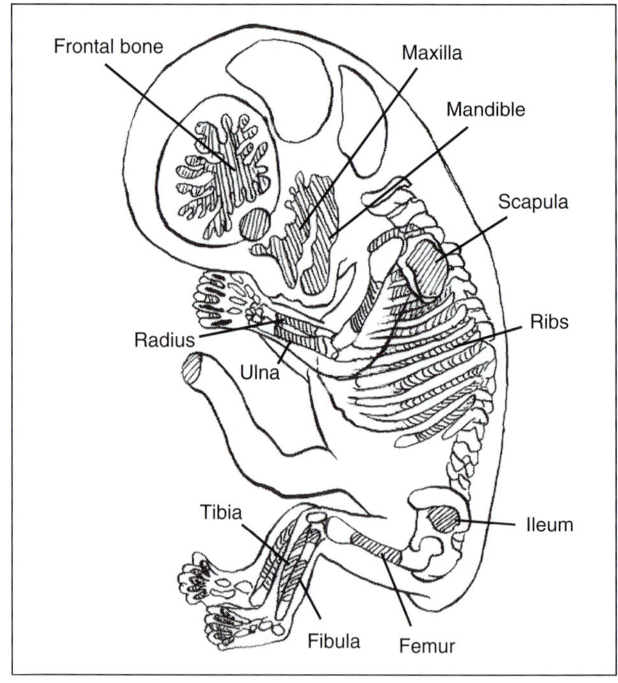

FIGURE 3.1 Embryonic bony development.

calcium that is visualized on a radiograph, allowing the interpreter to determine the age of the bone of an individual (Figures 3.3 and 3.4).

ARTICULATIONS

Most of the joints in the body are of the diarthrotic type, commonly referred to as synovial (sĭn-ō´vē-ăl)

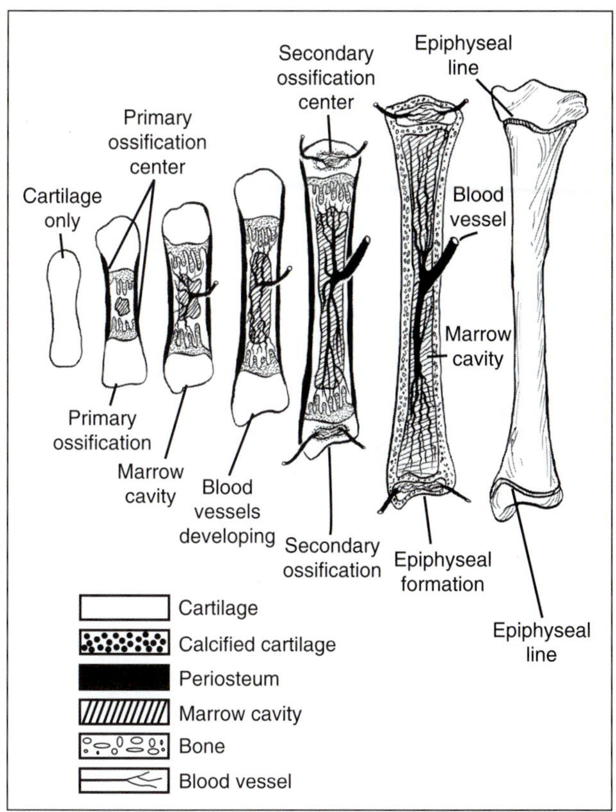

FIGURE 3.2 Development of a long bone.

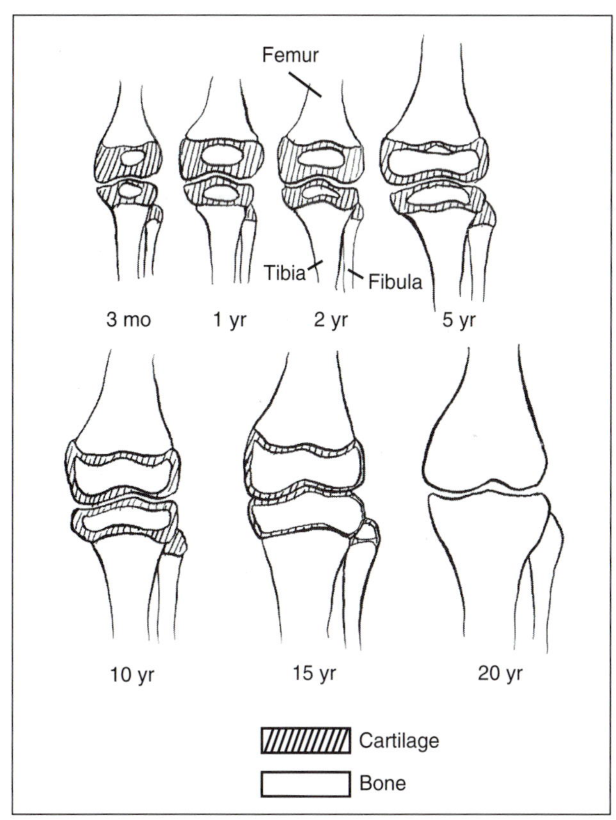

FIGURE 3.4 Ossification of the knee.

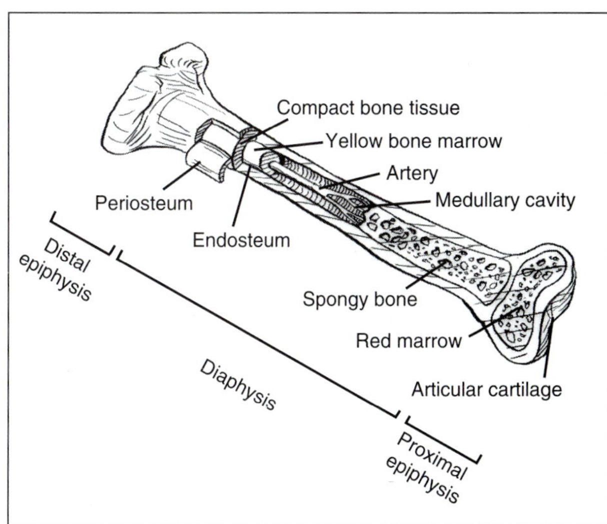

FIGURE 3.3 Structure of a long bone.

joints. All these joints feature a number of similar ingredients, with various modifications, but the major common feature is the presence of a synovial cavity between the articulating bones.

The basic structure of all synovial joints include:

- Articular cartilage, hyaline in nature, that covers the ossifying bones
- A joint capsule, strong and fibrous surrounding the joint. The fibers and capsules are continuous with the periosteum.
- A synovial membrane lines the joint capsule but does not cover the articular cartilage on the bone ends. This membrane produces the synovial fluid that acts as a lubricant for the joint.
- The joint is reinforced by ligaments that can lie within the joint itself or outside the articulations, along with muscles.
- In certain joints, notably the knee, disks of fibrocartilage are wedged into the joint cavity, separating the two bones (Figure 3.5).

THE VERTEBRAL COLUMN

The vertebral column is composed of a series of 26 discrete bones called vertebrae. Each vertebral body is composed primarily of cancellous bone covered by a thin layer of compact bone.

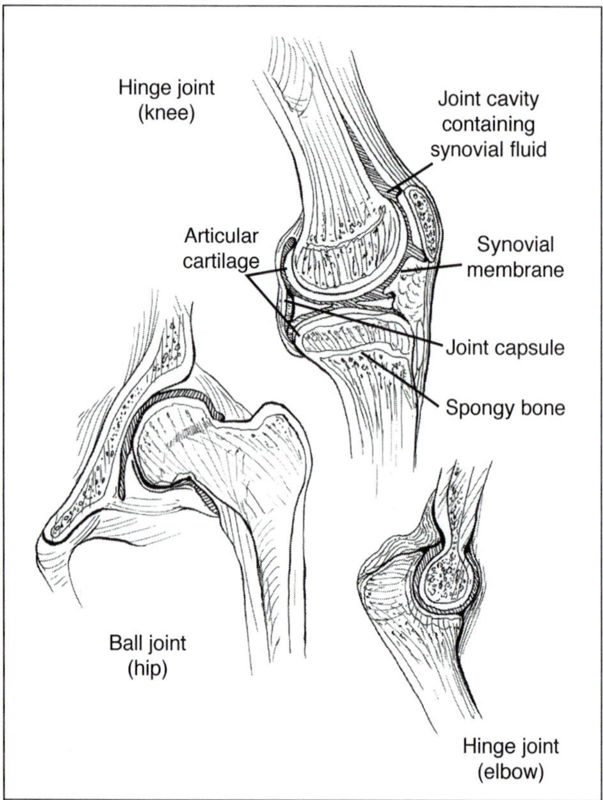

FIGURE 3.5 Diarthrotic joints.

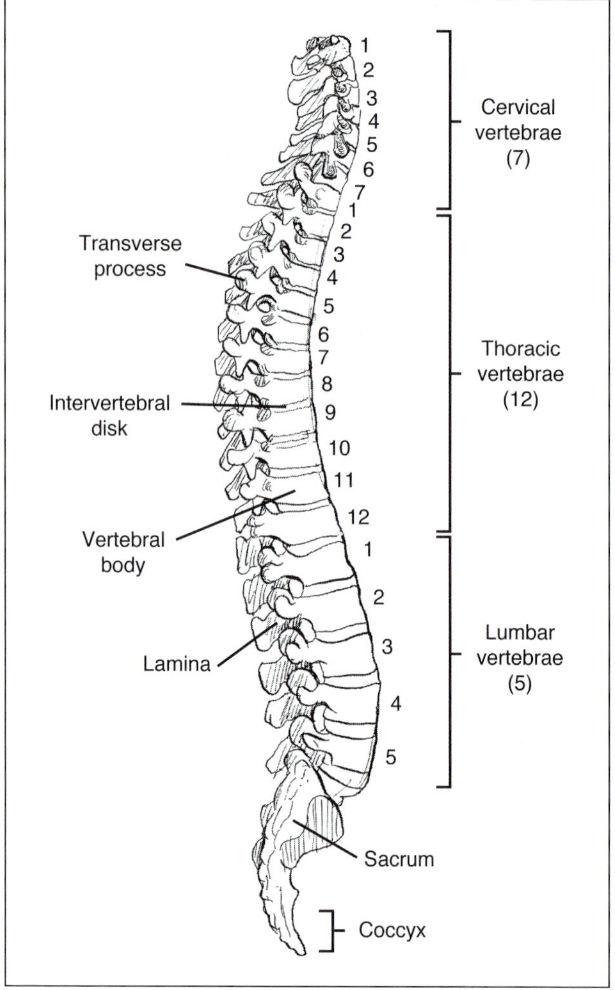

FIGURE 3.6 The vertebrae.

The vertebrae are connected by a number of ligaments including the longitudinal ligaments passing along the anterior and posterior aspects of the vertebral bodies. Between adjacent vertebrae is an intervertebral disk composed primarily of fibrocartilage in the center of which is a mucoid nucleus pulposus.

The five distinct regions of the column are cervical (7), thoracic (12), lumbar (5), sacrum (1), and coccyx (1) (Figure 3.6). The natural curves of the vertebral column are classified as primary and secondary curves. The primary curves are the sacral and thoracic curves, present at birth and kyphotic (kī-fŏt´ĭk) in nature (curving away from the body). The secondary curves are the cervical and lumbar curves, lordotic (lor-dŏt´ĭk) in form (curving in toward the body). These secondary curves develop as the child lifts the head at 3 months for the cervical configuration; the lumbar curve develops at about 6 months of age when the child moves more actively.

The long axis of the vertebral column is neither left nor right as dictated by the **notochord** in early embryonic development. However, there is a primary forward curvature of the complete vertebral column, which often increases with age.

Procedures

ARTHROGRAPHY

Arthrography is the radiologic examination of the synovial joint space, using an injection of contrast medium, which can be positive (chemical compound) or negative (air). The areas most commonly studied using this technique are the knee and hip, although occasionally the shoulder, temporomandibular joints, wrist, and elbow are examined in this way. Before any arthrogram, plain radiographs of the affected joint must be taken. The examination is a simple one, usually performed in the radiology department. Localized asepsis is required and frequently an aspirate is taken of the synovial fluid and sent to the pathology department for the following analyses to assess any microscopic pathology of the knee:

- Microscopy
- Cytology
- Crystal analysis
- Biochemistry

The correct positioning of the needle is important to ensure a smooth flow of the contrast material used.

A complementary, nonimaging study sometimes performed is the **arthroscopy** (ăr-thrŏs´kō-pē). This is the study of the joint space via an arthroscope. Occasionally, minor surgery such as partial **meniscectomies** (mĕn´´ĭ-sĕk´tō-mēs) are performed through an operating arthroscope. Arthroscopy is performed when a negative arthrogram is performed on a patient with persistent symptoms, and conversely, arthrography is performed to visualize areas not well demonstrated with an arthroscope, such as the popliteal space, the posterior medial meniscus, and the tibial surface of the menisci. Arthroscopy is also considered more invasive than an arthrogram.

ARTHROGRAPHY OF THE KNEE

Arthrography of the knee is often performed using the double-contrast technique.

Applied Anatomy Knee arthrography is most commonly used to assess the condition of the soft tissue regions of the knee joint. Figures 3.7 and 3.8 identify areas of major interest. The knee is the largest joint in the body and is a hinge or diarthrotic type, providing flexion and extension of the leg with slight rotation around the tibia.

Indications

- Cartilage, capsular injuries
- Ligament injuries, menisci injuries
- Loose bodies that are formed by the ossification of cartilage debris (often as a result of an old injury) or crumbling articular surfaces or detachment of **osteophytes.**
- Joint rupture
- Baker's cyst, which is a communication between the posterior aspect of the knee joint and the gastrocnemius bursa. If it is palpable this popliteal cyst is called a Baker's cyst.
- Synovial disease, **synovitis**

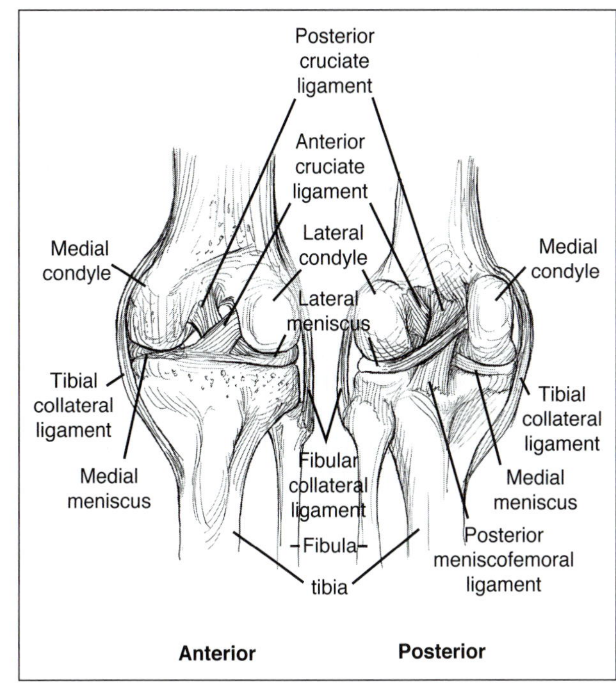

FIGURE 3.7 Anterior view of the right knee.

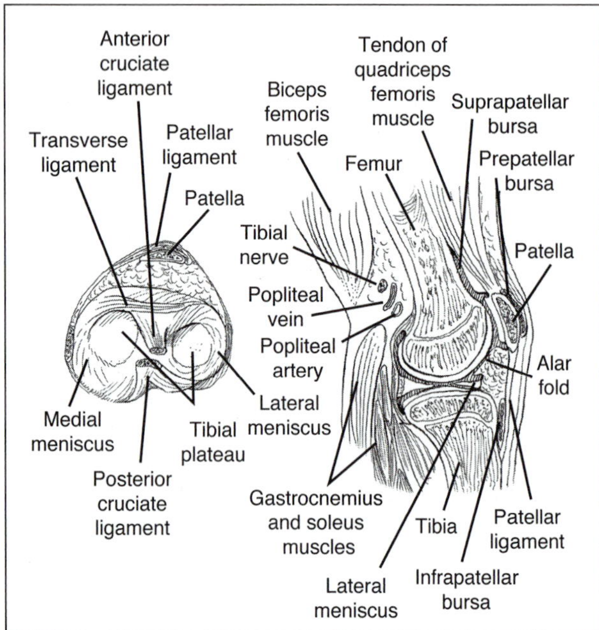

FIGURE 3.8 Lateral and superior views of the knee.

Contraindications

- Skin infections. A skin puncture could lead to infection being tracked into the joint space.
- Bleeding tendency or anticoagulant therapy. Prolonged bleeding into the joint space can cause serious joint problems.
- Allergy to contrast (although reactions are rare due to slow absorption of small doses)

Equipment This procedure is usually performed in a general duty fluoroscopy room. It is a sterile procedure requiring aseptic technique localized to the area of injection only. The fluoroscopy unit should have a small focal spot (0.3 mm). It should also have a spot film device or other method of acquiring the image (such as high-resolution video).

Other equipment:

- Translucent sponges to support the limb
- Sterile tray contents:
  —1 medicine cup
  —1 set forceps
  —Needles (18 or 21 and 25 gauge)
  —Syringes, 5 mL and 20 mL
  —Sterile towels and drapes
  —Gauze pads
- Sterile disposable gloves
- Local anesthetic
- Antiseptic solution
- Curved cassette

Contrast Media

- Water-soluble, nonionic contrast agent (positive). It is absorbed or excreted from the system in a few hours.
- Air (negative). There is no allergy risk, but there is poorer visualization than the positive contrast media. There is a slight risk of an air embolus, and it can take up to 4 days to be completely absorbed by the tissues.
- Occasionally a small quantity of epinephrine 1/1000 (0.3 mL) can be added to decrease resorption of contrast, decrease effusion, and provide a longer coating time to surface.

Radiation Protection

- Shielding of gonads
- Minimum number of radiographs taken

Preliminary Radiographs

- A projection of the knee joint with the leg extended and supported to place the tibial plateau perpendicular to the film
- Lateral view of the knee, flexed at right angles, and with the tibial plateau perpendicular to the film
- Intercondylar view, so that the knee is flexed over a curved cassette, with the knee at approximately 135°. The central ray must be perpendicular to the tibia (Figure 3.9).

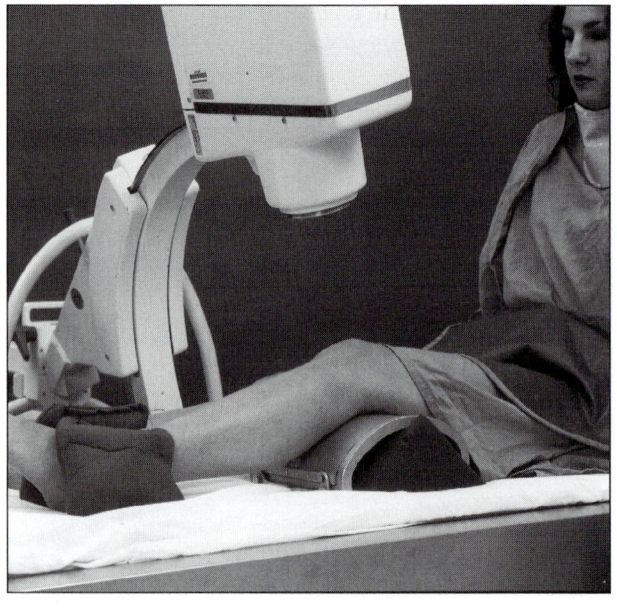

FIGURE 3.9 Intercondylar view.

Patient Preparation

- The patient is usually an outpatient and no sedation is required.
- The knee may need to be shaved if body hair is present in the area of the injection.
- The patient needs reassurance. The injection of air produces an odd sensation in the joint space and if the patient is made aware of this sensation he or she does not react to it adversely.

Procedure Sequence

- The patient is supine with the leg extended and relaxed.
- Using sterile technique, the skin and underlying soft tissues are anesthetized at a point 1 to 2 cm posterior to the midpoint of the medial border of the patella, using the 25-gauge needle.
- An 18- or 21-gauge needle is inserted posterior to the patella and angled approximately 30° anteriorly to facilitate entry into the joint space.
- Any effusion is aspirated for diagnostic examination.
- Positive contrast medium is injected into the knee joint. If the contrast moves away rapidly from the needle, that is a good indication that the contrast is flowing correctly into the joint space. Room air is then injected until a fullness is felt by the patient. This can cause a mild discomfort. Epinephrine (adrenaline) may be injected with the contrast media to reduce the speed of absorption of contrast by the synovial membrane.
- The needle is removed and the patient asked to gently exercise the knee. It is not necessary for the knee to become weight-bearing.
- The patient is placed prone with support under the thigh (Figure 3.10).

Procedure Radiographs Using a spot film device, a number of radiographs are taken of the meniscus. The leg is gradually rotated from prone through to supine to demonstrate all aspects of the medial meniscus.

- A projection with patient prone demonstrates posterior portion of medial meniscus
- 30° lateral anterior oblique
- 45° oblique view demonstrates middle portion of medial meniscus
- 60° lateral posterior oblique
- 90° lateral view demonstrates anterior portion of medial meniscus

These views are then reversed, beginning with the patient supine to demonstrate the lateral meniscus.

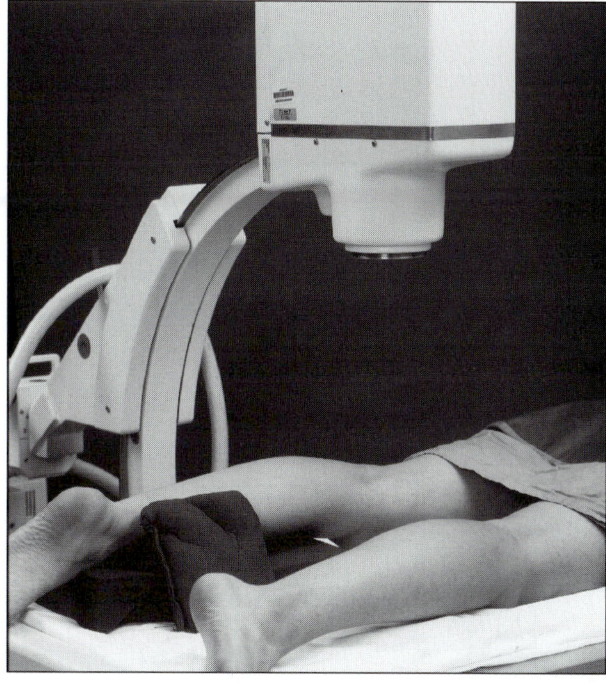

FIGURE 3.10 Postinjection positioning.

Stress is applied appropriately to open up the joint space, during the exposure.

- **Valgus** (văl´gŭs)—direction for the medial meniscus (Figures 3.11 and 3.12)
- **Varus** (vā´rŭs)—direction for the lateral meniscus (Figures 3.13 and 3.14)

Conventional radiographs are sometimes taken as indicated by the preliminary radiographs (Figures 3.15 and 3.16).

Alternative Radiographs

- Delay radiographs at 30 minutes to determine whether there is leakage of contrast into any other areas, indicating a tear.
- Lateral view tomography
- Medial and lateral stress views for detection of collateral ligament damage

Postprocedure Care A contrast synovitis can occur, with pain commencing about 4 to 6 hours after injection and subsiding after 12 hours. (Joint infection would have a later onset.) It is therefore common for the patient to experience discomfort for 1 to 2 days. The patient should be instructed to attempt to rest the limb and reduce movement for 1 to 2 days.

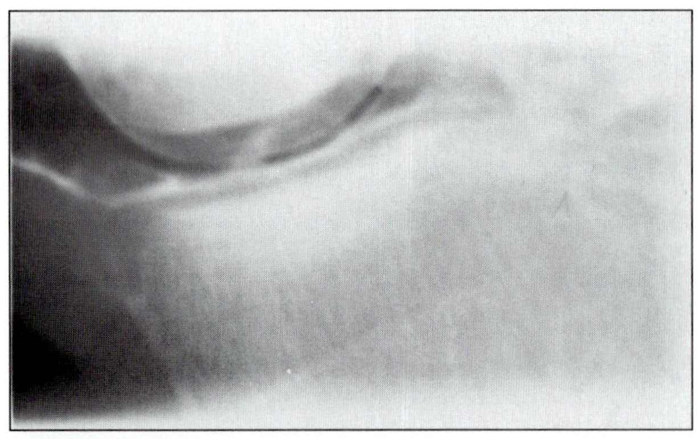

FIGURE 3.11 Medial meniscus.

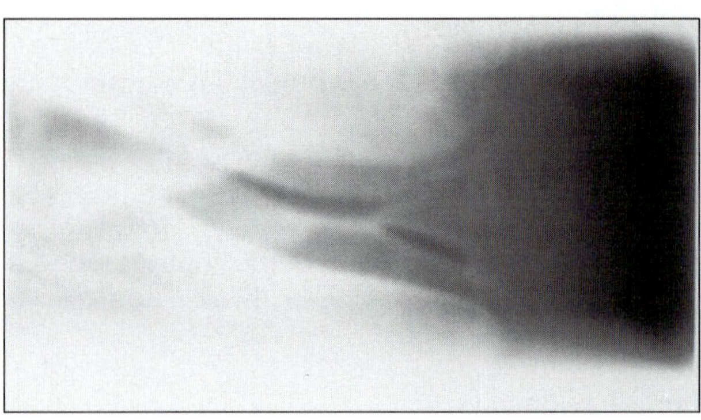

FIGURE 3.14 Lateral meniscus.

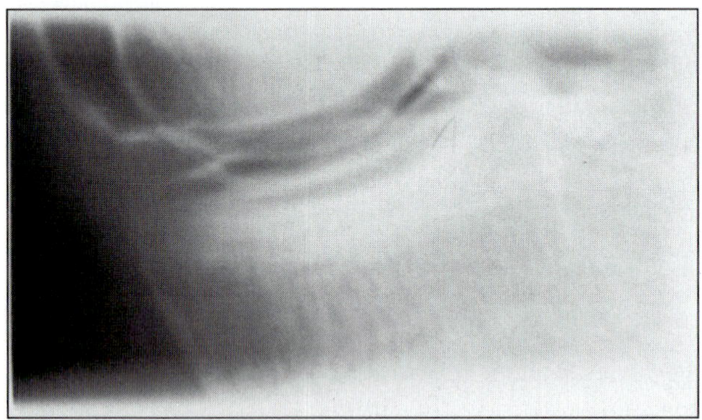

FIGURE 3.12 Medial meniscus.

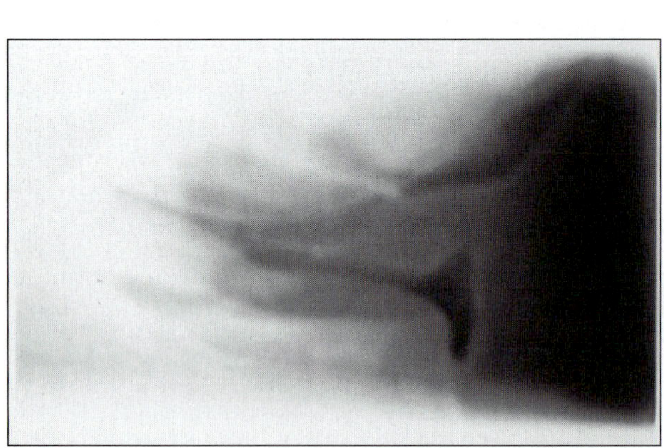

FIGURE 3.13 Lateral meniscus.

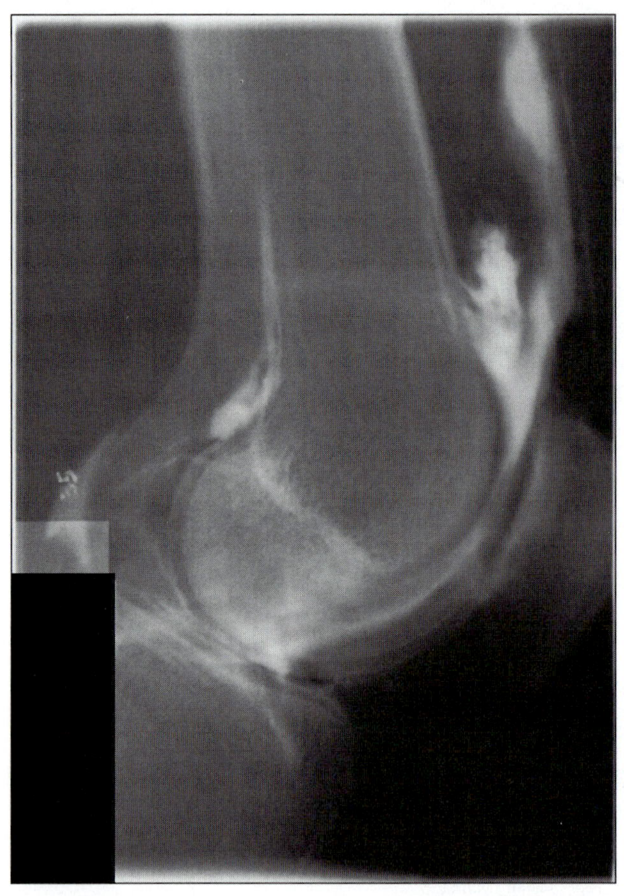

FIGURE 3.15 Lateral view of the knee with magnification.

Common Pathologies

- Baker's cyst
- Ligament tear
- Meniscal tear (Figure 3.17)
- **Prosthesis** check (Figures 3.18 and 3.19)

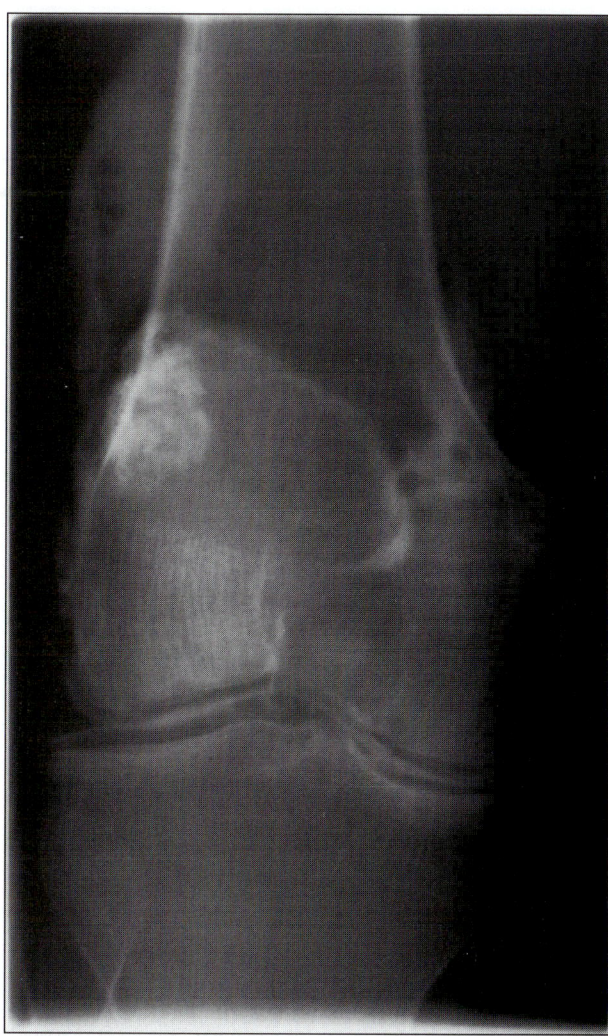

FIGURE 3.16 AP projection of the knee with magnification.

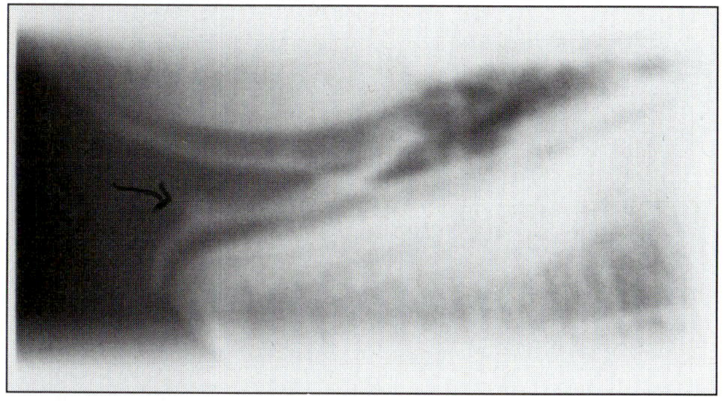

FIGURE 3.17 Meniscal tear.

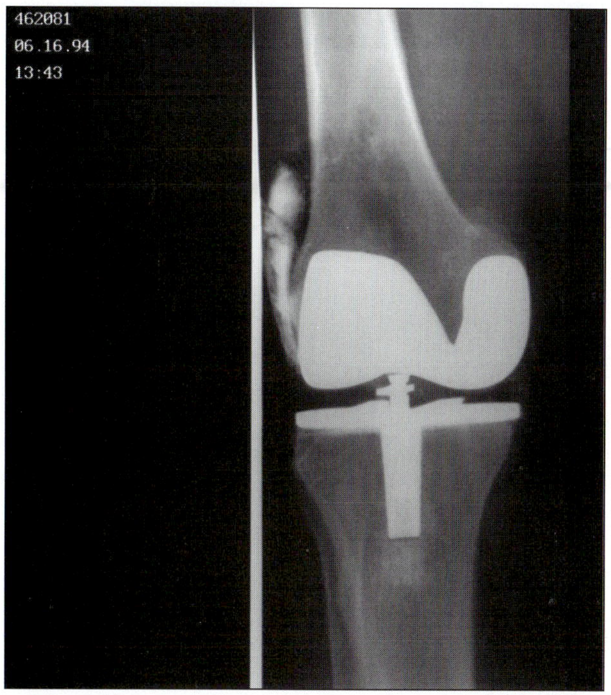

FIGURE 3.18 AP projection to check for prosthesis loosening.

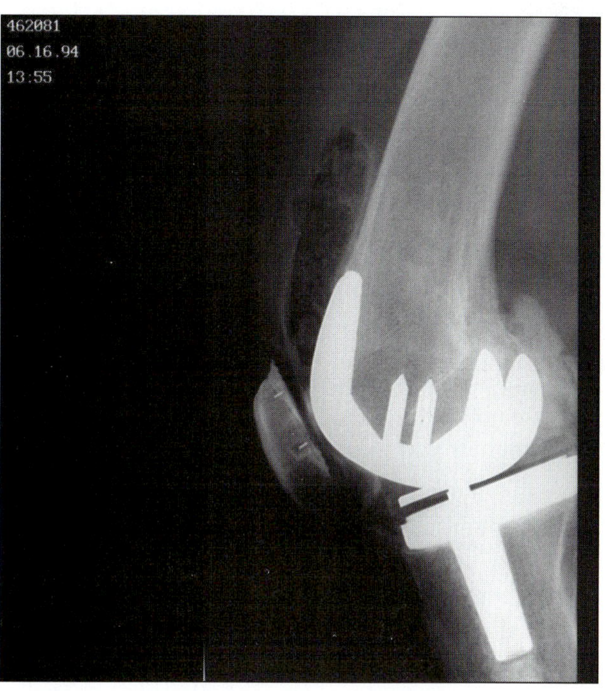

FIGURE 3.19 Lateral view to check for prosthesis loosening.

ARTHROGRAPHY OF THE HIP

Hip arthrography involves visualization of the upper third of the femur and this acetabular region of the pelvis. The hip joint is a diarthrotic ball and socket joint that allows flexion, extension, adduction, abduction, rotation, and circumduction. It is comprised of the femoral head and acetabulum (ăs´´ē-tăb´ū-lūm) of the iliac bone.

Applied Anatomy See Figure 3.20.

Indications

- Congenital dislocation of the hip (CDH)
- Loose bodies
- Loosening of prosthesis
- Perthes' disease—osteochrondritis of the epiphysis of the head of the femur
- Rheumatoid or osteoarthritis (to evaluate articular cartilage)

Contraindications

- Infection (sepsis)
- Allergy to contrast
- Bleeding problems

Equipment Fluoroscopy unit and conventional radiographic unit (the same equipment as for the knee arthrogram)

Contrast Media Water-soluble, ionic or nonionic compound (positive)

Radiation Protection Where possible, the gonads should be protected. It is important to keep fluoroscopy to the minimum, particularly in children with congenital dislocation, because it is likely they will require recurrent radiographic studies.

Preliminary Radiographs

- AP projection of the hip joint (Figure 3.21)
- Lateral view of the hip joint (Figure 3.22)
- For children with congenital dislocation, an AP projection of the pelvis with slight inversion of the lower limbs as well as a bilateral frog-leg view are often required.

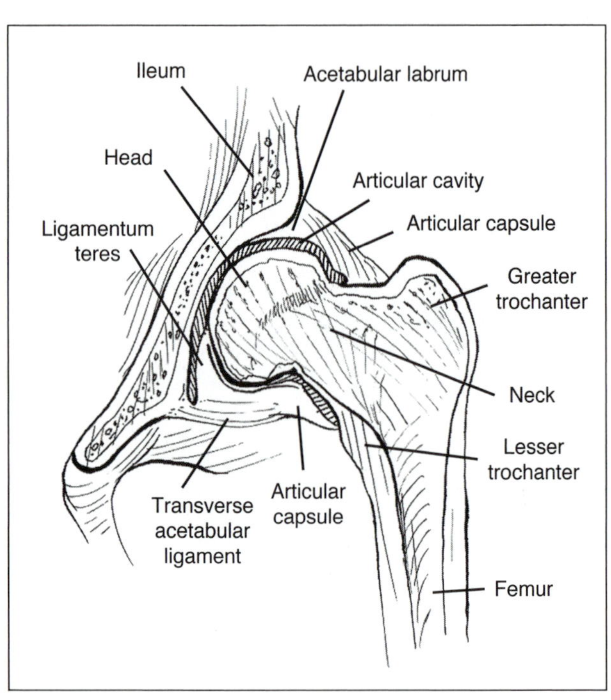

FIGURE 3.20 Anatomy of the hip.

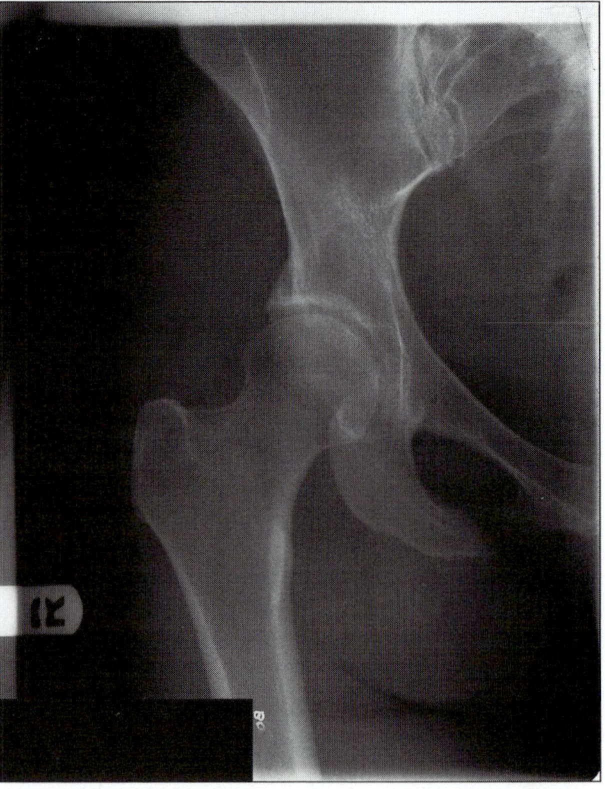

FIGURE 3.21 AP projection of the hip.

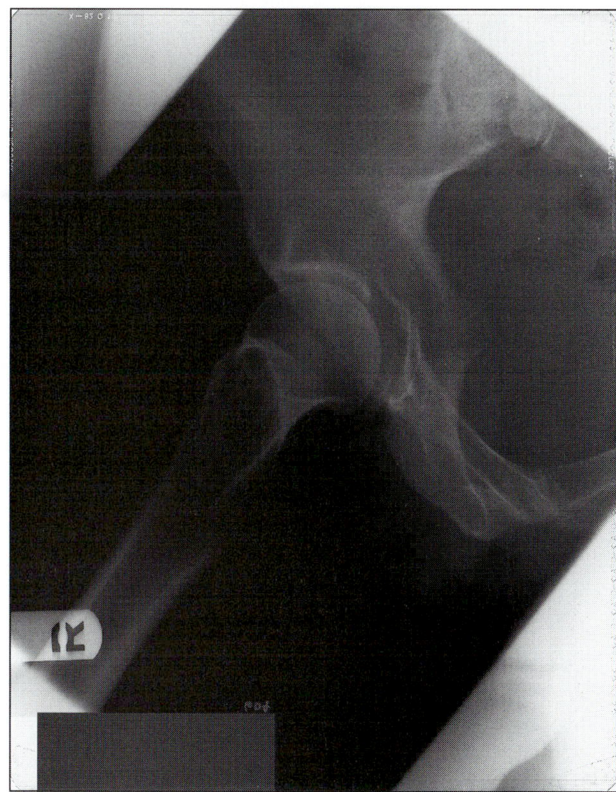

FIGURE 3.22 **Lateral view of the hip.**

Patient Preparation

- The injection area should be cleansed and shaved if necessary.
- The patient also requires reassurance and a sedative can be administered to patients experiencing extreme anxiety.

Procedure Sequence

- Patient lies supine on the fluoroscopy table. A hip that has 10° flexion, 10° abduction, and 10° internal rotation produces the maximum joint capacity. Frequently the joint position is arranged under fluoroscopy.
- Using sterile technique, a local anesthetic is applied to the region (approximately 3 cm inferior and at right angles to the midpoint of the inguinal ligament).
- A 22-gauge spinal needle is advanced medially and upward from the point described above. A "give" should be felt as the needle passes through the capsule.
- Correct positioning of the needle can be determined by injecting a small amount of contrast under fluoroscopy. (To reduce radiation, saline can also be injected. Incorrect placement of the needle would mean resistance to injection after a very few milliliters.)
- **Aspirations** for cultures should be performed at this time.
- After injection of contrast medium into the joint space (Figure 3.23), the needle is removed and the joint gently manipulated.
- Radiographs should be taken immediately because contrast is rapidly absorbed in this area.

Procedure Radiographs

- AP projection of the hip (Figure 3.24)
- AP projection of the hip with internal and external rotation
- AP projection of the hip with traction (Figure 3.25)
- Lateral view of the hip

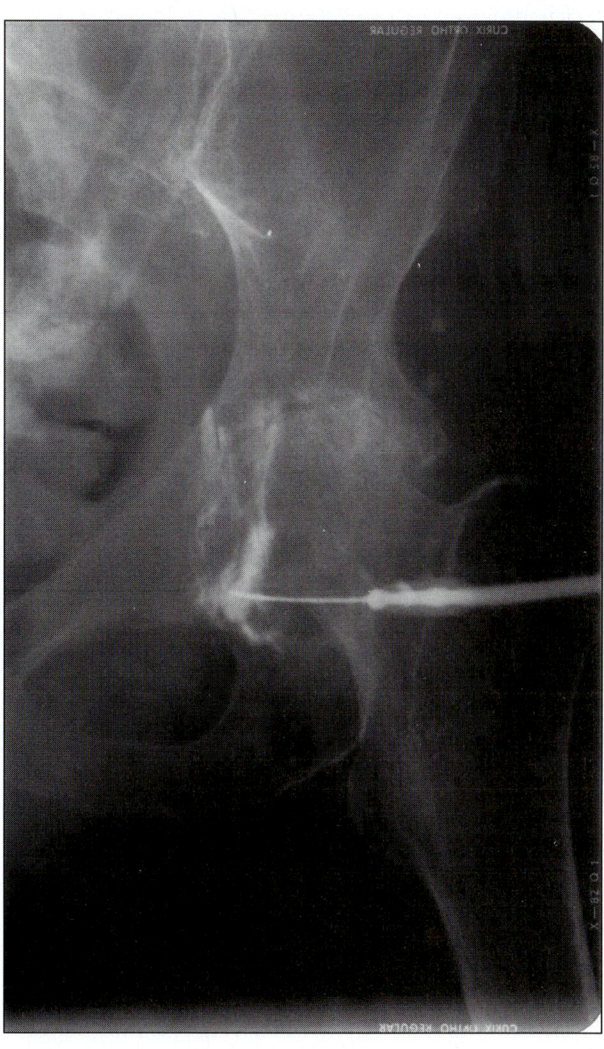

FIGURE 3.23 **Needle in position for hip arthrogram.**

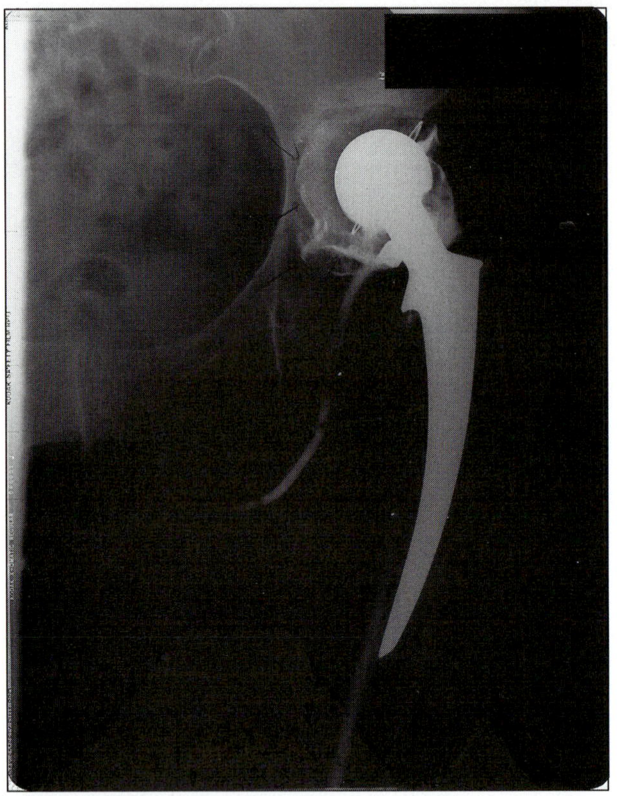

FIGURE 3.24 AP projection of hip and prosthesis.

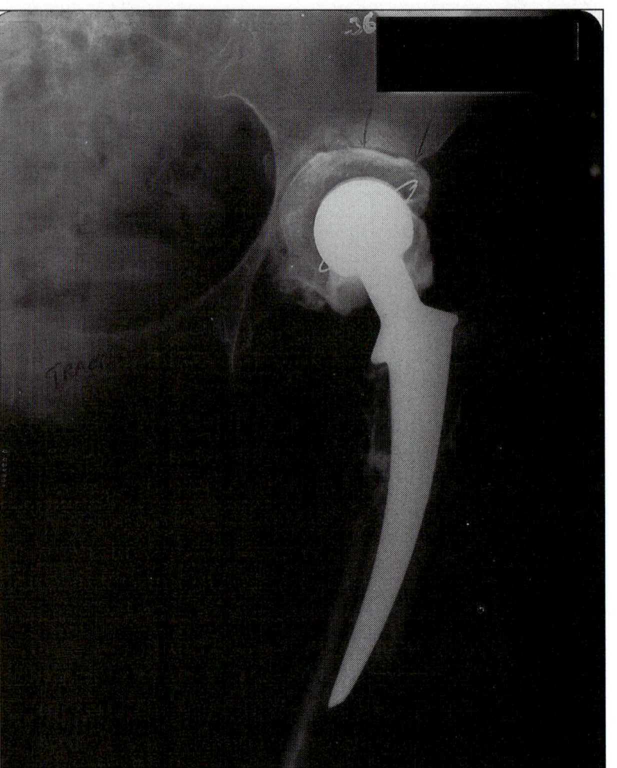

FIGURE 3.25 AP projection of hip with traction.

Alternative Radiographs

- Delayed films after 30 minutes.
- For prosthesis loosening, a subtraction technique can be used. A radiograph is taken with the needle in situ before injection and then a **mask** (reverse tone image) is made from this radiograph. Another radiograph is taken after 15 to 20 mL contrast has been injected. This technique will subtract out the prosthesis and glue to visualize any leakage of contrast around the prosthesis.

Postprocedure Care

- Bed rest for 1 to 2 days.
- This investigation is sometimes carried out under general anesthetic and in this case the patient is admitted into the care facility. Care should be taken to note for allergic or synovial reactions (same as for knee arthrography).

Common Pathologies

- Perthes' disease (Figure 3.26)
- Loose bodies, sign for synovial osteochondromatosis.
- Infection due to prosthesis

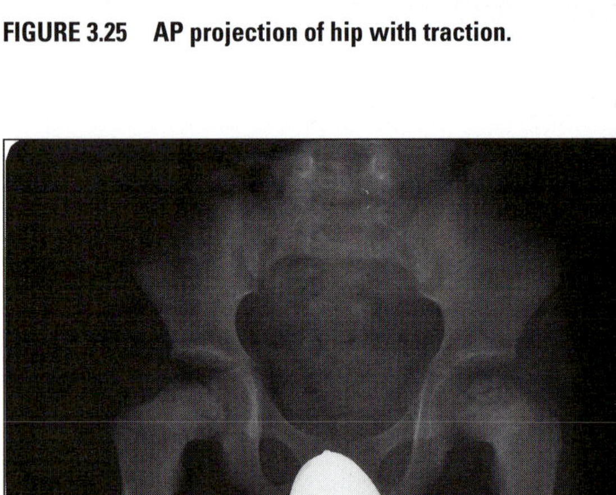

FIGURE 3.26 Bilateral Perthes' disease.

ARTHROGRAPHY OF THE TEMPOROMANDIBULAR JOINT

A positive contrast medium is injected into the joint space to allow the joint to be evaluated functionally and dynamically.

Applied Anatomy The bony structures of the temporomandibular joint (TMJ) are comprised of the articular temporal surfaces, the condyle of the mandible, and the articular disk and capsule. It is interesting to note that the articular surfaces are made up of collagen rather than hyaline cartilage. It is a hinge and gliding type of joint (Figure 3.27).

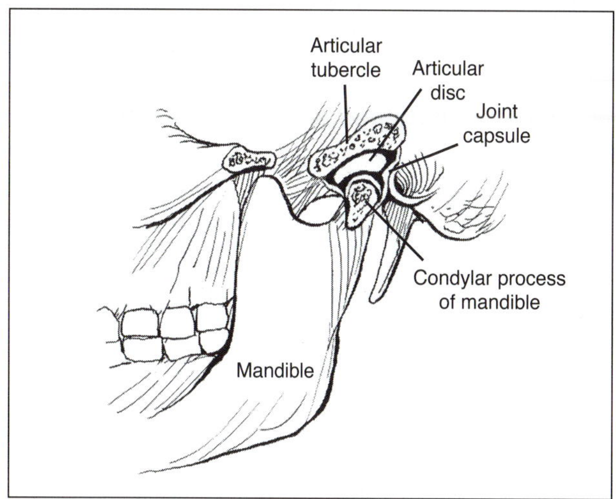

FIGURE 3.27 Anatomy of temporomandibular joint (TMJ).

Indications

- Subluxation of the TMJ with a partial dislocation of the joint, generally occurring only during movement
- **Aplasia** (ă-plā´zē-ă), hypo- and hyperplasia of mandibular condyle
- Fracture
- Ankylosis (ăng´´kĭ-lō´sĭs) or abnormal immobility or consolidation of a joint
- Arthritis
- Degenerative joint disease

Contraindications

- Allergy to contrast
- Bleeding tendency
- Acute infection

Equipment Fluoroscopy with fine focal spot and high-resolution video

Contrast Media Water-soluble, ionic or nonionic compound (positive)

Radiation Protection Protection to the gonads and thyroid, where possible

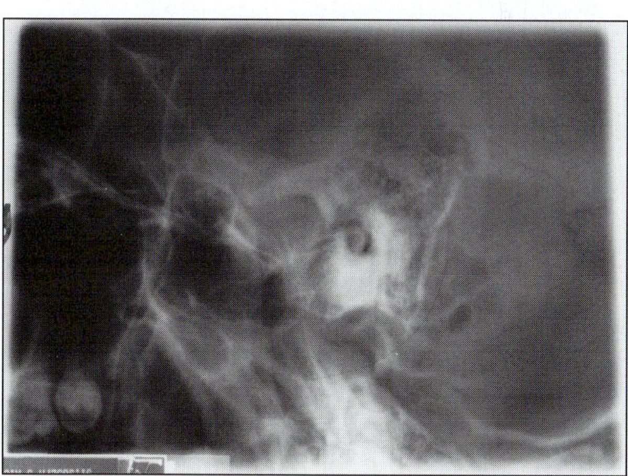

FIGURE 3.28 Open mouth—lateral view.

Preliminary Radiographs

- Lateral view of the TMJ with mouth open and closed (Figures 3.28 and 3.29).
- 30° fronto-occipital to show joints
- Submentovertical to show joints
- Panoramic tomography (occasionally)

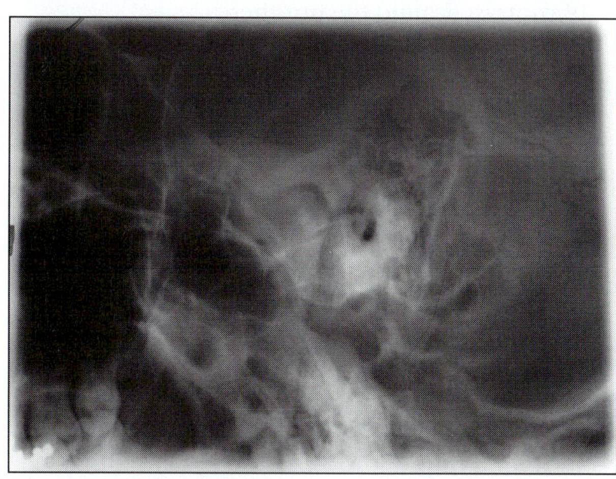

FIGURE 3.29 Closed mouth—lateral view.

Procedure Sequence

- The patient lies in the lateral decubitus position on the fluoroscopic table with the side to be examined uppermost.
- Using sterile technique, local anesthetic is administered to the area.
- A 25-gauge needle is guided into the inferior joint space with the aid of fluoroscopy (Figure 3.30) and

1 mL contrast medium is injected (more than this would cause painful overextension). A very small quantity of epinephrine can be added to reduce resorption of contrast and provide a longer coating time. The patient is often asked to slowly open and close the mouth to ease the introduction of the needle into the joint space (Figure 3.31).
- After correct placement and injection, the needle is removed and the patient asked to open and close the mouth while a fluoroscopic image is videotaped.
- This procedure can be repeated for the superior joint space if needed.

Procedure Radiographs

- Lateral TMJ with open and closed mouth
- AP and lateral autotomograms (Patient moves jaw open and shut during the exposure.)

Alternative Radiographs

- Lateral tomography (Figure 3.32 A and B)

Postprocedure Care

- Discomfort for 1 to 2 days is usually resolved by use of an analgesic.
- Ice can be administered to the affected joint for several hours.
- Persistent pain beyond 2 days could indicate infection and should be treated.

Common Pathologies

- Ankylosis
- Arthritis
- Degenerative disease
- Dysfunction of joint movement

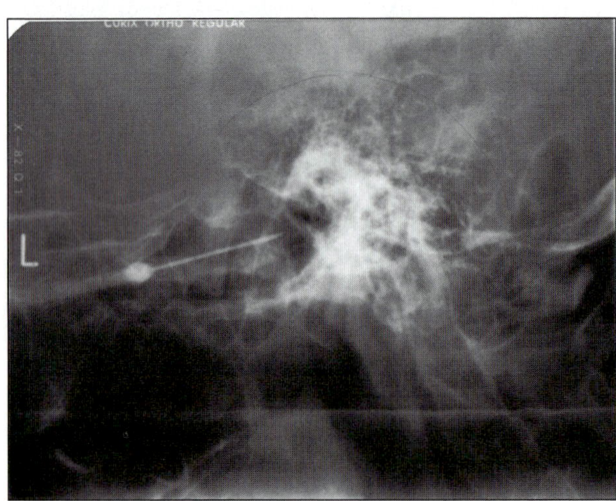

FIGURE 3.30 Needle inserted into TMJ.

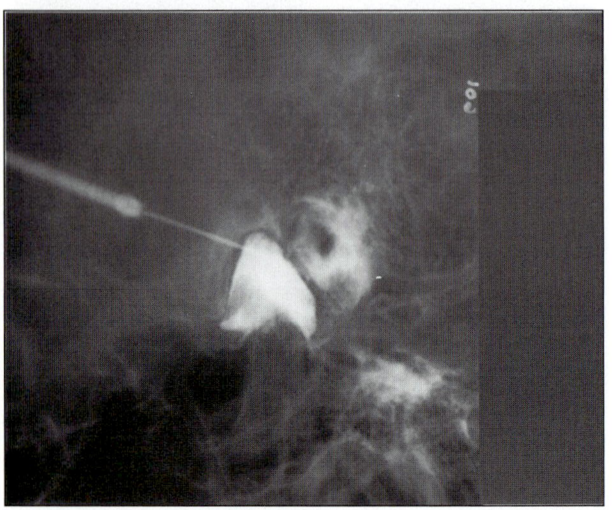

FIGURE 3.31 Contrast medium in TMJ.

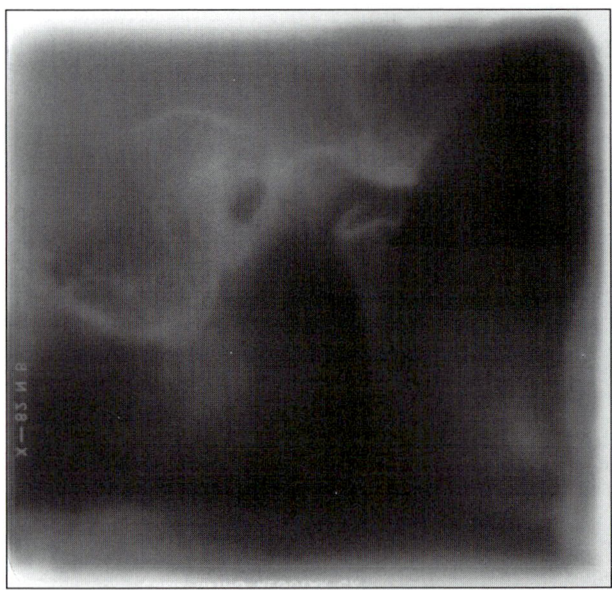

A

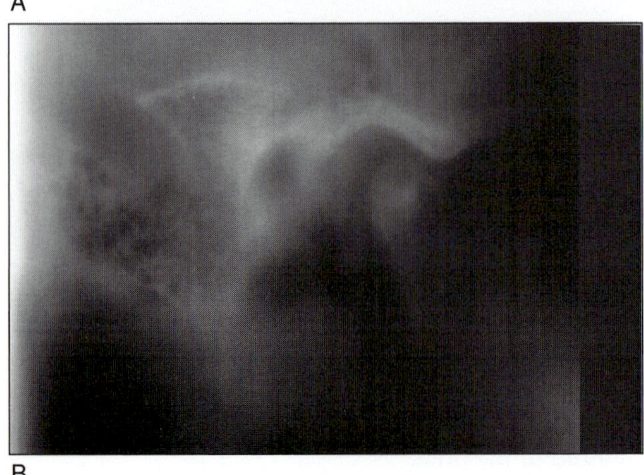

B

FIGURE 3.32 A and B Lateral tomography of TMJ.

ARTHROGRAPHY OF THE SHOULDER

Indications

- Rotator cuff or long head of biceps tears
- Foreign bodies

Contrast Media Often double contrast, using

- Low osmolarity water-soluble contrast medium
- Air

Preliminary Radiographs

- AP projections with internal and external rotation
- An axial view demonstrates the inferior aspect of the joint capsule

Procedure Sequence

- The patient lies supine on the fluoroscopy table with the hand supinated to rotate the long head of the biceps away from the injection point.
- The affected shoulder is closest to the operator.
- The arm lies alongside the body.
- Local anesthetic is applied to an area 1 cm inferior and 1 cm lateral to the coracoid process.
- A 21- or 22-gauge needle is inserted into the synovial sac under fluoroscopic control.
- The position is checked by the injection of a small amount of contrast medium during fluoroscopy and then the remainder of the contrast and the air (about 8–10 mL) is injected.
- The needle is removed and the shoulder rotated and manipulated gently to circulate the contrast media

Radiographs Taken

- AP projections in internal and external rotation (Figure 3.33)
- Axial view
- Views as needed can be taken with the spot film device or overhead tube.

Postprocedural care Patient should be advised of localized discomfort for 1 or 2 days.

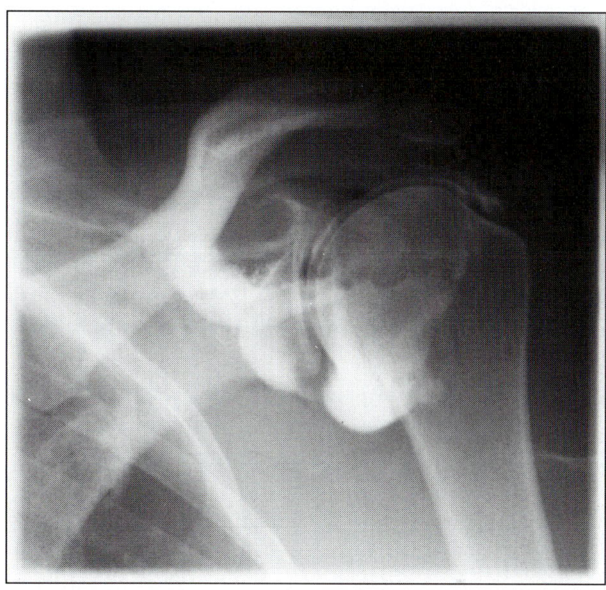

FIGURE 3.33 Arthrogram of the shoulder.

OTHER ARTHROGRAPHIC STUDIES

Elbow, ankle, and wrist arthrograms are occasionally done, using the same basic technique as identified.

Elbow Arthrography This is usually done to look for loose bodies. A double-contrast examination is performed with air and positive contrast injected just proximal to the radial head. Conventional AP and lateral views are taken.

Ankle Arthrography Pathologies demonstrated in this examination are usually ligament injury, loose bodies, a rupture, or osteochondral defects. Contrast (usually positive) is injected directly into the joint space from a point just lateral to the medial malleolus.

Other Imaging Modalities

COMPUTED TOMOGRAPHY

Joints can be imaged using CT. Movement can be kept to a minimum and radiation factors can be kept fairly low if bone is the primary area of interest. The usual reason for scanning is to visualize the extent of a lesion within a joint area and both limbs are generally included in any scan to determine symmetry and bony involvement of any lesion (Figures 3.34 and 3.35). It is important that slices encompass the entire area of concern. Slice thickness will vary according to the area and pathology presented.

Contrast is sometimes injected into the joint to be imaged to enhance the soft tissue areas to visualize ligament tearing. Three-dimensional reconstruction, if available, can be used to visualize the bony aspects of an articulation. Any foreign body, particularly a prosthesis, will affect the success of a reconstruction. This imaging method is particularly helpful in the examination of the femoral head within the acetabulum. It is often able to visualize fracture fragments or changes to the bone due to aseptic necrosis. Associated soft tissue pathologies can sometimes be well defined, such as an aneurysm or hematoma swelling (Figure 3.36).

Tarsal joints are well demonstrated on CT and three-dimensional reconstruction. CT is used to demonstrate degenerative changes that may not be apparent on plain radiographs. CT arthrography can be performed, using single- or double-contrast technique. Generally, less contrast is required than for the conventional procedure. Positioning is sometimes difficult due to the constraints of the gantry; however, CT can provide a dual purpose by having windows set for bone and for soft tissue.

CT is becoming frequently more used in the area of trauma, with units dedicated to emergency cases in some larger centers. Three-dimensional reconstruction of fractured bones is sometimes useful in determining the exact position of fragments and as a template for reconstructive surgery. The examples here demonstrate the detail that can be obtained from taking a number of slices that are then processed into a three-dimensional image (Figures 3.37 and 3.38).

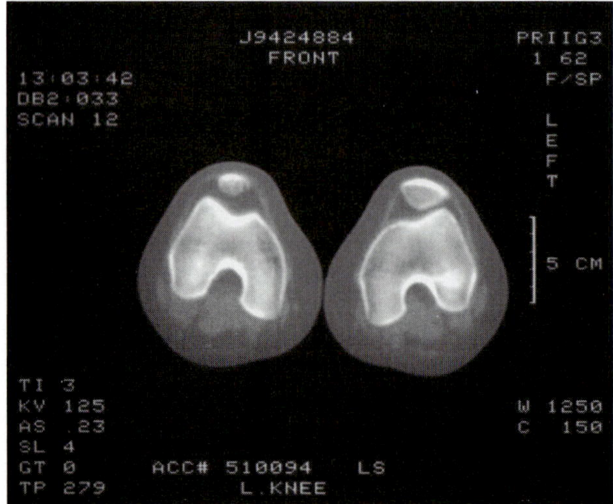

FIGURE 3.34 CT of the knee.

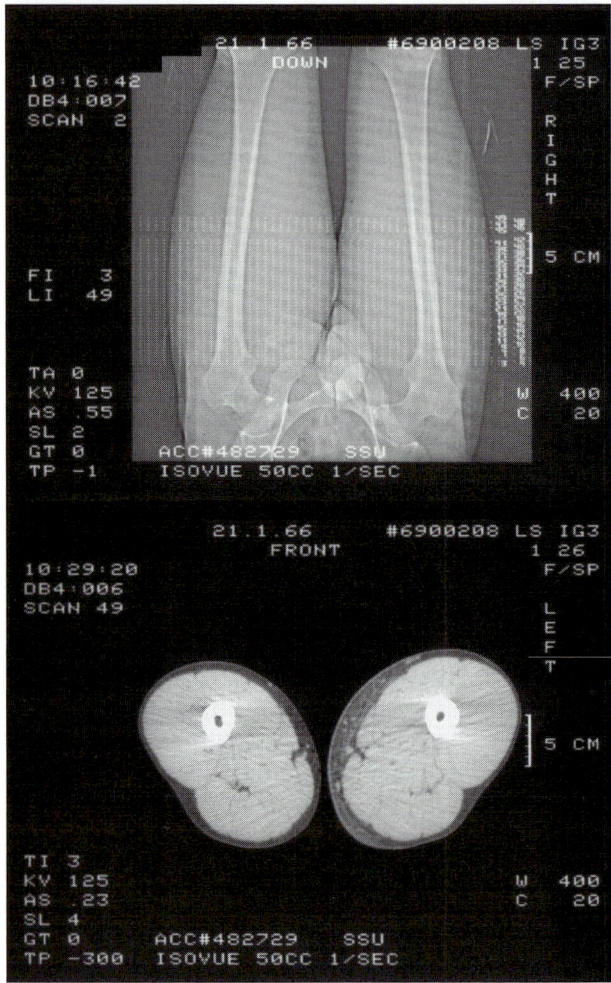

FIGURE 3.35 Bilateral CT of the femur.

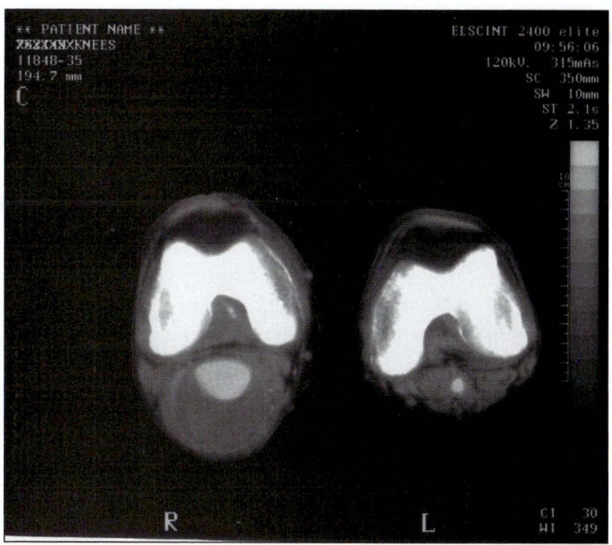

FIGURE 3.36 Aneurysm in the knee.

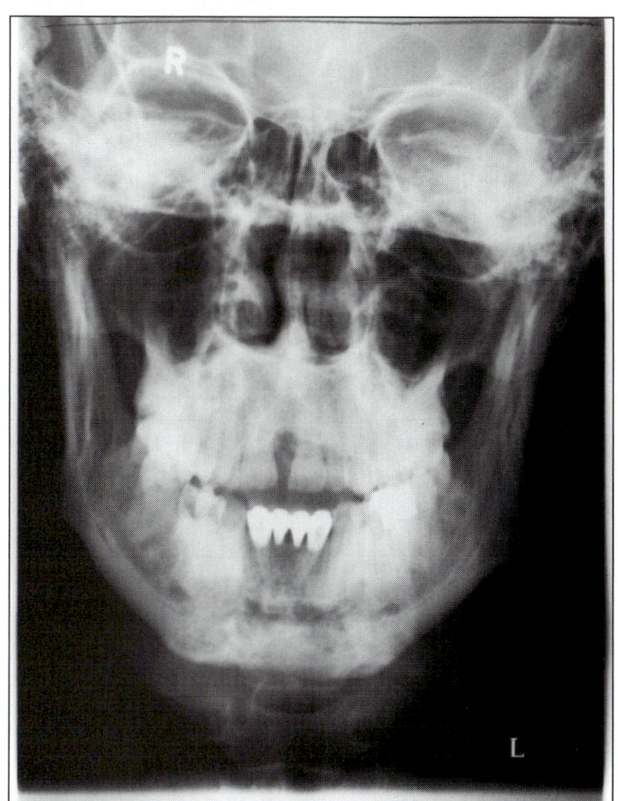

FIGURE 3.37 Plain radiograph of facial bones.

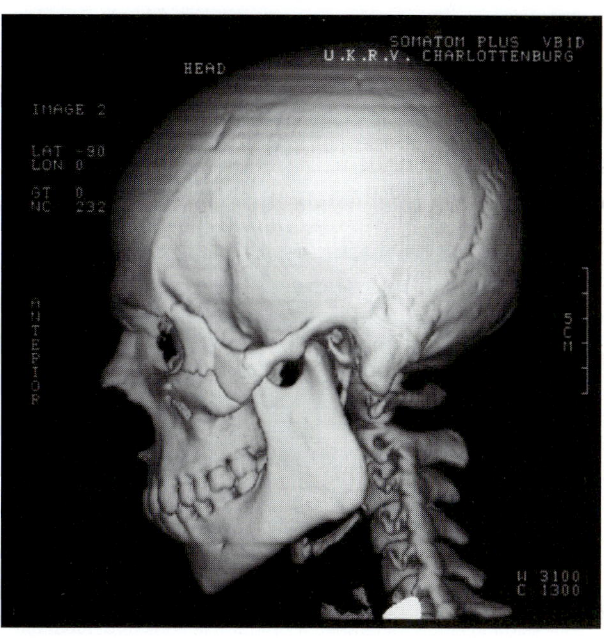

FIGURE 3.38 Three-dimensional image of CT reconstruction.

MAGNETIC RESONANCE IMAGING

This modality has the ability to produce outstanding studies of bone, providing extensive morphologic information. It is being used extensively in sports medicine, rheumatology, and all aspects of orthopedics because of its unique ability to assess soft tissue as well as osseous tissue. It is beyond the scope of this book to identify all the studies for which MRI can be used, but listed in Table 3.1 are some of the advantages as well as disadvantages to MRI in examining the musculoskeletal system.

TABLE 3.1 ADVANTAGES AND DISADVANTAGES OF MRI

Advantages

- Completely noninvasive
- Good differentiation between normal structures such as fat, marrow, bone, fibrocartilage, ligaments, tendons, nerves, and blood vessels
- Good demonstration of pathologies such as fluid collection (as in cysts, necrosis), increased tissue water content (tumor, edema, inflammation, hemorrhage), lesions and neoplasms

Disadvantages

- Costly examination
- Not as readily accessible as conventional imaging methods
- Not suitable as a screening tool (too expensive)
- Examinations take a long time
- Not as suitable as CT to demonstrate cortical bone because there are no mobile protons (see Chapter 2, Introduction to Specialized Imaging)
- Some materials used for orthopedic repair and prosthesis are magnetic materials
- Conventional radiography still produces excellent results!

MRI OF THE KNEE

Knee MRI has virtually replaced arthrography (wherever it is available). MRI has not replaced arthroscopy but is often used as a complementary examination because it is able to visualize articular and osseous structures not always seen during arthroscopy. The comparative advantage of arthroscopy lies in its ability to better evaluate cartilage and to repair damaged areas.

An MRI can evaluate many more structures besides the menisci and cruciate ligaments and yet is at least as accurate, if not more so, than arthrography in demonstrating these anatomic areas. The greatest contribution that MRI provides is its ability to determine truly normal structures. It provides a 100% negative predictive value. This reduces the number of invasive arthroscopic studies required.

Applied Anatomy See Figure 3.39.

Indications

- Ligament, meniscal injuries
- Effusions
- Doubtful knee condition (previous radiographs/ arthrograms not conclusive)
- Acute injury of confusing etiology
- Degenerative disease

Contraindications

- Trauma (plain radiographs still better and easier to perform)

Equipment

- MRI scanner. New smaller units for extremities can be used.
- A surface wrap-around coil is used.

Contrast Media None

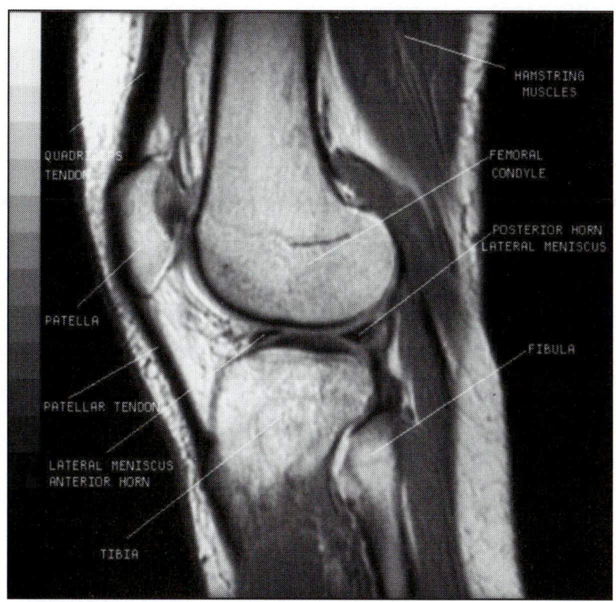

FIGURE 3.39 Lateral MRI of the knee.

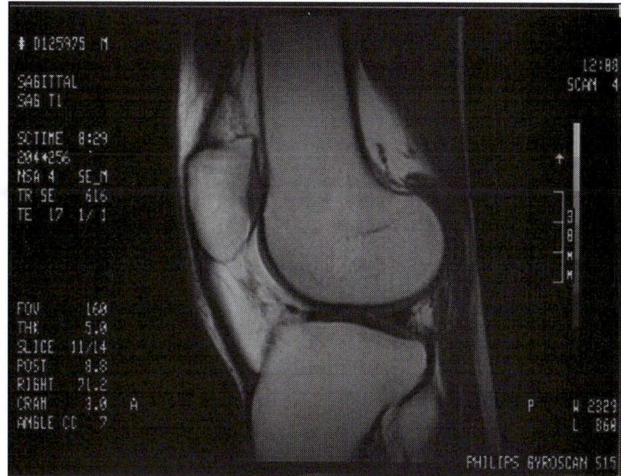

FIGURE 3.40 T1 lateral MRI of the knee.

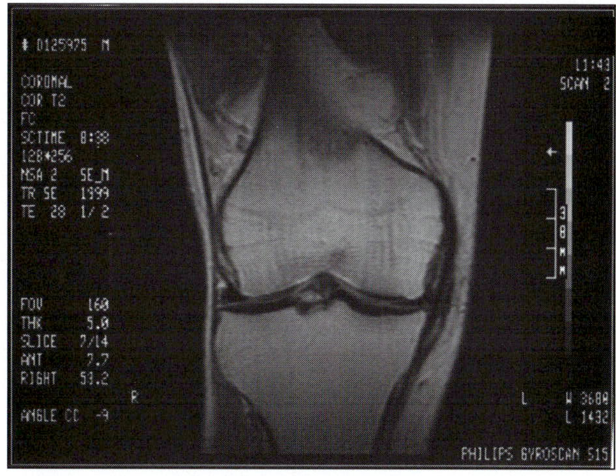

FIGURE 3.41 T2 anterior MRI of the knee.

Radiation Protection Not applicable

Preliminary Radiographs AP and lateral view of the knee

Patient Preparation

- A questionnaire should be completed that identifies any occupations that might have created the possibility of foreign or metallic objects (such as welding), previous surgeries or prostheses.
- Usually no other preparation required, although mild sedation if the patient is extremely agitated

Procedure Sequence

- The patient is imaged supine. The knee is extended and externally rotated about 10° to 20°.
- T1 and T2 studies are taken.

Procedure Images

- T1 visualizes the intramedullary abnormalities (Figure 3.40).
- T2 visualizes the ligaments and cartilage (Figure 3.41).
- The anterior cruciate ligament is seen as a thin solid dark band.
- The posterior cruciate ligament is seen as a thick dark band.

New developments are improving the speed and quality of knee imaging. Fast three-dimensional Fourier transform MRI scanning provides greater specificity and a quicker time (8–16 minutes).

Postprocedure Care None other than that associated with pathology presented

Common Pathologies

- Ligament, meniscal injuries
- Meniscal degenerative disease (particularly in older patients over 40)
- Effusions

MRI OF OTHER JOINTS

Hip

Arthrography is still the examination of choice for determining infections, intra-articular loose bodies, and synovitis. CT provides good imaging of fractures and generally MRI is only used when less expensive imaging methods cannot provide all the information for patient management. It can differentiate different types of infection, for example, osteomyelitis, cellulitis, and abscess.

Temporomandibular Joint

Arthrography remains the best examination to document meniscal abnormalities and joint mechanics. MRI is useful in determining soft tissue injury because it avoids the bony artifacts presented by CT when imaging this area. There also appears to be a higher incidence of claustrophobia with TMJ sufferers (up to 50%), making MRI less attractive as an examination of choice. New open sided designs will help eliminate their problem.

Ankle and Shoulder Joints

MRI is useful in assessing soft tissue mass and trauma, visualizing bony lesions, and evaluating tendons. However, plain radiography, arthrography, and CT all provide this information and MRI is not always the examination of choice.

ULTRASOUND

Although bone detail is not well visualized with ultrasound, joint integrity and pathologies such as congenital dislocations can be well visualized using ultrasound. Musculoskeletal ultrasound is a rapidly growing field because of its noninvasive quality and economics of use. This is particularly useful in children where the noninvasive nonionizing study is preferred.

The acetabular morphology can be assessed either by scans along various planes or by dynamic study, where the hip is flexed and adducted and the femur pushed and pulled in and out of the pelvis (Figure 3.42).

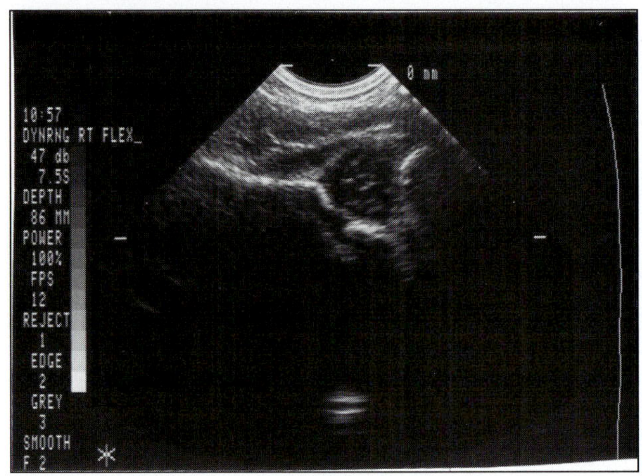

FIGURE 3.42 Ultrasound of pediatric hips.

RADIONUCLIDE IMAGING

This modality can be used to identify an aggravated synovial membrane or the presence of a bony lesion. Uptake of the **radionuclide** (^{99m}Tc-methylene diphosphonate or other ^{99m}Tc-labeled diphosphonate) will demonstrate a "hot spot" where there is inflammation or abnormal growth (Figures 3.43 and 3.44).

Radionuclide scanning has also proven useful in the determination of prosthetic loosening (of the hip joint). Loosening creates a high degree of sensitivity and therefore uptake will occur in the presence of movement of the prosthesis. This scan provides a noninvasive, low-dose study, but should not be done until 6 to 8 months after prosthetic surgery because the scan will read positive up until that time due to the natural healing process occurring during that time.

SPECT imaging can provide three-dimensional images as well as slices through areas of bone where there is abnormal activity to provide better localization.

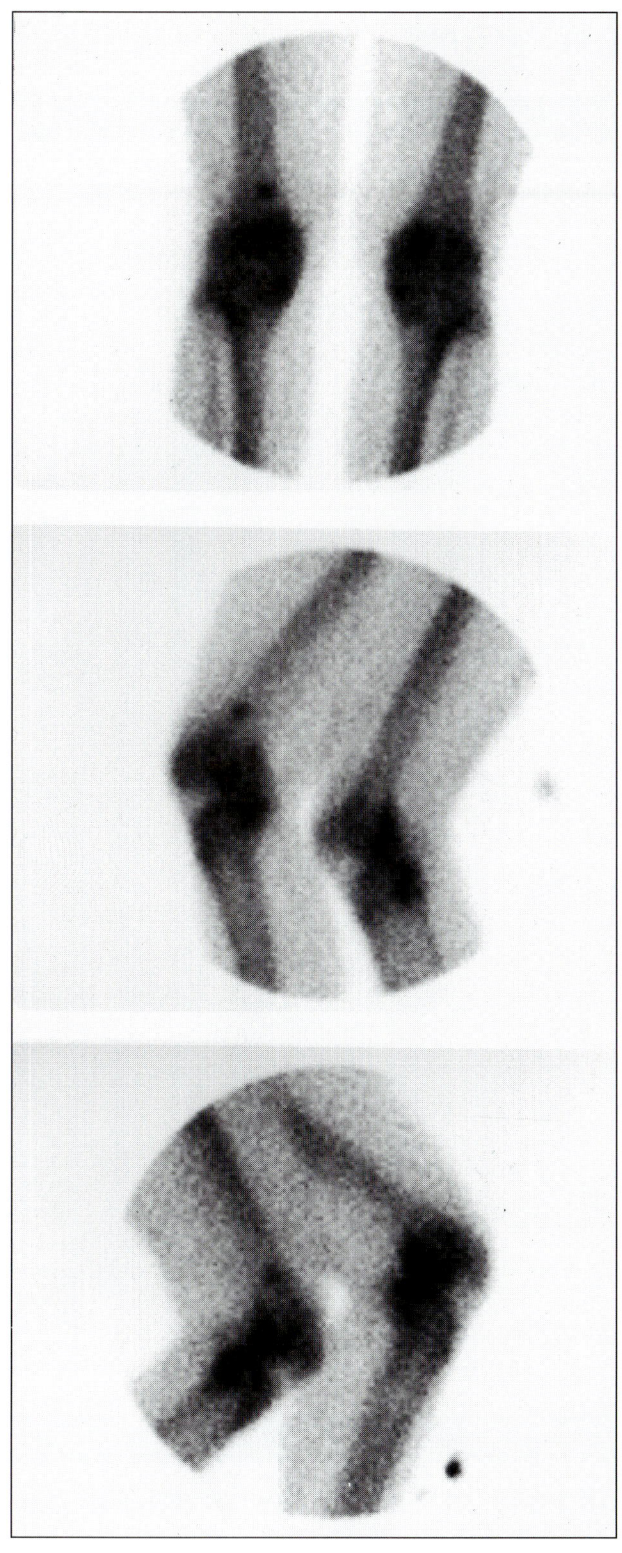

FIGURE 3.43 Normal knee scan.

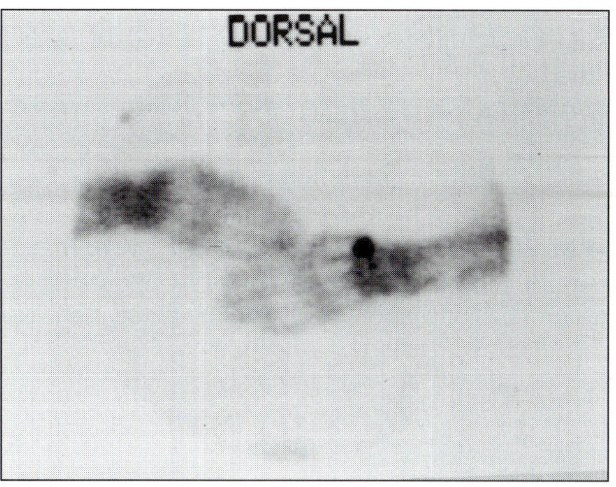

FIGURE 3.44 "Hot spot" in left scaphoid area.

Other Specialized Skeletal Studies

METASTATIC SURVEY

Skeletal **metastases** (mĕ-tăs´tă-sēz) can develop asymptommatically as a result of a primary tumor. Surveys are carried out when metastases are suspected but not known. (When distribution of metastases are diagnosed, conventional radiographs of affected areas are requested.) A radionuclide scan has now become the usual first step in diagnosis. Radiographs can identify whether there is underlying non neoplastic disease (i.e., Paget's or degeneration), but radiographs reveal some metastatic changes later than radionuclide scan. Conversely, advanced metastatic changes may appear as a normal scan. For this reason, the radiographic and radionuclide studies are sometimes performed as an adjunct to each other. It is important to remember that if the scan is performed first, sufficient time must elapse before the radiographs can be performed because the radionuclide could compromise the radiograph.

The Radiographic Survey The exact radiographs may differ from one clinical site to another but every survey should contain radiographs of the skull, long bones, and spine, each area only requiring one view (e.g., lateral of the skull).

The Bone Scan (Radionuclide Imaging) An IV injection of a radionuclide, followed by an entire body scan, will reveal any "hot spots" (Figure 3.45). These are areas of increased activity and indicate an abnormal lesion. It may not necessarily indicate a metastatic lesion. SPECT can be useful to locate individual lesions within joints. Depending on the known condition of the patient, conventional radiographs may be required.

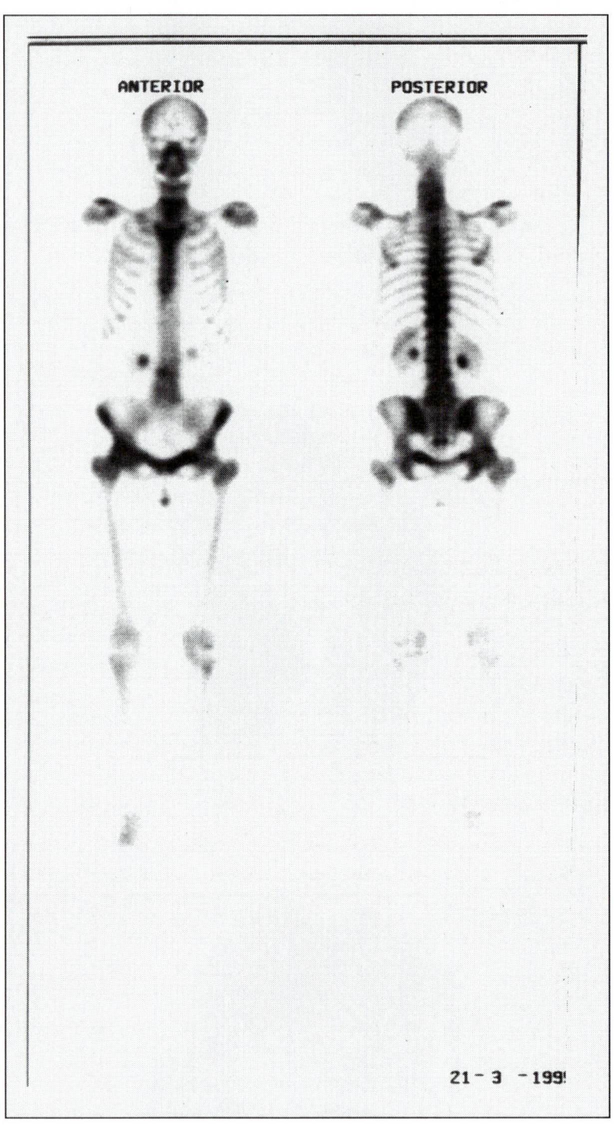

FIGURE 3.45 Whole body scan.

LONG BONE MEASUREMENT

The bones usually measured in this study are the lower extremities and several methods are used. Conventional radiography still remains the most reliable and accurate way to determine the difference in leg length. The most frequently used method is orthoroentgenography.

ORTHOROENTGENOGRAPHY (or´´thō-rĕnt-gĕn-ŏg´ră-fē)

Introduction This procedure reduces the risk of distortion by providing separate images of three articulations (hip, knee, ankle) on one film, by centering directly above the joint and taking three separate images. It is important that the patient remain immobilized in the supine position and that the articulation points are clearly identified by marking them on the skin surface.

Indications

- Congenital abnormalities
- Growth deficiencies

Equipment

- Conventional tabletop radiographic unit
- A 100-cm film in one long cassette or three cassettes laid beside each other. Separate cassettes can be used in the Bucky tray with exposures taken of each articulation provided the patient does not move.
- Metal ruler

Radiation Protection Gonadal protection is important because this procedure is often performed on children.

Procedure Sequence

- Both legs are positioned on the long film and cassette, to include all three lower limb joints.
- A radiograph is taken of each articulation. The first articulation is taken, collimating directly over the joint, then the tube moved so that the centering point is again above the joint space. This is repeated a third time. Neither patient nor film must move between exposures.
- A metal ruler placed longitudinally beside each joint during the exposure will allow accurate measurements to be taken.

Procedure Radiographs One 100-cm film on which are AP projections of the hip, knee, and ankle joints, or three radiographs of each joint and adjacent long bones. When attached and overlapped correctly, they will produce the same results.

SCOLIOSIS STUDIES

Scoliosis is a lateral curvature of the spine. Scoliosis has a number of causes including congenital abnormality or disease of the vertebral bodies, but the majority develop in childhood or adolescence from an unknown origin and are termed idiopathic scoliosis. Frequently, the entire vertebral column is involved because an initial curve is often followed by a compensatory curve in another section of the spine (Figure 3.46).

Conventional radiography continues to be the imaging of choice because it allows for accurate measurements of the degree of curvature and a sequence of radiographs during treatment can trace changes to the curves.

Procedure Radiographs

- Ideally, a long film and cassette are used (100 cm) and a single exposure made of the entire vertebral column in the AP projection. This exposure can be taken erect or supine. Occasionally both are requested.
- A lateral view is also sometimes requested.
- AP projections of a single curve with the patient bending to each side are sometimes required in an initial study of the scoliosis. This demonstrates degree of movement between vertebral bodies.
- A number of factors must be considered when taking the radiographs:

1. Compensating aluminum filters can be used to provide an even exposure.
2. Every attempt must be made to protect the gonadal area and breast tissue in young girls because these radiographs are often repeated through life.
3. All vertebral bodies must be included.
4. The epiphysis of the iliac crest must be demonstrated to determine bone age, and therefore, the effectiveness of treatment.
5. Collimation should be open enough to include ribs and pelvis because these will show increasing distortion if the disease is allowed to progress.

Alternative Radiographs

- It is sometimes important to visualize the L5–S1 articulation in the lateral aspect and a lumbar scoliosis makes this a difficult task. One method is to take two lateral views of this area, with the patient lying first on one side and then the other. The central ray should be at right angles to the L5–S1 space and this will generally require a caudad angulation of between 5° and 10° for scoliotic patients. (Observe body habitus for exact angulation.)
- The resultant two radiographs will provide information to accurately determine disk space height between L5 and S1.

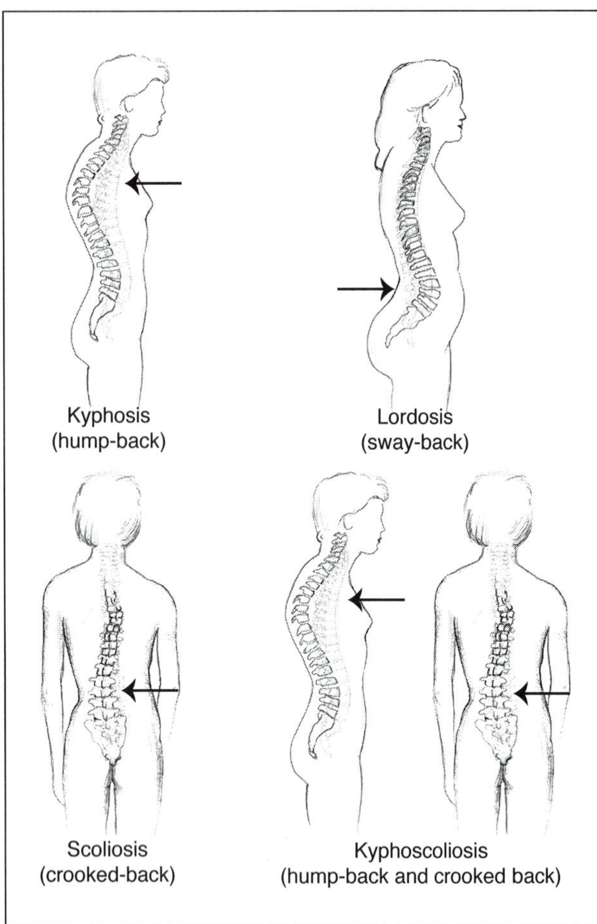

FIGURE 3.46 Abnormal scoliosis.

- Some studies indicate that radiation dosage can be reduced if the spine is radiographed in the PA projection. As well as digital computed radiography, very fast rare earth screens should be considered. The combination of these two will significantly reduce dosage to the sternum.
- There have been several attempts to introduce scoliosis screening programs into schools, for students in the high-risk ages between 11 and 14, but the risk incurred with radiation has stopped this procedure. Usually a single radiograph was performed when a preliminary positive diagnosis has been made from a physical assessment. A PA standing radiograph is taken to confirm degree of curve.

Other Imaging Methods Digital or computed radiography has been shown to significantly reduce exposure to the individual. The digital format allows for a very broad range of exposure latitude, allowing visualization of structures with wide differences in density. For example, the increased latitude would allow the lumbar vertebrae to be visualized without overexposing the cervical vertebrae. Studies have also indicated that dose can be reduced up to 50% without any compromise to image quality.

MRI can be used to determine any underlying pathologies or spinal cord involvement. MRI studies are generally only done on patients with atypical signs of scoliosis that indicate that the disease cause is other than idiopathic.

BONE DENSITY MEASUREMENT

The use of radiation to determine bone density has been extensively researched in an effort to produce a quantitative analysis that can detect early metabolic bone changes. It is becoming an increasingly common method of measuring calcium content of bone in pre- and postmenopausal women. A conventional radiograph is thought to detect changes only after there has been a 30% drop in mineral content. It is occasionally useful to measure cortical width of a bone in established osteoporosis, but this would be of little use in treating the progression of metabolic bone changes.

Several methods are now available:

- Quantitative CT (QCT)
- Single photon **Absorptiometry** (ăb-sorp´´shē-ŏm´ĭ-trē) (SPA)
- Dual photon absorptiometry (DPA)
- Dual x-ray absorptiometry (DXA)

Indications

- Osteoporosis
- Osteomalacia
- Hyperparathyroidism
- Agromegaly
- Cushing's disease
- Paget's disease
- Bone age
- Approaching menopause; as a screening tool

Quantitative CT This is a noninvasive method of providing an accurate assessment of trabecular mineral density. The area most commonly used is the lumbar region.

Procedure Sequence

- A single 8 to 10-mm slice is made through four lumbar vertebrae and the average CT number of the anterior trabecular bone is determined.
- The actual mineral density is determined by comparing these figures with the calibration standard.

NOTE: There are no absolute standards. These are calibrated for each CT scanner. Comparisons can therefore differ.

Radiation Protection Low-dose protocols are encouraged and the dose is estimated at 2000 Sv, with an effective dose equivalent of 50 Sv (roughly equivalent to a dental x-ray.)

Other Imaging Methods

Single Photon Absorptiometry Energy from a radionuclide source is passed through the measurement site and the transmitted fraction is detected. The usual body part used is the distal radius.

Dual Photon Absorptiometry This is used when it is necessary to measure the axial skeleton.

Dual X-ray Absorptiometry A dual energy x-ray source is used. Recent equipment has reduced doses and this has raised the possibility of using this technique for a screening protocol for women at high risk for osteoporosis. The patient's lateral lumbar spine is scanned and a computer analyzes the results (Figure 3.47).

Ultrasound Investigators have been examining the ability to measure the mineral content of the calcaneous by broad-band ultrasound attenuation. The calcaneous is used because it offers a large, relatively flat area of trabecular bone.

MRI It may become useful for measuring mineral density. It is considered too costly at present to use as a screening tool.

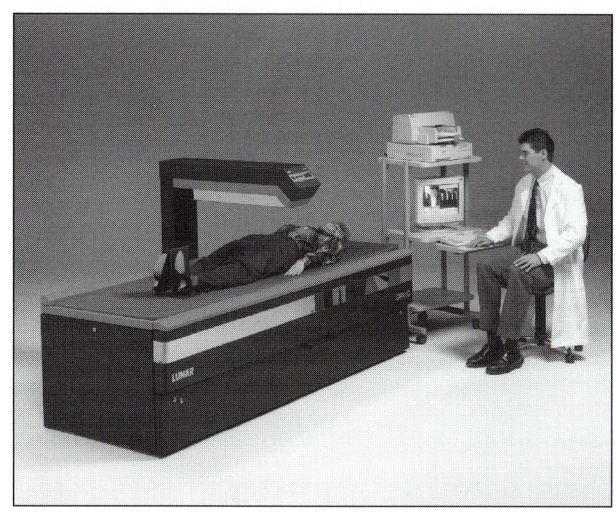

FIGURE 3.47 Densitometry equipment (Courtesy of Lunar Corporation, Madison, WI).

BONE AGE

The bone age of an individual can be determined by studying the development of epiphyses. Charts accurately define skeletal maturation and at what chronological time various epiphyses should normally appear. The most common radiograph taken to calculate bone age is the PA projection of the wrist and hand of a child (Figure 3.48).

The normal development times are as follows:

- Epiphysis of distal radius—secondary centers appear at 3 to 18 months
- Epiphysis of distal ulna—secondary centers appear at 4 to 9 years
- Carpal bones
  —Hamate—birth to 6 months
  —Capitate—birth to 6 months
  —Navicular—2.5 to 9 years
  —Triquetral—6 months to 1 year
  —Lunate—6 months to 9.5 years
  —Pisiform—6.5 to 16.5 years
  —Multangular, greater—1.5 to 10 years
  —Multangular, lesser—2.5 to 9 years
- The neonate knee (this is the most accurate assessment) (Figure 3.49).
- The epiphysis of the iliac crest. This area is considered the last bony structure to ossify and it is important to include this area when estimating whether there will be any future changes to spinal development.
- Occasionally, an AP projection and lateral view of the infant skull are taken to demonstrate closure of fontanelles and sutures.
- A lateral view of the sella turcica is requested in **amenorrhea** (ă-mĕn´´ō-rē´ă) to estimate developmental age (Figure 3.50).

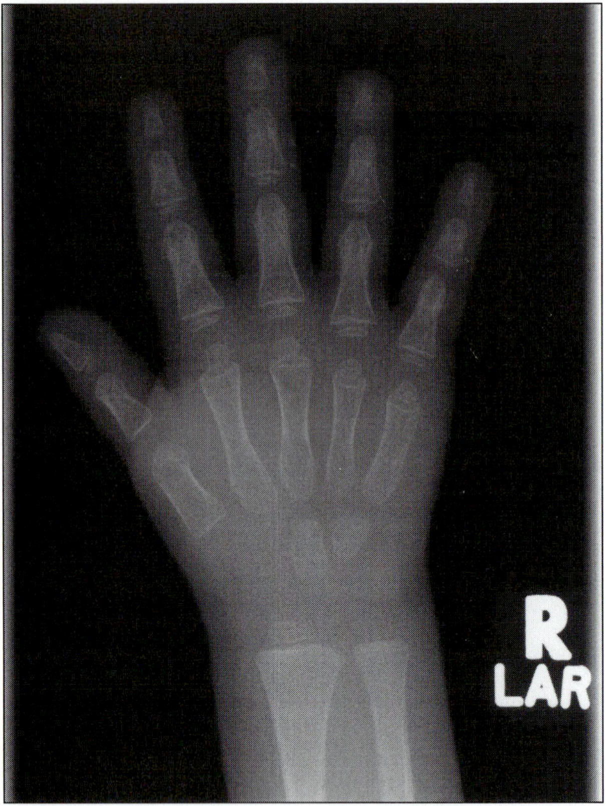

FIGURE 3.48 Wrist and hand of 18-month-old child.

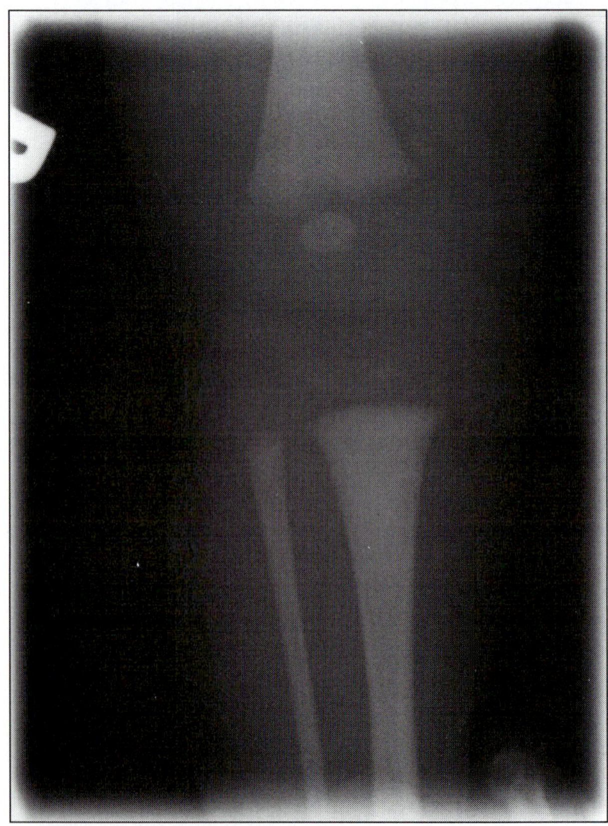

FIGURE 3.49 Knee of neonate.

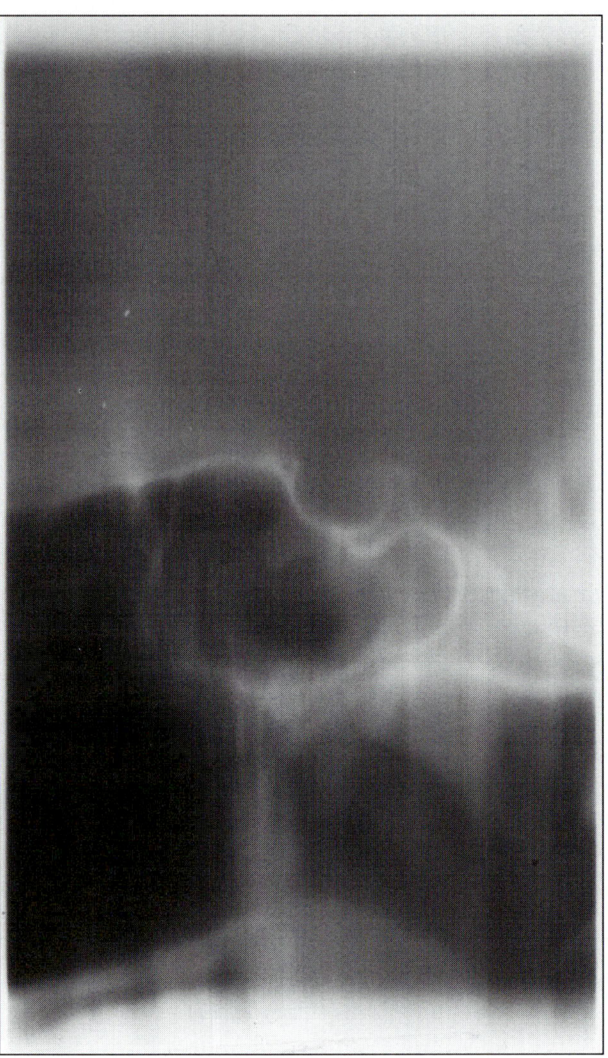

FIGURE 3.50 Lateral tomograms of sella turcica.

Interventional Procedures

BONE BIOPSY

Bone biopsies are sometimes carried out under fluoroscopic control. A needle is placed within a defined lesion and then withdrawn with a bore of bone. Larger needles are being replaced by smaller ones that have a motorized drilling attachment. Lesions that have caused considerable destruction can be biopsied using a standard fine needle. Areas being biopsied may include long bones and vertebral bodies. Radiographs are not usually taken.

Radiography of the musculoskeletal system forms a significant part of the clinical imaging performed in any department. Film radiography is well established and demonstrates many pathologies and pathologic conditions. However, in some instances the use of digital radiography is highly advantageous. The processing of a digital image can allow the operator to visualize bone or soft tissue injury from a single exposure. The ability to manipulate the image after exposure ensures a quality image together with a reduction in dose. Certain other features such as edge enhancement can accentuate pathologies such as hairline fractures. Fine detail is only possible with very high-resolution images and magnification is not a technique of choice when using a digital image to determine any subtle pathologies such as hyperparathyroidism. However, there is some indication that digital radiography can be used in arthographic studies of very small areas, using a small field and subtraction techniques.

Review Questions

1. Discuss the advantages of the MRI scan of the knee over conventional arthrography of the knee.

2. In what ways might MRI be a disadvantage in the imaging of joints.

3. Discuss the relative merits of arthrography versus arthroscopy.

4. Describe the type of stresses applied to joints during arthrography and indicate the reasons for this type of manipulation.

5. For the following conditions, suggest the primary imaging diagnostic study followed.
   a. congenital dislocation of the hips in a 1-year-old child
   b. 57-year-old man with known prostate cancer for general check of condition
   c. 27-year-old athlete for a suspected torn meniscus
   d. 52-year-old postmenopausal woman for suspected osteoporosis

6. Describe the type of contrast medium (media) commonly used for arthrography.

7. Which part of the skeleton is imaged to best demonstrate completion of ossification?
   a. lateral skull
   b. PA wrist of teenager
   c. iliac bone
   d. AP knee of infant

8. Which of the following would *not* reduce radiation dosage to the patient during a scoliosis study?
   a. PA projection of the spine
   b. collimated lateral view of L5–S1 articulation
   c. computed digital radiography
   d. rare earth screens

CASE STUDY

A 24-year-old male athlete has had a series of injuries to his left knee and has been referred to the imaging department for assessment. Describe the critical pathway that would be prescribed to assess his condition. Include three different types of imaging and one nonimaging procedure. What special care must be taken with this patient? List some of the more common sports injuries that occur to the knee.

References and Recommended Reading

Andrew, E. R., Bydder, G., Grifiths, J., Iles, R., & Styles, P. (1990). *Clinical magnetic resonance imaging and spectroscopy.* Chichester, UK: Wiley.

Ballinger, P. W. (1995). *Merrill's atlas of radiographic positioning and radiologic procedures* (8th ed.). St. Louis: Mosby-Year Book.

Barnes, P. D., Brody, J. D., Jaramillo, Akbar, J. U., & Eman, J. B. (1993). Atypical ideopathic scoliosis, MR imaging evaluation. *Radiology, 186,* 247–253.

Berland, L. L. (1987). *Practical CT technology and techniques.* New York: Raven Press.

Berquist, T. H. (1990). MRI of the foot and ankle. *Seminars in Ultrasound, CT and MRI, 11(4),* 324–325.

Chapman, S., & Nakielny, R. (1993). *A guide to radiological procedures* (3rd ed.). London: Bailliere and Tindall.

Cope, C., Burke, D., & Meranze, S. (1990). *Atlas of interventional radiology.* Philadelphia: Lippincott.

Crues, J. V., Mink, J., Levy, T. L., et al. (1987). Meniscal tears of the knee. Accuracy of MRI Imaging. *Radiology, 164(2),* 445–448.

Dalinka, M. (1980). *Arthrography. Comprehensive manuals in radiology.* New York: Springer-Verlag.

Davies, A. M. (1991). The current role of computed tomographic arthrography of the shoulder. *Clinical Radiology, 44,* 369–375.

De Schepper, A. M. A., Degryse, H. R. M. (1989). *Magnetic resonance imaging of bone and soft tissue tumors and their mimics: a clinical atlas.* Dordrecht: Kluweer Academic Publishers.

Doyle, T., Hare, W., Thomson, K., & Tress, B. (1989). *Procedures in diagnostic radiology.* London: Churchill Livingstone.

Ensign, M .F. (1990) Magnetic resonance imaging of hip disorders. *Seminars in Ultrasound, CT and MRI, 11(4),* 288–306.

Eisenberg, R. L. (1992). *Radiology: An illustrated history.* St. Louis: Mosby-Year Book.

Eisenberg, R., & Dennis, C. (1990). *Comprehensive radiographic pathology.* St. Louis: Mosby.

Friedrich, J. M., Schnarkowski, P., Rubenacker, S., Wallner, B. (1993) Ultrasonography of capsular morphology in normal and traumatic ankle joints. *Journal of Clinical Ultrasound, 22*(3), 179–187

Fritz, R. C., & Stoller, D. W. (1992). Fat suppression MR arthrography of the shoulder. *Radiology, 185*(2), 614–615.

Gilula, L. A., & Palmer, A. K. (1993). Is it possible to diagnose a tear at arthrography or MR imaging? [Letter] *Radiology, 187*(2), 582.

Green, R. E., & Oestmann, J. W. (1992). *Computed digital radiography in clinical practice.* New York: Thieme Medical Publishers.

Griffiths, H. (1987). *Basic bone radiology.* Norwalk, Conn.: Appleton and Lange.

Grossman, L., Ellis, D., & Brigham, S. (1983). *The clinician's guides to diagnostic imaging.* New York: Raven Press.

Hodgson, K. (1993). Dual energy x-ray absorptiometry in the diagnosis and monitoring of post-menopausal osteoporosis. *Radiography Today, 59,* 677.

Kling, T. F. Jr., Cohen, M. J., Lindseth, R. E., & De Rosa, G.P. (1990). Digital radiography can reduce scoliosis x-ray exposure. *Spine, 15*(9), 880–885.

Kobayashi, S., & Takei, T. (1991). Venous air embolism during knee arthrography–A Case Report. *Archives of Orthopedic Trauma Surgery, 110*(6), 311–313.

Koster, G., Munz, D. L., & Kohler, H. P. (1993). Clinical value of combined contrast and radionuclide arthrography in suspected loosening of hip prosthesis. *Archives of Orthopedic Trauma Surgeries, 112*(5), 247–254.

Kulthanen, T., & Noiklang, P. (1993). Arthrography and arthrotomy of the knee in sports injuries. *British Journal of Sports Medicine, 27*(2), 87–89.

Lescreve, J. P., Van Tiggeln, R. P., & Lamoureux, J. (1989). Reducing the radiation dosage in patients with a scoliosis. *International Orthopedics, 13*(1), 47–50.

Lonstein, J. E. (1988). Natural history and school screening for scoliosis. *Orthopedic Clinics of North America 19*(2), 227–237.

Kreel, L., & Thornton, A. (1992). *Outline of medical imaging,* Oxford: Butterworth-Heinemann.

Manaster, B. J. (1990). Magnetic resonance imaging of the knee. *Seminars in Ultrasound, CT and MRI, 11*(4), 307–326.

Martensen, K. M. (1992). Alternate AP knee method assures open joint space. *Radiologic Technology, 64*(1), 19–23.

Miller, B. F., & Keane, C. B. (1983). *Encyclopedia and dictionary of medicine, nursing and allied health.* Philadelphia: Saunders.

Munk, P. L., Vellet, A. D., Levin, M. F., Romano, C. C., Lentle, B., & Bourne, B. B. (1994). Imaging after arthroplasty. *Canadian Association of Radiology, 45*(1), 6–15.

Nitzan, D. W., Dowick, F. M., Marmary, Y. (1991). The value of arthrography in the decision making process regarding surgery for internal derangement of the temporomandibular joint. *Journal of Oral Maxillofacial Surgery, 49*(4),

Pollei, S., & Schellhas, K. P. (1990). Magnetic resonance imaging of the temporomandibular joint. *Seminars in Ultrasound, CT and MRI, 11*(4), 346–361.

Pope, T. L. (1994). MRI of knee ligaments. *Seminars in Ultrasound, CT and MRI, 15*(5), 366–382.

Roatikainen, T., & Puranen, J. (1993). Arthrography for the diagnosis of acute lateral ligament injuries of the ankle. *American Journal of Sports Medicine, 21*(3), 343–347.

Resnick, D., & Pettersson, H. (1992). Skeletal Radiology. *NICER Series on Diagnostic Imaging.* London: Merit Communications.

Saxton, H. M., & Strickland, B. (1972). *Practical procedures in diagnostic radiology,* New York: Grune & Stratton.

Seeram, E. (1994). *Computed tomography. Physical properties, clinical applications and quality control.* Philadelphia: Saunders.

Snopek, A. M. (1992). *Fundamentals of special radiographic Procedures* (3rd ed.). Philadelphia: Saunders.

Stiles, R. G., Resnick, D., Sartoris, D. J., & Andre, M. P. (1988). Rotator cuff disruption: Diagnosis with digital arthrography. *Radiology, 168,* 705–707.

Sutton, D. A. (1993). *Textbook of radiology and imaging.* Edinburgh: Churchill Livingstone.

Timmerman, L. A., Schwartz, M. L., & Andrews, J. R. (1994). Pre-operative evaluation of the ulnar collateral ligament by magnetic resonance imaging and computed tomography arthrography. Evaluation in 25 baseball players with surgical confirmation. *American Journal of Sports Medicine, 22*(1), 26–31.

Watkins, G., & Moore, T. (1993). *Atypical orthopedic radiographic procedures.* St. Louis: Mosby-Year Book.

Weissman, B., & Sledge, C. B. (1986). *Orthopedic Radiology.* Philadelphia: Saunders.

Wojtowycz, M. (1995). *Interventional radiology and angiography, handbooks in radiology.* St. Louis: Mosby-Year Book.

SECTION III

DIGESTIVE SYSTEM

CHAPTER **4**

Gastrointestinal System

PATRICIA MCDONALD, MRT(R)
CYNTHIA COWLING, BSc, MEd, MRT(R), ACR

OBJECTIVES

At the completion of this chapter, the student should be able to:

1. List the procedures used in the diagnostic studies of the GI system.
2. Identify the major features of the anatomy of the GI system.
3. Describe the procedures used to demonstrate certain pathologies and anatomy.
4. Identify relevant equipment for each study and procedure.
5. Describe the types of contrast media used for each procedure.
6. Identify radiation protection methods used.
7. Describe the relevant procedure sequences.
8. List common pathologies visualized for each examination and procedure.
9. Describe the basic concepts of alternative imaging routines.
10. Discuss the benefits and problems of the various imaging modalities in the visualization of the GI system.
11. Describe the main radiologic interventions used to assist in the treatment of GI pathologies.

Introduction and Historical Overview

Examination of the GI tract began shortly after the discovery of x-rays and the first documented study was in March of 1896. However, although it became relatively easy to radiograph the tract (usually by using bismuth), it was generally uncomfortable and tedious for the patient and the equipment used was extremely primitive. Rubber hoses and egg-beater-like instruments were introduced into the stomach to distribute the bismuth. Operators spent long periods close to fluoroscopy screens watching the peristaltic movements of the tract and there were many reported cases of radiation burns and acute leukemia among the pioneers of these studies. During the early years of the 20th century there was an ongoing discussion on the merits of fluoroscopy or radiography and it was not until 1917 that fluoroscopy was determined to be the superior way of demonstrating the stomach and intestines. In 1919, more than 50,000 fluoroscopic examinations were carried out at The Mayo Clinic. A radiologist at the clinic was one of the first to recommend the use of protective aprons and gloves. In the 1920s, barium sulfate gradually became the contrast medium of choice and it was not until the 1950s that water-soluble contrast was used in some pathologic conditions.

The newer modalities have become increasingly important during the last few years. The noninvasive nature of ultrasound makes it the modality of choice for infants and children. CT is extensively used for staging tumors and visualizing other lesions and MRI will gradually play a larger role in the imaging of this entire area.

The roles of radiology, surgery, and internal medicine have become blurred as the use of radiology as a therapeutic tool becomes more evident. Conditions previously requiring surgery have been replaced by endoscopic and **percutaneous** (pĕr′′kū-tā′nē-ŭs) procedures. A patient today is just as likely to have a procedure in a gastric imaging center that not only demonstrates a pathology but that also helps to treat the condition.

Anatomy

The digestive system consists of the primary and secondary organs of digestion. The primary organs consist of a long muscular tube that begins at the lips and ends at the anal canal. The secondary or accessory organs of digestion are the salivary glands, liver, gallbladder, and pancreas, which all empty their excretions into the primary tube (Figure 4.1).

PRIMARY ORGANS

The mouth or oral cavity is bounded anteriorally by the lips, the floor by the tongue, and the roof by the hard palate and opens into the oral pharynx through the fauces. The esophagus is a muscular tube that originates at the laryngopharynx, extends through the esophageal hiatus of the diaphragm to the cardiac end of the stomach. Its venous drainage at the inferor end is into the splenic vein.

The stomach is located in the epigastric region of the abdomen, connected at its proximal end to the esophagus and at the distal, or pyloric end, to the duodenum. The passage of the gastric contents to the duodenum is regulated by the pyloric sphincter (Figure 4.2).

The small intestine consists of three separate divisions. The *duodenum* extends from the pyloric sphincter to the jejunum. It is a C-shaped structure that extends a total of about 12 inches. The second part receives the ampulla of Vater, formed by the union of ducts from the liver and the main pancreatic duct. The *jejunum* and *ileum* (small intestine) extend from the duodenum to the cecum of the large intestine where the ileum combines with the cecum to form the ileocecal valve.

The *large bowel* extends from the cecum to the anus. It consists of the ascending colon, hepatic flexure, descending colon, and rectum (Figure 4.3).

SECONDARY ORGANS

The salivary glands consist of the bilateral parotid (pă-rŏt′ĭd), and submandibular and sublingual glands. Salivary amylase from the first two glands enters the mouth through Stenson's and Wharton's ducts.

The liver and gallbladder are the site of bile formation. The gallbladder stores and concentrates the bile. All bile is collected in bile ducts, which empty into the hepatic ducts, which pass to the right of the cystic duct. The common bile duct proceeds from the cystic duct to the duodenum.

The pancreas is a soft gland consisting of a head, body, and tail. The head lies in the loop of the duodenum, the body behind the stomach, and the tail next

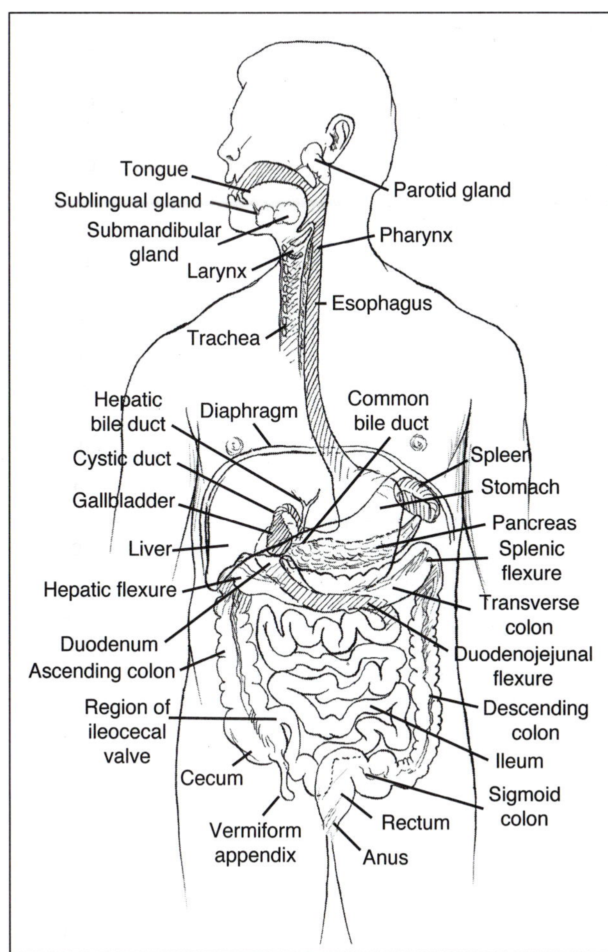

FIGURE 4.1 Anatomy of the digestive system.

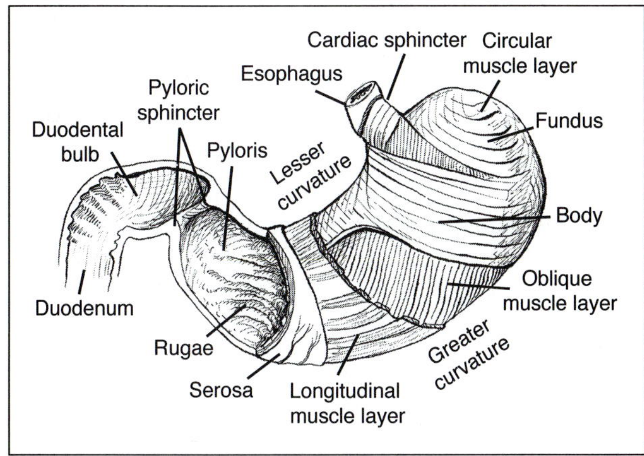

FIGURE 4.2 Anatomy of the stomach.

to the spleen. The pancreatic duct runs transversely from the tail to the head to enter the duodenum with the common bile duct as the ampulla of Vater or pancreatoduodenal duct (Figure 4.4).

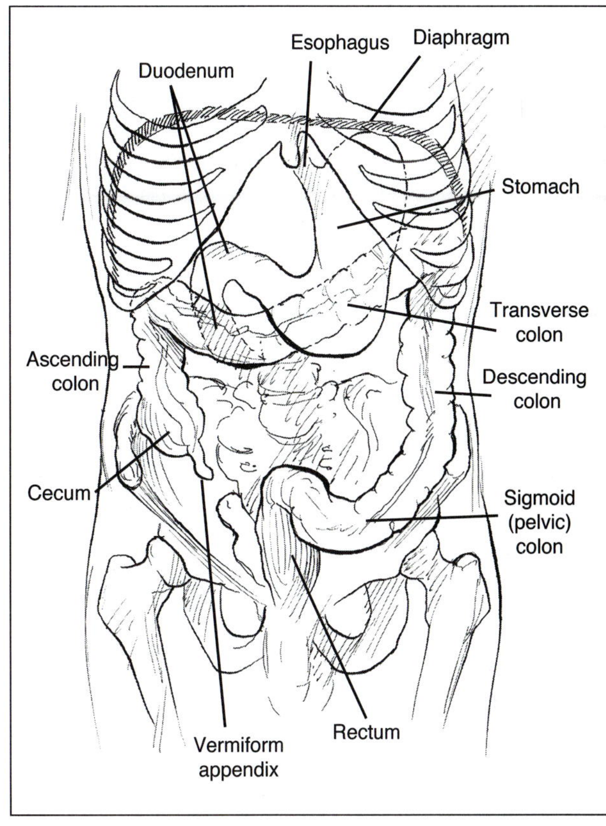

FIGURE 4.3 Anatomy of the large bowel.

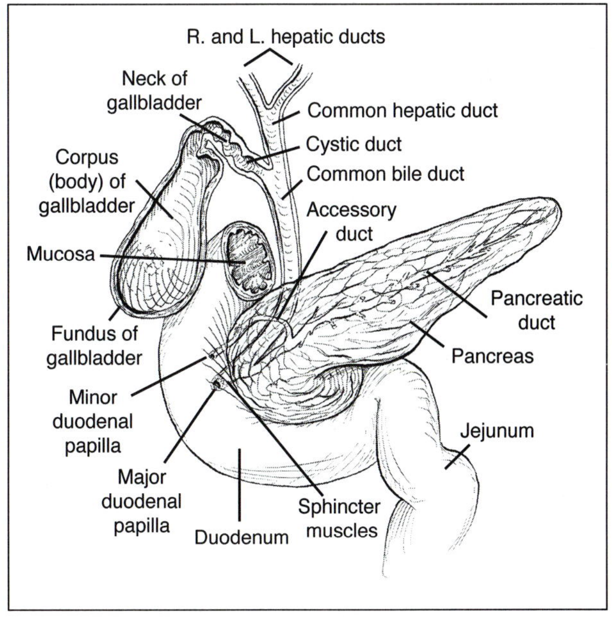

FIGURE 4.4 Anatomy of the duodenum.

Procedures

SIALOGRAPHY

Sialography (sī′′ă-lŏg′ră-fē) is the radiologic examination of the ducts of the salivary glands, after contrast media has been injected into these ducts. Although there are three pairs of salivary glands (the parotid, submandibular, and sublingual), the sublingual is not generally investigated in this way because the ducts are not easily cannulated.

Applied Anatomy Figure 4.5.

Indications

- Ductal obstruction due to stones within the duct (sialolithiasis)
- Ductal obstruction due to tumor or other extrinsic factors
- Inflammation of a duct (sialodenitis) or gland (sialodochitis)

Contraindications

- Severe infection of the glands
- Known allergies to contrast media

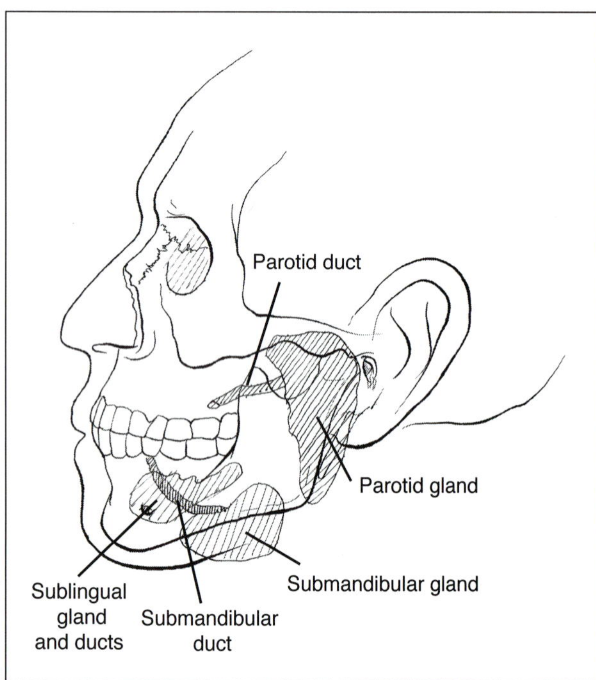

FIGURE 4.5 Anatomy of the salivary glands.

Equipment

- Ideally, a fluoroscopy unit with C-arm, magnification capabilities, and filming device
- Cannula for introduction of contrast (silver needle, angiocath, Lowman needle)
  —Connecting tubing
  —Dilators for duct
  —5-mL syringe
  —Overhead lamp
  —Gauze
  —Tape (to stabilize the connecting tubing)
  —Lemon wedge, lemon juice, or commercial mouthwash

Contrast Media Oily contrast medium provides a denser image, but for a normal study a water-soluble contrast medium such as Renografin is used.

Radiation Protection

- Fluoroscopy time kept to a minimum
- Gonadal and thyroid shielding

Preliminary Radiographs These can be taken if there is a suspected calculus. If not, a fluoroscopic scan will provide sufficient information.

1. Parotid
   - AP/posteroanterior(PA) projection of the mandibular ramus on the affected side
   - Lateral view of the affected side
2. Submandibular
   - AP/PA projection of the mandibular area on the affected side
   - Lateral view of the affected side
   - Lateral oblique view of the affected side
   - Occlusal (infrasuperior intraoral)

Patient Preparation

- The patient should be made aware of the discomfort of the procedure, because there is a sense of pressure when the contrast medium is injected.
- Dentures and any opaque items from the head and neck region, such as hairpins and jewelry, should be removed.
- Consent must be signed.

Procedure Sequence

- The patient is positioned supine on the radiologic table with the head resting comfortably on a radiolucent sponge. The head should be tilted back with the chin raised.
- An overhead lamp may be used to better illuminate the area of interest.
- The connecting tubing is joined to the cannula, and air in tubing is expelled after being connected to the syringe that contains the contrast medium.
- The duct being examined is located and cannulated (dilators may be needed to open up orifice of duct).
- Once the duct is cannulated, the patient is instructed to gently close the mouth (this holds the cannula in place).
- The connecting tubing may then be taped to the patient's cheek, out of the field of view.
- Under fluoroscopic guidance, a small amount of contrast media is then injected to ensure the cannula is in place and the duct in question is being filled.
- Radiographs are taken in various projections by either rotation of the C-arm or by the turning of the patient's head, while the contrast medium is being injected (approximately 1–2 mL or until entire duct is visualized).
- After the appropriate views are obtained with contrast medium within the duct, the cannula is removed and the patient is given lemon juice or mouthwash to rinse out the mouth (this act should expel contrast from the duct).
- Further radiographs are taken of the duct if retained contrast medium is seen under fluoroscopy.

Procedure Radiographs

- AP/PA projections, lateral and oblique views are done at the radiologist's discretion under fluoroscopic control after contrast has been injected into the duct and the duct under examination is entirely visualized (Figure 4.6).
- A tangential projection is sometimes taken with the the head in the AP position and slightly rotated away from the affected side and the central ray at right angles to the mandible.
- AP/PA projection is taken after the patient has sucked on the lemon to show how contrast has been expelled from the duct.

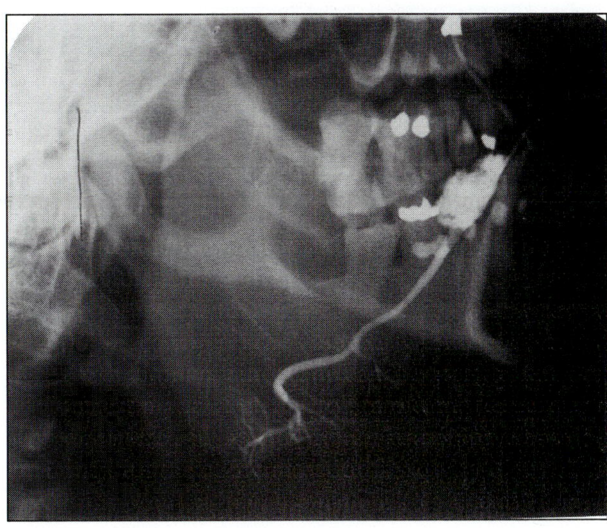

FIGURE 4.6 Submandibular sialogram.

Postprocedure Care

- Patients should be informed that they may have localized swelling for a few days after the procedure.
- The patient is encouraged to suck a lemon occasionally if contrast is retained in the gland.
- A warm cloth against the affected side may ease the discomfort.

Common Pathologies

- Sialolithiasis
- Sialodochitis
- Sialodenitis

SINOGRAM/FISTULOGRAM

This procedure is performed to locate and demonstrate the extent of a **sinus** or fistulous tract and its connection to any cavity or hollow viscera. This can be done by an injection of contrast media through an **orifice** on the abdominal wall or through a drainage tube already placed into the orifice.

Applied Anatomy The sinus or fistula can be present in any section of the GI tract.

Indications As indicated by clinical history

Contraindications None

Equipment

- Fluoroscopic unit with a spot film device /105 mm cine
- Fine catheter
- 20-mL syringe
- Blunt needle
- Gauze padding (4 × 4)

Contrast Media

- Water-soluble contrast
- If there is any suggestion that there is a connection with the pleural cavity, an oil-based contrast medium such as Dionosil is used.

Radiation Protection

- Gonadal shielding
- Minimum fluoroscopic time
- Appropriate collimation on tract and cavity site

Preliminary Radiographs AP projection (scout view) can be taken, centered over the cavity site before injection of contrast medium.

Patient Preparation None required

Procedure Sequence

- The patient is placed on the table so that the orifice of the sinus is easily accessible to the radiologist.
- The technologist removes the dressing and fills syringe with the contrast medium.
- A blunt needle is attached to the end of syringe.
- The filled syringe is attached to the catheter, which is then inserted into opening of sinus.
- Under fluoroscopic control, an AP projection is taken immediately before injection (Figure 4.7).
- A pad of gauze is placed over the orifice and the patient is asked to firmly place a gloved finger on the gauze. This should prevent a reflux of contrast medium back onto the skin.
- The contrast medium is injected under fluoroscopic guidance, the amount depending on the size of the sinus or fistula.
- Radiographs are taken as required by the radiologist (usually AP projection, both oblique views and a lateral view) (Figure 4.8).
- At the completion of the examination, the catheter is removed and a fresh sterile dressing is placed over the opening.

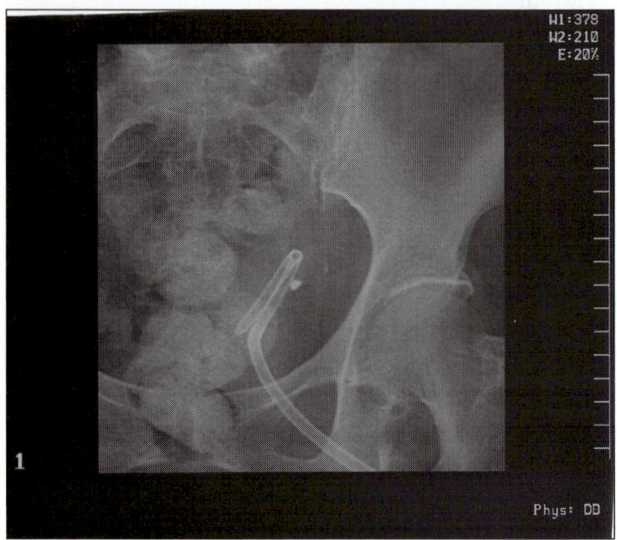

FIGURE 4.7 Catheter in place in fistula.

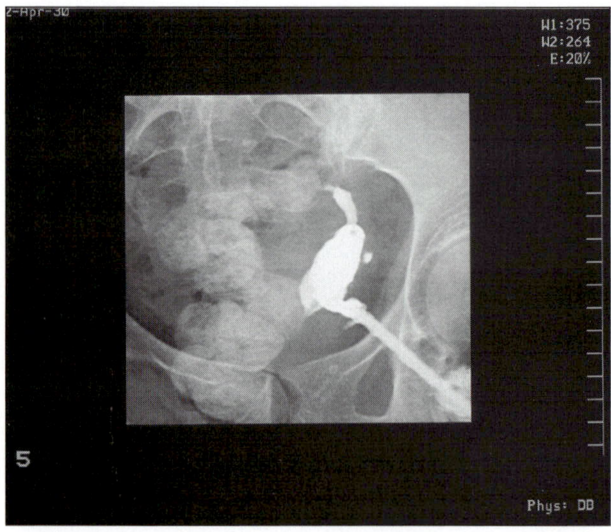

FIGURE 4.8 Sinogram with contrast medium.

NOTE: If patient already has a catheter in place, the injection is made through existing catheter and radiographs are taken of cavity size.

Postprocedure Care None specific to the procedure

LOOPOGRAM: COLOSTOMY INJECTION STUDY VIA STOMA

This examination demonstrates the large bowel proximal to a colostomy by the injection of a contrast medium through a **colostomy.**

Applied Anatomy See Figure 4.9.

Indications

- Perforation
- Obstruction
- Bleeding from **stoma**

Contraindications This examination is not recommended after recent colostomy surgery (1–2 weeks).

Equipment

- Fluoroscopic unit with spot film device
- Foley catheter
- Empty barium enema bag
- Clamp
- Gauze (4 × 4)

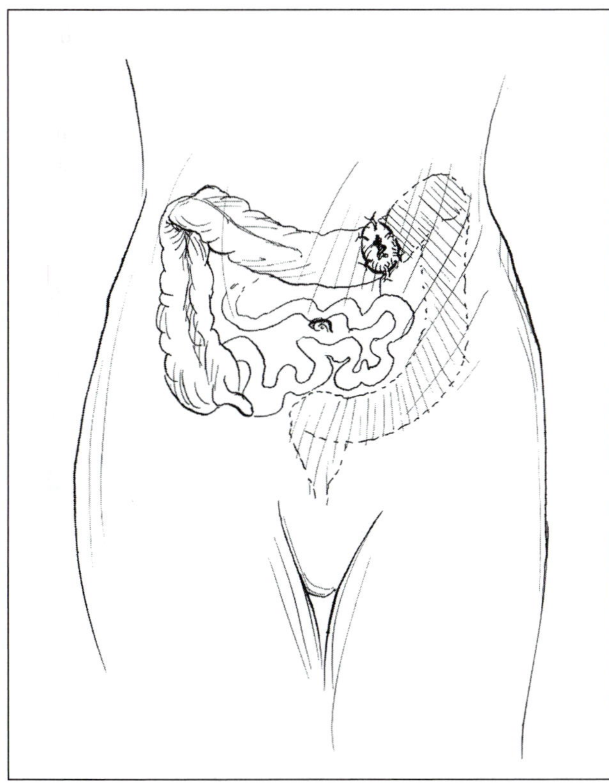

FIGURE 4.9 Example of colostomy.

Contrast Media Barium sulfate or a water-soluble contrast. If there is a suspicion of a perforation, a water-soluble contrast medium must be used.

Radiation Protection Fluoroscopic time kept to a minimum

Patient Preparation

- The patient is kept on fluids only, 24 hours before procedure.
- In an emergency this procedure can be performed without any preparation.

Procedure Sequence

- The enema bag is filled with a diluted solution of barium sulfate (200 mL barium with 1100 mL water) with a clamp near the end of the tubing.
- A Foley catheter is attached to the end of the enema tubing and the bag is hung on an IV pole ready to use.
- The patient lies supine on the fluoroscopy table.
- The Foley catheter is gently inserted a few centimeters through the colostomy and the balloon is inflated carefully in the bowel under fluoroscopic control.
- If a leakage of contrast medium occurs around the colostomy site, the patient is asked to apply light pressure over the colostomy site with gloved fingers and a gauze pad.
- With the technologist controlling the speed of flow, the contrast medium is allowed to run in through the catheter.
- Radiographs are taken under fluoroscopic control as the barium runs through the bowel.
- An overhead AP projection of the filled bowel may be requested (Figure 4.10).
- A radiograph of the draining stoma is taken just after the catheter has been removed.
- The patient lies on his or her side and the barium is allowed to drain into a container.

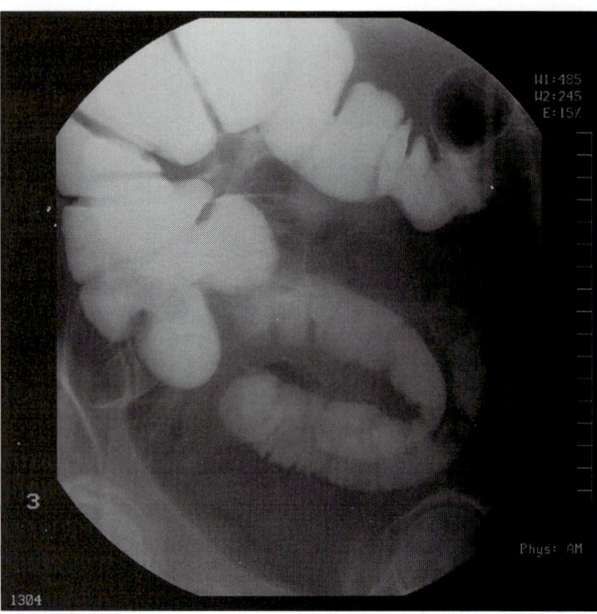

FIGURE 4.10 Loopogram.

- If no drainage views are required, then as much contrast as possible is drained back through the catheter into the bag.
- The catheter is then deflated and removed.

Postprocedure Care None specific to the procedure

HYPOTONIC DUODENOGRAM

This procedure demonstrates postbulbar duodenal lesions and pancreatic disease by **intubation** of the duodenum and use of **hypotonic** agents and contrast media.

Applied Anatomy The catheter is advanced via the esophagus and stomach into the bulb of the duodenum.

Indications

- This procedure is not frequently performed and is usually only done to demonstrate a tumor at the papilla of Vater.
- Duodenal lesions can be visualized.

Contraindications Presence of severe disease

Equipment

- Fluoroscopic unit with spot film device/105 mm cine
- Duodenal intubation tube (such as a small bowel enema tube) and guidewire
- Topical analgesia (anesthetic spray and gel)
- Hypotonic agent such as glucagon or Buscopan

Contrast Media Barium sulfate suspension

Radiation Protection Fluoroscopic time kept to a minimum

Patient Preparation Nothing to eat or drink after midnight before day of booking

Procedure Sequence

- The patient is seated in a chair or on top of the fluoroscopic table.
- The back of the throat and the inside of nostril is sprayed with a topical anesthetic spray to make passage of tube easier for patient and to lessen the gag reflex.
- The technologist should stand by patient's side to comfort the patient while the tube is being inserted because this is an uncomfortable procedure.
- The lower end of tube can also be coated with anesthetic gel.
- The tube is inserted transorally or transnasally into the pharynx.
- The patient is instructed to sip water through a straw as the tube is passed through the pharynx and esophagus into the stomach. This helps the tube to travel through the GI tract.
- The patient is placed supine once the tube has reached the stomach.

- A flexible guidewire is inserted into the tube and with fluoroscopic guidance carefully manipulated through the pylorus.
- The tube is advanced to the transverse duodenum and the guidewire is removed.
- The tube is secured to the side of the patient's nose with a piece of adhesive tape to keep it in position.
- The radiologist administers an intramuscular injection of Buscopan or glucagon (or any other chosen hypotonic agent) to stop the peristaltic movement of the duodenum.
- Within 3 or 4 minutes duodenal paralysis is obtained and the patient remains in this condition for about 20 minutes. A double-contrast examination of the duodenum can now be obtained without interference of peristaltic movement.
- The patient is turned onto the right side and about 100 mL of a barium mixture is injected through the tube.
- The patient then rotates into a supine left posterior oblique position and 150 mL air is injected through the tube.
- After the injection of barium and air, the radiologist takes the required radiographs under fluoroscopic guidance.
- The tube is removed at the completion of the examination.

Procedure Radiographs

- Spot films with compression on the abdomen are taken with the patient in a supine position. The compression prevents the contrast medium from moving into the small bowel.
- Right and left posterior oblique views are taken.

Postprocedure Care None specific to the procedure

Common pathologies

- Duodenal ulcers
- Duodenal strictures
- Pathologic duodenal indentations caused by other structures closely related to the duodenum (gallbladder, common bile duct, pancreas, parts of the liver)

With the introduction of more popular methods such as ultrasound, CT, endoscopy, and percutaneous transhepatic cholangiography to evaluate the duodenum, pancreas, and common bile duct, hypotonic duodenography is rarely used today.

ANGIOGRAPHY

(Covered in Chapter 7, Heart and Arterial System)

Other Imaging Modalities

COMPUTED TOMOGRAPHY

CT can be used extensively to demonstrate the small and large bowel in particular. Dilute barium or Gastrografin is frequently used to enhance the bowel loops providing no pathology is present that would contraindicate using contrast medium. It can also be used to visualize the salivary glands if a tumor is suspected and can be performed after the contrast medium has been injected. CT can also be used to determine the point of entry for biopsy needles, percutaneous catheters, and so on, but the less invasive choice of ultrasound is often preferred (Figure 4.11).

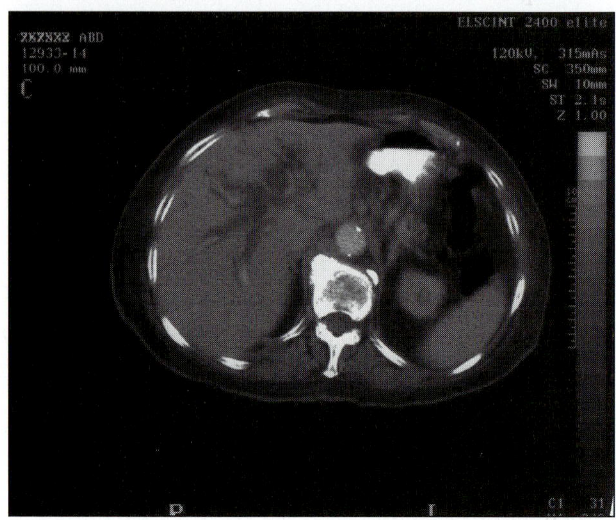

FIGURE 4.11 CT with contrast in the stomach.

MAGNETIC RESONANCE IMAGING

MRI of the digestive system is still in the development stages and therefore not considered a primary imaging modality for diagnosis of pathology in the GI tract.

Abdominal studies in MRI are limited because, despite many evaluations for an oral contrast agent to outline the GI tract in MRI images, no product has been approved for commercial sale. In the next few years continual research in this area should produce several different classes of contrast agents for clinical use.

The advent of the open concept magnet has encouraged research in the use of MR imaging for interventional procedures.

ULTRASOUND

Ultrasound has become one of the primary modalities used in many interventional procedures done today. It is used for both diagnostic and therapeutic purposes.

Some procedures, such as a biopsy, use only ultrasound for imaging during the procedure and can be done strictly in an ultrasound room. Other procedures, such as an abscess drainage, combine the use of a portable ultrasound machine and a fluoroscopic unit. The ultrasound image is essential for needle puncture and guidance into the cavity and fluoroscopy for guidewire and catheter placement.

Esophageal and stomach varices can be demonstrated by using a transcutaneous epigastric approach. It is possible to determine the layers of the stomach using this modality. Esophageal varices can also be demonstrated by using color Doppler ultrasound. The small and large bowel are occasionally examined to visualize significant malignancies. Ultrasound would generally be used in conjunction with other imaging modalities for most of the GI tract.

RADIONUCLIDE IMAGING

Radionuclide imaging is used extensively in the GI tract. It can be used to study GI reflux. A technetium colloid is mixed with orange juice or milk. The patient lies down and is scanned with the gamma camera. In adults, a compression band can be applied to the upper abdominal region to determine the effect of pressure on the cardiac sphincter area.

Radionuclides can be used to determine the rate of emptying from the stomach, but the variables that can affect this study, such as stomach contents, fat level, position of the patient, type of radionuclide, have made this a somewhat unreliable study, difficult to reproduce on the same patient.

Radionuclide imaging is the definitive imaging modality to demonstrate Meckel's diverticulum in children. A specific radionuclide, a pertechnetate, is used and administered IV as the patient lies beneath the gamma camera. Images are taken every 5 minutes up to 1 hour after administration. This study confirms whether a Meckel's diverticulum is the source of pain or bleeding in the GI region.

Gastric bleeding can often be first detected by an IV injection of a radionuclide and the imaging of activity in the abdominal area. Any increased activity could be a sign of gastric bleeding. Definitive positioning would then need to be performed using angiography.

Interventional Procedures

BALLOON DILATATION OF ESOPHAGUS

This procedure is done to eliminate strictures in the esophagus by dilatation with a balloon catheter.

Applied Anatomy See Figure 4.12.

Indications Narrowing in esophagus resulting from esophageal tumors, peptic strictures, or anastomatic strictures

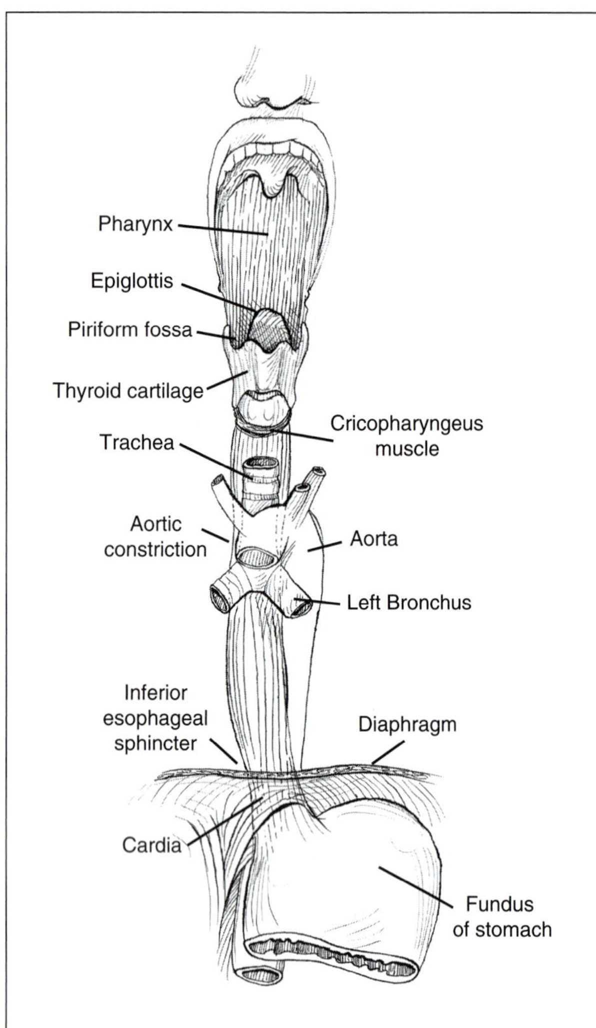

FIGURE 4.12 Anatomy of esophagus.

Contraindications Tracheoesophageal fistulas

Equipment

- Fluoroscopic unit with a spot film device
- Small bowel enema tube or nasogastric tube with a long flexible guidewire
- Balloon catheter (size of balloon varies with size of stricture)
- Mouthpiece (optional)
- Topical anesthetic spray

Contrast Media Water-soluble contrast medium

Radiation Protection

- Gonadal shielding
- Fluoroscopy kept to a minimum

Preliminary Radiographs Previous barium swallow demonstrating the esophagus

Patient Preparation

- The patient should have nothing to eat or drink for 6 hours before procedure.
- This procedure can be performed on an outpatient basis, but the patient should be admitted to a day bed unit in the hospital for preparation and postprocedure observation.
- An IV line is put in place before the procedure in case sedatives or **analgesics** need to be administered during the procedure.
- The patient is made aware of the procedure and asked to sign a consent form.

Procedure Sequence

- The patient is placed supine on table in a comfortable position.
- A sedative may be administered at this point if requested or if the patient shows signs of anxiety.
- The throat is sprayed with a topical anesthetic.
- A mouthpiece is put in place to make manipulation of catheter easier.
- With fluoroscopic guidance, the tube is then manipulated through mouthpiece and into the esophagus.

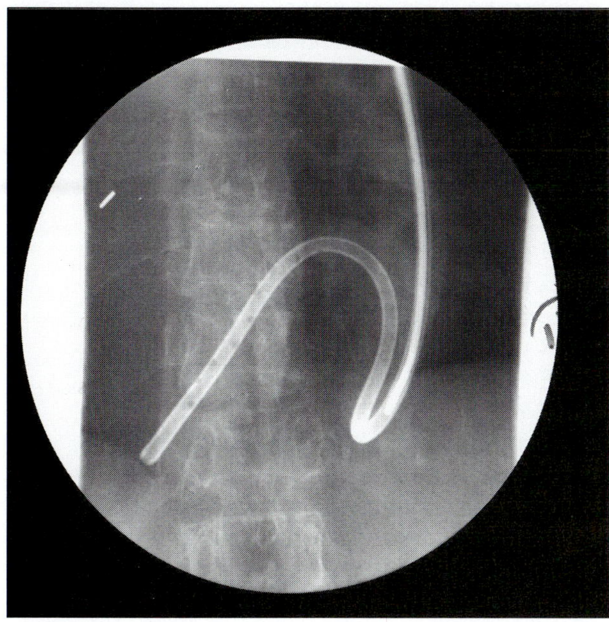

FIGURE 4.13 Catheter in place.

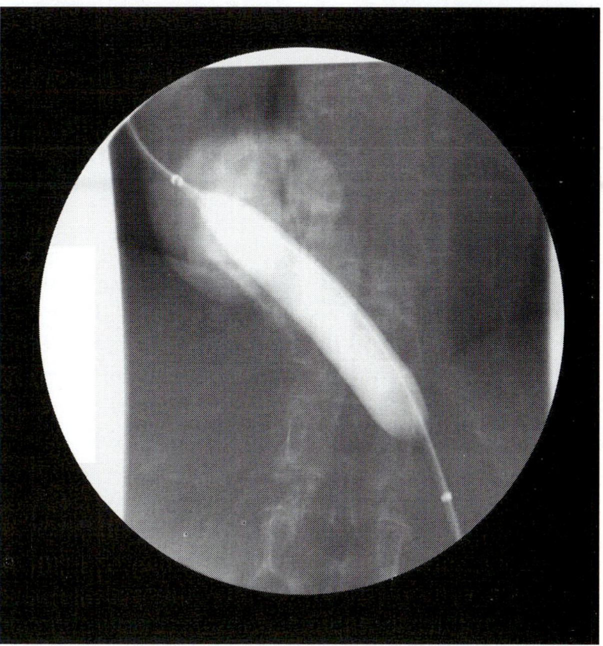

FIGURE 4.14 Balloon catheter inflated at stricture.

- Contrast medium may be injected to outline stricture area.
- A guidewire is inserted through the tube and manipulated beyond the stricture (Figure 4.13).
- The tube is then removed and the balloon dilatation catheter is passed over the guidewire.
- The balloon is positioned across the stricture and guidewire is removed.
- With a syringe filled with diluted contrast, the balloon is then inflated by hand until it appears fully inflated.
- It is left inflated for several minutes.
- Under fluoroscopic control, radiographs are taken of the inflated balloon to document position (Figure 4.14).
- If the stricture is very narrow it may be necessary to start with a very narrow balloon (6 mm) and gradually graduate to a larger balloon (up to 22 mm).
- After procedure is completed, the patient is moved onto a stretcher and returned to a day bed unit or room (if inpatient).

NOTE: This process is usually repeated on subsequent visits until the stricture is no longer apparent.

Postprocedure Care

- Vital signs should be taken at regular intervals for at least 4 hours after the procedure.
- The patient should have nothing to eat or drink for at least 4 hours after the procedure.
- The patient should be instructed to seek immediate help in an emergency department if he or she experiences a severe onset of pain after this procedure.

PERCUTANEOUS GASTROSTOMY AND JEJUNOSTOMY

This procedure involves the insertion of an enterostomy tube through the abdomen directly into the stomach and jejunum for the purpose of **enteral** feeding or decompression. This procedure is usually performed on patients with a functioning GI tract but who need long-term nutritional support or decompression. Traditionally this had been a surgical procedure requiring general anesthesia. However, since the early 1980s radiologists have been performing gastrostomy procedures in the diagnostic imaging department in a room equipped with fluoroscopic equipment and a portable ultrasound machine.

Applied Anatomy The catheter is introduced through the left upper quadrant of the abdomen and immediately into the stomach.

Indications

- For enteral nutrition
- **Dysphagia** caused by head and neck carcinoma, esophageal carcinoma, coma, dementia, trauma
- **Anorexia**
- For decompression
- Gastroparesis
- Paralytic ileus
- Mechanical obstruction in advanced malignancy

Contraindications

- Abnormal coagulation results (These should be corrected before procedure is attempted to reduce the risk of bleeding.)
- Gross **ascites** (ă-sī´tēz)
- Previous gastric surgery
- Enlarged liver with stomach lying below left lobe of liver
- Loops of large bowel lying between the skin and anterior wall of stomach

Equipment

- Fluoroscopic unit (preferably with a C-arm attachment) and hard copy image capabilities
- Portable ultrasound machine
- Basic sterile tray setup containing
  - 1 lap sheet
  - 6 green towels
  - 1 spinal towel
  - 1 small K basin containing
    - 2 medicine glasses, 1 for prep, 1 for hot water
    - 1 beaker, for local topical anesthetic
  - 1 medicine beaker for contrast
  - 2 small metal round basins
    - 1 for normal saline
    - 1 for drainage fluids
  - 1 each needles, 18, 22, and 25 gauge
  - 1 each forceps, artery, straight, curved
  - 1 nontoothed forceps
  - 1 knife handle
  - 1 needle driver
  - 1 pair of scissors
  - 1 #11 sterile blade
  - 4 × 4 gauze
- Puncture needle. Various needle sizes can be used ranging from 22 to 18 gauge. The usual choice is an 18-gauge, 15-cm two-part **trocar** needle.
- Straight guidewire (sometimes a stiffer wire such as an Amplatz is required)
- Dilators
- Feeding catheter. Various gastrostomy catheters are available ranging in size from 10.5 to 18 French. Usually a 12 French is used for initial placement and this can be replaced by a larger size when the need arises.

Contrast Media Water-soluble contrast medium

Radiation Protection

- Fluoroscopy time must be kept to a minimum.
- Because the radiologist is working close to the patient's skin surface, it is very important to use as much collimation as possible to prevent exposure to the hands.

Preliminary Radiographs

- A limited ultrasound study of the abdomen is performed with a portable machine in the procedure room. The patient is scanned while still on the stretcher to mark the inferior border of the liver. If the liver is enlarged and overlies the stomach, the procedure would be terminated at this stage.
- Fluoroscopy to localize transverse colon in AP and lateral projections

Patient Preparation

- The patient is generally admitted into the hospital as either an inpatient or day unit patient.
- IV access should be available in case IV sedation is required during the procedure.
- Recent coagulation results must be available before procedure.

- Patient must receive nothing by mouth (NPO) for at least 8 hours before the procedure.
- Informed consent must be signed by the patient or relative.
- A nasogastric tube should be placed into the stomach (this is needed for stomach distention during the procedure).

Procedure Sequence

- The patient is placed in a comfortable supine position such that the left side is accessible to the physician.
- The patient is prepped and draped in a sterile fashion.
- The physician determines the entry site (usually midbody of the stomach) and injects a local anesthetic into the skin and subcutaneous tissue.
- A small incision is made at the site with a scalpel.
- The needle (most popular choice is an 18-gauge, 15-cm two-part trocar needle) is inserted into the distended stomach using a sharp downward thrust and advanced until it is felt to move freely inside the stomach.
- Correct position of needle tip can also be confirmed by a small injection of contrast medium through the needle after removing the central trocar.
- A guidewire is then inserted through the needle into the stomach.
- If the tube is being used for decompression, the tract is dilated at this point and the final catheter is inserted.
- The guidewire is removed and the dressing applied.

Gastrojejunostomy

- Further manipulation of needle and guidewire is required.
- The needle shaft is angled toward the pylorus and a 0.038-inch (145-cm) straight guidewire is manipulated through the pylorus and the duodenojejunal flexure.
- The needle is removed and the tract is dilated to the size of the catheter being used.
- The feeding catheter is then inserted over the guidewire and advanced to the duodenal jejunal flexure.
- The guidewire can now be removed.
- The final position of the catheter is confirmed and documented by an injection of contrast into the catheter and a spot film taken.
- The catheter is then fixed to the skin and a dressing applied.

Postprocedure Care

- Vital signs are regularly assessed for 6 to 8 hours after the procedure.
- Development of any peritoneal signs should be carefully watched.
- The nasogastric tube can be removed after 24 hours.
- Feeding through gastrostomy tube can start in 24 hours and in 4 hours through jejunostomy tube.
- The patient should remain hospitalized overnight for observation after procedure is completed. (This may change in the near future as more interventional procedures are being done on an outpatient basis.)

Complications The following complications can arise after this procedure.

Major—frequency ranges from 0% to 6% of patients

- Peritonitis requiring laparotomy
- GI hemorrhage requiring transfusion
- Deep stomal infection
- External stomal infection
- Aspiration

Minor—frequency ranges from 4.4% to 15% of patients

- Superficial stomal infection
- Pneumoperitoneum
- Erosion of catheter through **viscus**

PERCUTANEOUS ABSCESS DRAINAGE

A catheter is inserted percutaneously for drainage of an intra-abdominal abscess or fluid collection. During the procedure a specimen of the fluid is usually collected and sent for laboratory analysis.

Applied Anatomy An abscess can develop in any fold of the peritoneum (Figure 4.15).

Indications

- Fever
- Persistent abdominal pain
- Presence of a fluid collection as demonstrated on ultrasound or CT

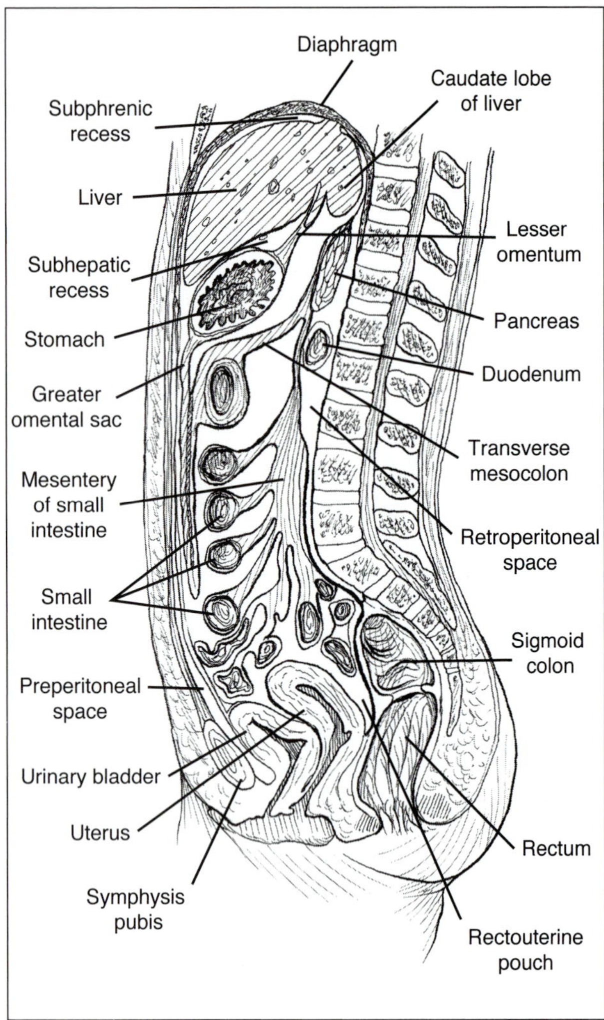

FIGURE 4.15 Folds of the peritoneum.

Contraindications

- Abnormal coagulation results
- Fluid and **electrolyte** depletion

Once these abnormalities are corrected, the drainage procedure can be performed. A safe access route in pelvic collections can sometimes be difficult because of surrounding bowel and adjacent organs. This would contraindicate the use of percutaneous catheter drainage in that area.

Equipment

- Portable ultrasound machine
- Fluoroscopic unit with hard copy capabilities
- Puncture needle (size varies depending on abscess size and location)
  - —Large collections—16-gauge sheathed needle
  - —Smaller collections—21-gauge needle
- Special needle that consists of a central 22-gauge needle with a stylet and a shorter outer 18-guage needle
- Catheter (selection depends on the size of collection, nature of the fluid, and margin of safety of the access route)
- For more viscous collections, a 12, 14, or 16 French catheter is necessary.
- For nonviscous fluid collection, an 8.3 or 10.3 French (pigtail) nephrostomy catheter can be used.
  - —0.038-inch 100-cm J-tipped guidewire
  - —Dilators
  - —Sterile tray setup
  - —Culture bottles
  - —Local anesthetic (lidocaine)

Contrast Media

- Water-soluble medium

Radiation Protection Fluoroscopy kept to a minimum

Preliminary Radiographs The area to be catheterized is scanned using sonography. In the pelvic area, because of the presence of other organs and fecal and air-filled bowel, CT is the modality of choice. These preliminary procedures demonstrate the presence of an abscess collection and help define its location and extent. This allows the radiologist to choose the most appropriate route and method of drainage.

Patient Preparation

- An informed consent must be signed by patient before any premedication is given.
- Patients are kept NPO 4 hours before procedure.
- Recent coagulation studies. Patients taking anticoagulants are temporarily taken off their anticoagulant before the drainage procedure to reduce the risk of bleeding.
- An IV line is put in place to allow for antibiotic therapy. The type of therpy depends on the etiology, position of the abscess, and condition of the patient.
- Premedication is given immediately before the start of the procedure.

Procedure Sequence

- This procedure is often performed using more than one imaging modality. Usually, the patient is asked to lie on the fluoroscopic table so that the site to be drained is easily accessible to the radiologist.
- The point of entry of the needle is determined by ultrasound scanning.
- The patient's abdomen is prepped and draped in a sterile fashion.
- The ultrasound probe is also draped with a sterile cover .
- The skin is injected with a local anesthetic.
- A small incision is made with a scalpel blade to accommodate the size of catheter being inserted.
- The angle and depth of insertion is determined by ultrasound or fluoroscopy (and sometimes CT) and the initial puncture is made with the inner 22-gauge needle.
- Under fluoroscopy a small amount of contrast is injected to confirm the needle position within the abscess.
- Once the needle is inserted into the collection, diagnostic aspiration is performed, the aspirated fluid evaluated, and samples sent for routine Gram stain and culture, as well as chemistry or cytology when indicated.
- A diagnostic sinogram using contrast media to determine the extent of the abscess should *not* be performed at the initial drainage stage because this could cause further complications.
- A fine J-tipped guidewire is then passed through the 18-gauge needle and carefully coiled into the cavity.
- The needle is removed and the tract dilated to the size of catheter being used.
- The catheter is then passed over the guidewire and into the cavity and the guidewire removed.
- At this point a sinogram can be performed and contrast medium is injected to outline the size and extent of cavity and to demonstrate any commications with the alimentary tract.
- At this point, as much **purulent** (pūr′ū-lĕnt) fluid as possible should be removed from the abscess.
- The catheter is then attached to a drainage bag and a dressing applied to hold catheter in place.

Postprocedure Care

- The patient is kept under observation as an inpatient and vital signs are regularly assessed for at least 24 hours.
- Antibiotic therapy is continued postprocedure.
- A sinogram is usually scheduled about 2 days after initial drainage to assess the condition of the abscess.
- When drainage from the abscess greatly decreases or ceases altogether, the patient is brought back for reassessment, either by fluoroscopy or by CT scanning, to determine the size of the cavity.
- If lack of drainage is due to tube blockage, the tube is changed (sometimes to a larger size if needed).
- If the abscess appears empty and the abscess well reduced in size, the tube is then removed and a sterile dressing placed over the wound.
- Complications to this procedure can include bleeding and sepsis.

Review Questions

1. Name the three pairs of salivary glands and give two reasons for performing a sialography procedure.

2. What would be a contraindication for using a barium sulfate solution to demonstrate the large bowel?

3. List three important patient preparations for any interventional special procedure.

4. In an abscess drainage procedure
   a. What three different modalities can be used?
   b. How does each one benefit the procedure?

5. Describe the way in which radiology of the GI tract has moved from diagnostic procedures to primary therapeutic procedures.

6. Percutaneous gastrostomy:
   a. requires a catheter introduced into the right upper quadrant of the abdomen
   b. always requires a general anesthetic
   c. is performed in patients with a paralytic ileus
   d. uses barium sulfate to outline the stomach

7. Which of the following is incorrect regarding the imaging of the GI tract?
   a. ultrasound can visualize esophageal varices
   b. MRI is the ideal modality for visualizing all sections of the GI tract
   c. meckel's diverticulum is best seen using radionuclide imaging
   d. barium sulfate is sometimes used with CT imaging of the GI tract

CASE STUDY

An elderly man is admitted to the emergency department complaining of a sudden onset of pain and blood in his stool. Suggest the imaging modalities used to determine his condition and state their priority.

References and Recommended Reading

Bell, S. D., Carmody, E. A., Yeung, E. Y., Thurston, W. A., Simons, M. E., Ho, C. S. (1945) Percutaneous gastrostomy and gastrojejunostomy: additional experience in 519 procedures. *Radiology 194*(3), 817–820.

Chapman, S., & Nakielny, R. (1993). *A guide to radiological procedures* (3rd ed.).London: Balliere Tindall.

Cope, C., Burke, D. R., & Meranze, S. (1990). *Atlas of interventional radiology.* Philidelphia: Lippincott.

Eisenberg, R. (1992). *Radiology, an illustrated history.* St. Louis: Mosby-Year Book.

Levine, M. S., Dachman, A. H. (1991). *Radiology of the esophagus.* Gastroenterology Clinicals of North America, *20*(4), 635–638.

Margulis, A. R., & Burhene, H. J. (1989). *Alimentary tract radiology* (4th ed.). St. Louis: Mosby.

Matzinger, F., Ho, C. S., Yee, A., & Gray, R. (1988). Pancreatic pseudocysts drained through a percutaneous transgastric approach: Further experience. *Radiology, 167*(2), 434–437.

Patten, R. M., Lo, S. K., Phillips, J. J., et al. (1993). Positive bowel contrast agent for MR imaging of the abdomen: Phase II and III clinical trials. *189*(1), 277–283.

Rainer, Ch. O., & Higgins, C. B. (1986). *New developments in imaging.* New York: Thieme.

Stark, D. D., & Bradley, W. G. (1992). *Magnetic resonance imaging* (Vol. 2). St. Louis: Mosby-Year Book.

Yeung, E. Y., & Ho, C. S. (1993). Percutaneous radiologic drainage of pelvic abscess. *Annals of the Academy of Medicine, 22*(5) 663–669.

CHAPTER 5

Hepatobiliary System

DENNIS A. BAIR, AS, RT (R)(CV)(ARRT)
PAMELA BONNERT, RDMS

OBJECTIVES

At the completion of this chapter, the student should be able to:

1. Describe the procedures used in the studies of the hepatobiliary system.
2. Describe the normal anatomy of the hepatobiliary system.
3. List the major indications and contraindications to procedures performed on the hepatobiliary system.
4. List the complications of the procedures performed.
5. Identify the relevant equipment.
6. List relevant contrast media types.
7. Identify relevant radiation protection methods used.
8. List relevant radiographs/images for each procedure.
9. Describe relevant patient preparation.
10. Describe relevant procedural sequences.
11. List alternate radiographs/images.
12. Describe relevant postprocedure care.
13. List common pathologies of the hepatobiliary system.
14. Identify other relevant imaging modalities.
15. Describe basic concepts of relevant alternative imaging routines.
16. Describe relevant interventional procedures.

Introduction and Historical Overview

According to Greek mythology, Prometheus stole fire from the gods and gave it to man. Zeus had Prometheus chained to the side of Mount Caucasus in punishment, where a vulture fed daily on his liver. Each day, Prometheus's liver would grow back only to be consumed again. It may have been the first recorded percutaneous approach to the liver.

Imaging of the hepatobiliary system dates back to 1924 when Graham and Cole reported radiographic visualization of the gallbladder. The first operative cholangiogram was performed in 1932 by Mirizzi. Postoperative or T-tube cholangiography soon followed. The technique of percutaneous transhepatic cholangiography (PTHC) was developed for direct nonoperative or postoperative visualization and evaluation of the hepatobiliary system. It was first described by Burkhardt and Mueller in 1921. The technique caused frequent complications and was reserved for presurgical evaluation before a planned surgical intervention. In 1974, Okuda developed a thin, flexible 22-gauge needle that significantly reduced the rate of complication during PTHC. PTHC is now often performed in conjunction with percutaneous biliary drainage (PBD).

Anatomy

The hepatobiliary system includes the liver, gallbladder, and ducts that carry the **bile** from the liver and gallbladder to the second part of the duodenum (Figure 5.1).

Bile is produced by the hepatic cells of the liver. The bile enters canaliculi (kăn′′ă-lĭk-ū-lī) to drain into bile ducts at the periphery of each liver lobule. The bile is ultimately collected into the right and left hepatic ducts, which emerge from the right and left lobes of the liver at the porta hepatis.

These two ducts unite to form the common hepatic duct from which arises the cystic duct after a distance of 3 to 4 cm. The cystic ducts convey bile from the common hepatic duct to the gallbladder where it is stored and concentrated.

Below the cystic duct the common bile duct curves posterior to the duodenum to combine with the main pancreatic duct to form the ampulla of Vater (hepatopancreatic ampulla). The ampulla opens into the descending (second) part of the duodenum, its orifice protected by the sphincter of Oddi.

The spincter will relax (open) when fatty gastric acid contents enter the duodenum. In response to chyme (kīm), the hormone cholescystokinin, released from duodenal cells, will elicit contraction of the gallbladder and opening of the sphincter of Oddi. This action is supplemented by the vagus nerve.

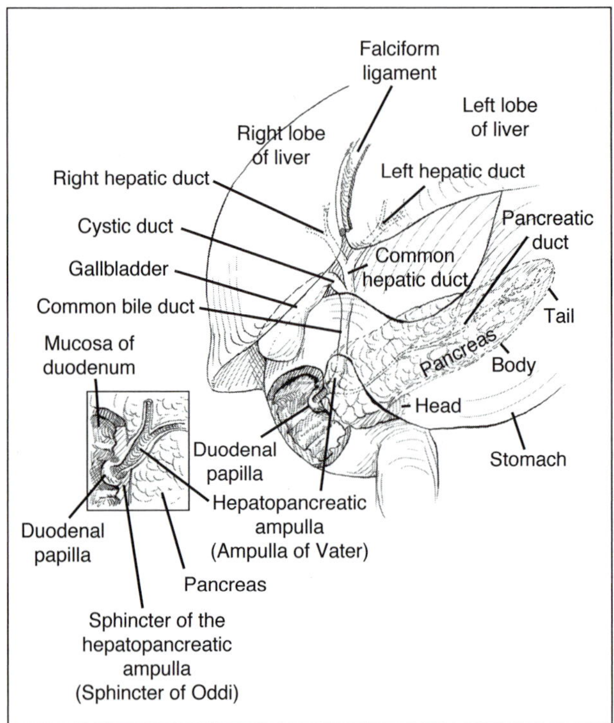

FIGURE 5.1 Normal anatomy of the biliary system.

Procedures

OPERATIVE CHOLANGIOGRAPHY

Operative cholangiography is performed in the operating suite to visualize the biliary tree after surgical intervention has been done. A small catheter is placed intraductally through the cystic duct remnant and contrast medium is injected.

Indications

- Patients undergoing surgical removal of the gallbladder for relief of **cholelithiasis** (kō´´lē-lĭ-thī´ă-sĭs)
- Operative extraction of **choledocholithiasis** (kō-lĕd´´ō-kō-lĭ-thī´ă-sĭs)

Contraindications Contrast media allergies—reactions are rare but possible.

Equipment

- Conventional portable x-ray unit with grid-cassette film or conventional C-arm with spot film device
- All other equipment supplied by surgical team

Contrast Media 60% or 76% water-soluble ionic contrast media

Radiation Protection

- Adequate collimation
- Minimize fluoroscopy time and number of radiographic exposures

Preliminary Radiographs AP projection of the right upper quadrant

Patient Preparation

- It is critical for the anesthesiologist to suspend respiration during exposures.
- The patient is managed by the surgical team.

Procedure Sequence

- Using an aseptic technique, the cassette is placed under the area to be imaged, with the center point identified by the surgeon. Wherever possible, the overhead tube or C-arm, suitably draped, is moved into position.
- After the operative catheter is in place and the biliary system is filled with contrast material, radiographic exposures are initiated.

Procedure Radiographs AP of the right upper quadrant after complete opacification of the common hepatic and common bile ducts

Alternate Radiographs

- Left posterior oblique (LPO) view of 30°
- Right posterior oblique (RPO) view of 30°
- Cranial or caudal views with the operative table tilting to show stone movement within the ducts

Postprocedure Care Per postoperative orders

Common Pathologies

- Normal operative cholangiogram (Figure 5.2)
- Operative cholangiogram with stones (Figure 5.3)

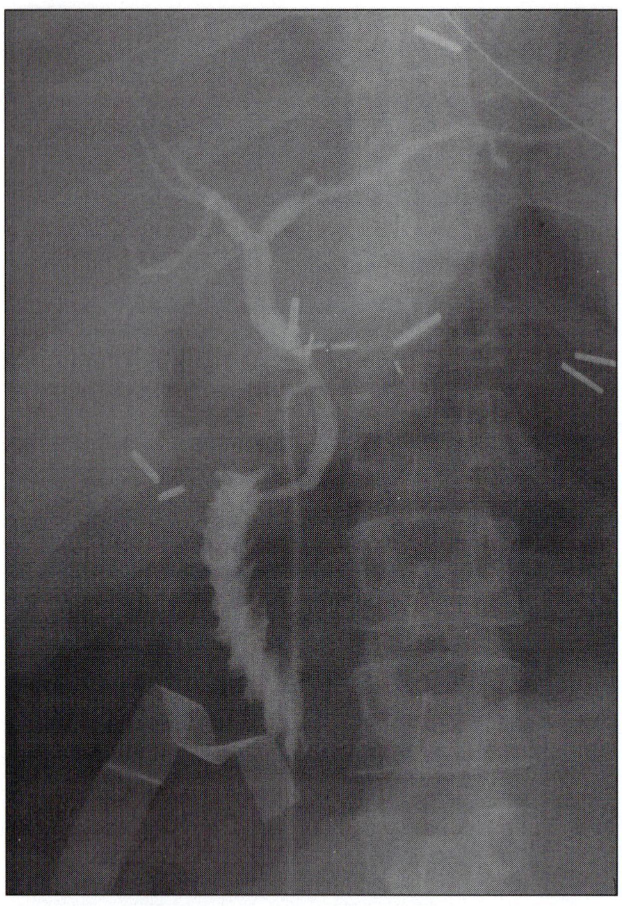

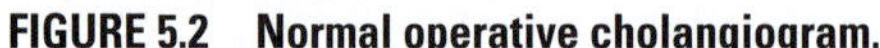

FIGURE 5.2 Normal operative cholangiogram.

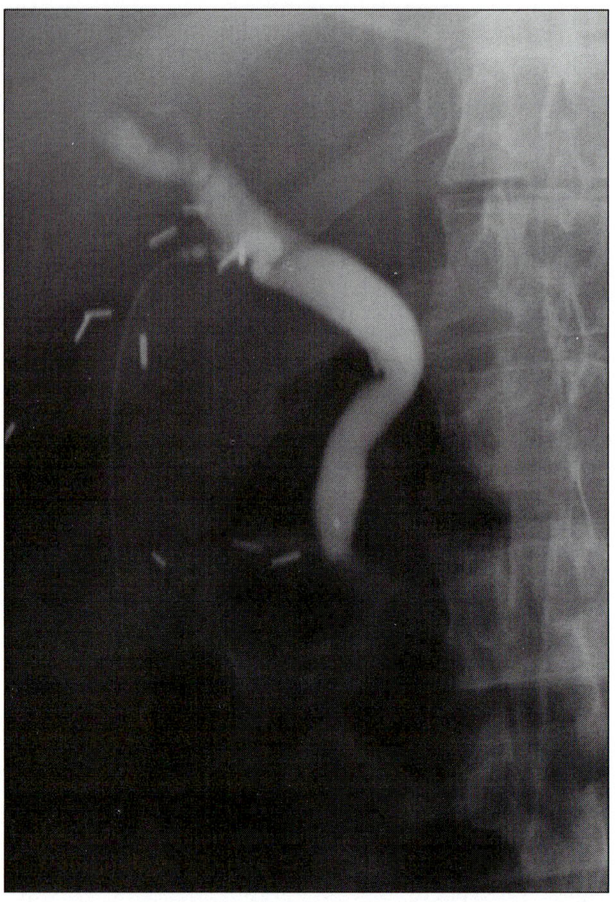

FIGURE 5.3 Operative cholangiogram with stones.

POSTOPERATIVE CHOLANGIOGRAPHY

T-tube cholangiography is performed via a surgically placed catheter. Contrast medium is injected through the catheter and the biliary tree is visualized.

Indications Postoperative evaluation of hepatobiliary system specifically for stones, narrowings, and **obstruction**.

Contraindications Contrast media allergies—reactions are rare but possible.

Equipment Conventional fluroscopic unit with tilt table and spot film device

Contrast Media 60% or 76% water-soluble ionic contrast media

Radiation Protection

- Adequate collimation
- Minimize fluoroscopy time and number of radiographic exposures

Preliminary Radiographs AP projection of the right upper quadrant

Patient Preparation

- Allow 4 to 6 weeks postoperative to allow for T-tube tract maturation.
- Unclamp T-tube before injection.
- Use catheter tip syringe or Luer lock syringe with adaptor.

Procedure Sequence

- The patient is placed on the fluoroscopy table with the left side elevated and the opening of the T-tube clearly identified.
- The syringe containing the contrast material is attached via the Luer lock and a small amount of contrast medium is injected under fluoroscopic control to ensure the patency of the T-tube tract.
- After the biliary system is sufficiently filled, single radiographic exposures are initiated using the spot

film device and the patient positioned at the request of the attending physician

Alternate Radiographs

- Left anterior oblique (LAO) view of 30°
- Right anterior oblique (RAO) view of 30°
- Cranial or caudal views with anterior obliquity to show any stone movement within the ducts

Postprocedure Care

- Reclamp T-tube and place a new sterile dressing over tube site if it is to remain in place.
- The patient is usually an outpatient by this time and will be asked to watch for signs of sepsis and pancreatitis.

Common Pathologies

- Normal T-tube cholangiogram (Figure 5.4)
- T-tube cholangiogram with stones (Figure 5.5)

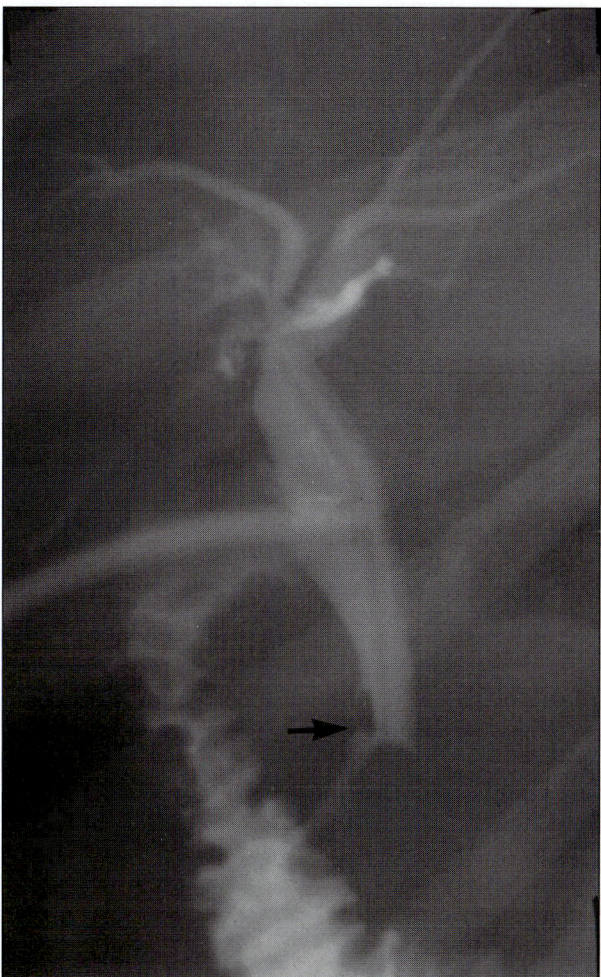

FIGURE 5.5 T-tube cholangiogram with stones.

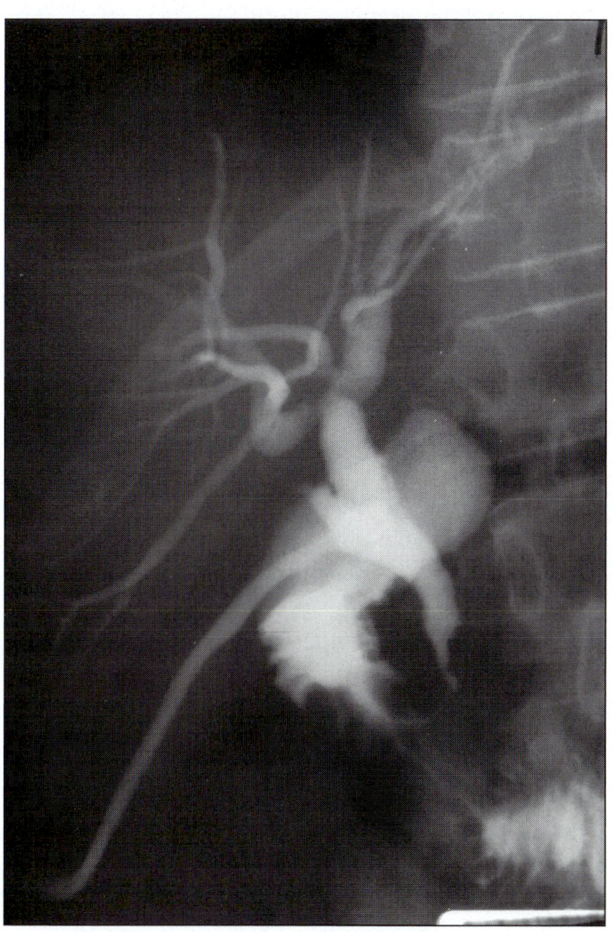

FIGURE 5.4 Normal T-tube cholangiogram.

ENDOSCOPIC RETROGRADE CHOLANGIOPANCREATOGRAPHY (ERCP)

ERCP is performed through an endoscope placed in the mouth of the patient and manipulated through the upper GI tract to the area in the duodenum known as the ampulla of Vater. A small catheter is placed through the endoscope into the biliary tree, contrast medium is injected, and the biliary tree is visualized.

Applied Anatomy The biliary tree, duodenum, and pancreas (see Figure 5.1).

Indications

- **Intrahepatic** or **extrahepatic jaundice**
- Tumors—primary, metastatic, or pancreatic
- Pancreatic disease
- Gallbladder disease
- Pre- and postoperative evaluation
- Interventional procedures

Contraindications

- Acute pancreatitis
- Life-threatening conditions
- Contrast media allergies—reactions are rare but possible.

Equipment

- Flexible endoscope
- Catheters
- Conventional fluoroscopic unit with spot film device

Contrast Media 60% or 76% water-soluble ionic contrast media

Radiation Protection

- Adequate collimation
- Minimize fluoroscopy time and number of radiographic exposures.

Preliminary Radiographs AP projection of the abdomen

Patient Preparation

- Fasting of patient at least 6 hours before the procedure
- History of medications currently being taken, any heart or lung conditions or other major diseases and history of any drug allergies

Procedure Sequence

- The patient is placed onto table in the left lateral recumbent position.
- IV administration is set up, primarily to be used in the event of a reaction.
- Mild sedation can be administered at this point.
- Blood pressure and oxygen saturation (pulse oximetry) should be monitored at this time and periodically throughout the procedure.
- A flexible endoscope is inserted via the mouth and manipulated into duodenum, the lower manipulations being carried out under fluoroscopic control.
- The ampulla of Vater is catheterized by the endoscope using fluoroscopic control.
- The appropriate duct is selectively catheterized and contrast media injected to demonstrate the biliary tree.

Procedure Radiographs Spot film exposures after complete opacification of duct being injected

Alternate Radiographs Various oblique views with cranial or caudal angulation to optimize duct visualization

Postprocedure Care

- Monitoring of vital signs per institutional postoperative nursing standard
- Observation for possible complications of endoscopy

Common Pathologies

- Normal ERCP (Figure 5.6)
- ERCP with stones (Figure 5.7)
- ERCP with tumor (Figure 5.8)

NOTE: The use of other imaging modalities, particularly ultrasound, has reduced the use of ERCP, which is an uncomfortable and invasive procedure for patients who are often very sick at the time.

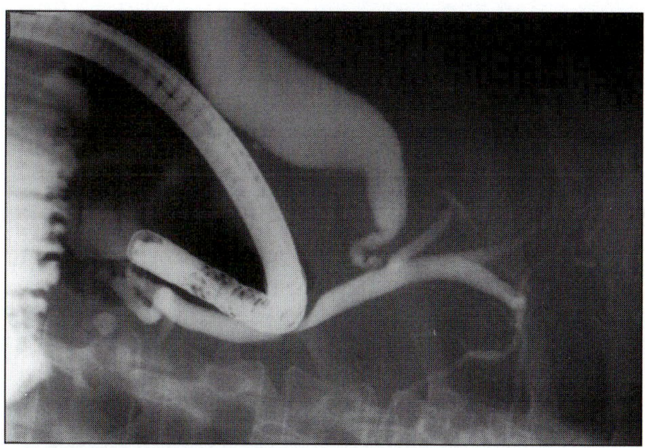

FIGURE 5.6 Normal ERCP.

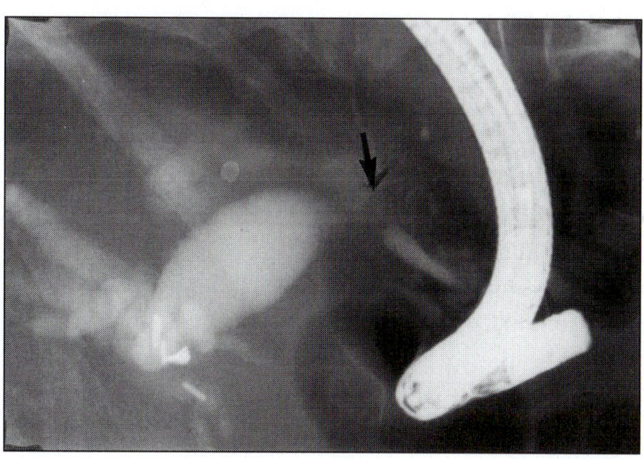

FIGURE 5.8 ERCP with tumor.

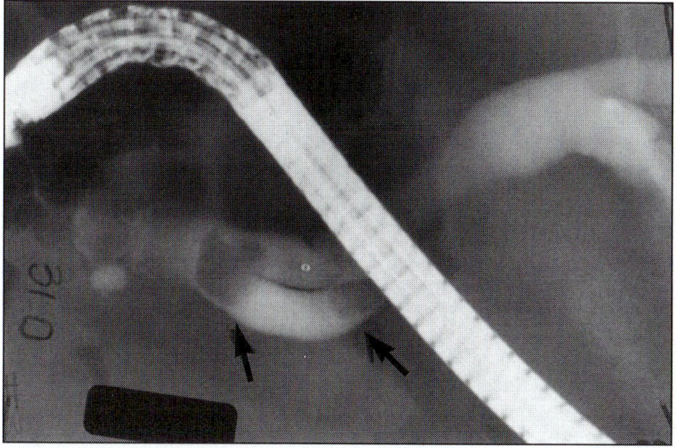

FIGURE 5.7 ERCP with stones.

PERCUTANEOUS TRANSHEPATIC CHOLANGIOGRAPHY (PTHC)

PTHC is performed to evaluate the biliary system through a small-gauge needle placed percutaneously in the the biliary ductal system.

Indications

- Reveal intrahepatic and extrahepatic choledocholithiasis
- Differentiate between different types of jaundice
- Diagnose abnormalities such as biliary atresia, choledocal cysts, and abcesses
- Evaluate postoperative surgical intervention

NOTE: Due of the possibility of biliary peritonitis and sepsis in the presence of **stricture** or obstruction, PTHC should be performed in conjunction with percutaneous biliary drainage.

Contraindications

- Impaired coagulation. If this is not correctable an ERCP can be performed because this does not involve the puncturing of any vessels.
- Contrast media allergies—reactions are rare but possible.
- Asymptomatic jaundice, ascites, advanced cirrhosis, and hepatic tumors

Equipment

- Conventional C-arm with spot film device to obtain multiple projections
- 22-gauge Chiba type needle
- Connecting tube
- 1% Xylocaine, saline, and contrast media
- Syringes and drapes

Contrast Media 60% or 76% water-soluble ionic contrast media

Radiation Protection

- Adequate collimation
- Minimize fluoroscopy time and number of radiographic exposures.
- Keep operator's hands out of x-ray beam when advancing the needle.

Preliminary Radiographs AP projection of the right upper quadrant

Patient Preparation

- Broad-spectrum antibiotics should be administered intravenously at least 1 hour before procedure
- The patient is made fully aware of the procedure and a consent form is signed.

Procedure Sequence

- The patient is placed onto x-ray table in a supine position.
- The patient is prepared and draped in the usual prescribed methods using sterile technique. The preparation should include nipple line to iliac crest top to bottom and lateral border past midline from side to side.
- Sedation is administered as needed and vital signs monitored appropriately.
- The area around the right ninth intercostal region is anesthetized with 1% Xylocaine.
- A small skin incision is made with the scalpel.
- With the needle parallel to table, PTC needle is advanced quickly, near midline and slightly cephalad.
- Tubing is connected to the needle and syringe containing contrast medium.
- A small amount of contrast medium is injected as the needle is withdrawn until duct is opacified.
- If no duct is successfully entered, then additional punctures can be made.
- After the needle is in place within the duct, the biliary system is filled and radiographs are obtained using the spot film device.

Procedure Radiographs AP projection of the right upper quadrant after opacification of the entire biliary tree

Alternate Radiographs LAO and RAO views with caudal or cranial angulation as needed to view as aspects of the biliary system

Postprocedure Care

- Monitoring of vital signs per institutional nursing standards
- Watch for signs of cholangitis, pancreatitis, and sepsis.

Common Pathologies

- PTHC with dilated ducts (Figure 5.9)
- PTHC with common bile duct obstruction (Figure 5.10)

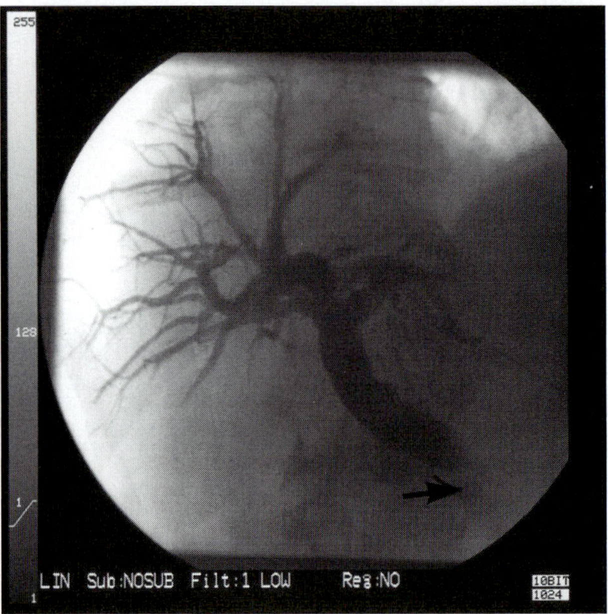

FIGURE 5.9 PTHC with dilated ducts.

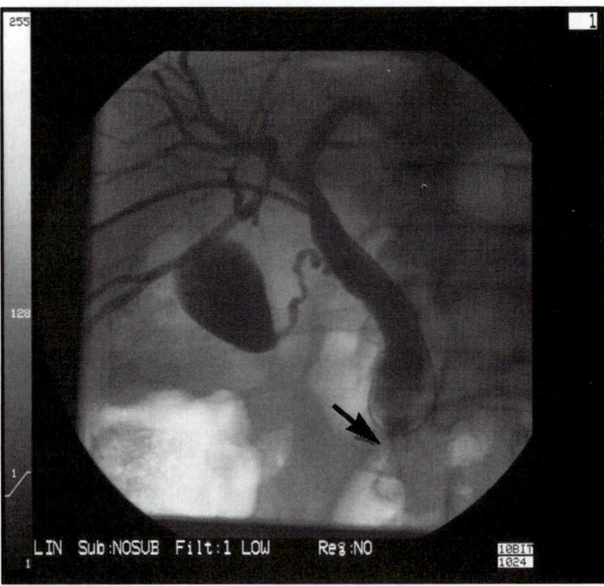

FIGURE 5.10 PTHC with common bile duct obstruction.

Other Imaging Modalities

COMPUTED TOMOGRAPHY

Although it is used often to evaluate the liver and pancreas, CT has a limited role in the direct diagnosis of the hepatobiliary system. It is useful in the diagnosis of choledocholithiasis, choledochal cysts, and tumors involving the biliary system. Some additional work is being done in the area of helical CT with the use of IV cholangiographic contrast media.

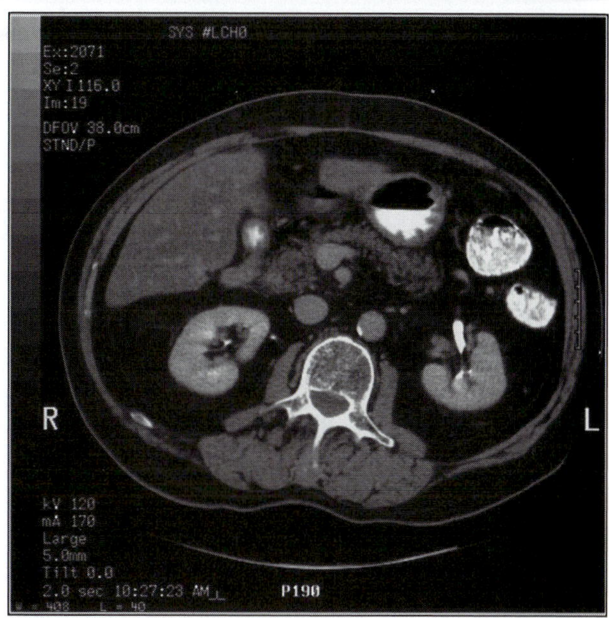

FIGURE 5.11 CT scan showing stones.

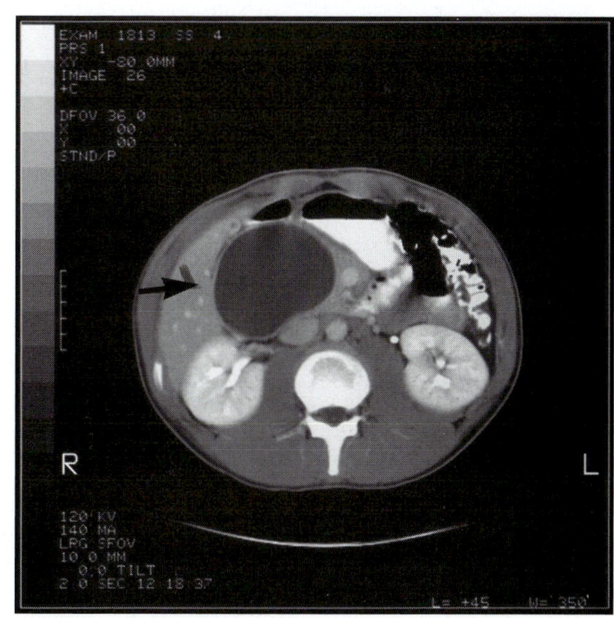

FIGURE 5.12 CT scan showing choledocal cyst.

Indications

- Choledocholithiasis
- Cholelithiasis
- Choledochal cysts
- **Cholecystitis**
- Obstructive jaundice
- Tumors involving the gallbladder, liver, biliary system, and pancreas

Contraindications Contrast media allergies

Equipment CT scanner

Contrast Media Routine oral contrast per institution standards, usually 1 hour before, to outline the digestive system

Radiation Protection Minimize the number of exposures when possible.

Preliminary Radiographs Scout of area to be scanned, standard of abdominal scan

Patient Preparation Refer to contrast media

Procedure Sequence Per standard of CT scan protocols for abdominal scans

Procedure Radiographs Standard 10-mm cuts throughout the abdomen

Postprocedure Care None

Common Pathologies

- Stones (Figure 5.11)
- Choledocal cyst (Figure 5.12)

MAGNETIC RESONANCE IMAGING

MRI has not yet become an everyday tool for examining the hepatobiliary system. Other imaging modalities such as ultrasound, ERCP, and standard percutaneous cholangiography are still used as primary tools of diagnosis. Some work has been done in the area of diagnosis of biliary atresia and in the imaging of hilar structures within the liver. Some advantages of MRI consist of it being noninvasive and not requiring the use of contrast media. Disadvantages may include demonstrating the dilation of ducts while visualizing the actual stricture or its length. Also, resolution of the area being imaged may be less than that of other imaging modalities.

ULTRASOUND

Ultrasound plays a leading role in the imaging of the hepatobiliary system. Often, it is the first imaging modality before ERCP and invasive studies such as PTHC. It has no known adverse side effects and does not require contrast media. Structures of the liver and surrounding biliary system can be imaged in many different planes as needed.

Indications

- Intrahepatic or extrahepatic obstructive jaundice
- Tumors—primary, metastatic, or pancreatic
- Pancreatic disease
- Gallbladder disease
- Pre- and postoperative evaluation
- Any of the above mentioned indications that may show choledocal cysts, biliary atresia, **sludge**, cholelithiasis, or **cholangitis**.
- Interventional drainage procedures performed under ultrasound guidance

Contraindications None

Equipment 3.5 to 5.0 MHz transducer with real-time ultrasound unit

Contrast media None

Radiation Protection Nonapplicable

Patient Preparation No food or drink for 6 to 8 hours before examination

Procedure Sequence

- Real-time examination in all standard planes (sagittal, transverse, and coronal)
- Oblique views as needed

Postprocedure Care None

Common Pathologies

- Sludge (Figure 5.13)
- **Pneumobilia** (Figure 5.14)
- Stones (Figure 5.15)
- Choledocal cyst (Figure 5.16)

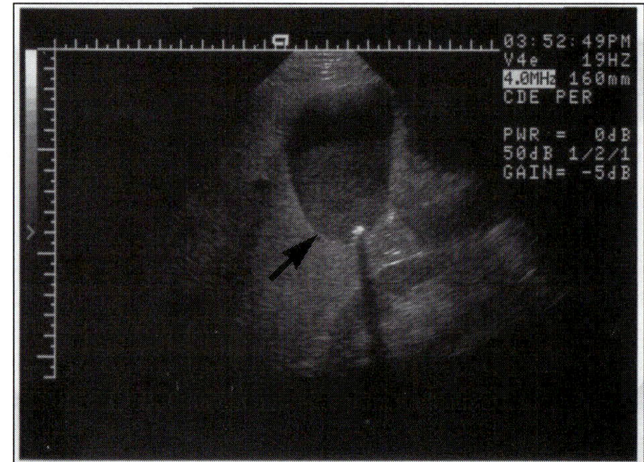

FIGURE 5.13 Sludge.

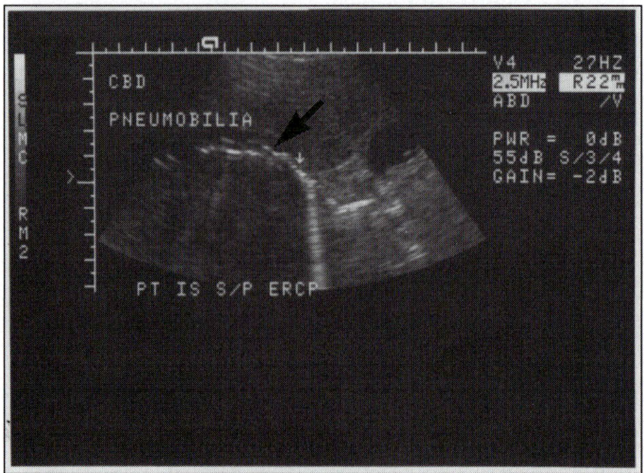

FIGURE 5.14 Pneumobilia.

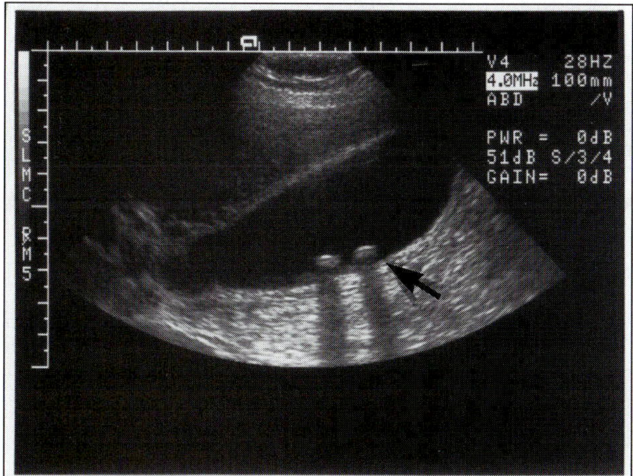

FIGURE 5.15 Stones.

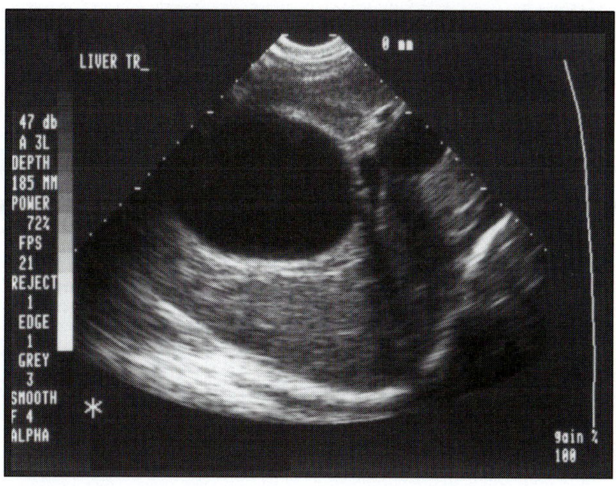

FIGURE 5.16 Choledocal cyst.

RADIONUCLIDE IMAGING

Cholescintography or IDA scan (iminodiacetic acid) is often performed as the first imaging modality to determine the structure and function of the biliary tree of a patient with suspected gallstones (cholecystitis). Several derivatives of the acid are used, the most common being HIDA ^{99m}Tc-diethyl-iminodiactic acid. Structural information is the primary focus of the IDA scan, but some functional information may be obtained when performed for specific problems. The speed at which the radionuclide is taken up provides a general indication of function. Nonvisualization of structures denotes pathologic conditions.

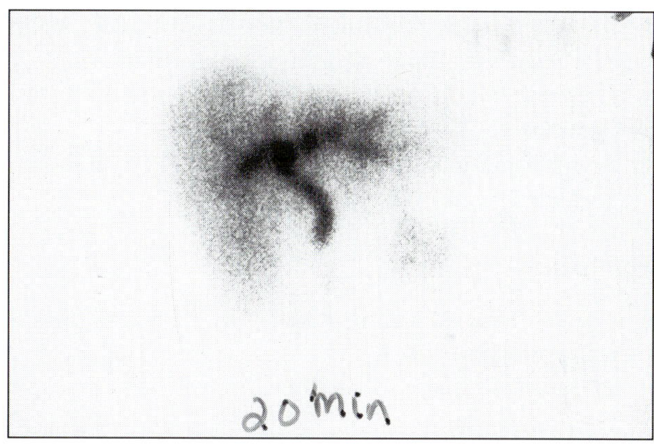

FIGURE 5.17 Normal IDA scan.

Indications

- Cholecystitis, acute or chronic
- Postoperative evaluation of bile leaks
- Biliary atresia
- Choledocal cysts

Contraindications

None

Common Pathologies

- Normal IDA scan (Figure 5.17)
- IDA scan with partial obstruction (Figure 5.18)

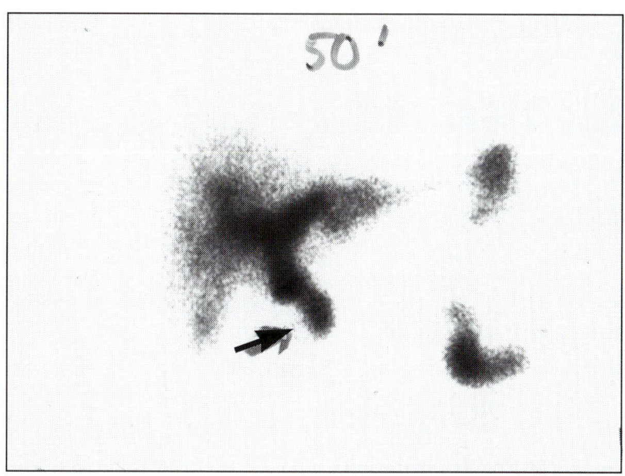

FIGURE 5.18 IDA scan showing partial obstruction of common bile duct.

Interventional Procedures

PERCUTANEOUS BILIARY DRAINAGE (PBD) AND DECOMPRESSION

All percutaneous interventional biliary procedures begin with the standard biliary drainage technique that is then modified to suit the needs for that particular procedure. After access is gained into the biliary system, additional angioplasty catheters, **stents,** or wire baskets can be used for their intended purposes.

Indications

- Biliary obstruction due to malignancy
- Cholangitis
- Postsurgical or traumatic biliary leak
- Palliation of unresectable obstructive lesions

Contraindications

- Impaired coagulation—if not correctable, then ERCP with drainage should be performed.
- Contrast media allergies—reactions are rare but possible.
- Asymptomatic jaundice, ascites, advanced cirrhosis, and hepatic tumors

Equipment

- Conventional C-arm with spot film device to obtain multiple projections
- 22-gauge Chiba-type needle
- Connecting tube
- 1% Xylocaine, saline, and contrast media
- Syringes and drapes
- High-torque guidewires, hydrophilic guidewires
- Biliary drainage catheters
- Fascial dilators

Contrast Media 60% or 76% water-soluble ionic contrast media

Radiation Protection

- Adequate collimation
- Minimize fluoroscopy time and number of radiographic exposures.
- Keep operator's hands out of x-ray beam when advancing the needle.

Preliminary Radiographs AP projection of the right upper quadrant

Patient Preparation

- IV broad-spectrum antibiotics are administered at least 1 hour before procedure.
- The patient is made fully aware of the procedure and a consent form signed.

Procedure Sequence

- The patient is placed onto the x-ray table in a supine position.
- The patient is prepared and draped in the usual prescribed methods using sterile technique. The area of prep should include nipple line to iliac crest top to bottom and lateral border past midline from side to side.
- Sedation is administered as needed and vital signs monitored appropriately.
- Topical anesthetic (1% Xylocaine) is injected around the right ninth intercostal region.
- A small skin incision is made with a scalpel.
- With needle parallel to table, the PTC needle is advanced quickly near midline and slightly cephalad.
- Tubing is connected to the needle and syringe containing contrast medium is connected to the tubing.
- A small amount of contrast medium is injected as the needle is withdrawn, until duct is opacified.
- If no duct is successfully punctured, then additional punctures are made.
- After the needle is in place within the duct, the biliary system is filled and radiographs are obtained. This provides the operator with a picture of the structure and also the presence of pathology.
- Once the obstructive area has been determined, a guidewire is inserted through needle and into the biliary system.
- The guidewire is advanced beyond the obstructed area if possible.
- Dilators are placed over the guidewire to gradually widen the tract.
- Biliary drainage catheter is inserted over the guidewire so that the distal end is placed in the duodenum and side holes of catheter are above and below the obstruction. The guidewire is then removed.

- A small amount of contrast medium is administered under fluoroscopic control to determine the position of the drainage catheter.

Procedure Radiographs AP projection of the right upper quadrant after opacification of the entire biliary tree

Alternate Radiographs LAO and RAO views with caudal or cranial angulation as needed to view aspects of the biliary system

Postprocedure Care

- Monitoring of vital signs per institutional nursing standards
- Watch for signs of cholangitis, pancreatitis, and sepsis.

Common Pathologies

- Biliary drainage, common bile duct obstruction (Figure 5.19)
- Biliary drainage, bilateral drainage catheters (Figure 5.20)
- Biliary drainage, access for radiation therapy (Figure 5.21)

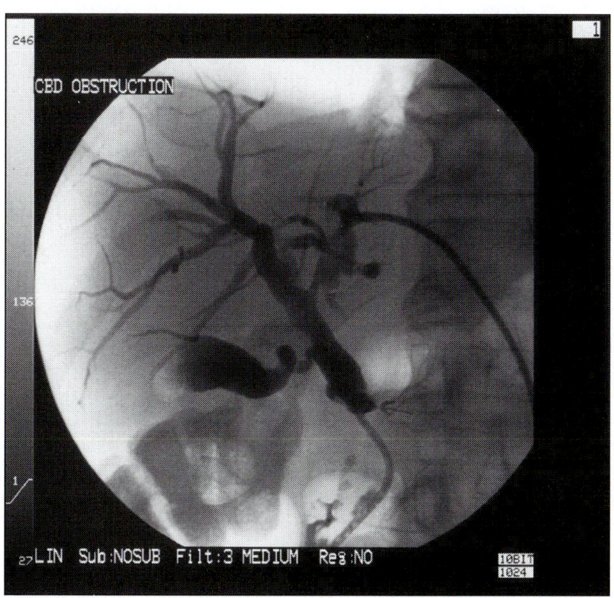

FIGURE 5.19 **Biliary drainage, common bile duct obstruction, left hepatic duct stenosis.**

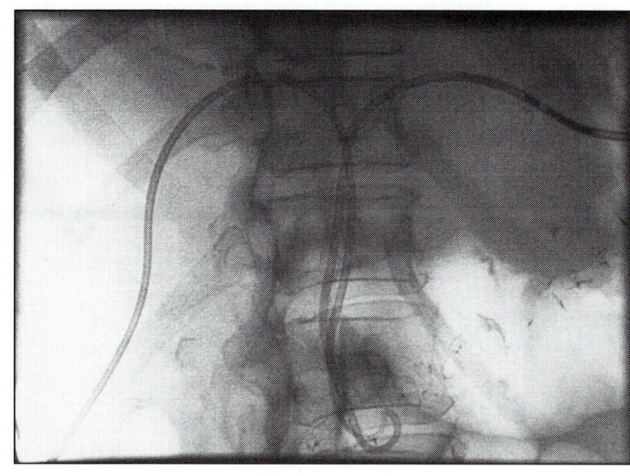

FIGURE 5.20 **Biliary drainage, bilateral drainage catheters.**

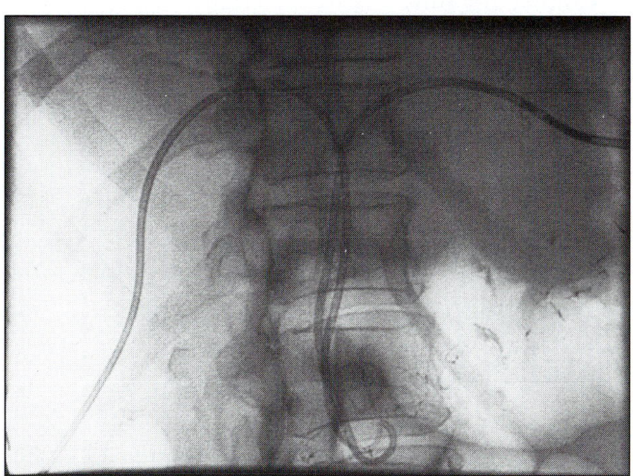

FIGURE 5.21 **Biliary drainage, access for radiation therapy.**

PERCUTANEOUS STONE EXTRACTION

Indications Biliary obstruction due to stones

Contraindications

- Impaired coagulation—if not correctable, ERCP with stone extraction should be performed.
- Contrast media allergies—reactions are rare but possible.
- Asymptomatic jaundice, ascites, advanced cirrhosis, and hepatic tumors

Equipment

- Conventional C-arm with spot film device to obtain multiple projections
- 22-gauge Chiba-type needle
- Connecting tube
- 1% Xylocaine, saline, and contrast media
- Syringes and drapes
- High-torque guidewires, hydrophilic guidewires
- Biliary drainage catheters
- Fascial dilators
- Various stone baskets or angioplasty catheters

Contrast Media 60% or 76% water-soluble ionic contrast media

Radiation Protection

- Adequate collimation
- Minimize fluoroscopy time and number of radiographic exposures.
- Keep operator's hands out of x-ray beam when advancing the needle.

Preliminary Radiographs AP projection of the right upper quadrant

Patient Preparation

- IV broad-spectrum antibiotics are administered at least 1 hour before procedure.
- The patient is made fully aware of the procedure and a consent form is signed.

Procedure Sequence

- The patient is placed onto x-ray table in a supine position.
- The patient is prepared and draped in the usual prescribed methods using sterile technique. The area of preparation should include nipple line to iliac crest top to bottom and lateral border past midline from side to side.
- Sedation is administered as needed and monitor vital signs taken appropriately.
- The area around right ninth intercostal region is anesthetized with 1% Xylocaine.
- A small skin incision is made with scalpel.
- With needle parallel to table, the PTC needle is advanced quickly near midline and slightly cephalad.
- Tubing is connected to the needle and a syringe containing contrast medium is attached to the tubing.
- A small amount of contrast is injected as the needle is withdrawn until duct is opacified.
- If no ducts are visualized, the procedure is repeated until a duct is punctured and seen under fluoroscopic control.
- After the needle is in place within the duct, the biliary system is filled with contrast medium and radiographs are obtained.
- Once the obstruction (stones) have been determined, a guidewire is inserted through the needle and into the biliary system. The needle is withdrawn.
- Dilators sequentially enlarge the tract.
- A biliary drainage catheter is inserted over the guidewire. Then the guidewire is removed and stone basket remover is threaded through the catheter.
- The stone basket is manipulated until stone(s) are trapped in the basket. The stones are either pushed through ampulla of Vater into duodenum or pulled out through the biliary drainage catheter. The biliary catheter will remain in place for a few days.

Procedure Radiographs AP projection of the right upper quadrant after opacification of the entire biliary tree

Alternate Radiographs LAO and RAO views with caudal or cranial angulation as needed to view aspects of the biliary system

Postprocedure Care

- Monitoring of vital signs per institutional nursing standards
- Watch for signs of cholangitis, pancreatitis, and sepsis.

Common Pathologies Percutaneous stone extraction (Figure 5.22)

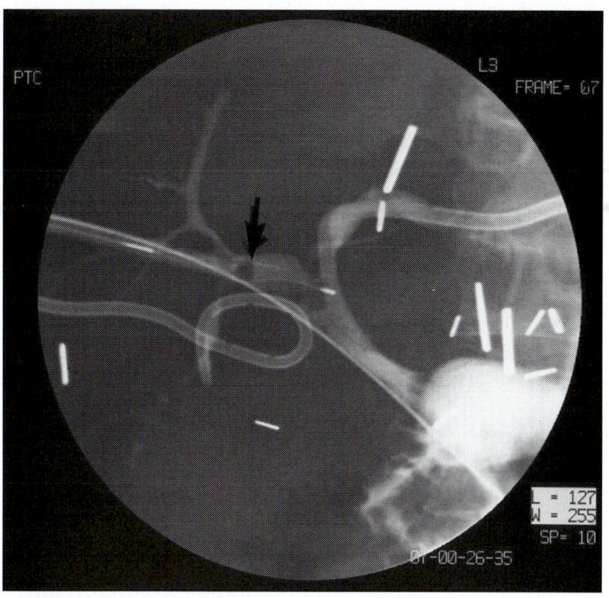

FIGURE 5.22 Percutaneous stone extraction.

PERCUTANEOUS BILIARY DILATATION

Indications

- Biliary obstruction due to malignancy
- Palliation of unresectable obstructive lesions
- Benign strictures

Contraindications

- Impaired coagulation—if not correctable, then ERCP with dilatation should be performed.
- Contrast media allergies—reactions are rare but possible.
- Asymptomatic jaundice, ascites, advanced cirrhosis, and hepatic tumors.

Equipment

- Conventional C-arm with spot film device to obtain multiple projections
- 22-gauge Chiba-type needle
- Connecting tube
- 1% Xylocaine, saline, and contrast media
- Syringes and drapes
- High-torque guidewires, hydrophilic guidewires
- Biliary drainage catheters
- Fascial dilators
- Angioplasty catheters

Contrast Media 60% or 76% water-soluble ionic contrast media

Radiation Protection

- Adequate collimation
- Minimize fluoroscopy time and number of radiographic exposures.
- Keep operator's hands out of x-ray beam when advancing the needle.

Preliminary Radiographs AP projection of the right upper quadrant

Patient Preparation The patient is prepared in the same manner as for the biliary drainage.

Procedure Sequence

- The procedure is the same as for the biliary drainage and stone removal procedures. Following the dilation of the tract with dilators, an angioplasty catheter is fed over the guidewire so that the balloon is placed within the obstruction or stricture and inflated as needed until the stricture is expanded.
- Following the angioplastic procedure, a biliary drainage catheter can remain in place for some time, with drainage holes placed at either end of the previous obstruction.

Procedure Radiographs AP projection of the right upper quadrant after opacification of the entire biliary tree and enlargement of the stricture

Alternate Radiographs LAO and RAO views with caudal or cranial angulation as needed to view aspects of the biliary system

Postprocedure Care

- Monitoring of vital signs per institutional nursing standards
- Watch for signs of cholangitis, pancreatitis, and sepsis.

Common Pathologies

- Percutaneous dilatation, predilatation (Figure 5.23)
- Percutaneous dilatation, balloon inflation (Figure 5.24)

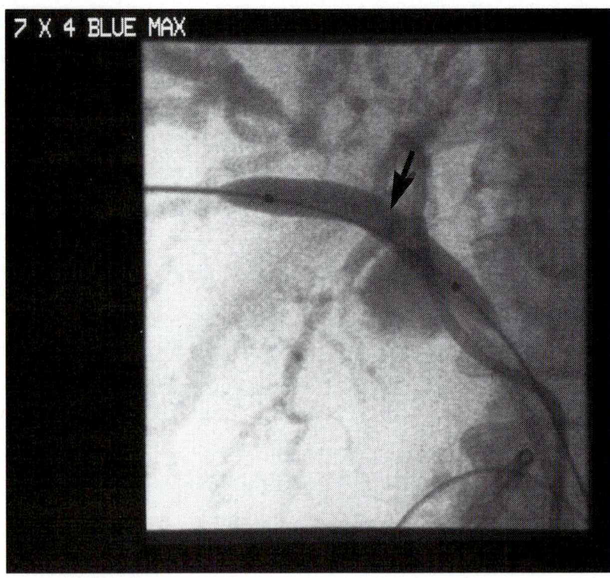

FIGURE 5.24 Percutaneous dilatation, balloon inflation.

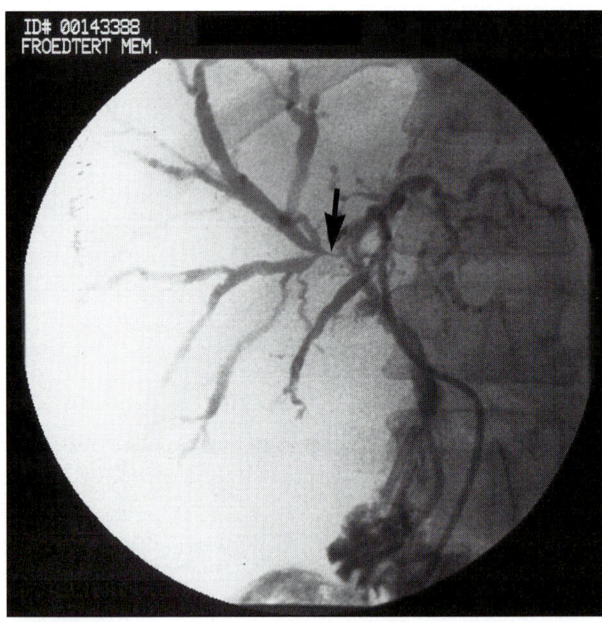

FIGURE 5.23 Percutaneous dilatation, predilatation.

PERCUTANEOUS STENT PLACEMENT

Indications

- Biliary obstruction due to malignancy
- Palliation of unresectable obstructive lesions
- Benign strictures

Contraindications

- Impaired coagulation—if not correctable, then ERCP with drainage should be done.
- Contrast media allergies—reactions are rare but possible.
- Asymptomatic jaundice, ascites, advanced cirrhosis, and hepatic tumors

Equipment

- Conventional C-arm with spot film device to obtain multiple projections
- 22-gauge Chiba-type needle
- Connecting tube
- 1% Xylocaine, saline, and contrast media
- Syringes and drapes
- High-torque guidewires, hydrophilic guidewires
- Biliary drainage catheters
- Fascial dilators
- Angioplasty catheters
- Metallic or plastic biliary stents (metallic stents are often used in radiology; plastic or metallic stents may be used during ERCP)

Contrast Media 60% or 76% water-soluble ionic contrast media

Radiation Protection

- Adequate collimation
- Minimize fluoroscopy time and number of radiographic exposures.
- Keep operator's hands out of x-ray beam when advancing the needle.

Preliminary Radiographs AP projection of the right upper quadrant

Patient Preparation The preparation is the same as for the biliary drainage and stone removal percutaneous procedures.

Procedure Sequence

- The procedure is the same as for the percutaneous procedures already described. Following the dilation of the tract by the use of dilators, stent catheter is inserted over the guidewire so that stent is placed proximal and distal to obstruction.
- The stent is deployed within the duct as per instructions.
- If angioplasty is needed to further expand the stent, the angioplasty catheter is inserted and the balloon inflated as needed.
- After dilatation biliary drainage catheter is inserted over guidewire and through the stent so that the distal end is placed in duodenum and side holes of catheter are above and below the obstruction.
- Follow-up cholangiogram is advised before biliary catheter removal.

Procedure Radiographs AP projection of the right upper quadrant after opacification of the entire biliary tree and after the insertion of the stent

Alternate Radiographs LAO and RAO with caudal or cranial angulation as needed to view aspects of the biliary system

Postprocedure Care

- Monitoring of vital signs per institutional nursing standards
- Watch for signs of cholangitis, pancreatitis, and sepsis

Common Pathologies Percutaneous stent placement (Figure 5.25)

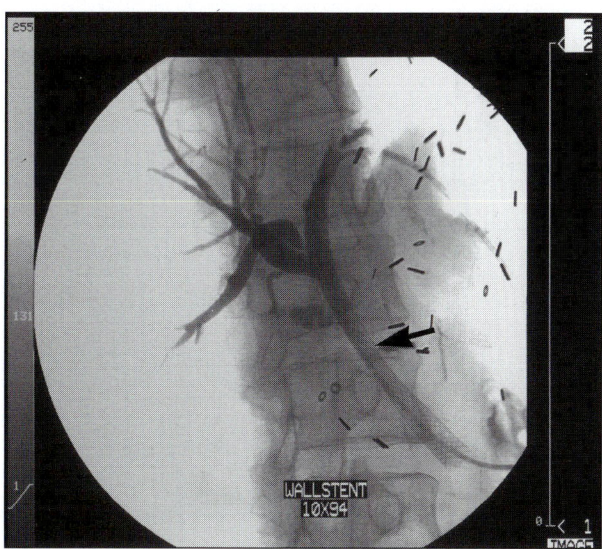

FIGURE 5.25 Percutaneous stent placement.

Review Questions

1. What are the contraindications to performing percutaneous biliary drainage?

2. What are some indications to performing percutaneous transhepatic cholangiography?

3. What are the nursing implications to performing percutaneous biliary dilatation?

4. Identify three other imaging modalities after cholangiography for evaluating the biliary system.

5. For percutaneous transhepatic cholangiography, identify the type of x-ray unit preferred. Explain what advantages this unit has over standard equipment.

6. Discuss the possibilities of a contrast reaction during cholangiography? Why are they rare in nature?

7. Biliary drainage should not be attempted on patients with:
   a. cholangitis
   b. cholecystitis
   c. metastatic disease
   d. asymptomatic jaundice

8. A T-tube cholangiogram:
   a. requires a general anesthetic
   b. requires supine and prone radiographs
   c. uses water-soluble ionic contrast media
   d. is contraindicated in the presence of biliary stones

CASE STUDY

A patient is admitted into the emergency department with signs and symptoms of acute cholelithiasis. Describe the imaging procedures that might be performed and the order in which they might take place. Describe how procedures carried out in the imaging department could relieve the patient of his symptoms.

References and Recommended Reading

Ballinger, P. W. (1995). *Merrill's atlas of radiographic positions and radiological procedures* (8th ed., Vols. 1, 2, and 3). St. Louis: Mosby-Year Book.

Casteneda-Zuniga, W. R. (1988). *Interventional radiology.* Baltimore: Williams & Wilkins.

Cope, C., Burke, D., & Meranze, S. (1989). *Interventional radiology.* Gower Medical Publishing.

Curry, R. A., & Tempkin, B. B. (1995). *Ultrasonography: An introduction to normal structure and functional anatomy* Philadelphia: Saunders.

Ferrucci, J. T., et al. (1985). *Interventional radiology of the abdomen* (2nd ed.). Baltimore: Williams & Wilkins.

Goldberg, H. I. (1994). Helical cholangiography: Complementary or substitute study for endoscopic retrograde cholangiography. *Radiology, 192,* 615–616.

Hall-Craggs, M. A., et al. (1993). M R cholangiography, clinical evaluation in 40 cases, *Radiology, 189,* 423–27.

Kandarpa, K., & Aruny, J. E. (1996). *Handbook of interventional radiologic procedures* (2nd ed.). Boston: Little, Brown.

Kawamura, D. M. (1992). *Diagnostic medical sonography.* Philadelphia: Lippincott.

Mettler, F. A., & Guiberteu, M. J. (1991). *Essentials of nuclear medicine imaging* (3rd ed.). Philadelphia: Saunders.

Rose, J. S. (1983). *Invasive radiology, risks and patient care.* Chicago: Year Book Medical Publishers.

Sandler, M. P., et al. (1989). *Correlative imaging.* Baltimore: Williams & Wilkins.

Siegel, J. H. (1992). *Endoscopic retrograde cholangiopancreatography.* Philadelphia: Raven Press,

Snopek, A.M. (1992). *Fundamentals of special radiographic procedures* (3rd ed.). Philadelphia: Saunders.

Tortora, G. J., & Anagnostakos, N. P. (1990). *Principles of anatomy and physiology* (6th ed.). New York: Harper & Row.

Tortorici, M. R., & Apfel, P. J. (1995). *Advanced radiographic and angiographic procedures.* Philadelphia: F. A. Davis.

Wojtowycz, M. (1993). *Interventional radiology and angiography, handbooks in radiology.* Chicago: Year Book Medical Publishers.

SECTION IV

VASCULAR SYSTEM

CHAPTER 6

Angiographic Procedures and Equipment

CYNTHIA COWLING, BSc, MEd, MRT(R), ACR

OBJECTIVES

At the completion of this chapter, the student should be able to:

1. Define angiography and other associated terms.
2. Describe the main types of radiographic equipment found within an angiographic suite.
3. List the features of film changers.
4. List the features of pressure injectors.
5. Describe the main components and function of a digital subtraction angiographic system.
6. Describe the procedure used in a percutaneous needle puncture.
7. Define and describe the Seldinger technique.
8. Discuss the use of catheters and guidewires in an angiographic procedure.
9. Describe the process of a femoral artery puncture.
10. Identify the best contrast agent materials suggested for angiography.
11. Describe the pre- and postangiographic care of the patient.
12. Describe the main types of interventional procedures associated with angiography.
13. Relate the use of angiography with interventional procedures.

Introduction and Historical Overview

The first angiogram was performed only months after Roentgen's discovery, when two physicians injected chalk into an amputated hand and created an image of the arteries. Unfortunately, in the absence of safe contrast media, angiography experiments were restricted to amputated limbs. In 1919, sodium iodine was first used for urologic studies and this substance was used in angiography. By 1924, several in vivo arteriograms had been performed. Moniz published his classic work on cerebral angiography in 1928 and in 1929, Don Santos described his work on lumbar arteriography. With the contrast media better established, the next problem was how to keep it in the vessels or to image it before it disappeared. To avoid multiple injections, the first film changers were devised in 1932 by Moniz and Caldas, allowing several radiographs to be taken in rapid succession. During this time, experiments were also being carried out with the use of catheters. In 1929, Forssman experimented on himself by having his own heart catheterized. However, it was not until the 1950s that angiography moved out of the surgical suite. The Scandinavians devised the Seldinger technique, which allowed percutaneous injections that did not require cut-down surgery.

Technical innovations continued to facilitate angiography—image intensification, three-phase generators, rapid film changers, automatic pressure injectors, and advanced catheter technology all helped to establish angiography as an essential diagnostic tool by the 1960s. Since that time, other technologies have been developed, which demonstrate the vasculature to a greater or less degree. CT, MRI, ultrasound, (particularly Doppler), and nuclear medicine are all used to image vessels and each has its advantages and disadvantages as discussed in following chapters. However, at this time, angiography, and its associated technology, digital subtraction angiography (DSA), is still considered the gold standard of vessel imaging when other modalities are inconclusive. Current developments such as CT and magnetic resonance angiography (MRA) may change this in the future. Vessel imaging is a constantly evolving area.

An important offshoot of angiographic imaging has been the development of interventional techniques that have created a therapeutic technology. Embolization, intra-arterial drug therapy, and transluminal angioplasty are among the procedures that have radically changed and broadened the scope of the diagnostic imaging department.

Angiography

Angiography is a general term used to describe the radiologic examination of a vessel by means of an introduced contrast medium, rendering the vessel visible radiographically. This term can be altered or prefixed to describe more accurately the type of vessel being examined.

The purpose of these examinations listed below is primarily to examine the structure and sometimes the function of the vessels. Dynamic imaging also provides for motion studies, if required. Heart function is a good example of this. Angiography is frequently performed now as a precursor to therapeutic procedures, assessing the condition of the vessel before the intervention.

Aortography: study of the aorta, either ascending or descending (thoracic or abdominal) (Figure 6.1)
Arteriography: study of any arterial system (e.g., abdominal, cerebral, femoral)

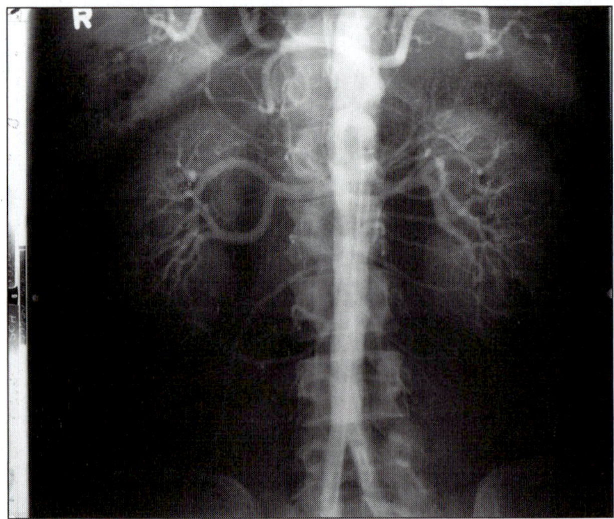

FIGURE 6.1 Abdominal aortography.

Venography: study of any venous system (e.g., peripheral venography of the leg [Figure 6.2])
Angiocardiography: study of the chambers of the heart and great vessels
Coronary arteriography: study of the vessels supplying blood to the heart (Figure 6.3)

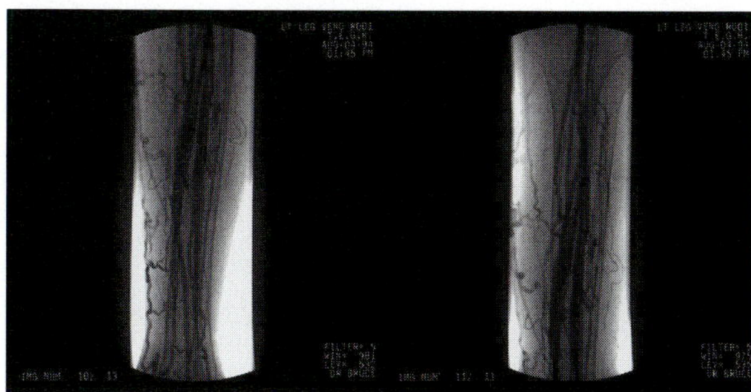

FIGURE 6.2 Leg venography.

Lymphangiography: study of the lymph vessels and nodes
Cholangiography: study of the biliary tract (covered in Chapter 5, Hepatobiliary System)

Additional definitions help to define further the type of examination.

Percutaneous: injected through the skin, either via needle puncture or via catheterization of a vessel
Selective angiography: study of a vessel that has been selected and catheterized via another main vessel. For example, mesenteric or renal arteries would be selected via the abdominal aorta.
Superselective angiography: study of vessels that have been selected from the branches of the main vessels. Catheterization of some of the smaller vessels in the head would be considered a super selected vessel and examination.

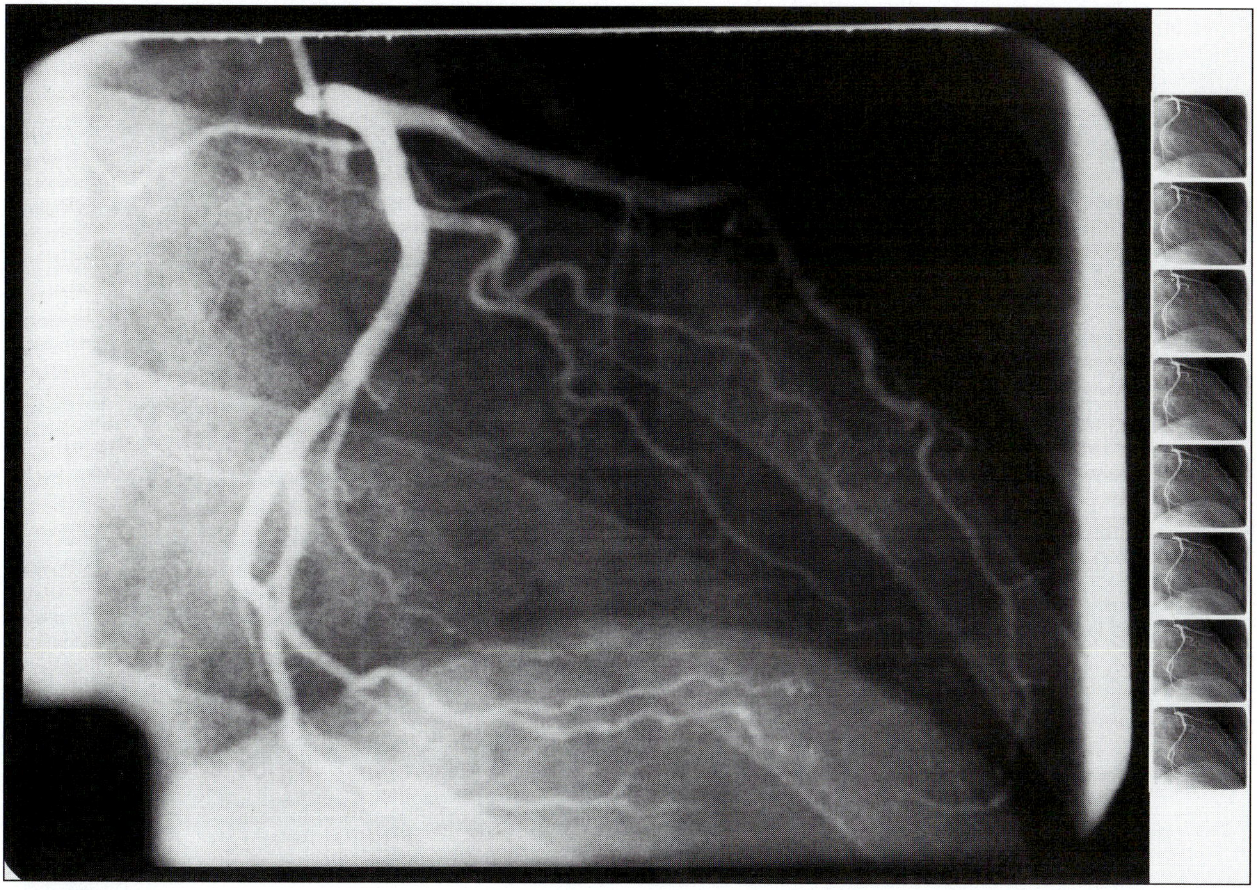

FIGURE 6.3 Coronary arteriography.

Angiographic Equipment

Vascular studies usually require a room or suite of rooms specifically designed to accommodate the sophisticated and accessory equipment needed to perform angiography and interventional procedures. The procedure room should be large enough to accommodate all of the equipment as well as radiologic and ancillary staff. Special procedures sometimes require a general anesthetic that necessitates extra equipment and staff. These procedures are also more hazardous to the patient and each room must be equipped to deal with emergencies that may occur. Ideally there should be anterooms for patient preparation and for storage. Remote computerized equipment should also be housed adjacent to the special room. Although there must be adequate protection for all operators and staff, there must at all times be clear access and view of the patient being examined (Figure 6.4).

The main features of the angiographic room are listed below. This equipment encompasses the needs of angiography, angiocardiography, and interventional procedures. For each examination accessory equipment may be needed. These will be added to the description of each procedure.

- **Generator**: This must be a three-phase or high-frequency 12-pulse machine and at least 1000 mA to accommodate the rapid, short, and high exposure values required in angiography. A constant potential generator is a definite advantage when requiring extremely short exposures such as those required in cine radiography in cardiac angiography. If there is **biplane** equipment, each tube should have its own generator. This allows each tube to work completely independently of the other with varying exposure values and times and the breakdown of one does not close the facility (Figure 6.5).
- **X-ray tube**: High-speed rotating anode tubes. The object of an angiogram is to produce the highest quality radiographs in the shortest time possible. Ideally, a small focal spot (0.3 mm) will produce the best detail. However, problems can occur where a tube rating can be exceeded because of the rapid succession of exposures needed. It is therefore more usual to have a 0.6-mm focal spot tube for general angiographic work and a smaller focal spot for **macroangiography**. Tube rating and cooling charts should always be adhered to.
- **Single or biplane image intensification units**: A C-arm or U-arm device is preferable for these procedures so that the equipment can be rotated rather than the patient when visualization of the catheter is critical. Biplane is particularly important in angiocardiography where simultaneous biplane visualization/exposures are needed to reduce the number of injections of contrast required (Figure 6.6).
- **Film changers** (See also Chapter 2): These are units that have the ability to move film in rapid succession, allowing for a number of exposures to be registered each on its own film. There are a number of makes, the most common at present being the Puck system (Siemens), which uses cut film (Figure 6.7). Older varieties have used continuous roll film, which has the advantage of fewer jams because there are no leading edges. However, the cassettes, often containing rolled film 14 inches

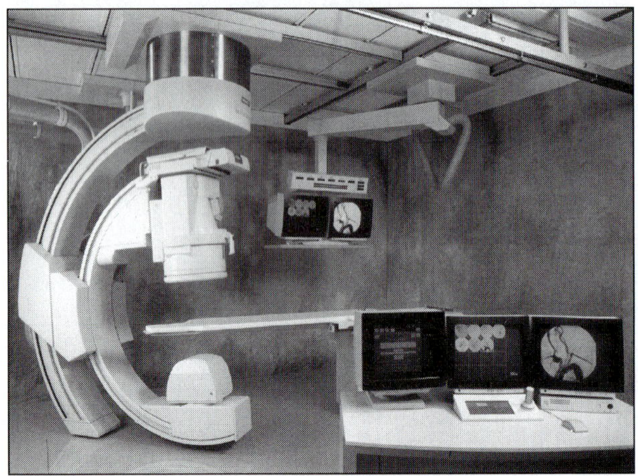

FIGURE 6.4 Special procedures room (Courtesy of Siemens Medical Systems).

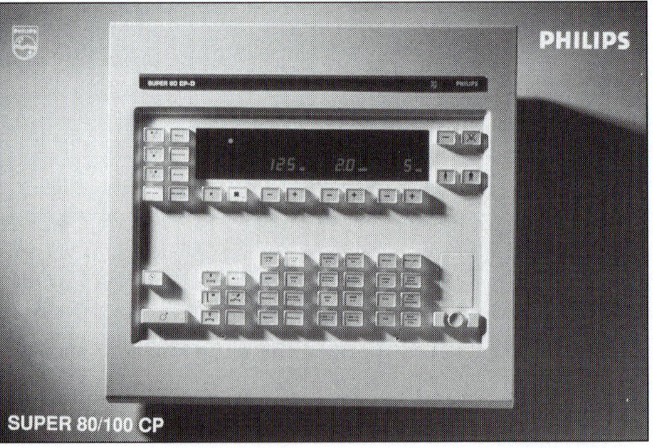

FIGURE 6.5 Generator (Courtesy of Philips Medical Systems, Shelton, CT).

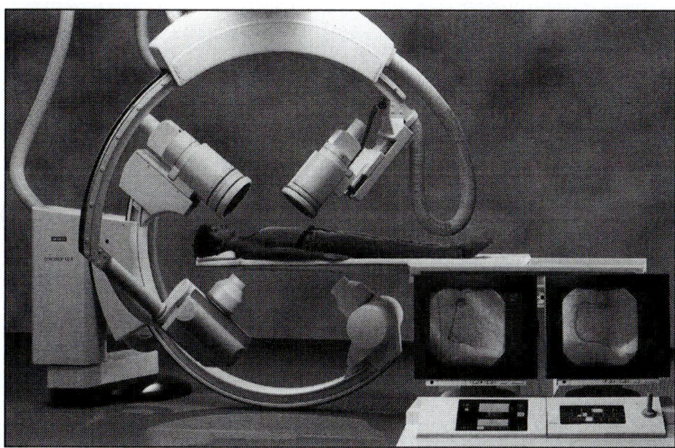

FIGURE 6.6 Biplane C-arm (Courtesy of Siemens Medical Systems, Iselin, NJ).

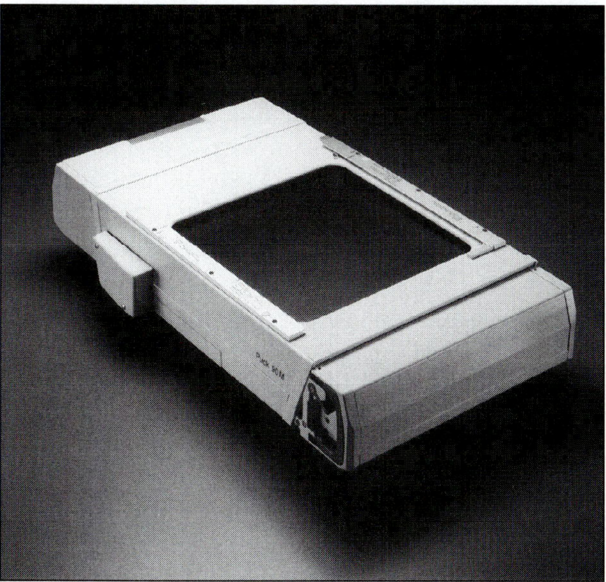

FIGURE 6.7 Puck film changer (Courtesy of Siemens Medical Systems, Iselin, NJ).

wide, are cumbersome and rarely used today. The Puck system and those like it are programmable, allowing the operator to vary the speed and the number of films passing through the changer. Speeds vary from 3 to 12 films per second, the speed required depending on the examination being carried out. These changers can also be single or biplane, allowing for simultaneous exposures. Film changers have five main features:

—**Supply magazine**. This is a light-tight box that can be filled with film in the darkroom and then attached to the film changer.

—**Transport mechanism**. This consists of a series of compression roller devices that moves the film from the supply magazine to a pair of intensifying screens and then to the receiving cassette.

—**Compression table**. This contains a pair of screens. As soon as the film is positioned between them, they compress the film and the exposure is automatically triggered. As soon as the exposure is complete, the compression is released and the film advanced to the receiving cassette.

—**Receiving cassette**. This is the magazine that holds the exposed film. When the examination is complete, the cassette is removed from the changer and taken to the darkroom to be unloaded. It is returned empty to the changer.

—**Program selector**: This allows the operator to set speeds and film quantity to suit the examination being undertaken. Programs can be designed to fit standard requirements of various procedures. Individual programs can be designed for patients who return for repeat examinations or for pathologies that have demonstrated the necessity for a different program; for example, pathologies requiring delay films.

- **Cine radiography**: Depending on the need, 35- to 105-mm can be used, usually at 25 frames per second. Images are recorded using a pulsed beam and can be single or biplane.
- **Fluoroscopy unit with TV monitor**: Single or biplane fluoroscopy units are available. Biplane is essential for angiocardiography and coronary angiography. A cesium iodide image intensifier is required (Figure 6.8).
- **Video equipment**: This has become an essential component of any angiographic suite. The video

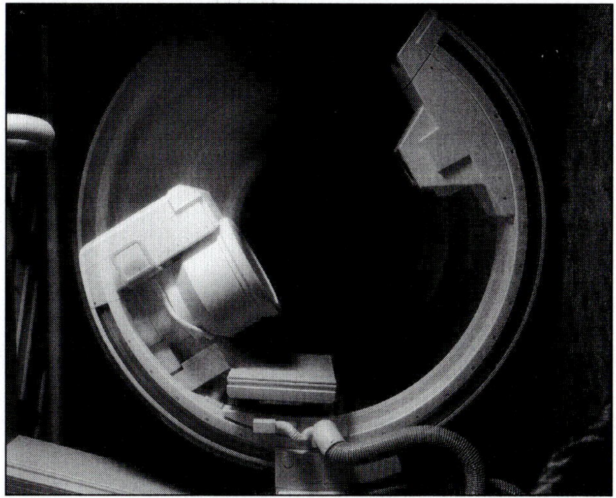

FIGURE 6.8 Close up of image intensifier (Courtesy of Philips Medical Systems, Shelton, CT).

imaging can be single or biplane and allows for instant replay of a procedure or contrast injection as well as a method of recording the images produced. The video is an indirect imaging system used in combination with image intensification and it simply records the intensified image as seen on the monitors. Audio track allows for a commentary during the examination if needed.

- **Other image recording devices**: Images can be stored and reproduced using a laser disk system. Radiographic information can also be acquired and stored in a digital format, allowing the resultant images to be manipulated (postprocessing). This is the fundamental principle of DSA.
- **Angiographic table**: Most tables in the angiographic suite are horizontal only but with moving or floating capabilities. It is important that during a procedure, a patient can be moved without actually being repositioned, particularly with the catheter in situ. Lateral and horizontal movements are essential and controls should be available remote from the table, such as a foot switch, to allow movement to take place during a procedure without jeopardizing the sterile technique. In examinations of the peripheral regions, the table should be able to move in programmed steps between exposures (see section on femoral arteriography for further information).
- **Pressure injector**: In most angiographic studies, contrast must be administered at a consistent speed, either faster, as in abdominal angiography, or slower as in lymphangiography (Figure 6.9). Pressure injectors today are motor driven and have the following major components:
  —**Control panel** where parameters for injections are set.
  —**Motor drive mechanism** is the electromechanical device that drives the plunger into the syringe at a specific pressure.
  —**Syringes** are always removable for sterilization purposes or are disposable.
  —**Heating system** maintains the contrast at near body temperature to reduce shock and lower the viscosity of certain contrast media. Pressure injectors can function in two ways. The pressure and speed required are calculated by a computation of patient variables (e.g., blood pressure) and catheter variables (e.g., size) or via a feedback mechanism to monitor the injection rate, so that the injection can be synchronized with the R wave impulses monitored from the patient using an ECG triggering device.

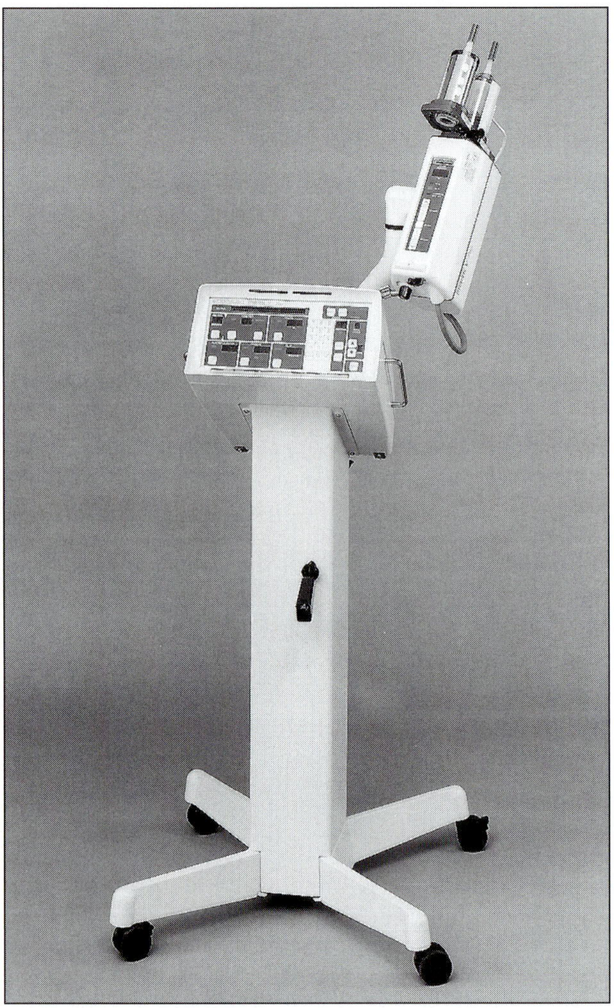

FIGURE 6.9 Pressure injector (Courtesy of MedRad Inc., Pittsburgh, PA).

- **ECG monitoring device**: This can be integral with the pressure injector or a separate system that monitors the ECG patterns during the procedure, essential in angiocardiography.
- **Pressure monitoring device**: Some examinations require the reading of intralumen pressures, particularly for cardiac catheter studies and certain angioplasty procedures (see further information under specific examination).
- **Resuscitation devices**: As well as an emergency drug supply, angiographic rooms should contain or have immediate access to a defibrillator, a ventilator bag, and endotracheal tubes. During some procedures, specialized staff such as an anesthetist or respiratory therapist are asked to be in attendance.

Digital Subtraction Angiography

This technique has been one of the first applications of digital radiography in common use (See also Chapter 2). A subtracted image is produced by the manipulation of digitally produced images, a mask, and a contrast-enhanced image. The image is taken from the image intensification system rather than the film system and allows for instant video replay of a continuously subtracted image (**real time**). There was a tremendous surge to integrate this technology in the 1970s, when it was thought that the technique would allow angiography to be performed using an IV injection, making it a less invasive procedure that could be done on an outpatient basis. However, problems of misregistration due to patient movement, particularly in the abdominal area, the need for larger amounts of contrast, and the superimposition of vessels made this procedure problematic. DSA was extremely helpful when used in conjunction with regular arteriography, as a screening tool, and to improve the quality of manually subtracted films. The rapid development of MRI and MRA may temper its use. It is, however, currently used consistently in angiographic suites. It allows for the use of lower doses of contrast and smaller catheters. Its resolution is not as fine as film, but for most screening purposes it is adequate. Its other main advantage is that because it subtracts electronically, it is more accurate than manual techniques. The storage of images allows for postprocessing manipulation to compensate for movement, misregistration, or poor exposure techniques. Its most frequent use is in the study of:

- Carotid stenosis (as a screening tool)
- As a guide during interventional procedures
- As a follow-up study after angioplasty or vascular surgery
- As an adjunct to arteriography, enabling the use of less contrast and smaller catheters (3 French)

DSA EQUIPMENT

Digital subtraction angiography requires more complex equipment than digital radiography, specifically because it has to manipulate a number of pulsed images and at the same time create a subtracted image using the first precontrast image as a mask.

- **Generator and tube**: The specialized nature of the angiographic tube and generator, designed to take a number of images in rapid succession, make it suitable for DSA without further modifications. Tube loading and heating curves are similar.
- **Image intensifier**: The digital image is taken from the television image produced during fluoroscopy. It is, therefore, vital that all the parts of the image intensification unit are suitable for digital fluoroscopy and thus digital subtraction. It is critical to create an environment where there are no major fluctuations in power because small differences can affect the quality of the subtraction. There must also be a high contrast ratio so that small variations in beam attenuation can be registered and used in the subtraction process.
- **TV camera**: A camera focuses on the image intensification image and scans it electronically. This is a vital section of the system. The camera must have properties that keep electronic noise to a minimum and a low lag to eliminate ghosting. The amount and quality of light reaching the TV camera are carefully controlled by a light diaphragm.
- **Image digitizer**: This turns the analog TV image into a digital image consisting of **pixels**, the number of which depends on the lines per inch of the TV image. The usual pixel numbers in an image are 512 × 512 or 1024 × 1024 (high resolution) (Figure 6.10).

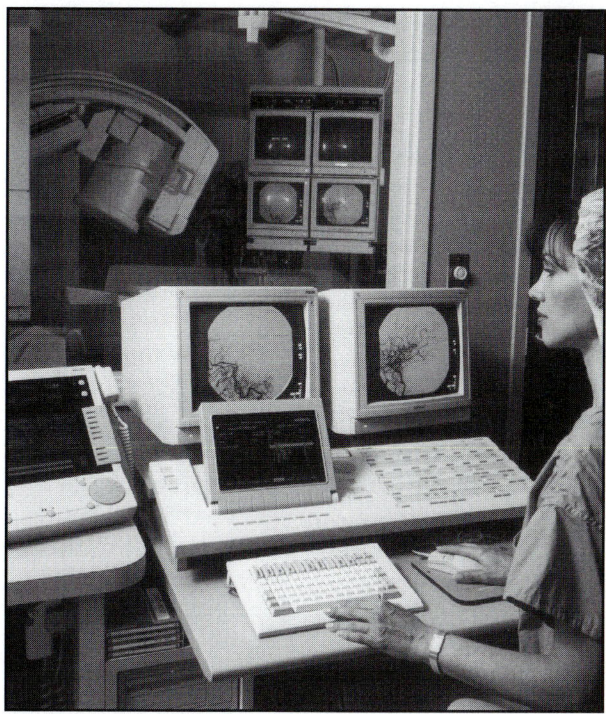

FIGURE 6.10 Image digitizer (Courtesy of Philips Medical Systems, Shelton, CT).

- **Image storage and processor**: This is the section of the computer that takes the acquired images, manipulates the subtraction, and then recreates an analog video image for visualization on a screen. Current technology allows for this to happen very quickly so that a real-time image is available as the procedure is being performed, that is, as the contrast is being injected.
- **Postprocessing image manipulation**: This is performed using the computer and images stored within it and is performed after completion of an examination to create the best image possible.
- **Multiformat camera**: A hard copy of the resultant analog image can be produced using this image processor (Figure 6.11).

The use of DSA requires a familiarity of the equipment by the radiographer. It is the responsibility of the radiographer to monitor and improve images during real-time imaging and to produce the highest quality images from postprocessing manipulation.

Other equipment specific to a procedure will be discussed in that section.

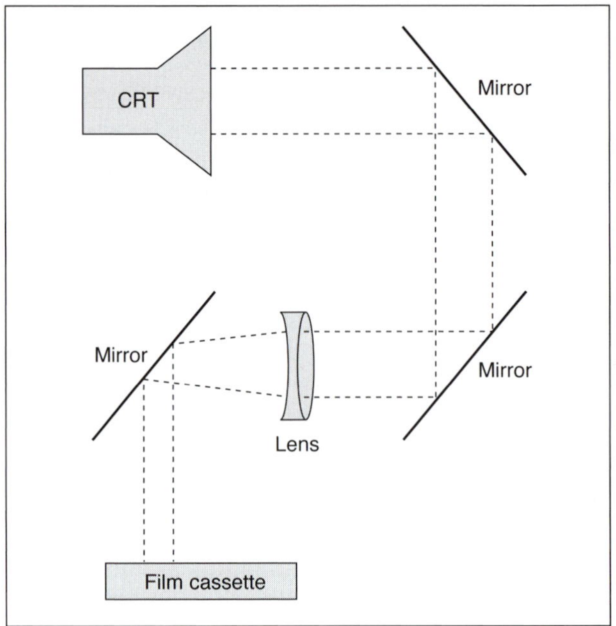

FIGURE 6.11 The configuration of a multiformat camera. Multiple images are obtained by moving the cassette after each exposure.

Injection Methods

Several methods are used for introducing contrast into arteries, veins, or lymph vessels. They can be subdivided into two main types, the direct puncture or the indirect catheter approach, the latter being the most common today.

PERCUTANEOUS NEEDLE PUNCTURE

A needle is placed directly within the **lumen** of the vessel and injection made via the needle in situ. The percutaneous needle used for a direct injection into the artery or vein will consist of two parts, a **cannula** (kăn′ū-lă) and **stilette** (stī-lĕt′), which will allow puncturing of the vessel, and then with the removal of the stilette, a passage for injection. Each needle will also have a connecting hub, usually a Luer-lok, to ensure a pressure-resistant attachment (Figure 6.12). A two- or three-way stopcock and transparent tubing must be ready for connecting onto the needle as soon as the vessel has been punctured.

In the past this approach has been used to visualize carotid and vertebral arteries, vessels of the extremities, and the abdominal aorta. This approach has largely been discarded in favor of the indirect catheter system, but it is still used for femoral arteriography and occasionally lumbar aortography. It is a system that can be used if the catheter method is not possible because of practical or pathologic or morphologic reasons.

The method for the arterial puncture is the same initially for the direct and indirect approach.

- A sterile field is provided and maintained around the puncture site.
- A local anesthetic is injected around the puncture site.
- A small incision is usually made 1 to 2 cm below the puncture site to facilitate needle entry.
- The artery is palpated and held in place by the fingers of one hand while the needle is guided and inserted by the other.
- Successful puncturing of the artery is noted by rapid, pulsing blood flow after removal of the stilette.
- A transparent connector attached to the hub of the needle allows visualization of the blood flow and then is used as a flushing system.
- As soon as the flow is visualized, the needle should be flushed with saline via the connecting tube and

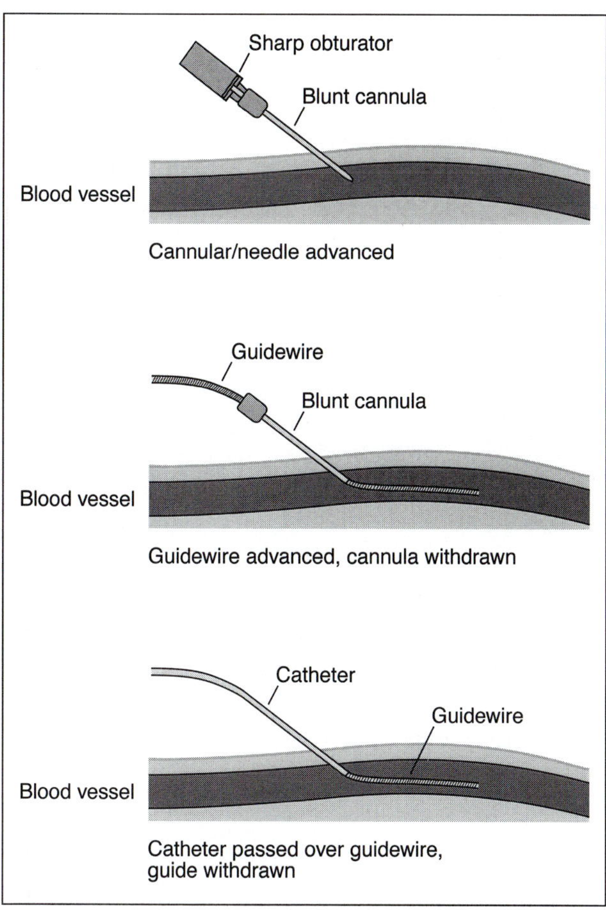

FIGURE 6.12 Seldinger technique.

then controlled by the stopcock. It is important to keep the needle and any tubing free of clotting and the system should be flushed occasionally throughout the procedure.

PERCUTANEOUS CATHETERIZATION—SELDINGER TECHNIQUE

This method of catheterizing the vessel is based on the work of the Swedish physician, Seldinger, and has come to be called the Seldinger technique. This method as follows allows for the introduction of a needle, guidewire, and catheter into a vessel. The two most common areas of insertion are the femoral artery and the axillary artery. Most arteries can be selected from these two entry points (see individual procedure descriptions) but occasionally the brachial, axillary, carotid, and lumbar aorta have been used as introducing sites (see Figure 6.12).

- Site is prepared as for direct puncture (Figure 6.13). A Seldinger or similarly designed needle is used to puncture the vessel as for the direct puncture (Figures 6.14 and 6.15).

The original Seldinger needle consisted of three parts, the blunt cannula, an inner needle, and a

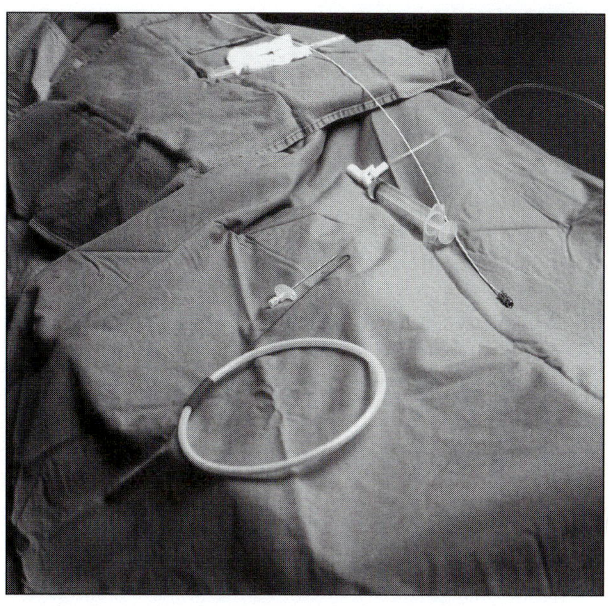

FIGURE 6.13 Seldinger needle and guidewire.

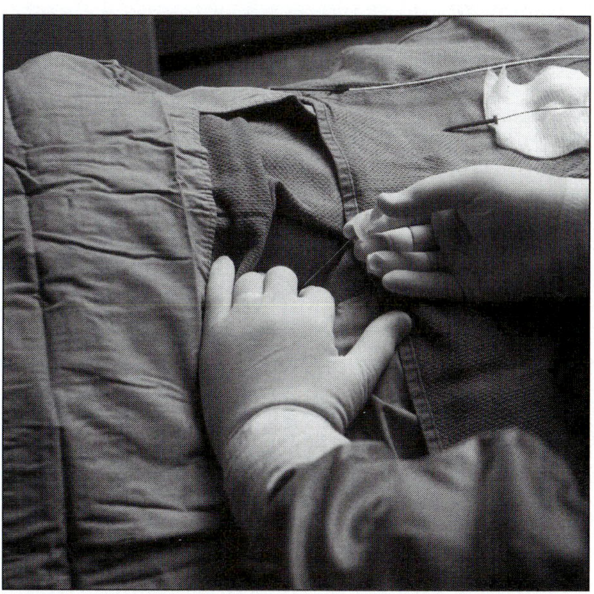

FIGURE 6.14 Femoral artery being punctured.

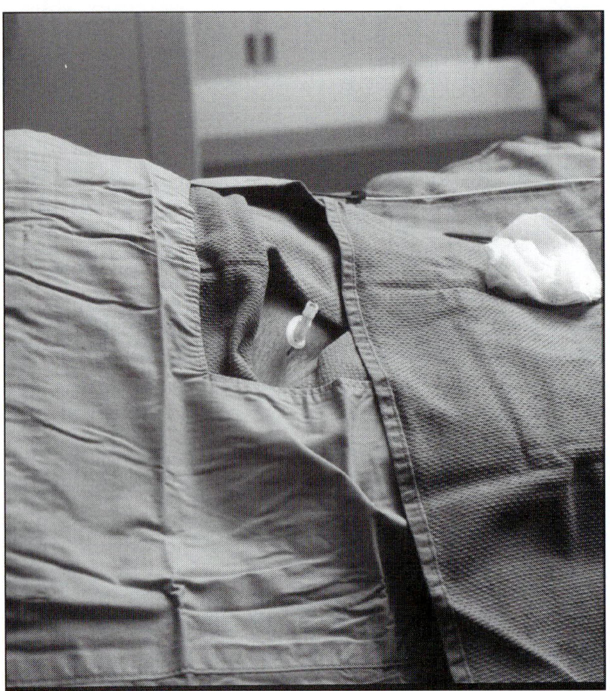

FIGURE 6.15 Needle in situ.

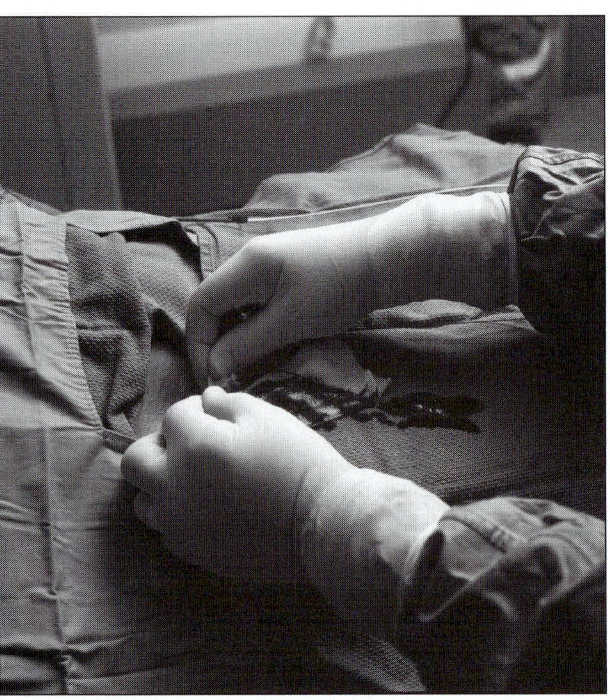

FIGURE 6.16 Blood spurting from puncture.

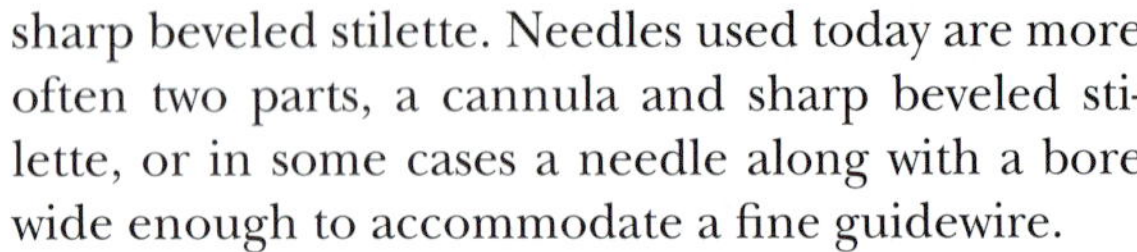

sharp beveled stilette. Needles used today are more often two parts, a cannula and sharp beveled stilette, or in some cases a needle along with a bore wide enough to accommodate a fine guidewire.

- As soon as blood is seen freely spurting from the needle cannula following removal of the stilette (Figure 6.16), a guidewire is introduced through the cannula and advanced 5 to 8 cm into the lumen of the vessel (Figure 6.17).
- The needle is removed and manual pressure maintained over the puncture site to prevent bleeding or **hematoma** formation.
- The guidewire is wiped with saline to prevent clot formation.
- The catheter is slipped over the guidewire and introduced carefully into the vessel by exerting gentle pressure while rotating slowly.
- Occasionally a short introducer or dilator is advanced over the guidewire and through the puncture site into the vessel before the catheter is introduced. It is gently moved back and forth to facilitate the entry of the catheter and then removed. This technique is not so necessary with thin-walled catheters.
- The guidewire is longer than the catheter and is moved forward under fluoroscopic control until it sits in the required position in the correct vessel.

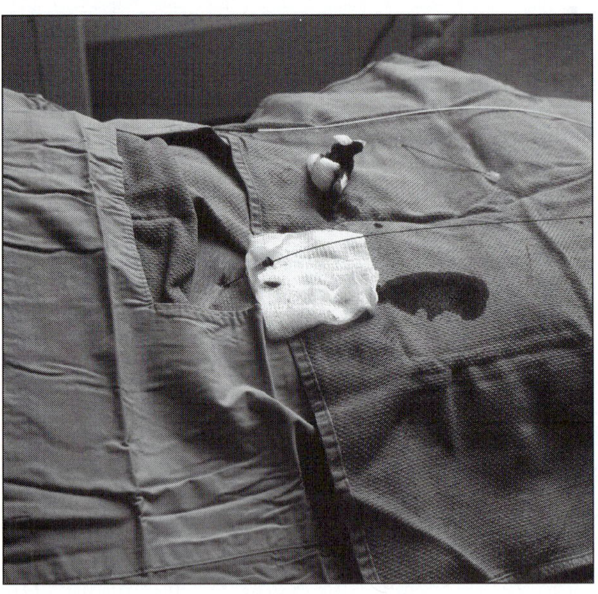

FIGURE 6.17 Guidewire inserted.

- The catheter is then advanced until its tip is exactly in position and then the guidewire is removed (Figure 6.18).
- The catheter can now be moved to any desired level. Different types of catheters allow for various

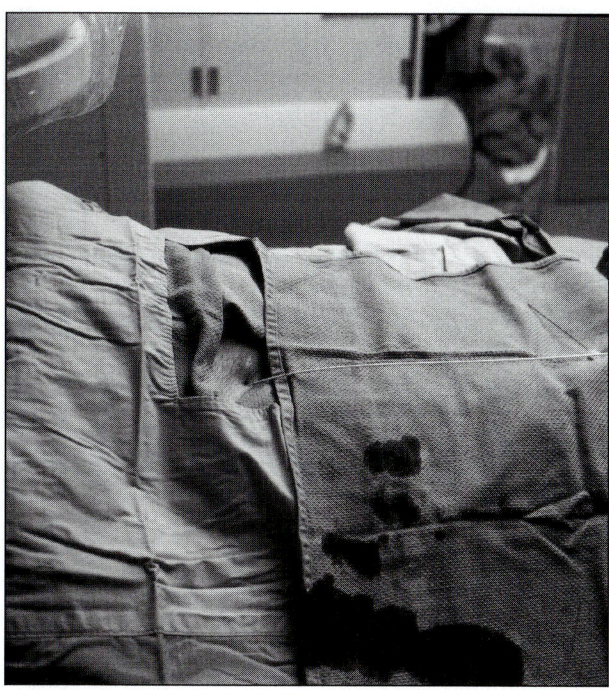

FIGURE 6.18 Catheter in place.

vessels to be selected (see individual descriptions under the catheter heading). The selecting of specific vessels may require the reintroduction of the guidewire.

- A small injection of contrast medium under fluoroscopic control assesses the position.
- Guidewires and catheters must be carefully swabbed with saline with each movement introduction or retraction.
- During the positioning and selection, there must be an infusion of saline either by a manual injection or by a saline drip attached via a three-way stopcock.

Selective and Superselective Catheterization

Catheters come in various styles and have been designed to fit into curves and origins of vessels. The various types of catheters and guidewires are described. The objective of these catheters is to facilitate their introduction into the required vessel. For instance, the renal arteries can be selected from the abdominal aorta. If different vessels are required to be selected during a single procedure, the original catheter can be removed by first replacing the guidewire through it, removing the catheter, and then replacing it with the required replacement catheter.

The term superselective is used to describe a procedure where a smaller vessel is selected from another selected vessel. A good example is the celiac axis and its branches . The celiac axis is selected from the aorta and then the gastroduodenal, hepatic, or splenic artery is "superselected" from the axis.

CATHETERS

Most catheters today are produced commercially, preformed with appropriate holes and Luer-lok end, and disposable. They are made of polyurethane, polyethylene, Dacron, or Teflon. Originally catheters were custom made in the angio suite, but this practice is rarely carried out now. If required, straight catheters can be molded by submerging in hot water, curving into the shape required, and then placed into cold sterile water. Catheters vary in length from 100 to 145 cm, the latter being able to select the aortic arch branches from a femoral artery insertion point. Most catheters are thin walled and 5 **French** size.

Common catheter types (Figure 6.19) include:

- Straight—end hole only
- Pigtail—catheter with a circular tip with multiple side holes to reduce whiplash and control contrast
- Sidewinder—catheter is curved to facilitate vessel selection
- Cobra—a variation in curvature to facilitate selection of vessels

Specialized catheters are used when the angiogram includes some intervention. The most common variety is the coaxial catheter, which consists of a standard introducing catheter, through which an inner catheter can be threaded to select secondary and tertiary branched vessels. These are often very fine (3 French) and sometimes difficult to visualize radiographically, but their fineness is needed to move into small vessels that may need to be embolized.

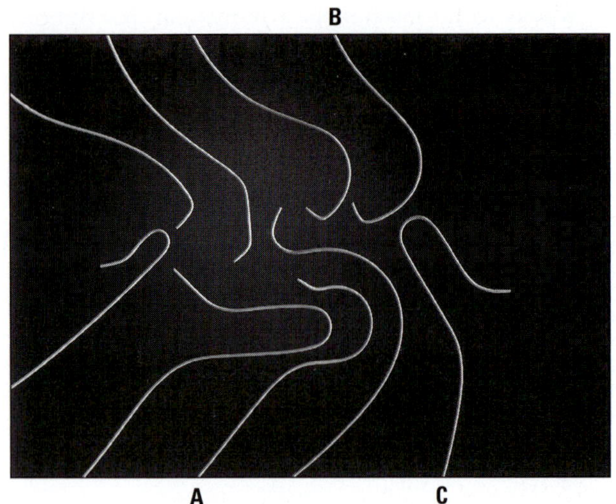

FIGURE 6.19 Varieties of catheters: (A) headhunter (B) cobra (C) sidewinder (Courtesy of Cook Incorporated, Bloomington, IN).

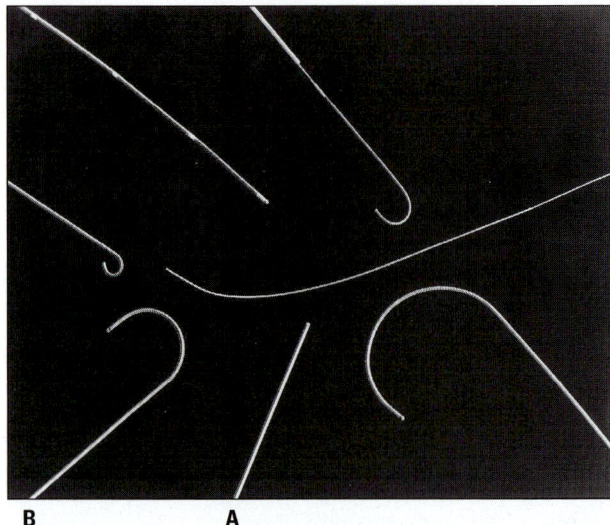

FIGURE 6.20 Varieties of guidewires: (A) straight-tipped (B) J-tipped (Courtesy of Cook Incorporated, Bloomington, IN).

The various shapes and end hole requirements are listed under the individual procedures.

GUIDEWIRES

A guidewire consists of a solid wire core, usually two straight wires, surrounded by a wire coil that is coated to reduce friction (Figure 6.20). Guidewires come in many sizes, metal types, and coatings and can be classified as follows:

- Introducing guidewires: These are standard guidewires that have either a straight end or a floppy, J-shaped tip. They should be Teflon coated to prevent friction as they pass through the polyurethane catheters.
- Exchange guidewires: These are generally long, 180 to 260 cm, and are used if catheters are being replaced during a procedure. They have a stiff body and a soft flexible tip to prevent vascular perforation.
- Long floppy-tipped guidewires: These guidewires have soft, variable-length ends that allow catheterization of **tortuous** or atherosclerotic vessels and for superselection. The length of the floppiness can be controlled by moving one of the internal core wires.
- **Torque** (tork) guidewires: These are specialized guidewires that allow for the careful selection of arteries of the brain, heart, abdomen, and extremities.

Puncture Sites

Several sites are used during angiography. The most common area is the femoral artery.

FEMORAL ARTERY PUNCTURE

- Provides access to aorta, left ventricle, and all branches
- Lower complication rate
- Not recommended if a femoral artery aneurysm is suspected
- Extreme **tortuosity** may inhibit advancement of catheter into the aorta or even iliac vessels. Alternative approaches or the use of DSA should be considered.

Technique

- Patient lies supine on angiographic table.
- Where possible the asymptomatic side is used. This leaves untouched any area that may need surgery in the future.

- The puncture site is located by finding the femoral pulse.
- The puncture site is prepared using aseptic technique. (The groin area may need to be shaved initially.)
- Local anesthetic is administered to either side of the artery to the periosteum.
- A small incision is made with a scalpel at the puncture site to ease entry of the catheter.
- The needle is aimed 45° **cephalically** at a point just distal to where the femoral artery becomes the external iliac artery. It is important not to puncture too deep into the groin because it will be difficult to stem bleeding and thus prevent a hematoma occurring at the site.
- The artery is immobilized by the fingers of one hand and a stab is made that should traverse both walls of the artery.
- At this point the needle should be pulsating.
- The stilette is removed, the needle flattened slightly so that it sits along the skin surface and then the needle is withdrawn until a pulsating blood flow is achieved.
- The Seldinger technique is then used.

The saline drip used to flush the system can be heparinized by using 2500 units in 500 mL of 0.9% saline. This reduces the risk of clotting. However, it is important that if bleeding at the puncture site continues for more than 5 minutes after removal of the catheter, attempts should be made to neutralize the effects of the heparin by administering protamine sulfate.

- At the completion of the procedure, the catheter is removed and manual pressure exerted on the puncture site for about 5 minutes. A pressure bandage can also be placed over the area after this time.
- The puncture site must be carefully observed for at least 4 hours. The use of larger catheters, greater than 5 French, will require a longer observation period.
- Bed rest should occur during this period.
- Vital signs, particularly peripheral pulses, must be taken periodically, up to 24 hours.

AXILLARY ARTERY PUNCTURE

- Because this site has a higher degree of risk, it should only be considered if the femoral approach is not possible.
- The patient lies supine with the arm fully extended and abducted.
- The axillary pulse is localized, just distal to the axilla.
- The site is prepared as for the femoral injection, using aseptic technique.
- The needle is directed cephalically along the long axis of the humerus.
- The Seldinger technique is used and the remainder of the procedure is as for the femoral puncture.

Other sites include the brachial artery and the translumbar approach.

IV PUNCTURE FOR DIGITAL SUBTRACTION ANGIOGRAPHY

This method is used when arterial catheterization is not possible and when fine vessel detail is not needed. It is a useful procedure to assess the patency of grafts and the procedure is less hazardous.

- Before the procedure, an antiflatulent can be administered to reduce abdominal gas and help reduce subtraction artifacts, if the abdomen is the area to be imaged.
- The patient lies supine on the table, with the arm extended.
- A suitable vein is chosen within the antecubital fossa.
- Using aseptic technique, the puncture site is prepared.
- The vein is punctured and a guidewire introduced through the needle.
- The needle is withdrawn and a 5 French pigtail catheter advanced over the guidewire.
- The two are then advanced to lie either in the superior vena cava or right atrium.
- The catheter is flushed, as in arterial catheterizations.
- The guidewire is removed before contrast is injected.
- Abdominal compression can be used to reduce subtractions errors.
- Separate injections of contrast are needed for each view needed to obtain suitable masks.
- The guidewire is reintroduced before the catheter is retracted to straighten out the pigtail end.
- At the completion of the procedure, firm pressure is applied over the puncture site.

Contrast Media

When Moniz began his work in angiography, thorium dioxide (Thorotrast) was used. This contrast was retained in the body and its radioactivity gave rise to long-term malignancies. Today, contrast agents in angiography are all organic iodine solutions. These contrast media have been found to be **nephrotoxic** during the excretory process and can create uncomfortable sensations. The latest contrast agents have a low osmolarity and this has proven to be relatively painless with fewer side effects. The osmolarity of the newer contrast agents such as iohexol is much closer to that of normal plasma. (See Chapter 1, Introduction to Diagnostic and Interventional Procedures, for chemical composition and properties of contrast media.)

Care for the Patient in Angiography

Angiography is an examination that is not without risks and it is important that patients are made aware of these by their physician when the procedure is first ordered. A number of less hazardous imaging modalities can demonstrate the vasculature and any angiographic team receiving the patient for an examination must assume that the patient's physician has made an informed decision regarding the necessity for this examination.

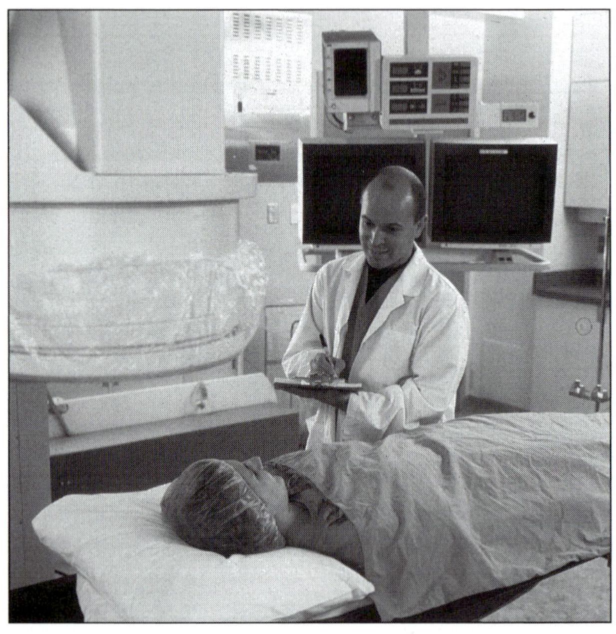

FIGURE 6.21 Explaining the procedure to patient.

Patient Preparation

- Before the procedure, the patient is admitted to the hospital for careful observation. This may be as an inpatient or as a day patient, depending on the severity of the patient's condition and the procedure to be done.
- Vital signs and peripheral pulses should be taken to serve as a baseline for postangiographic care.
- Anticoagulant therapy should be assessed and careful note made of prothrombin time to ensure that it is within normal limits. Administration of these drugs should be withheld for 4 hours before the procedure and resumed after 24 hours postprocedure.
- The procedure must be explained and an informed consent signed. The patient's fears should be alleviated as much as possible. A composed patient reduces the risk of complications (Figure 6.21).
- Once the consent form has been signed any premedication prescribed can be administered. The usual medications include:
  —Atropine—to inhibit a vasovagal reaction
  —Demerol (meperidine hydrochloride)—analgesic
  —Valium (diazepam)—muscle relaxant and sedative
- Patient should fast for 4 to 8 hours before the procedure. Fluid intake is recommended for patients with renal disease.
- The puncture site is shaved.

Complications in Angiographic Procedures

Contrast Media Intra-arterial complications are rarer than with an IV injection of contrast. Apart from reactions covered in Chapter 1, Introduction to Diagnostic and Interventional Procedures, some specific reactions can occur.

- Hotness and pain at injection site are reduced by the low-osmolarity contrast agents.
- A **chemotoxic** affect can occur. Sodium or meglumine salts can affect the ECG. Sodium can produce **neurotoxic** effects.
- Acute renal failure is extremely rare but can occur if there has been significant dehydration, the recent administration of nephrotoxic drugs, and high doses of contrast medium.

Catheter/Procedure Technique

- Hematoma
- Hemorrhage
- Arterial thrombus, due to trauma to the artery wall; this can happen for several reasons:
  —Large catheters
  —Frequent catheter changes
  —Prolonged time in the arteries
  —Rough handling and maneuvering of the catheters
  —Rough-surfaced catheters, specifically polyurethane
- Heparinization of the saline, heparin-bonded catheters, and guidewires and repeated wiping of these during use, by gauze soaked in heparinized saline
- Infection at puncture site caused by nonsterile technique

Other rare complications can include:

- Arteriovenous fistula formation
- Embolus production, atherosclerotic or air
- Artery dissection
- Catheter knotting and impaction
- Guidewire breakage

Postangiographic Care

- Bed rest for 4 to 12 hours depending on the procedure
- Observation of puncture site
- Vital signs taken, including peripheral pulses
- **Hydration** encouraged
- Resumption of any drug therapy when assessed to be safe

Interventional Procedures

Several angiographic interventional procedures are closely associated with angiography. All of them require a preliminary angiogram as a map to the vasculature and they frequently require a follow-up angiogram to assess the success of the procedure. The basic procedures are the same. Specific variations are covered in the appropriate chapters.

PERCUTANEOUS TRANSLUMINAL ANGIOPLASTY (PTA)

Angioplasty is a procedure that seeks to improve blood flow and supply by widening a vessel. The most common vessels it is used for are iliac, femoral, renal, and coronary arteries. The original procedure used a telescoping device that gradually enlarged the lumen, but the width attainable was restricted by the size of the puncture through which these dilators had to pass. The advent of Gruntzig's balloon catheter resolved this problem.

Applied Anatomy (Figure 6.22)

Indications

- Stenosis of a vessel due to atherosclerotic deposits
- Discrete or "focal" stenoses are the most easily treatable. (Specific indications are discussed under each system.)

Contraindications Diffuse atherosclerotic disease. It is difficult to resolve the occlusion that affects the entire length of a vessel and attempts to perform angioplasty can result in the production of an embolus, with extremely serious effects. It is therefore essential that any prospective PTA candidate has a preliminary angiogram to decide whether PTA or perhaps surgery is the best method of treatment.

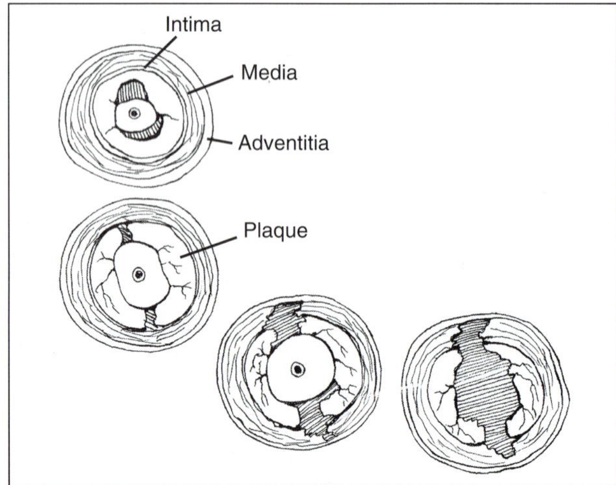

FIGURE 6.22 Action of angioplasty on anatomy of vessel (Courtesy of Cook Incorporated, Bloomington, IN).

Equipment

- Fluoroscopy unit with hard copy image capabilities, digital subtraction
- Catheters: Gruntzig-type catheters are the most used. They have a double lumen, one for the guidewire and one for the balloon and inflation channel. They come in varying lengths, from 80 cm to 120 cm, and can be straight or curved, the choice depending on the vessel to be selected and widened. The balloon's inflated size can vary as well, from 2 to 10 mm (Figure 6.23).
- Guidewires
- Sterile tray to include needles for Seldinger percutaneous approach
- Optional pressure measuring equipment

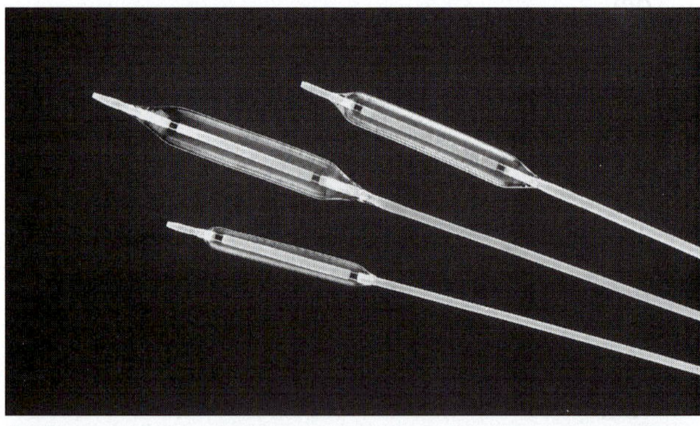

A

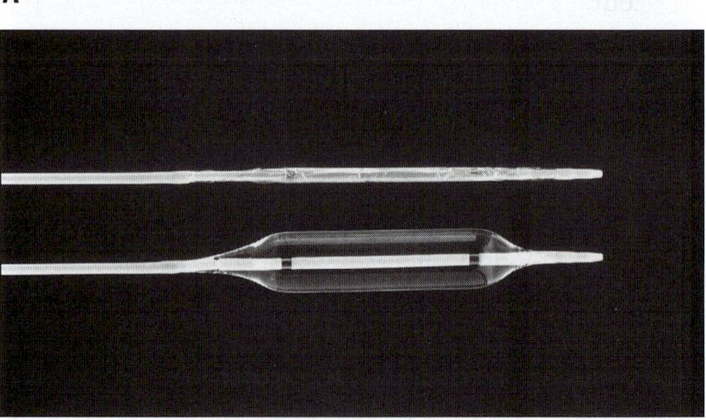

B

FIGURE 6.23 (A) Balloon catheters (B) Preinflated and inflated catheters (Courtesy of Cook Incorporated, Bloomington, IN).

Contrast Media A water-soluble nonionic contrast medium may be used incidentally to confirm the placement of the catheter. The balloon can be inflated with contrast.

Radiation Protection Fluoroscopy time kept to a minimum, by use of a pulsed image and video image freeze frame.

Preliminary Radiographs An angiogram should be performed before this procedure to assess the condition of the vessel.

Patient Preparation

- This is an inpatient procedure.
- The patient must be made aware of all the risks and complications and sign a consent form before any premedications are administered.
- There must be close cooperation with the vascular surgeon, who should be in attendance or reachable during this procedure in case of a surgical intervention being required.
- The patient's vital signs should be taken, particularly blood pressures proximal and distal to the stenosis (only possible with extremities).
- Anticoagulant therapy can be administered depending on the condition of the patient. Heparin is the drug of choice. This heparinization should continue during the procedure. If necessary, its effects can be reversed by using protamine.
- Aspirin and dipridamole can also be administered before the procedure. These are platelet inhibitors and help to prevent platelet aggregation.
- The patient is sedated before the procedure.
- Patient is NPO for 4 hours before the procedure.
- Nifedipine can be given sublingually 30 minutes before the procedure. It is a vasodilator and reduces the risk of vascular spasm during the procedure.

Angioplasty Procedure Most angioplasty procedures use the femoral artery as their percutaneous approach and the catheter is introduced using the Seldinger technique. Specifics of location are discussed under appropriate systems. The following describes the technique of balloon dilatation in generic terms.

- A guidewire is introduced via the Seldinger technique and advanced beyond the point of the stenosis. It is usually a soft-tipped variety to reduce the likelihood of an embolus being produced.
- A regular catheter is advanced and used to demonstrate the condition of the stenosed vessel by injecting a small amount of contrast under fluoroscopic control.
- A larger, more rigid guidewire is inserted into this catheter. This is to facilitate catheter exchanges (Figure 6.24).
- The initial catheter is removed and a balloon catheter inserted. The inflatable width and length of the balloon has been predetermined from the previous angiogram.
- The balloon catheter is moved into place so that the balloon fits as closely as possible to the length of the stenotic area. This reduces the degree to which the balloon would press into healthy tissue.
- The balloon is then slowly inflated by inserting about 10 cc of air through the syringe attachment (Figure 6.25).
- Inflation should last from between 15 and 30 seconds.
- If the balloon has to be moved to another stenotic site, it must first be deflated and then reinflated at the site.
- When the angioplasty is complete, the area is reexamined with a further flush of contrast to estimate the success of the procedure.
- Catheters are removed and pressure applied to the percutaneous site.

Procedure Radiographs Images can be taken using the fluoroscopy and video equipment, together with digital subtraction. Full angiograms are rarely performed.

Postprocedure Care

- The patient should be closely monitored for any changes in vital signs or neurologic signs, depending on the site being treated.
- The production of an embolus must be carefully screened for.
- Aspirin can be administered daily.

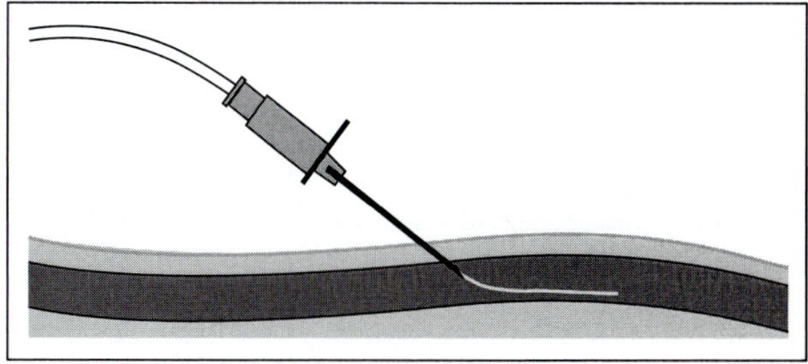

FIGURE 6.24 Introduction of guidewire (Courtesy of Cook Incorporated, Bloomington, IN).

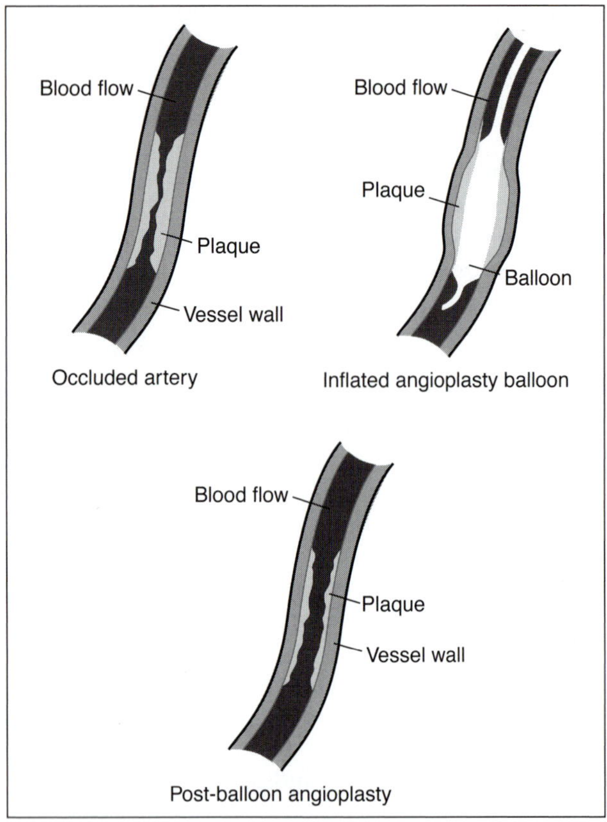

FIGURE 6.25 Three images of angioplasty.

- If there appears to be a connection between the patient's condition and smoking, the patient is strongly advised to stop.
- Angioplasty has a patency rate of between 5 and 10 years and certain drugs and lifestyle can prolong this time. Patients should be aware, however, that having the angioplasty does not prohibit the return of the atherosclerotic condition.

> It was originally thought that angioplasty simply pressed the atherosclerotic plaque against the wall of the vessel. It has now been determined that this could not, in fact, happen because the plaque has very little water content and is very firm. Instead, the angioplasty cracks the plaque and breaks down the intima and the lumen is enlarged by stretching the outer diameter of the artery.

Common Pathologies Stenosis of the femoral artery, before and after angioplasty

LASER ANGIOPLASTY

There has been significant interest in the development of a laser angioplasty catheter as a means to clear an occlusion. However, at this point there has been no definite indication of study that demonstrates that the vessels remain patent any longer than from conventional balloon angioplasty.

ATHERECTOMY

It has been felt that the success rate and length of patency time could be improved if, as well as breaking up the plaque, it could somehow be removed nonsurgically. Several catheters have been designed to attempt this—pulsating, rotating, ultrasonic—but at this time this has not replaced surgery, if the vessel does not or cannot respond to angioplasty.

VASCULAR STENTS

These are essentially tubes that can be placed within the newly opened vessel to keep it patent. They are still experimental but do hold the promise of prolonging the effectiveness of the angioplastic procedure.

THROMBOLYSIS

There are situations where occlusions are caused by thrombus (usually in a vein) and these can sometimes be treated by positioning a catheter at the occlusion and administering a thrombolytic agent. The use of streptokinase fell out of favor because of complications. Currently, studies are being performed to find agents that will dissolve the thrombus without jeopardizing the condition of the patient.

THROMBUS FILTERS

The main pathway for a clot to follow is from the leg via the inferior vena cava to the pulmonary artery where its effects can be devastating. Filters can be placed within the inferior vena cava to catch the clots. This procedure would only be performed on individuals with a history of recurring clot development.

EMBOLIZATION

It is sometimes desirous to produce an occlusion rather than reduce one and this procedure, called **embolization**, introduces a substance, either a mechanical device or chemical material, to produce a temporary or permanent occlusion. Although this procedure has only been used regularly within the last 20 years, the very first embolization occurred in 1904 when melted paraffin was injected into the external carotid arteries of patients suffering from tumors. However, it was not until the 1970s that embolytic agents were described and put to general use, Gelfoam in 1974 and detachable balloons also in 1974. Since that time there has been a proliferation of devices. Only those in general use are mentioned below.

There are three main reasons to perform this procedure:

1. To control bleeding, usually from the GI tract or GU tract or as a result of trauma
2. To reduce blood supply to tumors or organs or circulatory malformations
3. As a preoperative procedure to stem blood flow to a particular site

There are a number of ways that vessels can be embolized and they are discussed under the specific systems. However, there are three main types of embolizing materials:

1. Liquid: These can be a dextrose-alcohol mixture or quick-setting glues or a vasoconstrictor drug.
2. Particulate: Gelfoam is the most common example. It is a spongy substance that is produced as small or larger pellets.
3. Solid: These are mechanical devices that actually occlude the vessel, such as a detachable balloon, or a mechanism that when in place encourages the production of thrombus.

Although the effects can be temporary or permanent, all embolization devices should be considered irreversible, requiring a great deal of care and meticulous work if they are to be used in the treatment of a patient. The embolization substances can also be subdivided into temporary and permanent.

- Temporary: Vasoconstrictors such as pitressin and vasopressin can be injected via a catheter to provide temporary relief in the event of an acute bleed such as a GI bleed. Strictly speaking, they do not create an embolus.
- Gelfoam is a substance that does form a temporary embolism. It too can be used in the treatment of a GI bleed and will stay in place for several days, while hemostasis is maintained. Gelfoam is also used as a preoperative procedure to stem blood loss during surgery.
- Permanent: Detachable balloons placed in specific vessels with the flow of blood will form a permanent occlusion beyond which blood ceases to flow (Figure 6.26). Balloons are made from latex or silicone rubber and can be threaded through catheters as small as 5 French. The larger the balloon inflated diameter, the larger the catheter must be (5 French can accommodate a 3-mm balloon, a 9 French, 9-mm when inflated). This is used to occlude tumor circulation. The balloon can be used alone, or together with particulate material, where it serves as a stopper until the clot is permanently formed. The balloon is then removed.
- The Gianturco coil is a stainless steel spring with stranded nylon or woolen fibers attached to induce thrombosis. It is used for the embolization of larger

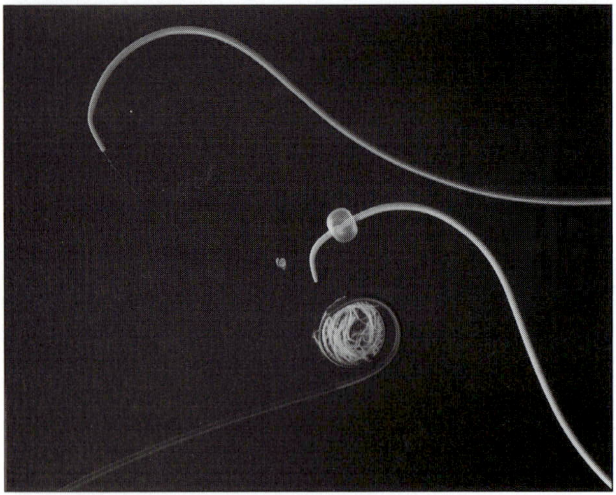

FIGURE 6.26 Detachable balloon (Courtesy of Cook Incorporated, Bloomington, IN)

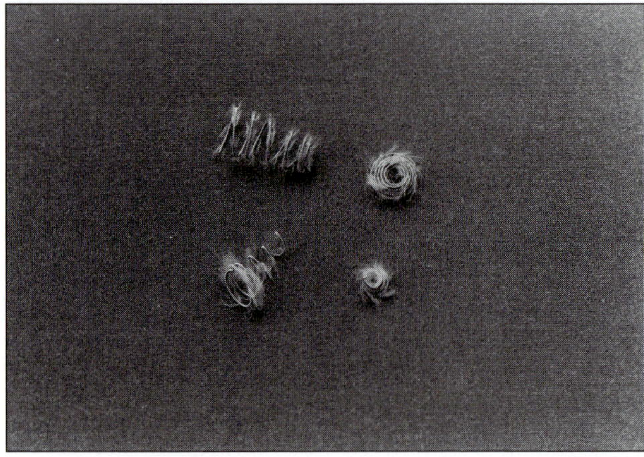

FIGURE 6.27 Gianturco coil (Courtesy of Cook Incorporated, Bloomington, IN).

vessels, but has been found not to always produce a complete thrombic embolus and has been replaced by the detachable balloon where possible (Figure 6.27).

Care for Embolization Patients Care will vary according to the procedure, the pathology, and the patient's condition but there are some general principles regarding aftercare and complications.

- Most embolizing occurs via a percutaneous puncture using the Seldinger tehnique and the usual care should be taken as for any postangiography patient.
- Tissue that has been infarcted (deprived of a blood supply) is often painful and sufficient analgesic should be provided to the patient.
- There must be careful observation of all surrounding tissues and vital signs to ensure that the clotting has not progressed beyond the site required.
- Patients tend to have a fever for up to 10 days after the procedure. This must be carefully monitored.
- Infarcted tissue has a tendency to become infected. This must also be carefully monitored.

The embolus can become dislodged or throw off sections that pass to the lungs. Again care and observation must be carefully maintained.

Angiography is performed throughout the vascular systems. The following chapters describe the main procedures performed and will refer to the generic techniques described in this chapter.

Review Questions

1. Describe the process of the Seldinger technique.

2. Discuss the various modes of collecting the imaged data. Suggest advantages and disadvantages to cut film, versus cine film, versus video, versus digital acquisition.

3. Describe the ongoing care needed for a patient during angiography, including possible emergency situations.

4. Which of the following is an essential feature of generators used in angiographic suites?

a. large focal spot
b. 500 mA
c. 1000 mA
d. falling load

5. The size of a 7 French catheter would be:

a. 0.66 mm
b. 2.31 mm
c. 1.9 mm
d. 3.33 mm

6. Pigtail catheters are designed specifically to:

a. prevent whiplash
b. inhibit contrast flow
c. prevent clots
d. select very small vessels

7. In the Seldinger technique

a. The catheter is introduced through the cannula.
b. A dilator is used to facilitate entry of the percutaneous needle.
c. The cannula must be reintroduced into the puncture site if catheters have to be replaced.
d. The stilette is removed when both walls of the artery have been traversed.

CASE STUDY

An emergency angiogram is proceeding in a fully equipped angiographic suite. During a series run using the cut film changer, you experience a jam. The patient is seriously ill and cannot be subjected to another angiogram. Describe what you might do in this situation.

___

___

___

___

___

___

___

___

___

___

___

References and Recommended Reading

Abrams, H. L. (1983). *Abrams' angiography:Vascular and interventional radiology* (3rd ed.). Boston: Little, Brown.

Ballinger, P. W. (1991). *Merrill's atlas of radiographic positions and radiologic procedures,* (7th ed.). St. Louis: Mosby-Year Book.

Castaneda-Zuniga, W. R., Tadavarthy, S. T. (1992). *Interventional radiology.* Baltimore: Williams & Wilkins.

Chapman, S., & Nakielny, R. (1993*). A guide to radiological procedures* (3rd. ed.). London: Bailliere Tindall.

Cope, C., Burke, D., & Meranze, S. (1990). *Atlas of interventional radiology.* Philadelphia: Lippincott.

Cope, C. (1990). *Interventional arterial catheterization techniques* (Cook Inc.). New York: Gower Medical Publishers.

Cullinan, A., & Cullinan, J. (1994). *Producing quality radiographs* (2nd edition). Philadelphia: Lippincott.

Curry, T. S., Dowdey, J. E., & Murray, R. C. (1990). *Christensen's physics of diagnostic radiology* (4th ed.). Philadelphia: Lea & Febiger.

Doyle, T., Hare, W., Thomson, K., & Tress, B. (1989). *Procedures in diagnostic radiology.* London: Churchill Livingstone.

Eisenberg, R. L. (1992). *Radiology, an illustrated history.* St. Louis: Mosby-Year Book.

Gibson, P. H. (1992). Balloon angioplasty versus surgery. *Radiology, 185*(3), 908–909.

Kereiakes, J. G., Thomas, S. R., & Orton, C. G. (1986). *Digital radiography selected topics.* New York: Plenum.

Lasjaunais, P., & Berenstein, A. (1987). *Surgical neuroangiography* (Vol. 1). Berlin: Springer-Verlag.

Lasjaunais, P. (1980). Nasopharyngeal angiofibromas: Hazards of embolization. *Radiology, 136,* 119–123.

Moodie, D. S., & Yiannikas, J. (1986). *Digital subtraction angiography of the heart and lungs.* Orlando, FL: Grune & Stratton.

Ouriel, K., Shortell, C. (1994). Acute peripheral arterial occlusion: Predictors of success in catheter-directed thrombolytic therapy. *Radiology, 193*(2), 561–566.

Seldinger, S. (1953). Catheter replacement of needle in percutaneous arteriography; new technique. *Acta Radiologica, 39,* 368–376.

Snopek, A. M. (1992). *Fundamentals of special radiographic procedures* (3rd ed.). Philadelphia: Saunders.

Sutton, D. A. (1993). *Textbook of radiology and imaging* (5th ed.). Edinburgh: Churchill Livingstone.

Tortorici, M. R. (1982). *Fundamentals of angiography.* St. Louis: Mosby.

White, R. I. (1984). Embolotherapy in vascular disease. *American Journal of Roentenology, 142,* 27–30.

CHAPTER 7

Heart and Arterial System

HOLLY ENGEL, RT (R)(CV)(ARRT), RCVT
MARY J. HAGLER, MHA, BA, RT (R)(N)(M)(ARRT)

OBJECTIVES

At the completion of this chapter, the student should be able to:

1. Describe the anatomy of the heart and major vessels.
2. Compare and contrast the different procedures for cardiac catheterization, abdominal arteriography, and peripheral arteriography.
3. Recognize indications as to why various studies are performed and contraindications as to why the study may not be advised for the patient.
4. List the imaging equipment and accessory equipment appropriate to each study.

5. Discuss alternate imaging modalities for angiography.
6. Explain the special needs of the cardiac patient in terms of pre- and postprocedure care.
7. Understand normal and abnormal radiographic anatomy.
8. Recognize the role and proper use of contrast agents.
9. Discuss the various types of interventional procedures and their applications.
10. Be able to apply radiation protection practices to protect the patient and cardiac catheterization laboratory staff.
11. Differentiate the use of catheter sheaths, different types of catheters, and guidewires.
12. Discuss the process of acquiring hemodynamic pressures.
13. Explain the imaging sequences taken in cardiac catheterization and potential alternative studies.
14. Identify alternative approaches for arteriography.
15. Describe catheter flushing procedures.

Introduction and Historical Overview

In 1844, Claude Bernard placed a **catheter** in both the right and left ventricles of the heart from both the jugular vein and the femoral artery. The subject was a horse and thus became the first successful cardiac catheterization patient. About one month after Roentgen announced his discovery of x-radiation in 1895, Haschek and Lindenthal injected chalk into the brachial artery of a corpse for the first **angiography** procedure. Both these events were the cornerstones to what we refer to today as cardiac and vascular angiography. Over the next 30 years the limitations of radiographic equipment and the lack of suitable contrast material hampered the advancement of angiographic research. In the 1920s and 1930s with the advent of the tungsten filament x-ray tube and the use of sodium iodide as contrast material, quality angiographic procedures were performed, but coronary and vascular angiography continued to have significant risks to the patients. With the development of the Seldinger technique for accessing the arteries and veins, angiography became a safer and more routine procedure in the 1950s. Also in the 1950s and 1960s, the use of rapid film changers and the development of improved catheters made angiography the standard in the diagnosis and treatment of vascular and cardiac disease.

Since then, the major emphasis of advances has been the development of **interventional procedures** such as **angioplasty**, atherectomy, thrombolysis, and stenting of affected arteries. With these new procedures it is possible to intervene with the course of certain disease processes without having to expose the patient to the higher risks of surgery or other invasive procedures.

The cardiac catheterization laboratory or the special procedures angiography suite provide radiographers with an environment unique in radiography, that of the medical team approach (Figure 7.1). The medical team approach ensures coordinated efforts of a highly qualified group of health care practitioners comprised of radiographers, nurses, cardiovascular technicians, and physicians. Each professional brings a special knowledge that is integral to the smooth functioning of the laboratory. It is also an environment where the necessity for cross-training and continuing education provides a challenging work atmosphere.

It should be noted that procedures may differ among laboratories or angiography suites. Physician preferences and patient anatomy and pathology dictate changes in selection of equipment, contrast media, filming sequences, and injection rates.

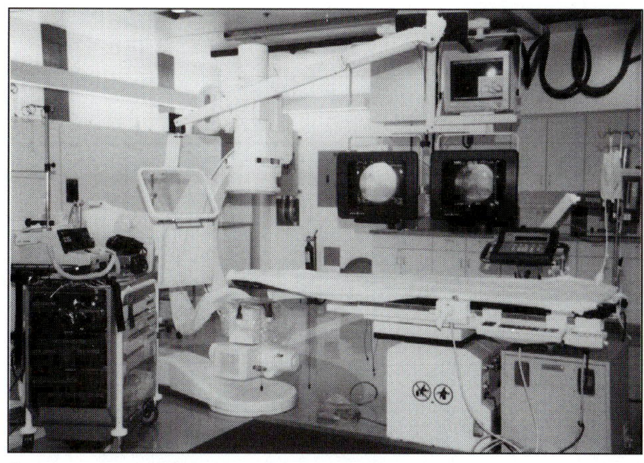

A

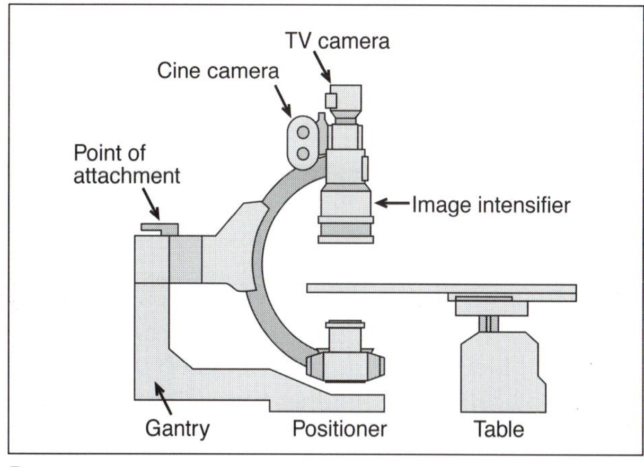

B

FIGURE 7.1 (A) Cardiac catheterization laboratory (B) Schematic of C-arm fluoroscope (Courtesy of GE Medical Systems).

Anatomy

CARDIAC ANATOMY

The heart is a hollow muscular organ that acts as a pump to circulate blood throughout the body. It lies obliquely in the center of the thoracic cavity and is about the size of a fist. The heart is divided into right and left halves, which are each divided into halves. This creates the four chambers of the heart, the right and left ventricles and the right and left atria (Figure 7.2). The right side of the heart receives unoxygenated blood from the veins of the body; the left side pumps oxygenated blood through arteries to the systemic system.

Blood is received into the right atrium from the superior and inferior vena cava and transported through the tricuspid valve into the right ventricle. As the right ventricle contracts, blood moves through the pulmonic valve and into the pulmonary artery. This vessel is identified as an artery even though it carries unoxygenated blood due to its classification as a vessel that leaves the heart. The main pulmonary artery then divides into the right and left pulmonary arteries, which branch to spread the blood to all lobular areas of the lung for oxygenation. After oxygenation occurs, the blood enters the left atrium, through the four pulmonary veins and travels through the mitral valve and into the left ventricle. The left ventricle then contracts and sends the blood through the aortic

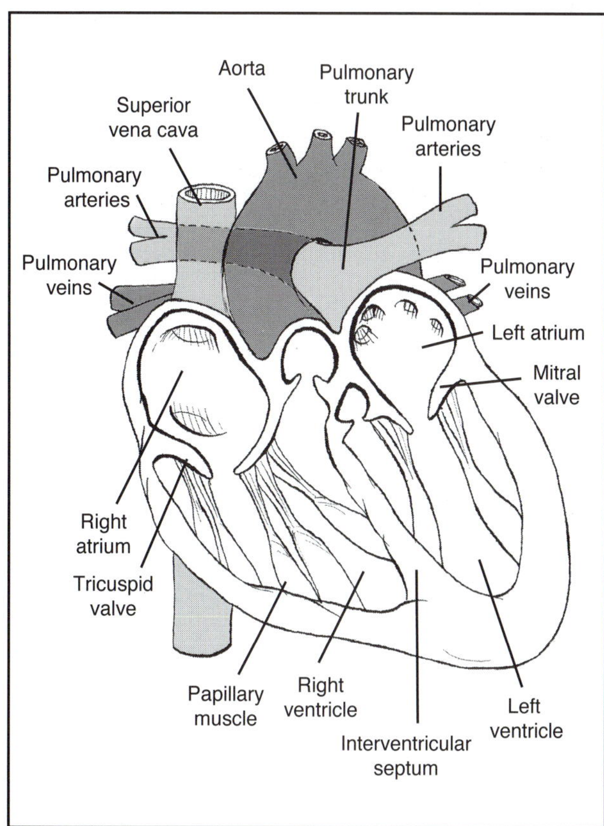

FIGURE 7.2 Chambers of the heart.

valve and to the rest of the body (Figure 7.3). Because the left ventricle must pump the blood to a large area, and the systemic resistance is much higher, the ventricle has a much larger chamber than the others and it has a thicker muscular wall to acheive this. The valves of the heart act as blood flow directors by preventing blood from backing up, or regurgitating, into a chamber it has already flowed through, thus keeping the blood moving in the right direction (Figure 7.4). Blood is kept flowing by the rhythmic contraction (systole) and dilation (diastole) of the heart.

As the blood leaves the heart it travels through the aortic valve into the ascending aorta. The aortic valve is a tricuspid structure where the coronary arteries arise from two of the three cusps. In normal anatomy, the left main coronary artery arises from the left cusp, and the right coronary artery arises from the right cusp. The third cusp is termed noncoronary because no artery arises from it.

The left main artery divides into two arteries, the left anterior descending (LAD) and the circumflex. The LAD travels to the anterior portion of the heart and wraps around the apex giving off branches called diagonals along the way. These branches will feed the free wall of the left ventricle and the right ventricle. The circumflex artery wraps posteriorly giving off branches called obtuse marginal (OM) branches that feed the posterior free wall of the heart.

The right coronary artery (RCA) is a single artery that travels to the inferior portion of the heart. The

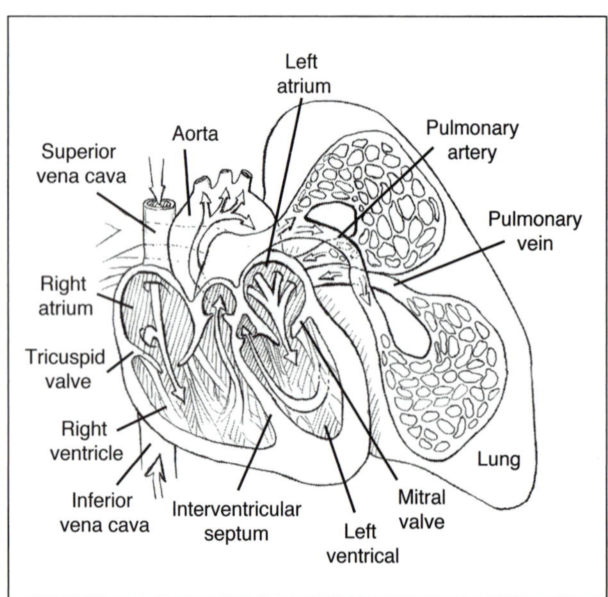

FIGURE 7.3 Blood flow pathways of the heart and lung.

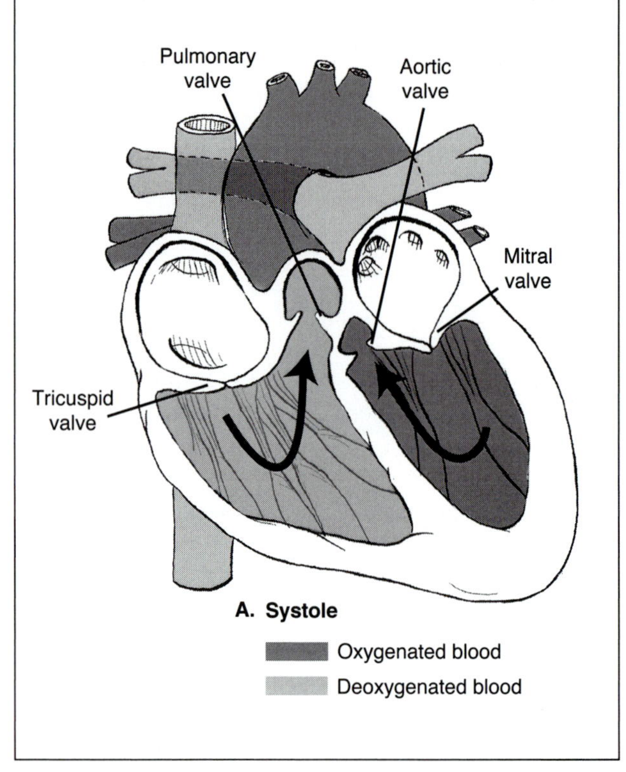

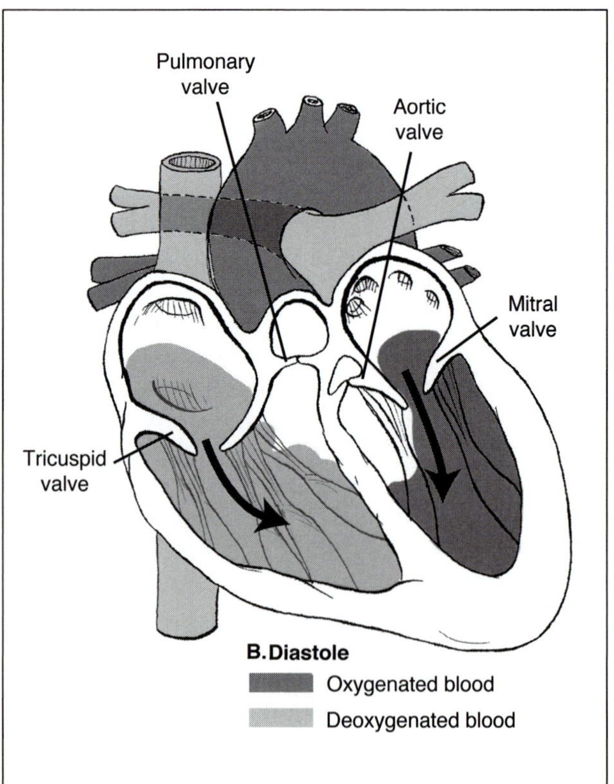

FIGURE 7.4 Valves during (A) systole and (B) diastole.

RCA feeds both the inferior wall of the left ventricle and portions of the right side of the heart, but also feeds the sinoatrial node and the atrioventricular node, which are the pacemakers of the heart (Figure 7.5).

Blood is returned to circulation by the coronary veins. The three major veins are the anterior interventricular, posterior interventricular, and the left marginal veins. These veins will normally join to form the coronary sinus, which empties into the right atrium.

ABDOMINAL ANATOMY

The aorta is the largest artery in the human body. As it extends through the abdomen, the aorta branches to supply the organs and tissues located in the abdomen (Figure 7.6). The first major branch is the celiac axis, which arises anteriorly from the aorta at about the level of T12 (Figure 7.7). As it exits the aorta, the celiac axis trifurcates into the left gastric, hepatic, and the splenic arteries. The left gastric artery travels upward and toward the left to feed the distal esophagus, the lesser curvature of the stomach, and the anterior and posterior walls of the stomach. The hepatic artery travels to the right and divides into the right and left hepatic arteries after the branch of the gastroduodenal artery (Figure 7.8). The gastroduodenal artery then divides to feed the anterior and pyloric areas of the stomach, duodenum, and pancreas. The right and left hepatic arteries supply the various lobes

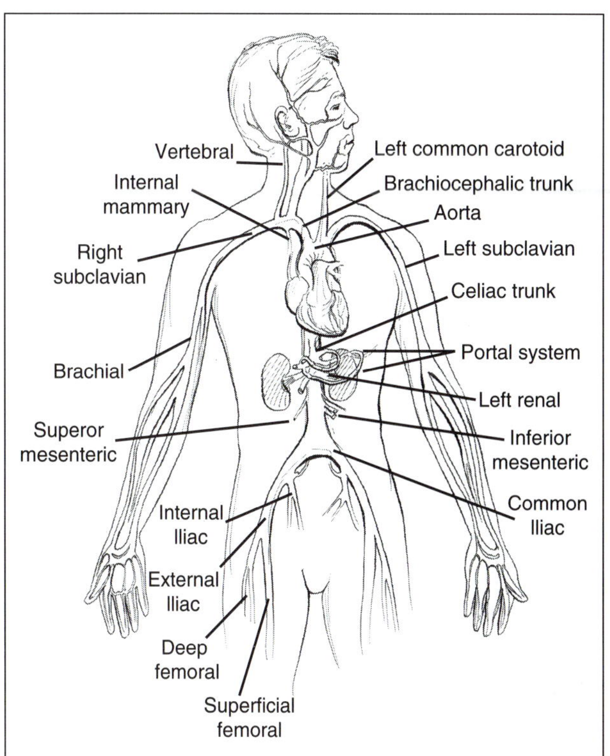

FIGURE 7.6 Basic arterial anatomy of the body.

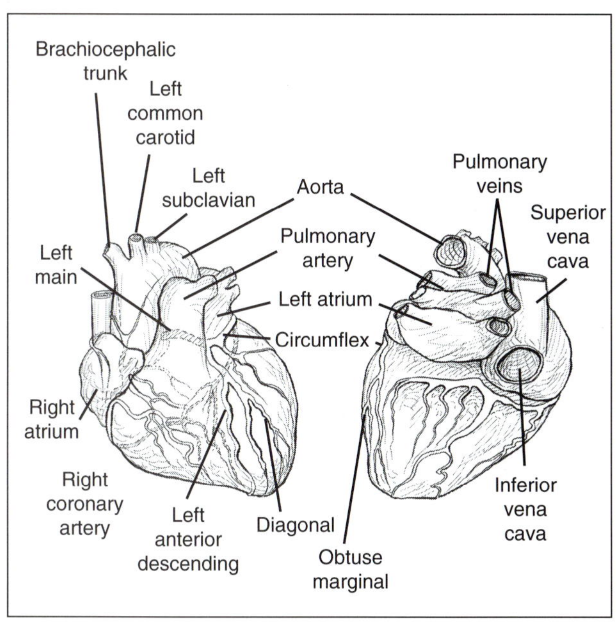

FIGURE 7.5 Coronary arteries of the heart.

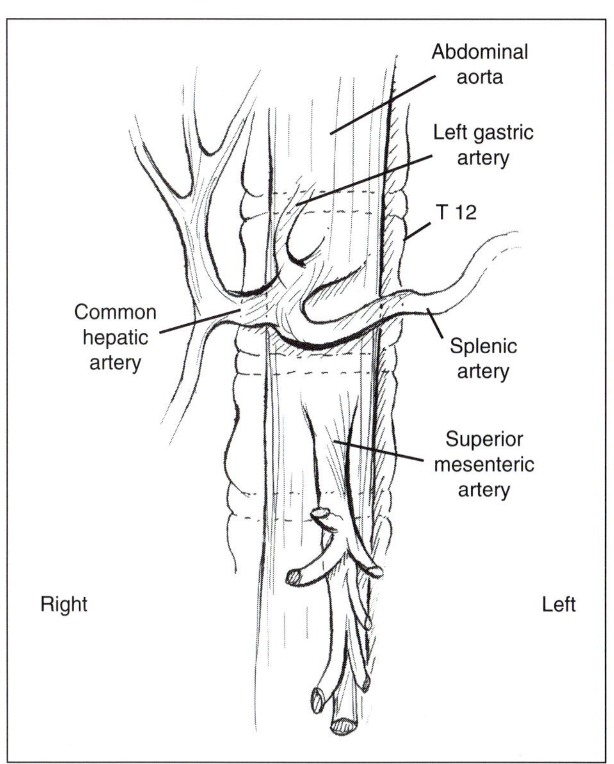

FIGURE 7.7 Celiac axis anatomy.

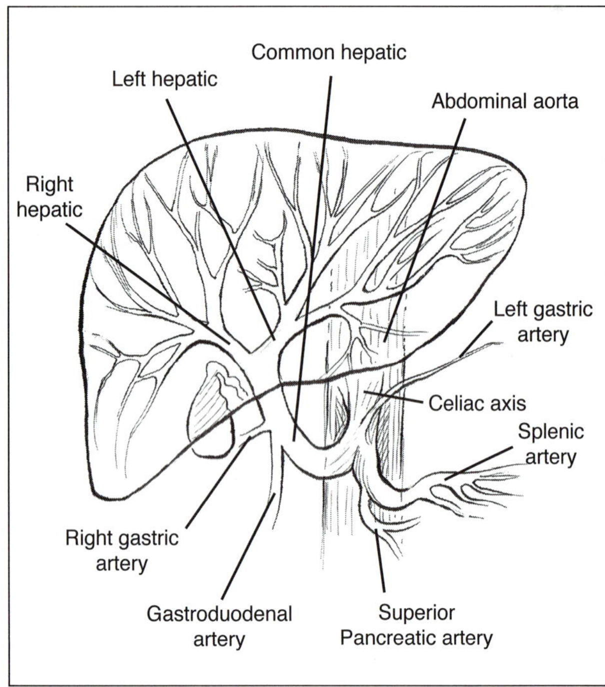

FIGURE 7.8 Hepatic arterial anatomy.

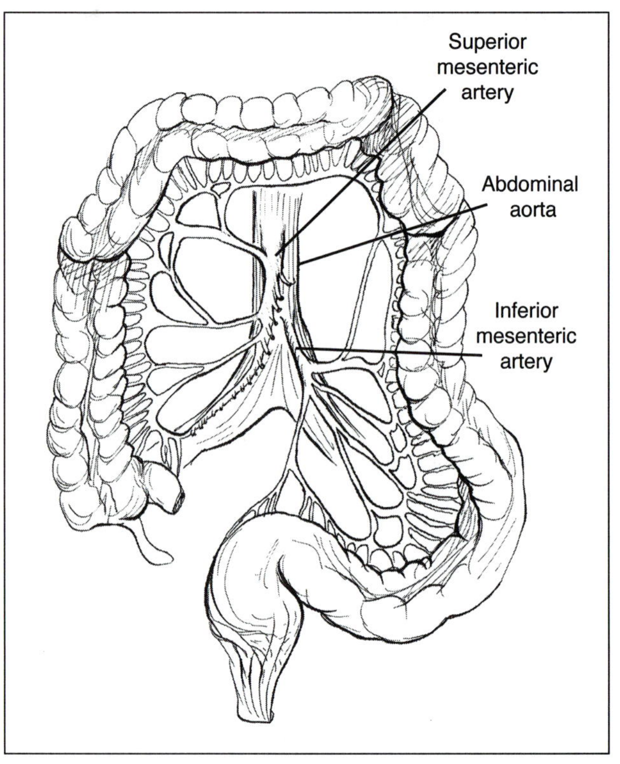

FIGURE 7.9 Mesenteric arteries.

of the liver. The splenic artery is the longest and travels to the left behind the stomach to the spleen where it divides into two or three branches that enter the spleen.

The superior mesenteric artery is the next artery to arise from the aorta. It exits anteriorly at the level of L1 and travels downward to feed the small intestine, cecum (sē´kŭm), ascending portion of the colon, and approximately one-half of the transverse colon (Figure 7.9). The inferior mesenteric artery arises from the aorta at the level of L3 just above the bifurcation of the aorta. It passes downward and to the left and feeds the remaining half of the transverse colon, the descending colon, sigmoid colon, and rectum.

The renal arteries arise from both sides of the aorta at the level of L1–L2 between the superior and inferior mesenteric arteries and travel transversely to each kidney (Figure 7.10). In approximately 30% of the population there are two arteries feeding each kidney in which case all four arteries must be visualized. As the renal artery travels to the kidney, the artery branches into an anterior and a posterior branch, which divide into interlobular arteries that transport blood to the glomeruli, tubules, and capillaries where waste products are filtered from the blood. This filtered blood is returned to the heart through the renal veins and the inferior vena cava.

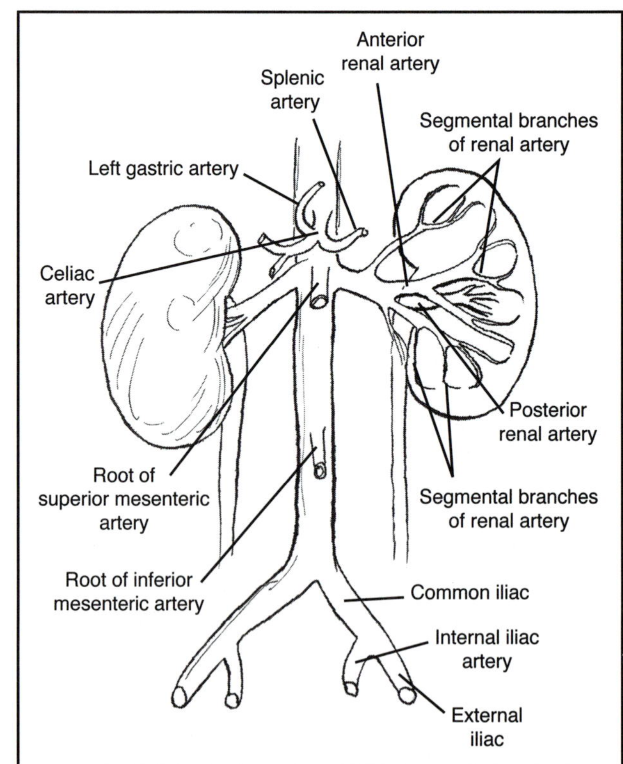

FIGURE 7.10 Renal arterial anatomy.

PERIPHERAL ANATOMY

Upper Extremity

As the ascending aorta travels over the aortic arch, three arteries branch off (Figure 7.11). The first is the innominate-brachiocephalic artery, which supplies blood to the right arm and to the right side of the brain. The innominate artery divides into the right common carotid and the right subclavian artery. The second arterial branch gives rise to the common carotid artery. The third branch of the aorta is the left subclavian artery. As the subclavian artery reaches the border of the first rib, it then becomes the axillary artery. After several branches, the axillary artery becomes the brachial artery at the lateral border of the teres major muscle and travels to the level of the elbow. At this point the brachial artery will divide into the radial and ulnar arteries and travel to the wrist, giving off small branches along the way.

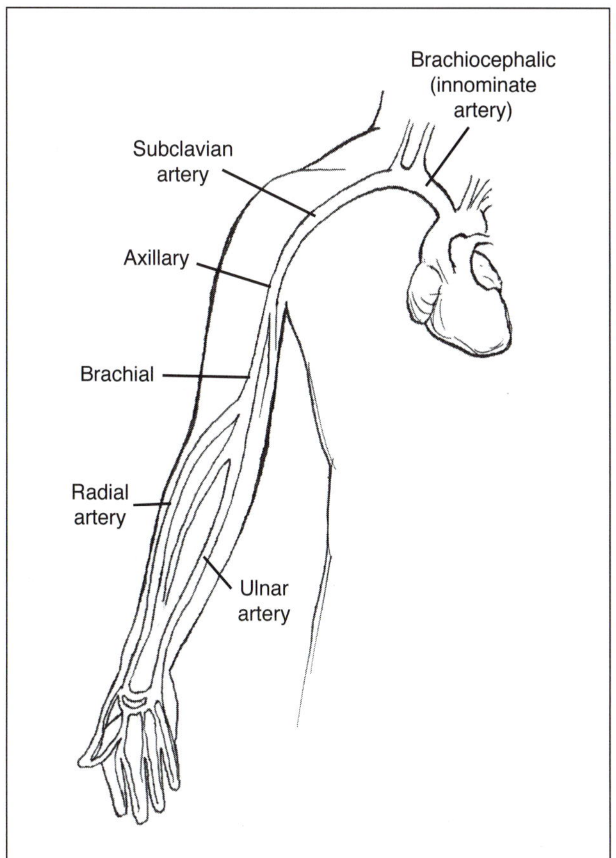

FIGURE 7.11 Upper limb arterial anatomy.

Lower Extremity

At the level of L4, the descending aorta bifurcates into the right and left common iliacs (Figure 7.12). These arteries then bifurcate into the internal and external iliac arteries where the internal arteries supply the pelvis and pelvic organs. The external arteries continue to become the right and left femoral (fĕm´or-ăl) arteries, which supply the lower extremities. At this same point, the profunda femoris (deep femoral) and the profunda circumflex arteries branch. The femoral artery continues to the level of the knee and becomes the popliteal (pŏp´´lĭt-ē´ăl) artery, which then trifurcates into the anterior tibial, posterior tibial, and peroneal arteries. These arteries then continue to form the arteries that supply blood to the foot.

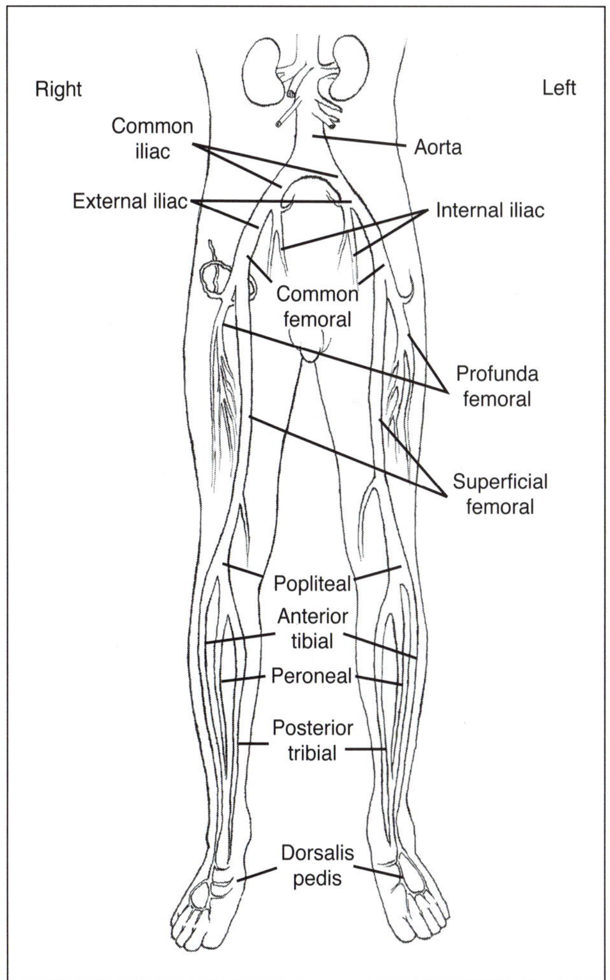

FIGURE 7.12 Arterial anatomy of the pelvis and lower limb.

Procedures

GUIDELINES

Radiation Protection

Because radiation protection is essential to all imaging procedures, the appropriate use of time, distance, and shielding precautions are similar to the many procedures covered in this chapter. The following guidelines are recommended:

- Use of minimal fluoroscopic exposure time
- Maximized distance from the source of radiation for staff
- Use of lead shielding/barriers
- Frame rate of cine is a determinant of radiation exposure to the patient; the faster the frame rate, the higher the dose.
- Field size limits

Patient Preparation

Angiography is an invasive procedure requiring careful preparation of the patient. The parameters of patient preparation are common to all angiographic studies. The following parameters should be carefully followed:

- Informed consent
- NPO for 4 to 8 hours before examination
- Patent IV access
- Preoperative medications as indicated in Chapter 6, Angiographic Procedures and Equipment
- Establishing ECG monitoring
- Baseline vital signs with documentation on the patient's chart
- Vascular access site prepared with an antiseptic solution such as Betadine or Septison
- Patient draped with a sterile drape extending from neck to feet
- **Fenestrated** (fĕn´ĕs-trāt´´ĕd) drape applied to the puncture area

Postprocedure Care

The relatively high risk that occurs with all venous or arterial imaging studies mandates similar postprocedure care.

The following postprocedure care is recommended for all arterial studies:

- If a **catheter sheath** remains in place, a heparin IV drip is established in a brachial vein.
- If the sheath is removed, manual or mechanical pressure is maintained to the puncture site until **hemostasis** is achieved.
- The patient's vital signs are monitored and documented.
- Bed rest for 6 to 8 hours is required.
- Detailed instructions, such as keeping the affected leg straight, holding the affected groin when coughing or sneezing, restricting the head of the bed to 20° to 30°, and encouraging fluid intake are given to the patient.

CARDIAC CATHETERIZATION

Cardiac catheterization is the procedure using insertion and passage of small plastic catheters into arteries and veins to the heart to obtain radiographic and fluoroscopic images of the coronary arteries and cardiac chambers.

ANGIOCARDIOGRAPHY

Angiocardiography is a general term referring to the study of the chambers of the heart or pulmonary artery. Selective angiocardiography is divided into **right**- and **left**-sided **heart** catheterization. The left selective angiocardiography procedure can also be referred to as left ventriculography. Right heart catheterization is used to record and evaluate **intracardiac** pressures.

Applied Anatomy

(See Figure 7.12.)

Indications

- **Cardiomyopathy** (kăr´´dē-ō-mī-ŏp´ă-thē)
- Congenital heart abnormalities
- Valvular heart diseases
- Preoperative evaluation

Contraindications

- The only absolute contraindication is the refusal of a mentally competent patient to consent to the procedure (Grossman, 1980).
- Absence of a pulse in a limb precludes **percutaneous** needle puncture in that limb
- Conditions that must be controlled prior to elective catheterization: hypertension, ventricular irritability, fever, uncontrolled congestive heart failure, electrolyte imbalance, sepsis, recent cerebral vascular accident, acute GI bleed, pregnancy

Equipment

- Fluoroscopic imaging equipment with television monitor, multifilm imaging, cine, video tape or video disk, similar to that of arterial angiography discussed in Chapter 6, Angiographic Procedures and Equipment
- Pressure injector
- Prepared sterile tray, preferably disposable
- Computer-controlled **hemodynamic pressure monitoring** device (Figure 7.13)
- **Swan-Ganz** pulmonary catheter
- Pigtail catheter (Figure 7.14)

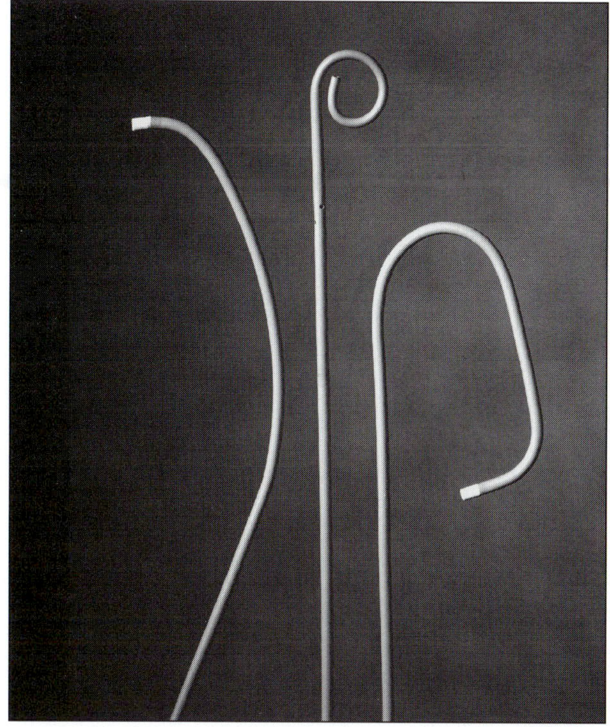

FIGURE 7.14 From left to right: Judkin's right, pigtail, Judkin's left coronary catheters (Courtesy of SCIMED/Boston Scientific Corporation, Maple Grove, MN).

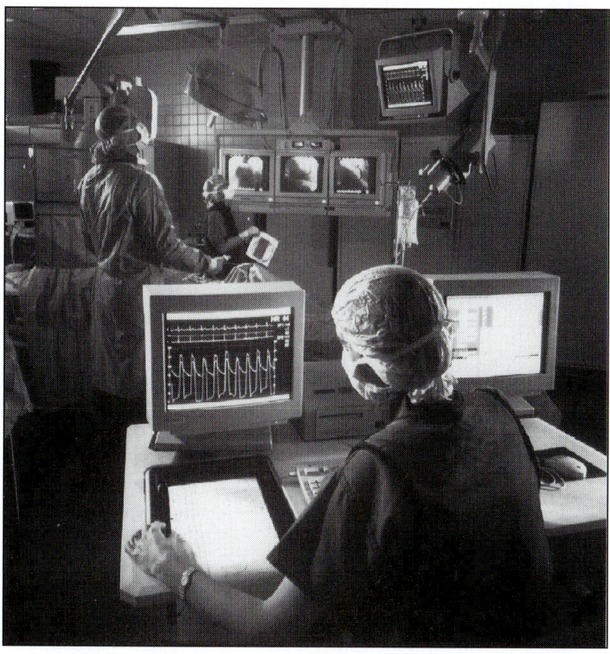

FIGURE 7.13 Pressure monitoring device (Courtesy of Mennen Medical Corporation, Clarence, NY).

- Guidewire
- Catheter sheath sometimes inserted after the percutaneous puncture
- **Manifold** (Figure 7.15)
- Emergency tray equipment for cardiac resuscitation

Contrast Media

- Ionic (Hypaque 76, Conray 50) or nonionic (Omnipaque or Optiray) contrast of 30 to 60 mL to the left ventricle
- Contrast under pressure is necessary to completely fill the relative large volume of the left ventricle.

Preliminary Radiographs Scout radiographs are generally not performed for cardiac catheterization.

Procedure Sequence

- The sterile manifold system is flushed to remove any air.
- The Seldinger technique is used for the percutaneous femoral puncture.

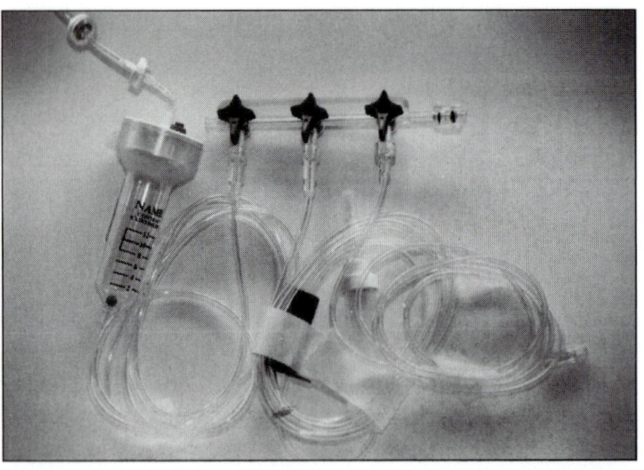

FIGURE 7.15 Three gang manifold with contrast-saving device.

- A catheter sheath may be inserted after the percutaneous puncture.
- The Swan-Ganz catheter is advanced through the right femoral vein into the right side of the heart.
- Pressure recordings are made in each chamber of the heart (Figure 7.16).
- A pigtail catheter is advanced through the aorta and across the aortic valve into the left ventricle where hemodynamic pressure recordings are made.
- The left ventricle is injected and filmed.
- Pressure recordings are made while the pigtail catheter is moved from the left ventricle into the aorta (Figure 7.17).

After completion of this procedure, coronary arteriography is performed.

Procedure Radiographs

- During the pressure injection of contrast, a 30°, RAO orientation of the heart is filmed (Figure 7.18).
- Cine fluorography from 15 to 60 frames per second is commonly used to evaluate heart wall function, valvular regurgitation, and cardiac **ejection fractions**.
- A 60°, LAO orientation is sometimes imaged to best demonstrate the lateral and septal wall motion of the left ventricle.

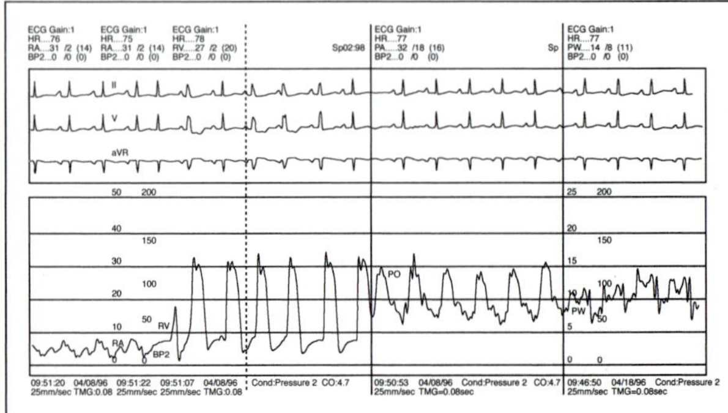

FIGURE 7.16 Hemodynamic tracing of the right heart.

Common Pathologies

- Valvular **stenosis**
- Valvular insufficiencies
- Cardiomyopathy
- Myocardial infarction
- Congenital defects: septal, atrial, ventricular, patent **foramen ovale**, tetralogy of Fallot
- Transposition of the great vessels

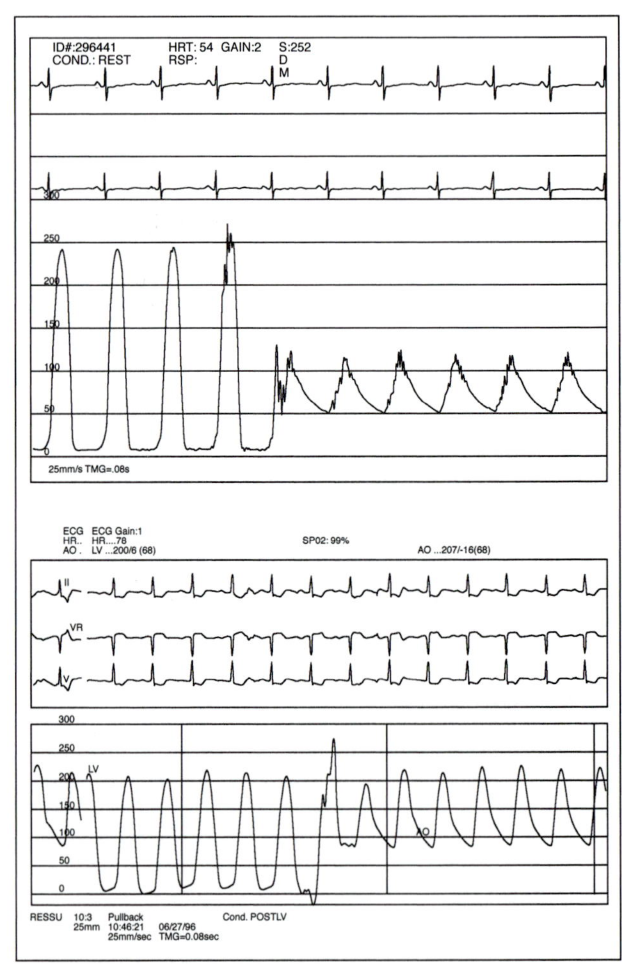

FIGURE 7.17 Aortic valve pullback pressures.

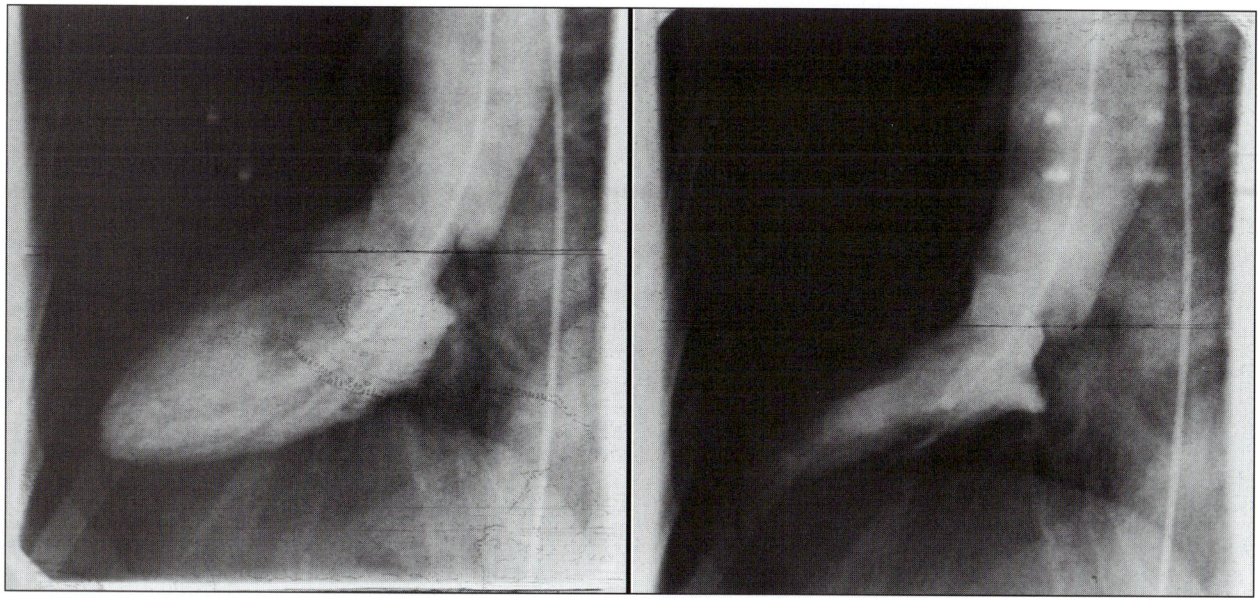

FIGURE 7.18 Left ventricle in diastole (left) and systole (right).

CORONARY ARTERIOGRAPHY

Coronary **arteriography** is the selective injection of the arteries that supply blood to the heart.

Applied Anatomy (See Figure 7.5)

Indications

- Chest pain of uncertain origin
- Coronary artery disease
- Preoperative evaluation

Contraindications See angiocardiography list.

Equipment

- Fluoroscopic imaging equipment with television monitor, multifilm imaging, cine, video tape or video disk, similar to that of arterial angiography discussed in Chapter 6, Angiographic Procedures and Equipment
- Prepared sterile tray, preferably disposable
- Guidewire
- Catheter sheath
- Computer-controlled hemodynamic pressure monitoring device (see Figure 7.13).
- Judkin's right and Judkin's left catheters, Amplatz bypass graft or multipurpose (Figure 7.19).
- Emergency tray equipment

Contrast Media Ionic or nonionic contrast 7 to 10 mL, hand injected

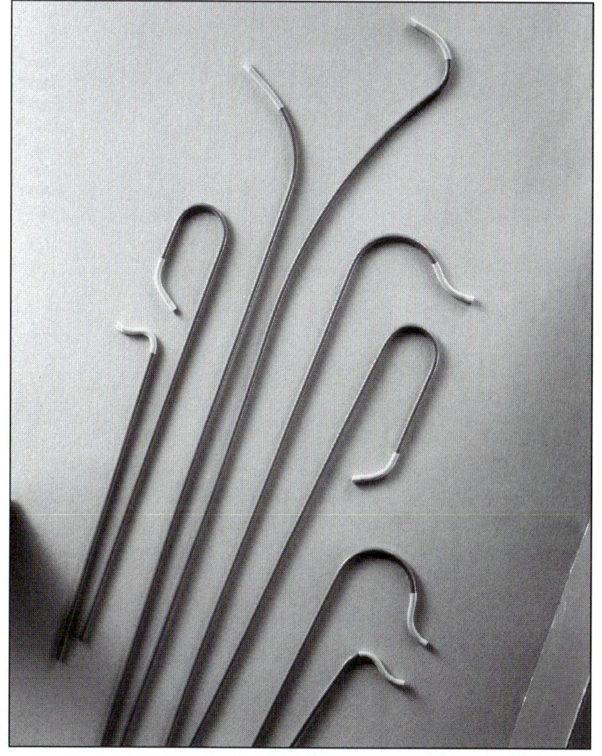

FIGURE 7.19 From left to right: Amplatz right II, Amplatz left I, Judkin's left 6, Amplatz left II, multipurpose HS, multipurpose B II, Judkin's left 3.5, and Amplatz right I (Courtesy of SCIMED/Boston Scientific Corporation, Maple Grove, MN).

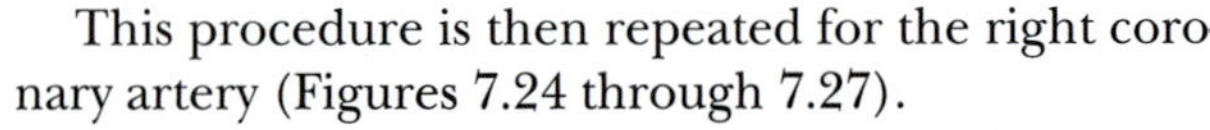

Procedure Sequence

- Usually follows angiocardiography.
- The ostium of the left coronary artery is cannulated with the Judkin's left catheter.
- The left coronary artery system is filmed.
- The **ostium** of the right coronary artery is cannulated with the Judkin's right catheter.
- The right coronary artery system is filmed.
- When it is determined that no additional films are necessary, the catheter is removed from the sheath.

Procedure Radiographs Common imaging orientations for the left coronary artery are AP, RAO (Figures 7.20 and 7.21), LAO with either 15° to 30° caudal or cephalad angulation (Figures 7.22 and 7.23).

This procedure is then repeated for the right coronary artery (Figures 7.24 through 7.27).

The table is **panned** (moved longitudinally and laterally) to adequately demonstrate the entire coronary artery and branches.

Common Pathologies

- Coronary arteriosclerotic disease (Figure 7.28)
- **Coronary bridging**
- Coronary spasm
- Collateral blood flow (Figure 7.29)
- Acute occlusion of coronary artery

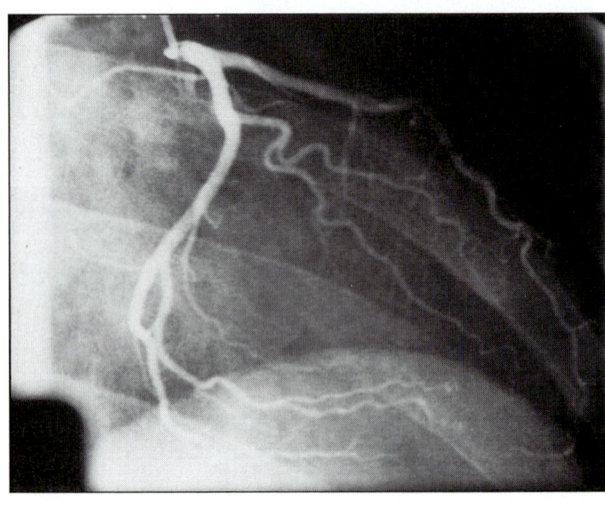

FIGURE 7.20 Left coronary angiogram, RAO.

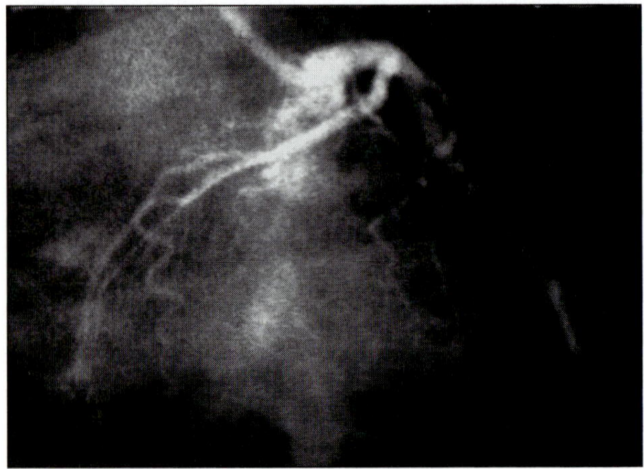

FIGURE 7.22 Left coronary angiogram, LAO.

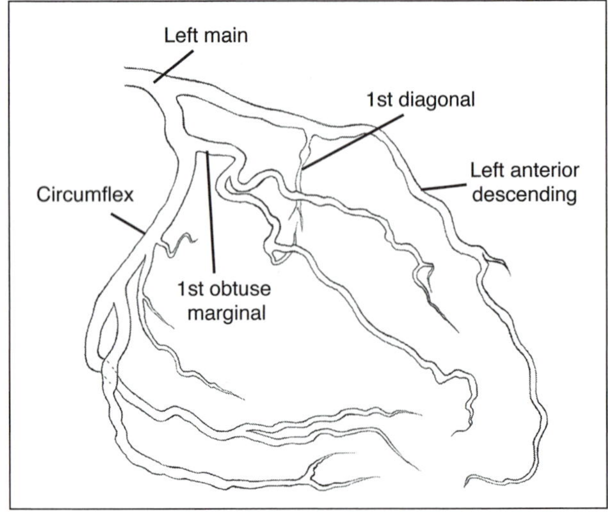

FIGURE 7.21 Left coronary angiogram with related anatomy, RAO.

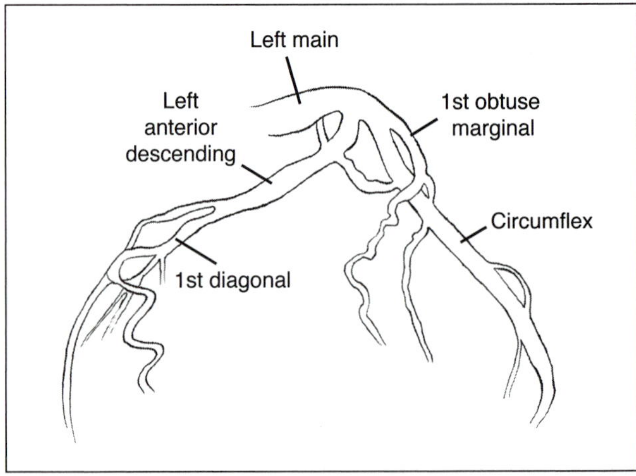

FIGURE 7.23 Left coronary angiogram with related anatomy, LAO.

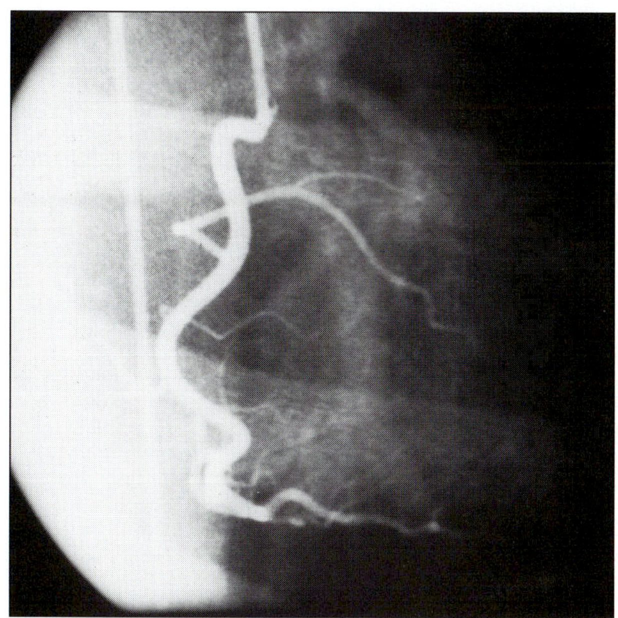

FIGURE 7.24 Right coronary angiogram, RAO.

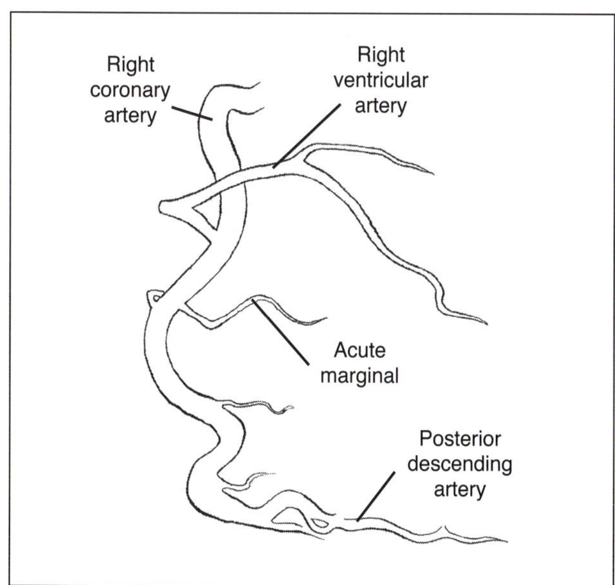

FIGURE 7.25 Right coronary angiogram with related anatomy, RAO.

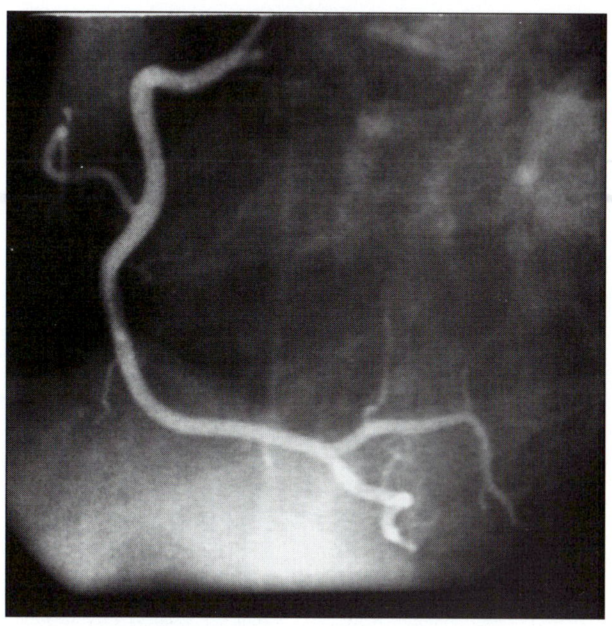

FIGURE 7.26 Right coronary angiogram, LAO.

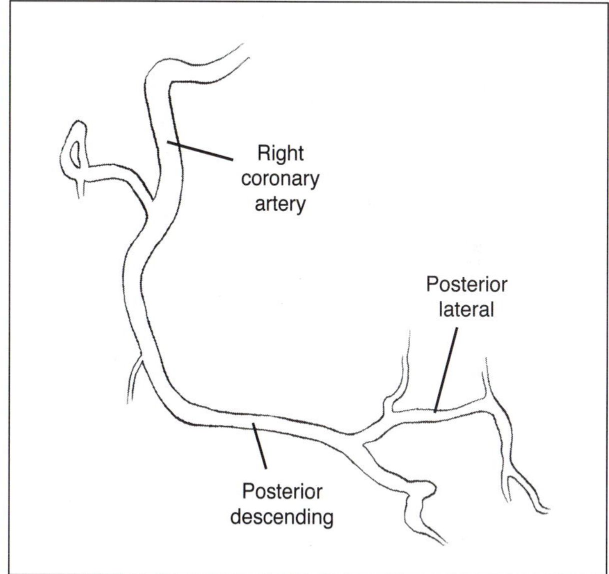

FIGURE 7.27 Right coronary angiogram with related anatomy, LAO.

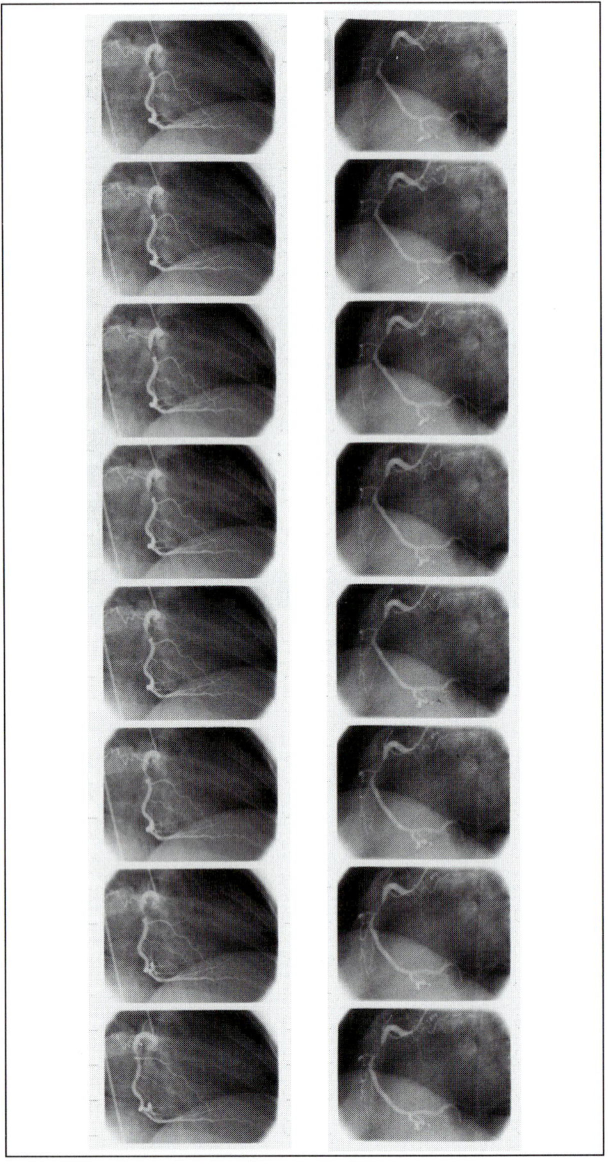

FIGURE 7.28 Coronary arteriosclerotic disease.

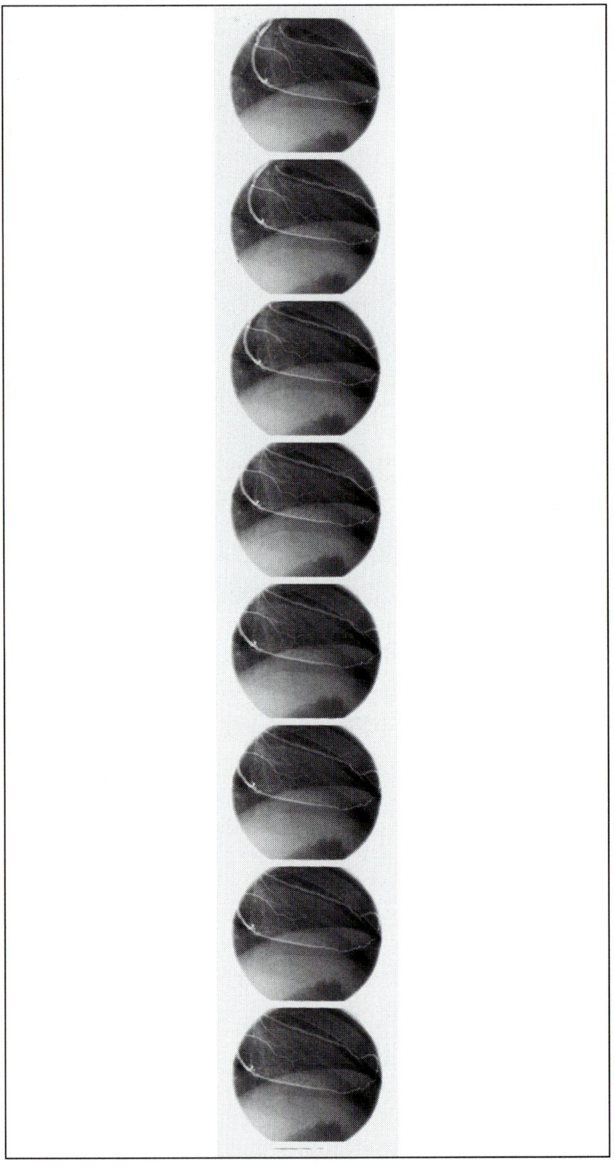

FIGURE 7.29 Collateral blood flow when main artery is occluded.

ASCENDING AORTOGRAPHY

Ascending aortograms are performed following left ventriculography (vĕn-trĭk′′ū-lŏg′ră-fē). This procedure differs from aortic arch studies by limiting the area of interest to that part of the aorta extending from the aortic valve to the innominate artery (Figure 7.30).

Indications

- Locate coronary artery bypass grafts
- Aortic insufficiency
- Aortic dissection or aneurysm

Equipment See angiocardiography.

Contrast Media Forty to 60 mL of ionic or nonionic contrast with pressure injection

Procedure Sequence

- A pigtail catheter is placed distally to the aortic valve.
- The ascending aorta is filmed.
- When it is determined that no other films are necessary, the catheter is pulled.

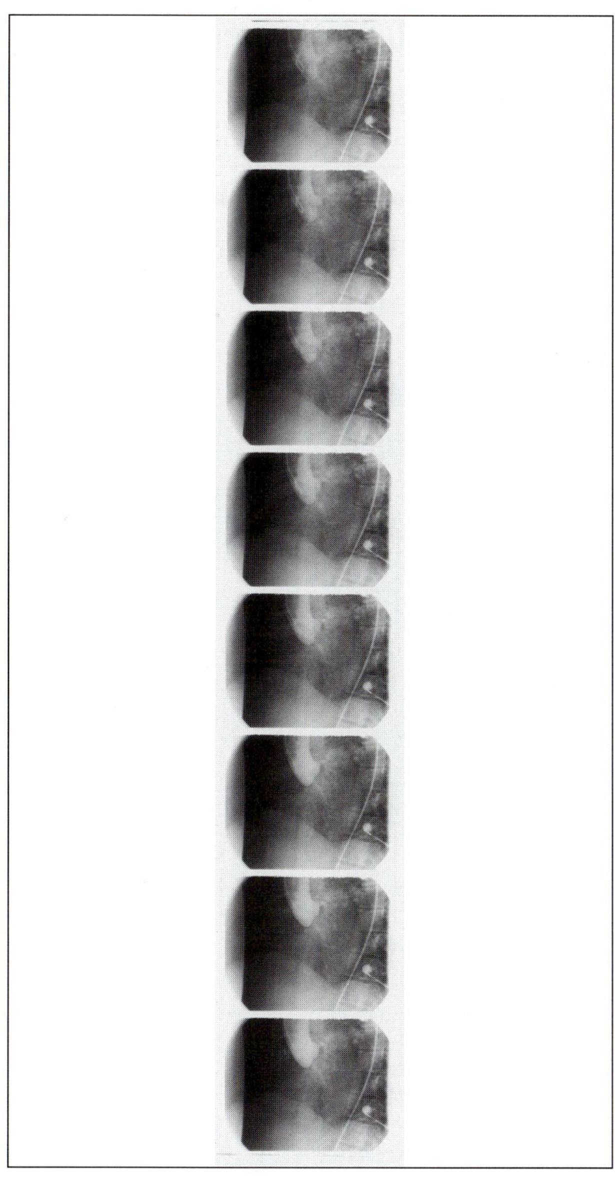

FIGURE 7.30 Ascending aortogram.

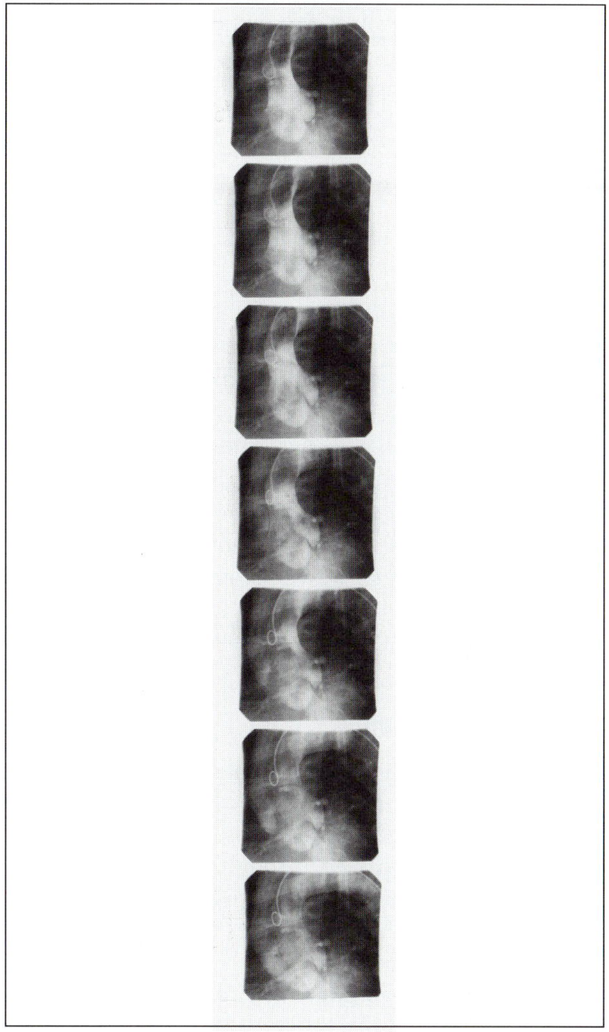

FIGURE 7.31 Ascending aortic dissection.

Procedure Radiographs Generally, the filming orientation of ascending aortography is 30° to 50° LAO on 35-mm cine film.

Common Pathologies

- Aortic insufficiency
- Ascending aortic dissection or aneurysm (Figure 7.31)

PULMONARY ANGIOGRAPHY (ARTERIOGRAPHY)

Pulmonary angiograms are obtained following cardiac angiocardiography or may be performed as a separate procedure.

Applied Anatomy (Figure 7.32)

Indications

- Pulmonary emboli
- Pulmonic stenosis
- Anomalous pulmonary venous drainage

Equipment

- See angiocardiography.
- The use of either a balloon-tipped flotation catheter (Berman catheter) with side holes only or a Grollman pigtail catheter with a 90° angle is common.

Contrast Media Ionic or nonionic contrast with pressure injection

Procedure Sequence

- A venous approach is performed via the right femoral vein.
- A Seldinger technique is used.
- The catheter is passed through the vena cava into the right atrium through the right ventricle and is placed into either the right or left pulmonary artery for selective injection.
- The venous system of the lung of interest is filmed.

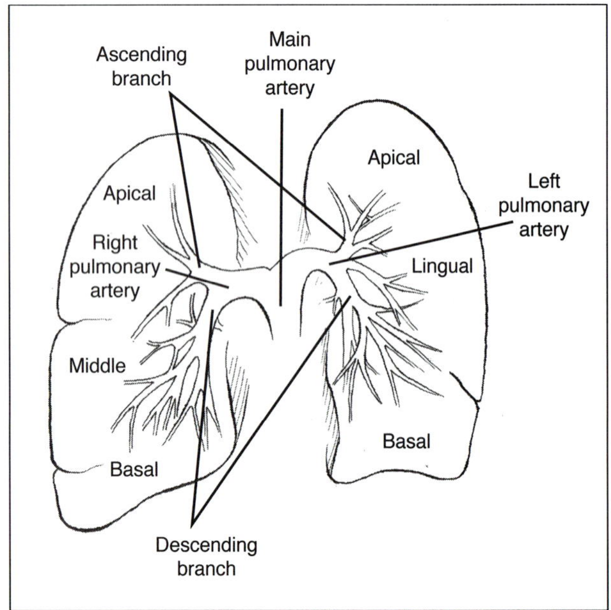

FIGURE 7.32 Pulmonary anatomy.

Procedure Radiographs

- A scout film of the chest consisting of a 30° LAO is common.
- Use of biplane radiographic studies is recommended with long filming sequence intervals of over 10 seconds for pulmonary angiography (Figures 7.33 and 7.34).

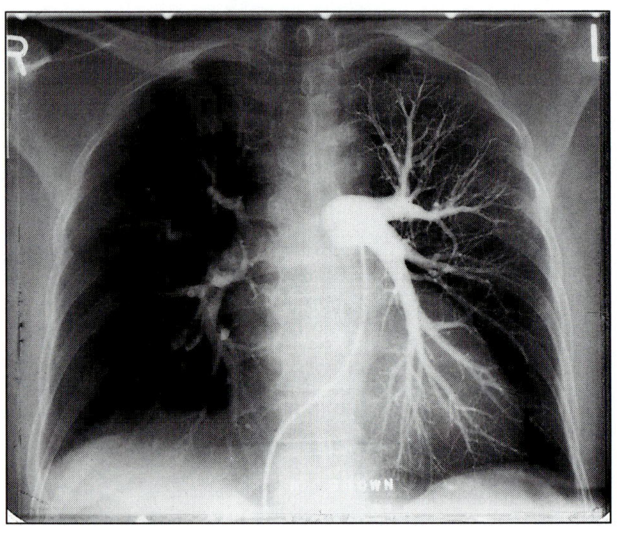

FIGURE 7.33 PA pulmonary angiogram.

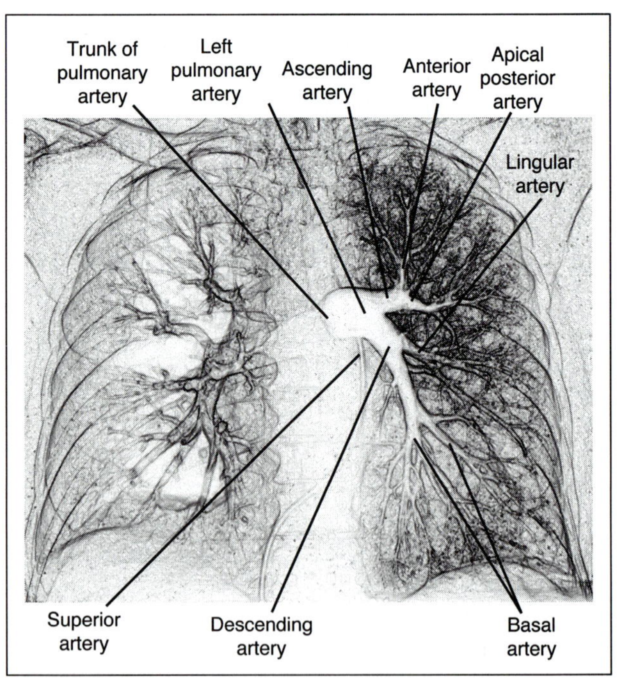

FIGURE 7.34 Pulmonary angiogram anatomy.

Common Pathologies

- Pulmonary emboli (Figure 7.35)
- Pulmonary hypertension

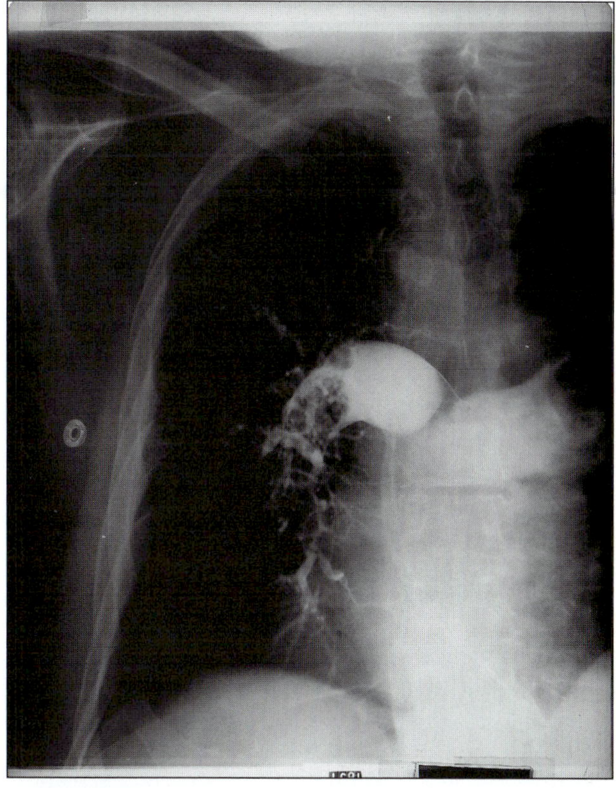

FIGURE 7.35 Pulmonary emboli radiograph.

Abdominal Arteriography

Abdominal arteriography is divided into selective and nonselective studies. Nonselective abdominal arteriography is commonly used as a screening study in which the specific origins of each artery arising from the abdominal aorta can be localized. Common selective studies consist of the celiac axis, superior mesenteric, inferior mesenteric, and renal arteries.

DESCENDING ABDOMINAL AORTOGRAPHY

Abdominal aortography is one of the most common procedures performed in angiography. This study provides information for basic anatomy and subsequent selective localization of the arterial trees arising from the abdominal aorta.

Applied Anatomy (Figure 7.36)

Indications

- Abdominal aorta aneurysm
- Obstructive diseases of the aorta (requires a brachial approach)
- Screening for gross abnormal disease processes

Contraindications

- Femoral arteriosclerosis will preclude femoral approach.
- Severe hepatorenal disease

Equipment

- Fluoroscopy is used to confirm the position of the catheter.
- Biplane radiography with rapid film changer
- Digital subtraction angiography (DSA)
- Pressure injector
- Disposable sterile tray
- Pigtail catheter

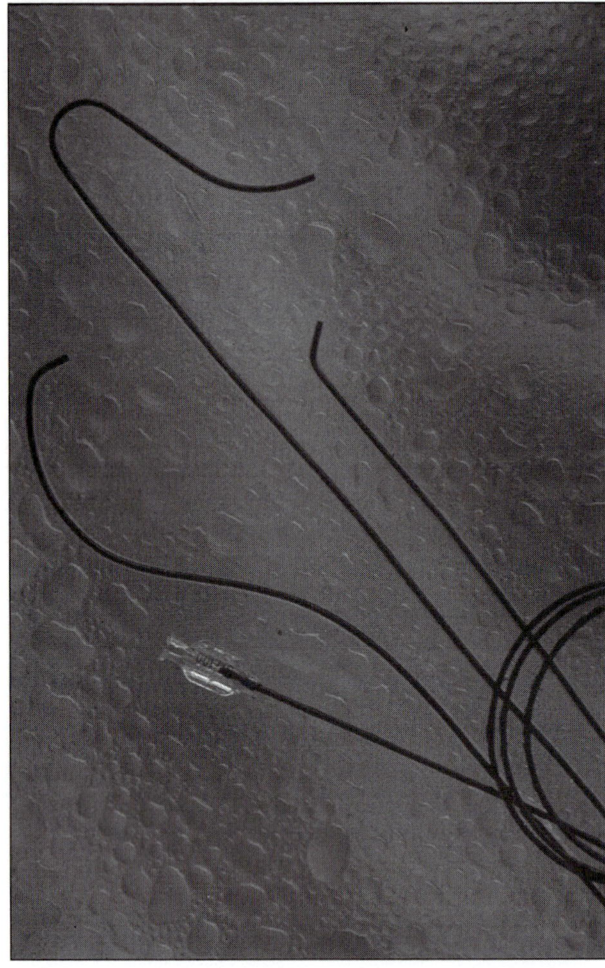

FIGURE 7.36 Selective abdominal catheters from right to left: Cobra 2, sidewinder, and headhunter (Courtesy of Medi-tech/Boston Scientific Corporation, Natick, MA).

- Guidewire
- Catheter sheath
- Emergency tray equipment

Contrast Media

- Nonionic contrast, such as Optiray or Omnipaque or ionic contrast such as Hypaque 76 or Conray 60
- Using DSA, 20 to 30 mL of contrast
- Serial filming 40 to 60 mL is used

Preliminary Radiographs

- AP projection scout of the abdomen.
- A dorsal decubitus position radiograph is taken if an abdominal aneurysm is suspected.

Procedure Sequence

- A femoral approach is used with a Seldinger technique.
- A pigtail catheter is inserted into the aorta and placed either at the level of T12 or L1 or L2 level.
- Filming of the descending aorta is performed.
- After films have been evaluated, the catheter is removed from the sheath.

Procedure Radiographs

- Either serial or digital radiographs are obtained in the AP projection.
- Manual subtraction techniques may be used (see box at end of chapter).

Common Pathologies

- Descending aortic aneurysm)
- Dissection of the descending aorta
- **Occlusion**
- Aortic stenosis

TRANSLUMBAR AORTOGRAPHY

The translumbar is a seldom used, alternative approach to gain access to the descending abdominal aorta. The patient lies prone on the table for a flank insertion approach. A 6- to 8-inch, 18-gauge, translumbar needle is inserted percutaneously and placed into the abdominal aorta. At this point either contrast can be injected through the needle or a catheter may be inserted for administration of contrast. This approach limits the examination to the abdominal aorta because a translumbar needle either with or without a catheter cannot be used for selective visceral angiography.

CELIAC AXIS ARTERIOGRAPHY

Because the celiac (sē´lē-ăk) artery trifurcates, celiac studies are referred to as celiac axis arteriography. Studies that demonstrate the common hepatic, left gastric, and splenic arteries, which originate from the celiac artery, are referred to as superselective studies. The use of the term superselective indicates a study that extends to the next level of bifurcation or in this case, trifurcation of the arterial tree.

Applied Anatomy (See Figures 7.7 and 7.8)

Indications

- GI bleed
- Vascular abnormalities
- Portal hypertension
- Hepatic trauma

Contraindications Femoral arteriosclerosis will preclude femoral approach.

Equipment

- See descending aortography.
- Cobra 2 catheter or use of the headhunter, sidewinder, or a Judkin's right catheter (Figure 7.36)

Contrast Media

- Ionic or nonionic contrast may be used.
- The amount of contrast ranges from 10 to 40 mL depending on the size of the vessels.

Preliminary Radiographs A scout of the AP abdomen is obtained.

Procedure Sequence

- A femoral approach is used with a Seldinger technique.
- A Cobra or other similar catheter is passed through the aorta and advanced to the level of T12, where the celiac axis is engaged.
- A hand injection of a small amount of contrast is used to confirm the correct placement of the catheter.

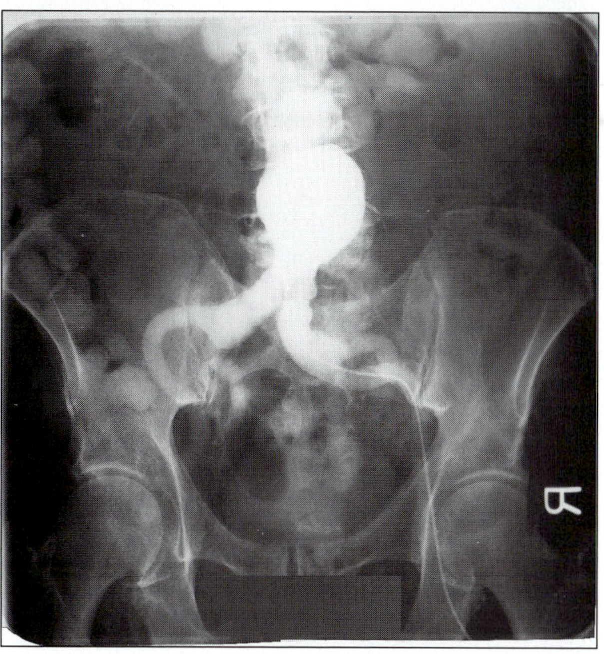

FIGURE 7.37 Vascular narrowing of celiac axis.

- Films of the celiac axis are obtained (Figure 7.37).
- After films have been evaluated, the catheter is removed from the sheath.

Procedure Radiographs Either serial or DSA filming is used. DSA is not optimal due to the necessity of longer run times and the presence of bowel motion.

Common Pathologies

- Active GI bleed
- Obstruction of the portal vein
- Cirrhosis of the liver
- Ruptured spleen
- Tumors
- Aneurysms
- Vascular narrowing
- AV malformations

SUPERIOR MESENTERIC ARTERIOGRAPHY

Selective angiography of the superior mesenteric artery (SMA) identifies abnormalities of the vessel structures that supply the small bowel, cecum, ascending colon, and midtransverse colon. Extravasation of contrast media is indicative of acute GI bleed.

Applied Anatomy (See Figure 7.9)

Indications

- GI bleed
- Vascular abnormalities

Contraindications Femoral arteriosclerosis may preclude femoral approach.

Equipment See celiac axis arteriography.

Contrast Media Ten to 20 mL of ionic or nonionic contrast may be used depending on the size of the vessels.

Preliminary Radiographs A scout of the AP abdomen is obtained.

Procedure Sequence

- A femoral approach is used with a Seldinger technique.
- A Cobra or other similar catheter is passed through the aorta and advanced to the level of L1, where the superior mesenteric artery is engaged.
- A hand injection of a small amount of contrast is used to confirm the correct placement of the catheter.
- Films are taken of the SMA during contrast injection (Figure 7.38).
- After films have been evaluated, the catheter is removed from the sheath.

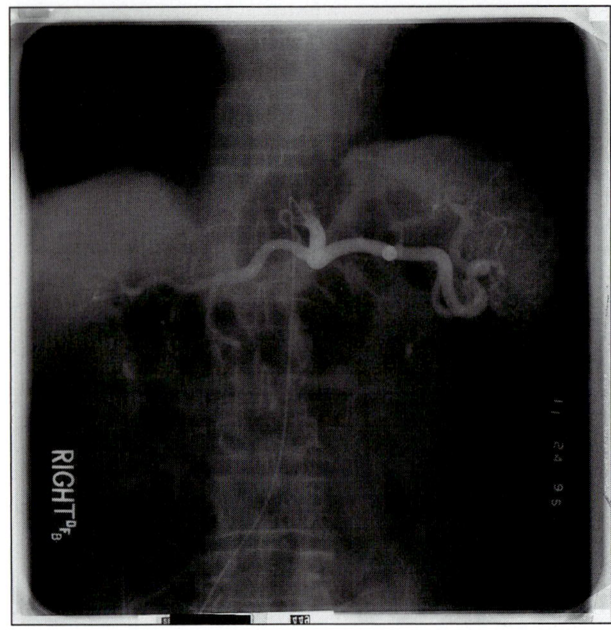

FIGURE 7.38 SMA angiogram depicting tumor.

Procedure Radiographs See celiac axis arteriography.

Alternative Radiographs/Images Endoscopy or radionuclide scanning is used as a screening examination to locate the source of hemorrhage in patients with suspected GI bleeds.

Common Pathologies

- Active GI bleed
- Arterial occlusion
- Tumors

INFERIOR MESENTERIC ARTERIOGRAPHY

Selective angiography of the inferior mesenteric artery (IMA) identifies abnormalities of the vessel structures that supply the transverse colon, descending and sigmoid colon, and rectum. Extravasation of contrast media is indicative of an acute lower GI bleed.

Applied Anatomy (See Figure 7.9)

Indications

- GI bleed
- Vascular abnormalities

Contraindications None

Equipment See celiac axis arteriography.

Contrast Media

- Ionic or nonionic contrast may be used.
- The amount of contrast ranges from 15 to 30 mL depending on the size of the vessel.

Preliminary Radiographs A scout of the AP abdomen/pelvic area is obtained.

Procedure Sequence

- A femoral approach is used with a Seldinger technique.
- A Cobra or other similar catheter is passed through the aorta and advanced to the level of L3, where the IMA is engaged.
- A hand injection of a small amount of contrast is used to confirm the correct placement of the catheter.
- Radiographs with contrast are taken of the IMA (Figure 7.39 A and B).
- After films have been evaluated, the catheter is removed from the sheath.

Procedure Radiographs

- Serial filming of low abdomen/pelvis area.
- Longer run times are necessary due to amount of filling required.

Alternative Radiographs/Images

- Endoscopy
- Radionuclide scanning

Common Pathologies

- Active GI bleed
- Arterial occlusion
- Tumors

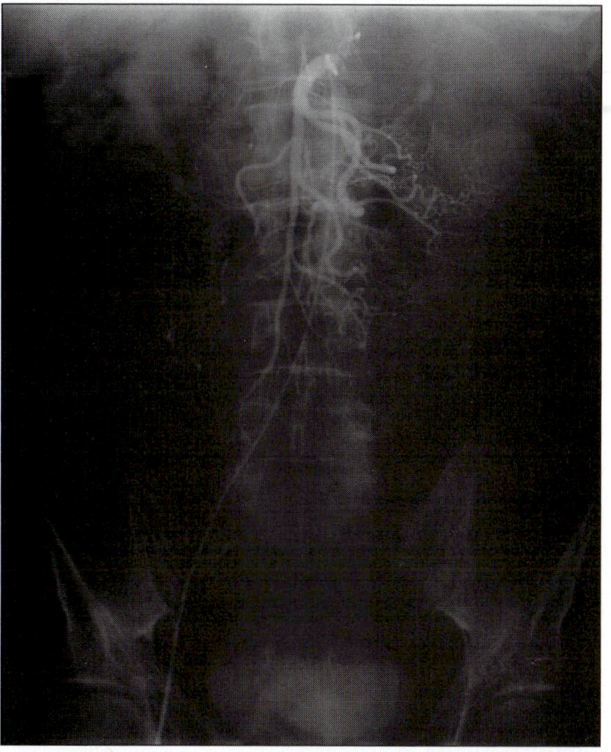

A

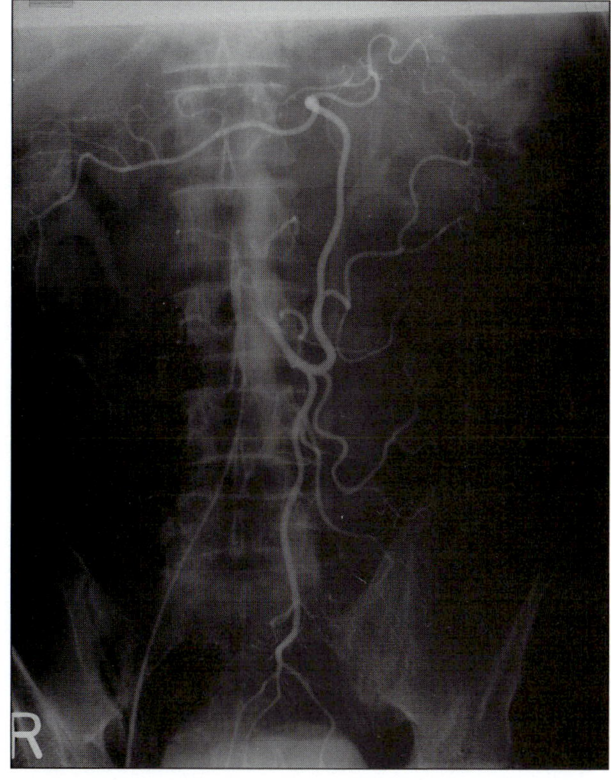

B

FIGURE 7.39 Occlusion of IMA.

RENAL ARTERIOGRAPHY

Renal arteriography is a selective vessel abdominal study. In addition to obtaining films, blood samples from the venous system are occasionally collected and analyzed for **renin** content. Renin is an enzyme produced by the kidneys. Elevated renin is sometimes an indicator of hypertension.

Applied Anatomy (See Figure 7.10)

Indications

- Hypertension
- Preoperative evaluations of renal masses
- Evaluation for renal transplant
- Visceral trauma

Contraindications

- Severe renal disease
- Femoral arteriosclerosis will preclude femoral approach.

Equipment See celiac axis arteriography.

Contrast Media

- The use of ionic contrast media is avoided due to the increased incidence of renal injury.
- A pressure-injected or hand-injected volume of nonionic contrast may be used.
- The amount of contrast ranges from 10 to 12 mL. Variation in the range of contrast is indicative of differences in vessel sizes.

Preliminary Radiographs A scout of the AP abdomen is obtained.

Procedure Sequence

- A femoral approach is used with a Seldinger technique.
- A Cobra or other similar catheter is passed through the aorta and advanced to the level of L1 or L2, where the renal artery is engaged.
- A hand injection of a small amount of contrast is used to confirm the correct placement of the catheter.
- After films have been evaluated, the catheter is removed from the sheath.

Procedure Radiographs

- Either serial or DSA filming is used.
- Films are obtained in the AP projection and 20° LPO and RPO positions.

Common Pathologies

- Renal artery stenosis (Figure 7.40)
- Fibromuscular hyperplasia (Figure 7.41)
- Renal cyst
- Occlusion of a branch of the renal artery
- Renal tumor (Figure 7.42)

> When formatting subtraction films, a radiographic image of the area of interest without contrast must be obtained to provide manual subtraction masks. In a serial run, the first film should have no contrast to provide this mask for manual subtraction films.

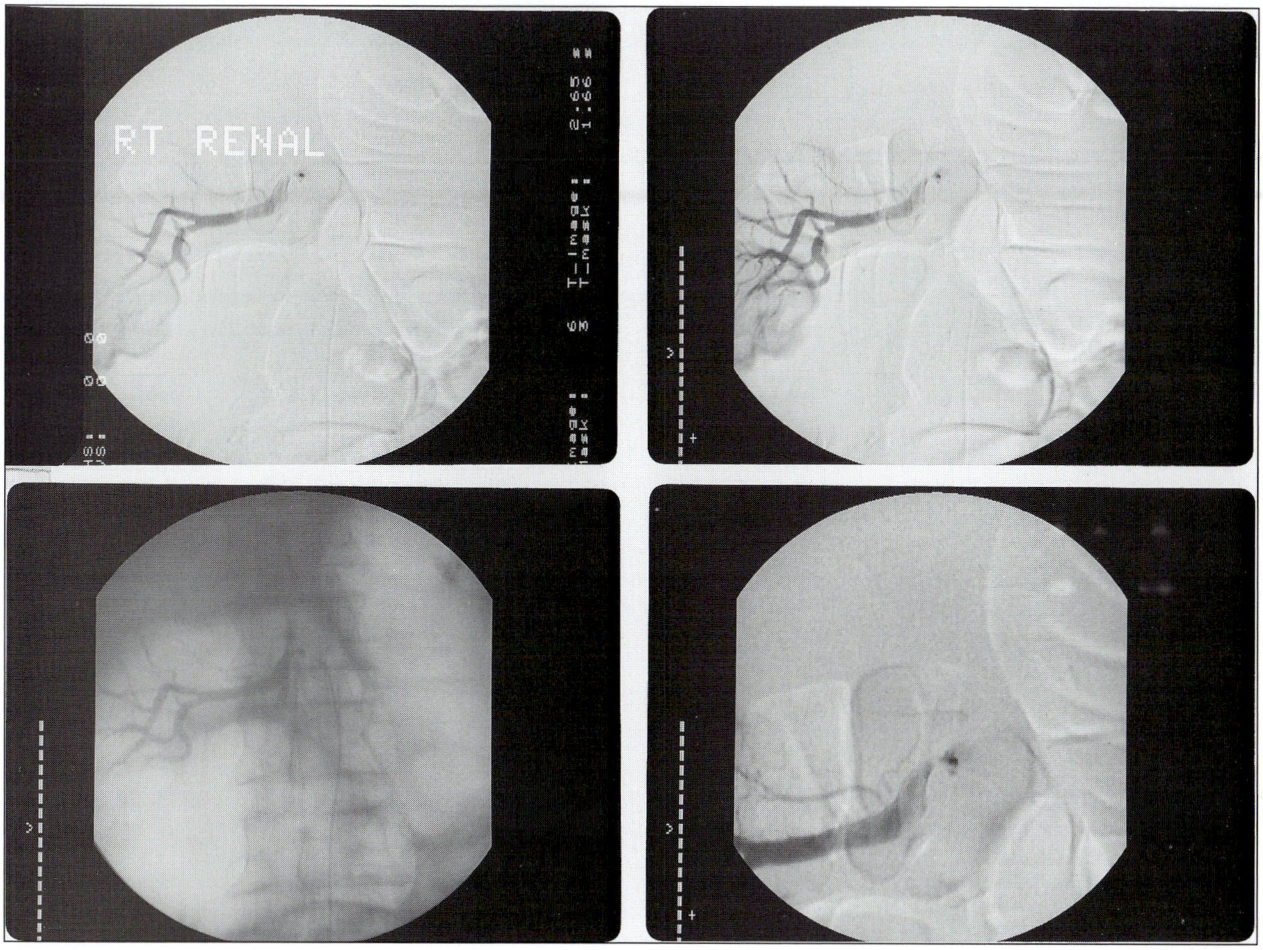

FIGURE 7.40 Renal artery stenosis.

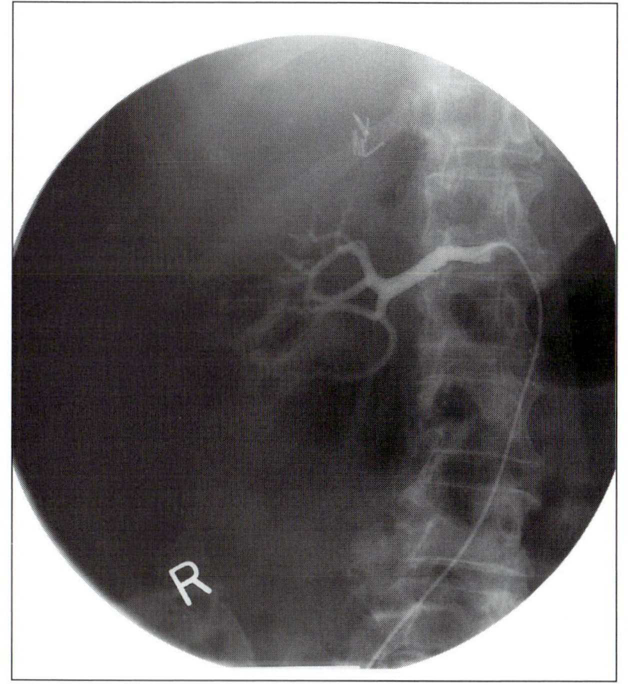

FIGURE 7.41 Demonstration of fibromuscular hyperplasia.

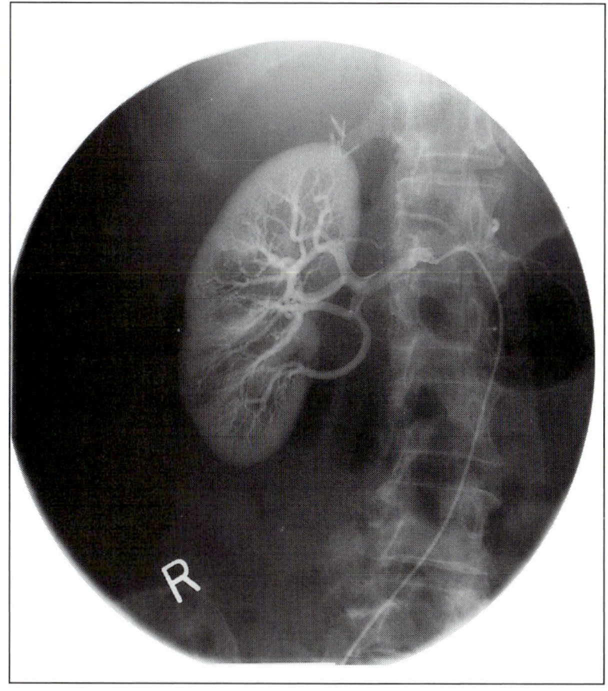

FIGURE 7.42 Renal tumor.

UPPER LIMB ARTERIOGRAPHY

Upper limb arteriography, although performed less often than lower limb arteriography, is a valuable tool in the diagnosis and treatment of upper extremity disease or trauma. Because there is not a common artery to select, upper limb arteriography is limited to unilateral studies. Because of this limitation of access, each side must be approached as separate studies.

Applied Anatomy (See Figure 7.11)

Indications

- Trauma
- Diminished or absent upper extremity pulses
- Persistent cold hand(s)
- Pain of unknown origin

Contraindications None

Equipment

- Digital or serial filming
- Pressure injector
- Disposable sterile tray
- Pigtail catheter or a straight catheter with side holes
- Catheter sheath
- Guidewire
- Emergency tray equipment
- If available, a long, 14 × 30 inch (35 × 76 cm) cassette may be used to image the entire upper limb.

Contrast Media

- The use of ionic contrast media is avoided due to the increased incidence of patient motion.
- The amount of nonionic contrast ranges from 15 to 20 mL.

Preliminary Radiographs A scout film of the AP projection of the upper limb is obtained.

Procedure Sequence

- A femoral approach is used with a Seldinger technique.
- The catheter is passed through the aorta to the innominate artery for a study of the right upper limb.
- For a study of the left upper limb, the catheter is passed through the aorta directly to the left subclavian artery.
- A small test injection is made to confirm proper catheter location and to evaluate blood flow.
- Films are obtained of the upper extremity.
- After films have been evaluated, the catheter is removed from the sheath.

Procedure Radiographs

- An AP projection of the upper limb of interest
- Multiple injections are needed to visualize the entire upper limb.

Common Pathologies

- Obstructed artery
- Aneurysm
- Arterial dissection
- AV malformation
- Traumatic injury
- Arterial sclerotic disease (Figure 7.43)

PERIPHERAL ARTERIOGRAPHY

Peripheral arteriography refers to studies of the arterial system of the upper or lower limbs. Patients with peripheral vascular disease will more commonly manifest symptoms in the lower limbs.

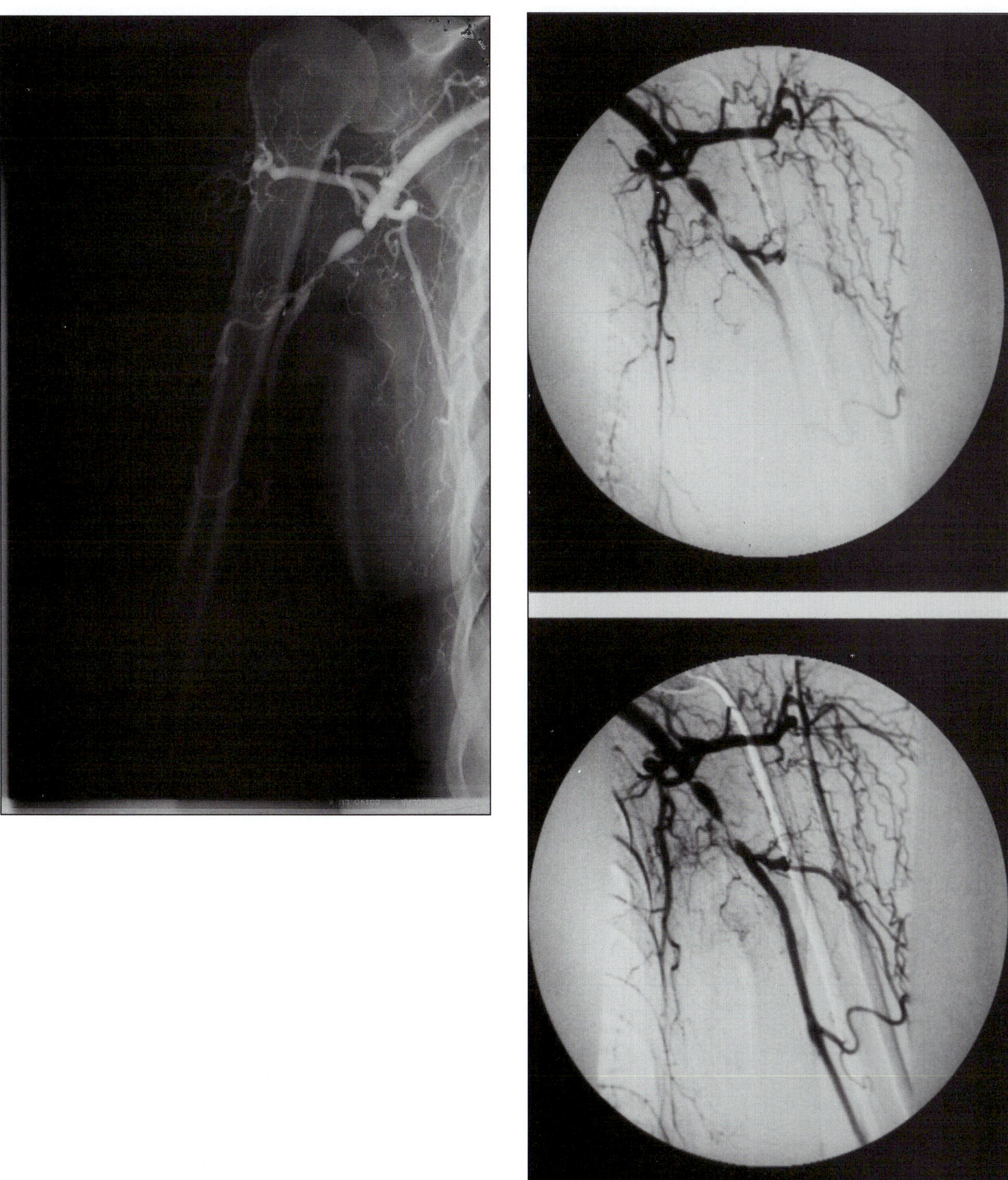

FIGURE 7.43 Demonstration of arteriovenous (AV) malformation.

LOWER LIMB ARTERIOGRAPHY

Lower limb arteriography is a common peripheral study. As opposed to upper limb studies, which require unilateral studies, angiographic studies of the lower limb result in bilateral studies of the legs with a single injection of contrast. Lower limb arteriography requires additional accessory equipment to adequately visualize the entire length of the lower limb. Abdominal aortography is frequently performed before lower limb angiography.

Applied Anatomy (See Figure 7.12)

Indications

- Pain in legs on exertion
- Arterial sclerotic disease
- Trauma
- Diabetic complications

Contraindications None

Equipment

- A serial film changer with a **stepping table** or a **long film cassette changer**
- DSA may be used.
- Fluoroscopy is used to confirm the position of the catheter.
- Pressure injector
- Disposable sterile tray
- Pigtail catheter
- Guidewire
- Catheter sheath
- Emergency tray equipment

Contrast Media

- 80 to 100 mL of nonionic contrast.
- The use of ionic contrast media is avoided due to the increased incidence of patient motion.

Preliminary Radiographs

- Scout film of the AP projection of the bilateral lower limbs
- An AP projection of the abdomen is also recommended because an abdominal aortogram commonly precedes lower limb arteriography.

Procedure Sequence

- A femoral approach is used with a Seldinger technique.
- An abdominal angiogram is performed.
- The pigtail catheter is pulled back to the level of the iliac bifurcation for a study of the lower limbs.
- A small test injection is made to confirm proper catheter location and to evaluate blood flow. This test injection aids in the determination of filming sequence and is used to configure the timing of the stepping motion of the table.
- Radiographs are obtained of the lower limbs.
- After films have been evaluated, the catheter is removed from the sheath.

Procedure Radiographs An AP projection of the lower limbs is obtained using a stepping table or a long film cassette changer.

Alternative Radiographs As indicated in trauma or if the area of interest is a single limb, an **antegrade** approach can be used for unilateral lower limb arteriography. The sheath and catheter are placed into the femoral artery and directed inferiorly. This results in lower contrast use for the patient. Only the affected lower limb is imaged.

Common Pathologies

- Obstructed artery (Figure 7.44)
- Aneurysm (Figure 7.45)
- Arterial dissection
- AV malformation
- Traumatic injury

> It is important to remember that all catheters need periodic flushing. Flushing usually is performed after insertion and guidewire removal, after bolus contrast injection, and intermittently to avoid **clot** formation.

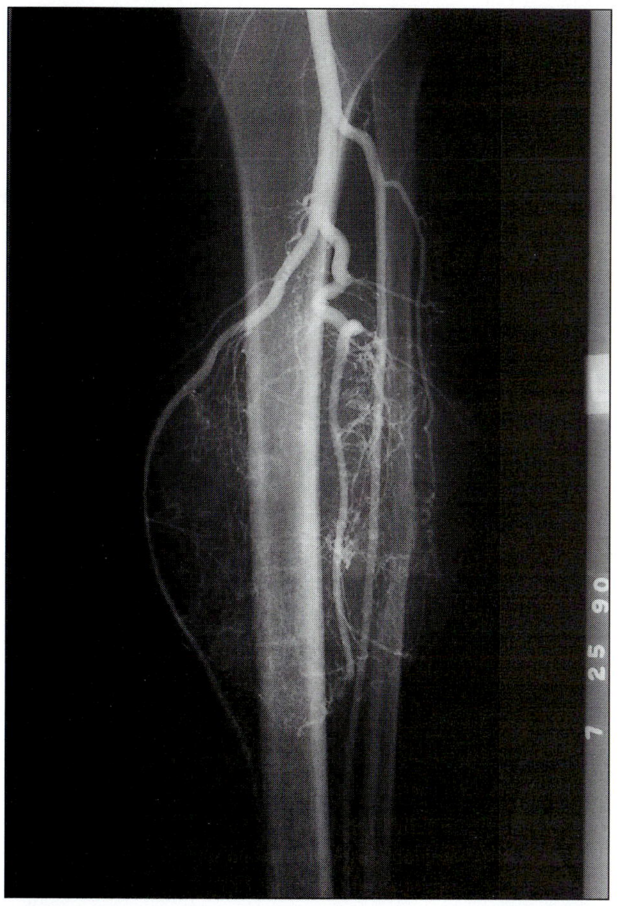

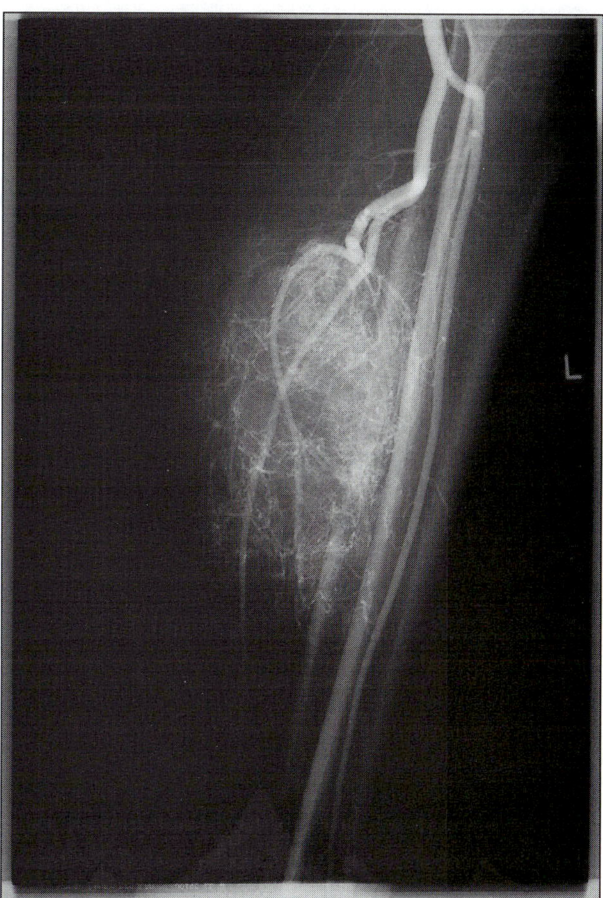

FIGURE 7.44 Lower limb arteriography demonstration of an obstructed artery.

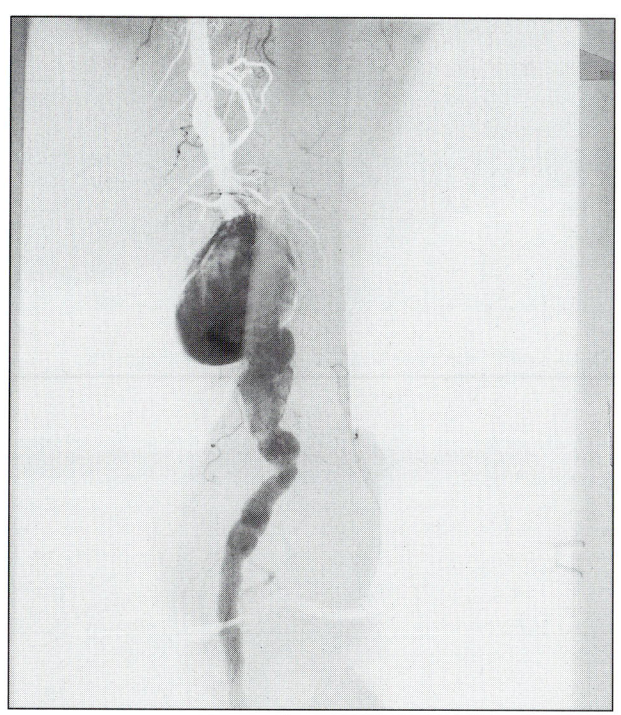

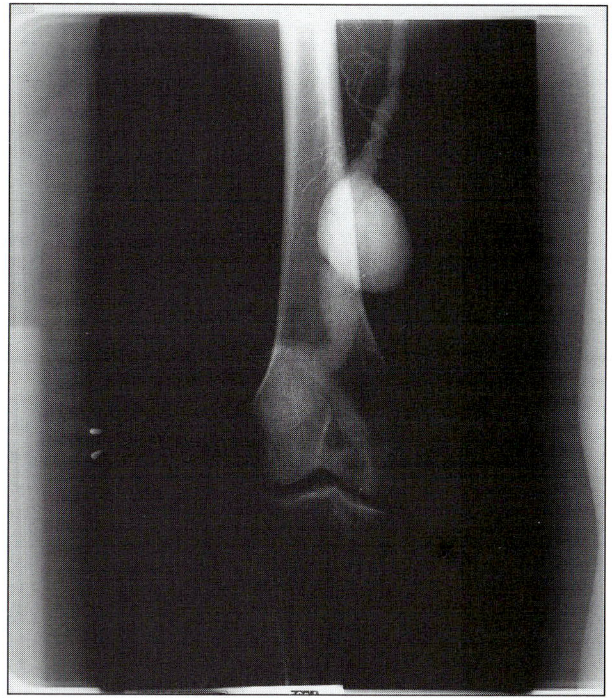

FIGURE 7.45 Femoral artery aneurysm.

Other Imaging Modalities

COMPUTED TOMOGRAPHY

Computed tomography can be useful as either a screening tool as, for instance, when the diagnosis of aortic aneurysm is suspected, or as a preliminary study before surgical or interventional repairs are performed. Aortic tears, aneurysms, and dissections (Figures 7.46 and 7.47) can be demonstrated or ruled out by simple CT measurement of the aorta. The ability to use CT as an initial, noninvasive diagnostic assessment eliminates the significantly higher patient risks of infection and the potential catheter dissection of angiography. CT is often more readily available and less complicated than angiography. These preliminary studies for vascular injuries can offer less risk and trauma to the already critical patient.

In CT angiography, a combination of bolus injections of contrast with helical CT imaging equipment is used to image vascular structures. This process allows image reconstruction without additional radiation dose to the patient and provides enhanced, three-dimensional images for diagnoses. Volume scanning, as helical CT is also termed, allows for the scanning of a volume of tissue rather than slices. With faster computers, constant table motion along with volume scanning, faster scan times result in the collection of large amounts of data in very short access times. One-second scan times are also made possible with the advent of slip-ring technology.

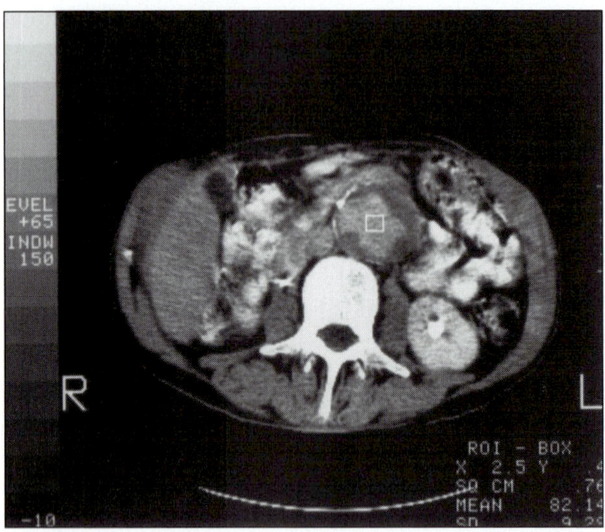

FIGURE 7.46 **CT of aortic dissection.**

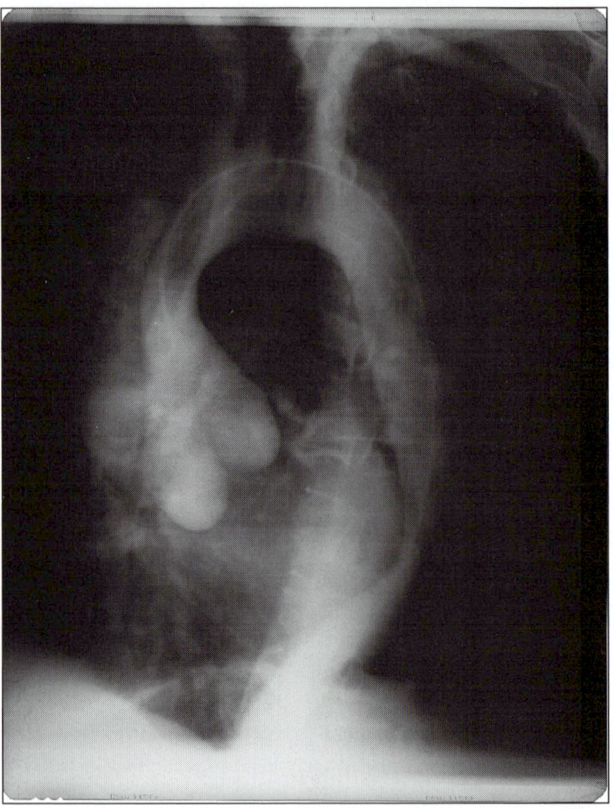

FIGURE 7.47 **Aortic arch angiogram of aortic dissection.**

MAGNETIC RESONANCE IMAGING

When used in conjunction with angiographic techniques, MRI is termed magnetic resonance angiography or MRA. MRA is recognized as an imaging tool that may eventually rival angiography in its ability to accurately pinpoint vascular disease. MRA has the capability to project vessels and structures in three dimensions without the use of ionizing radiation (Figure 7.48). Special pulse sequences permit the noninvasive demonstration of moving blood within vessels by two methods termed time-of-flight and phase-contrast MRA. Difficulties such as patient breathing motion limit some scans, such as cardiac gated studies, to the length of time patients can hold their breath.

Once perfected, MRA may potentially become a screening tool for coronary arteriography, abdominal angiography, and neurologic angiography.

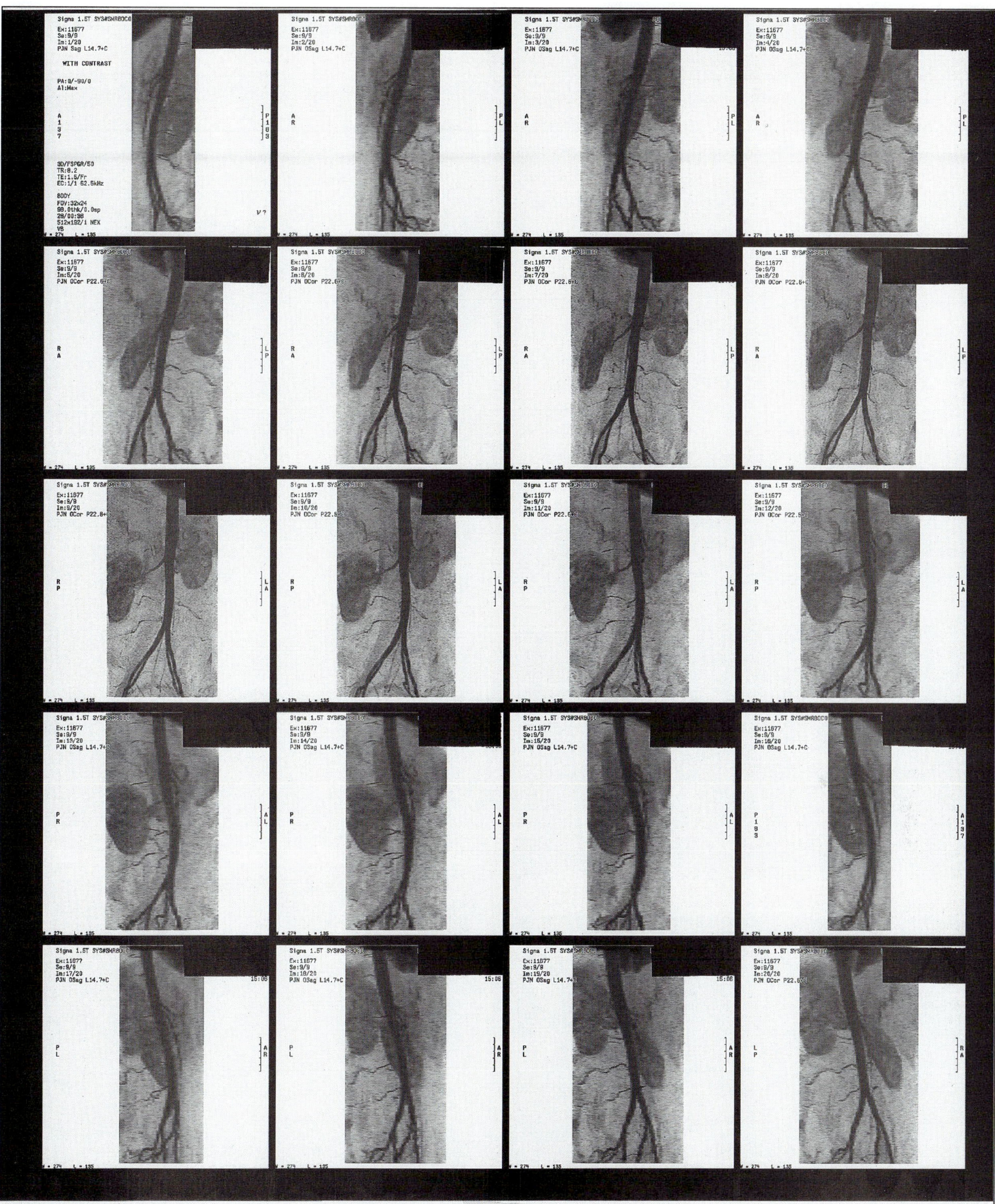

FIGURE 7.48 Magnetic resonance angiography.

ULTRASOUND

Ultrasonography or ultrasound imaging has become an important diagnostic screening tool, particularly in the heart and in peripheral arteries. Termed echocardiography when used on the heart, the two-dimensional, real-time study is used in cases of suspected cardiac valvular diseases, **cardiac tamponade**, and cardiac myopathy (Figure 7.49). With the advent of Doppler and color-flow Doppler, demonstration of the common carotid artery and its branches to detect obstruction or stenosis became a common screening examination (Figure 7.50). Mapping techniques, to demonstrate obstruction, allow for the imaging of vessels when the structure is not fully compressed by the sonographer.

Other vessels that may be imaged via ultrasound are femoral arteries and veins, subclavian artery and vein, the brachial artery and vein, and radial graphs.

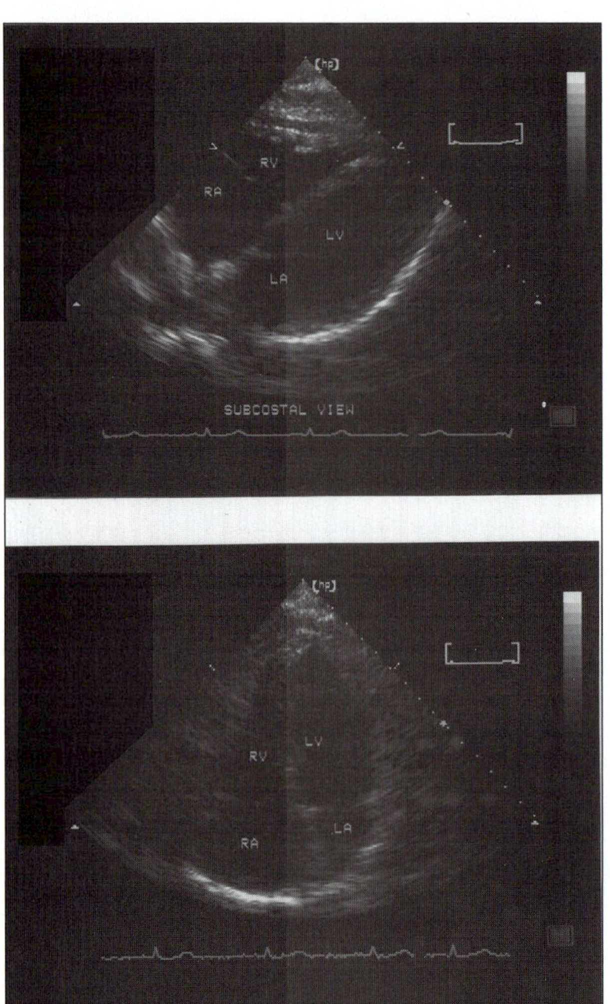

FIGURE 7.49 Echocardiography.

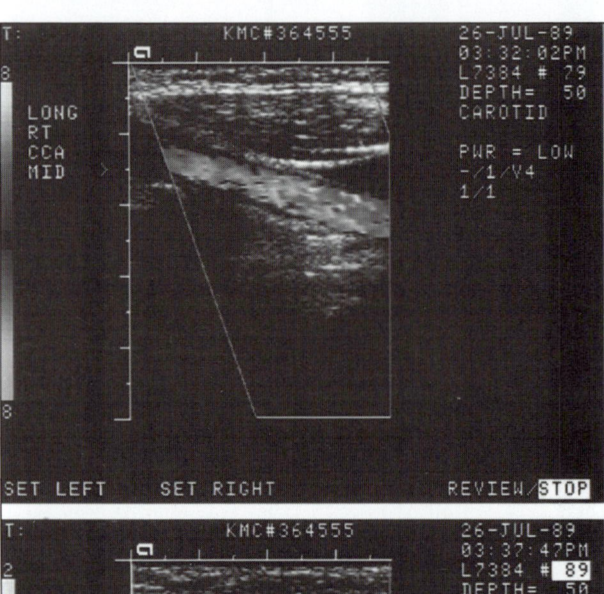

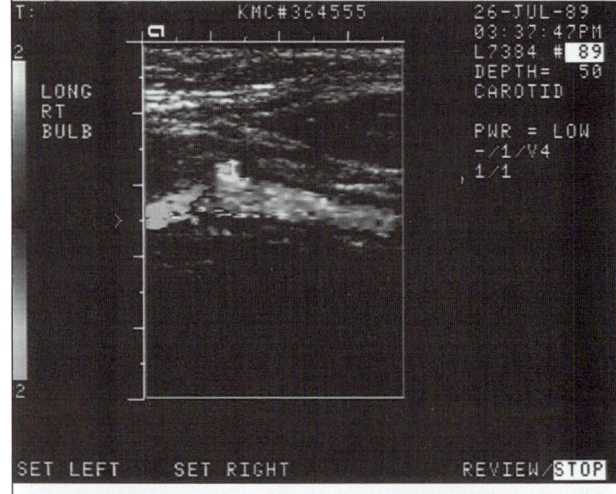

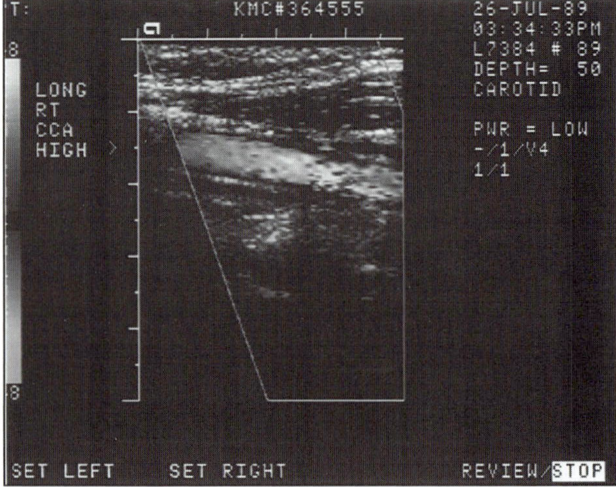

FIGURE 7.50 Color-flow Doppler of femoral artery.

RADIONUCLIDE IMAGING (NUCLEAR MEDICINE)

Nuclear medicine imaging provides the clinician with a range of noninvasive cardiovascular assessments. Cardiac scanning procedures include studies that range from cardiac uptake of technetium 99m stannous pyrophosphate, which produces an area of increased concentration on an image, a "hot spot" to thallium 201, which provides information about the heart and depends on a lack of uptake or concentration, that is, a "cold spot" (Figure 7.51).

Nuclear medicine cardiac assessments currently in practice are single photon emitted computed tomography (SPECT) ^{201}Tl cardiac perfusion studies. These studies include imaging protocols with the patient under stress conditions as well as delayed images at rest, termed redistribution scans. During the test the patient either exercises on a treadmill or is artificially stressed by the physician-guided injection of a pharmaceutical, which provides loading on the heart without the patient having to exercise. The use of an artificial stressor is advantageous to those patients who cannot tolerate treadmill performance. The patient is carefully monitored via ECG during this time. This study differentiates and defines the extent of damage of either **ischemic** (ĭs-kē´mĭk) or **infarcted** myocardial tissue.

With the advent of SPECT in nuclear medicine, more sophisticated imaging can be performed including three-dimensional reconstructions and computer-generated analyses. Other studies offered in the nuclear medicine department specific to cardiac assessments are acute myocardial infarct scanning (the "hot spot" study mentioned previously) and gated cardiac blood pool studies. Myocardial infarct studies are termed "acute" because the study will only accurately demonstrate acute conditions of myocardial infarct within 1 to 10 days of the initial event. Gated cardiac studies provide information about cardiac function in terms of assessing ejection fraction and wall motion of the heart.

Nuclear medicine studies of lung ventilation and perfusion demonstrating the presence or absence of pulmonary emboli (Figures 7.52, 7.53, and 7.54) contribute to information regarding the performance of pulmonary arteriography. Blood pool scans to determine acute GI bleeds are a screening assessment commonly used before abdominal angiography.

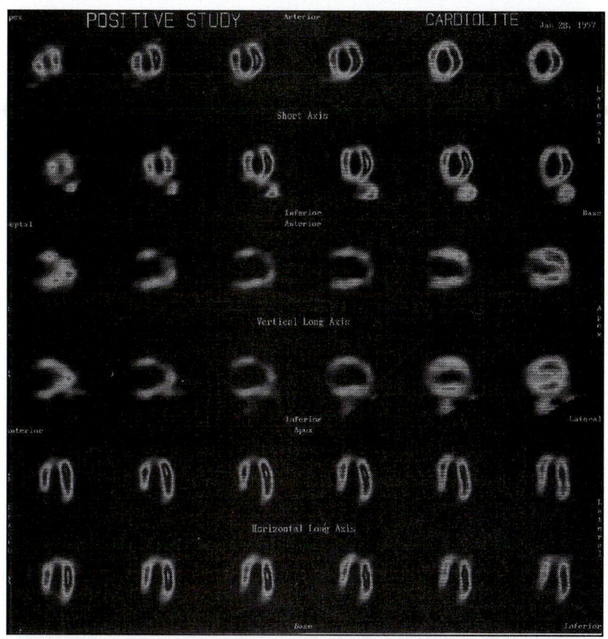

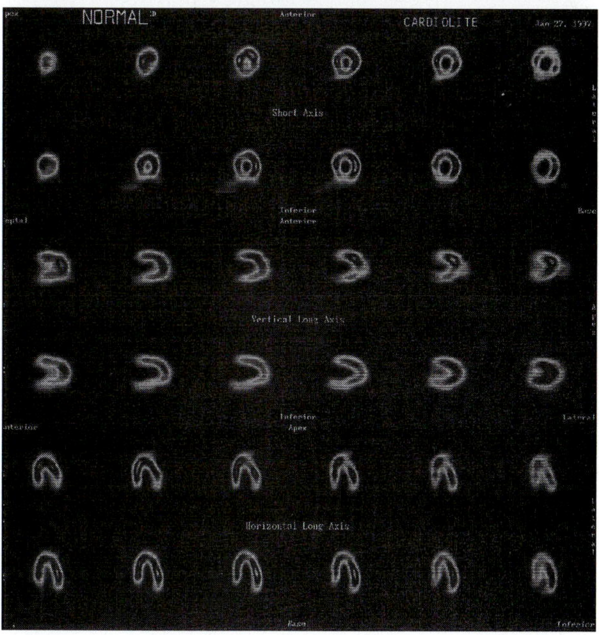

FIGURE 7.51 **Myocardial perfusion (thallium) nuclear medicine study.**

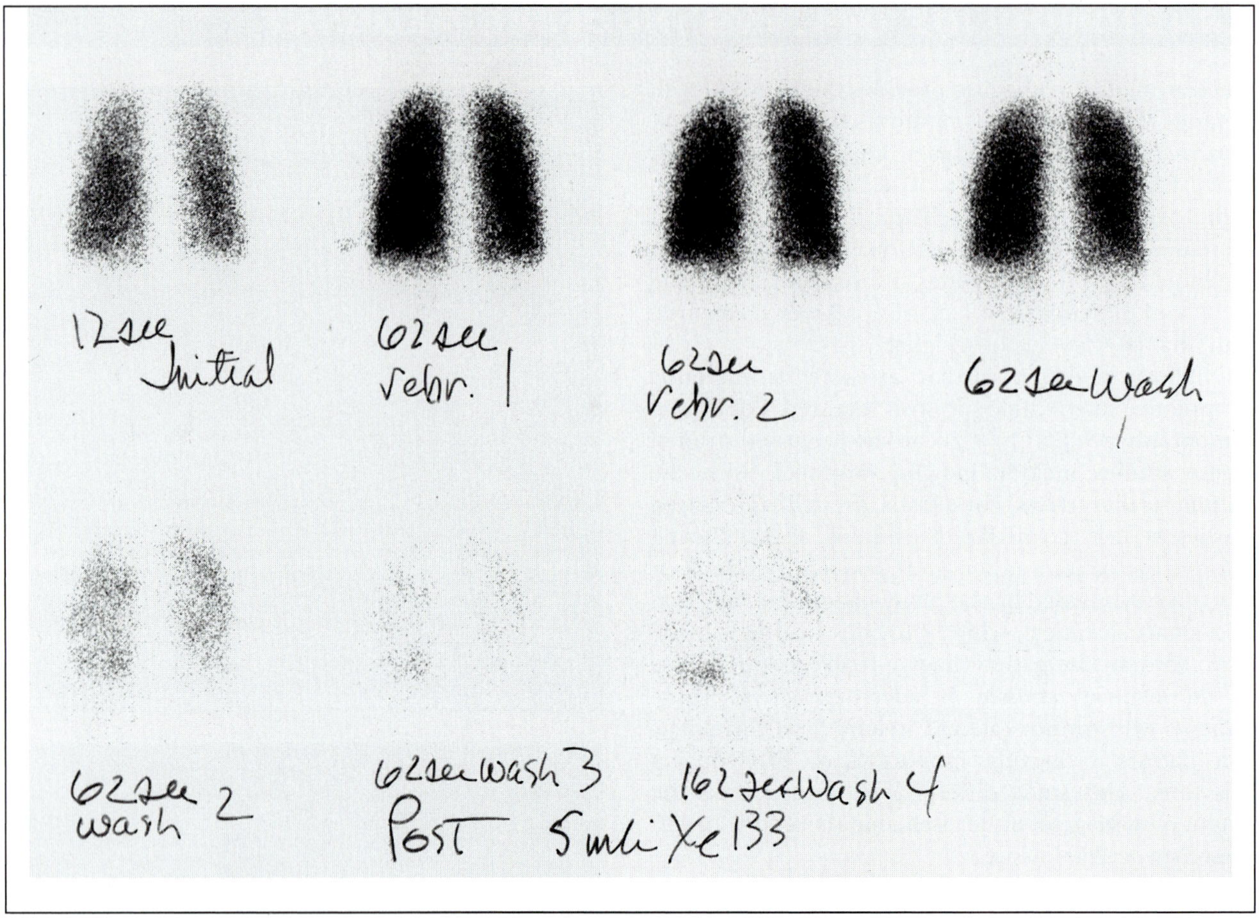

FIGURE 7.52 Ventilation lung scan.

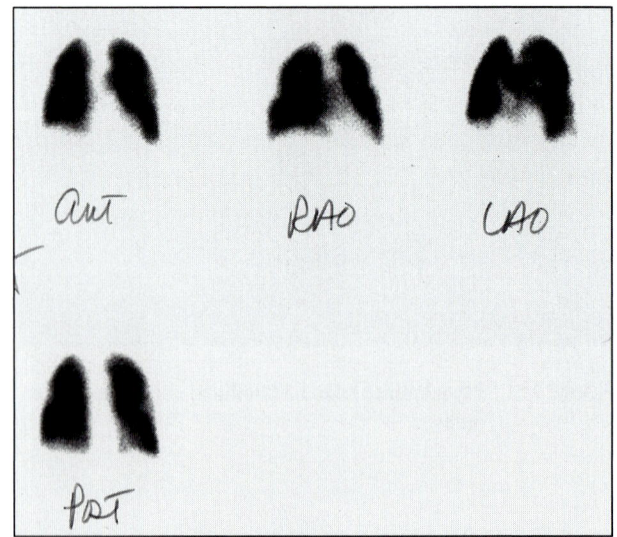

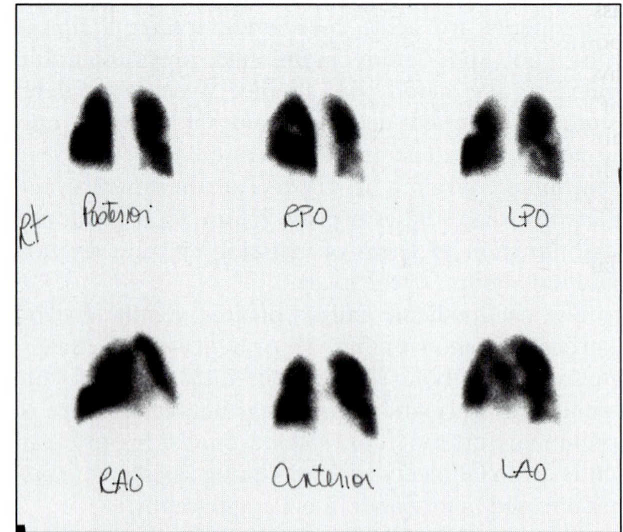

FIGURE 7.53 Perfusion lung scan.

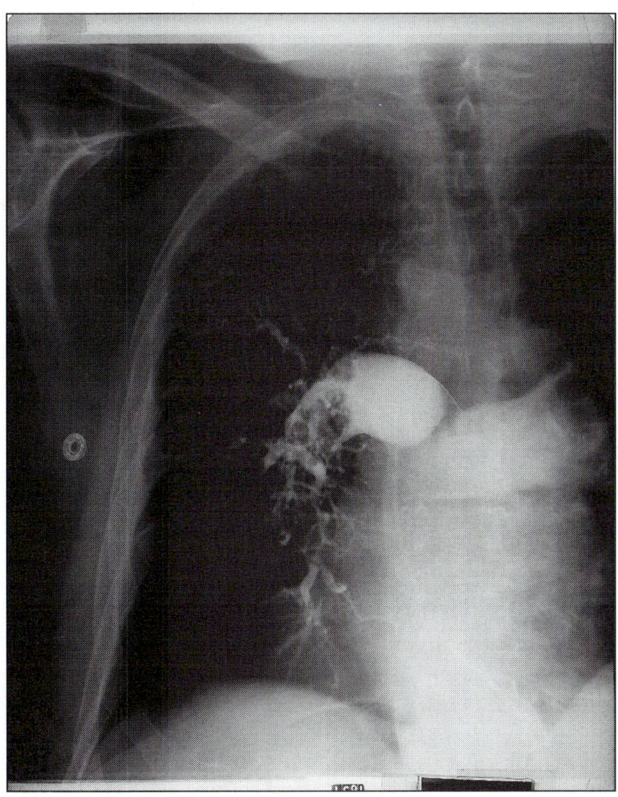

FIGURE 7.54
Pulmonary angiogram demonstrating pulmonary emboli.

POSITRON EMITTED TOMOGRAPHY (PET)

The use of PET allows for a noninvasive, radionuclide assessment of the physiologic distribution status of body elements such as carbon, oxygen, nitrogen, and hydrogen. Image reconstruction is similar to CT and SPECT. Due to its current high expense and low availability, PET use is limited. The extremely short half-life radionuclides used for scanning require cyclotron or accelerator production, which are relatively costly.

Diagnostic information from PET is somewhat similar to SPECT of myocardial perfusion imaging. PET, however, can provide metabolic information with increased sensitivity and specificity in coronary artery disease detection. This enhanced information provides more detailed information to physicians as to identifying patients who may benefit from percutaneous transluminal coronary angioplasty (PCTA) or bypass surgery.

Interventional Procedures

Prior to 1960, angiographic procedures were limited to diagnosing disease processes. In 1964, Dotter and Judkins performed the first percutaneous recannulization of a femoral artery, that is, the femoral artery originally was occluded and subsequently reopened. These early attempts were referred to as angioplasties and were actually angiographic procedures that intervened and repaired anatomic anomalies within the artery. The use of nonspecialized equipment and larger catheter sizes reduced the probability of long-term success. Early procedures were more prone to restenosis.

In 1972, transcatheter embolizations were performed. This procedure allowed for occlusion of specific arteries with the use of chemical, particulate, and mechanical means. The occlusion allowed for control of bleeding, reduction of vascular feeding of tumors and occlusion before surgical intervention.

In 1974, Gruntzig developed a specialized, double-**lumen** angioplasty balloon catheter. This design reduced procedural risk to the patient and increased the long-term patency of the vessel. With the discovery and subsequent use of these new catheters the possibility of recannulizing coronary arteries was possible.

In 1995, the use of stents was approved by the Federal Drug Administration in the United States and became a primary interventional procedure. Stents are wire scaffolds that provide physical structure to and prevent arteries from restenosing.

PERCUTANEOUS TRANSLUMINAL ANGIOPLASTY (PTA)

A complete discussion of angioplasty can be found in Chapter 6, Angiographic Procedures and Equipment. PTA refers to an interventional procedure that allows for the increase of blood flow through a formerly occluded or stenotic vessel that has been corrected through the use of a balloon catheter (Figure 7.55). PTA can be used for any peripheral artery as well as renal and coronary arteries. When the coronary artery is the subject of intervention, the procedure is termed percutaneous transluminal coronary angioplasty or PTCA. For a discussion of coronary angioplasty, see the next section.

Other interventional studies under current investigation are angioplasty studies of the carotid and cerebral arteries.

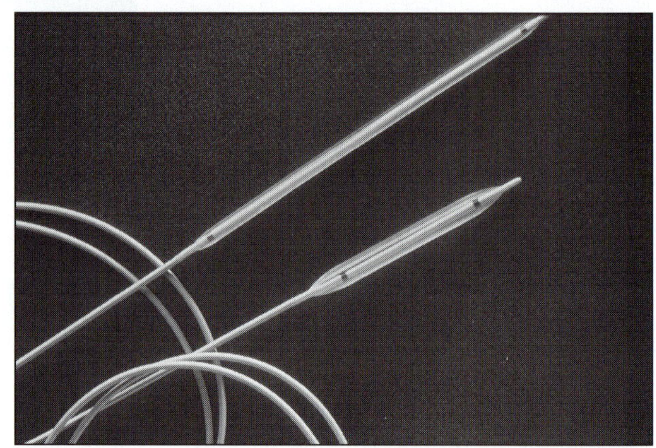

FIGURE 7.55 Peripheral balloon catheters used for PTA (Courtesy of Medi-tech/Boston Scientific Corporation, Natick, MA).

PERCUTANEOUS TRANSLUMINAL CORONARY ANGIOPLASTY (PTCA)

Percutaneous transluminal coronary angioplasty (PTCA) differs from PTA in that PTCA is specific to the coronary arteries. Smaller guidewires and catheters are used in PTCA. In all coronary angioplasties, a guiding catheter is used. This type of catheter has a large lumen to accommodate the passage of both the balloon catheter and guidewire (Figure 7.56). The guiding catheter also provides support when the balloon is advanced into the coronary artery.

After an angiogram has been performed resulting in a diagnosis recommending subsequent angioplasty for the patient (Figure 7.57), a larger guide catheter is inserted into the ascending aorta and into the affected arterial osteum. Through this catheter, a smaller catheter with a deflated balloon is inserted over a small (.014 inches) guidewire and positioned at the blockage or occlusion. A small amount of contrast is injected to confirm correct position of the balloon. Following this, the balloon is inflated with contrast (Figure 7.58). Contrast is used at this point so that the shape of the balloon can be seen on fluoroscopy. Also, filling the balloon with contrast replaces air in the balloon so that

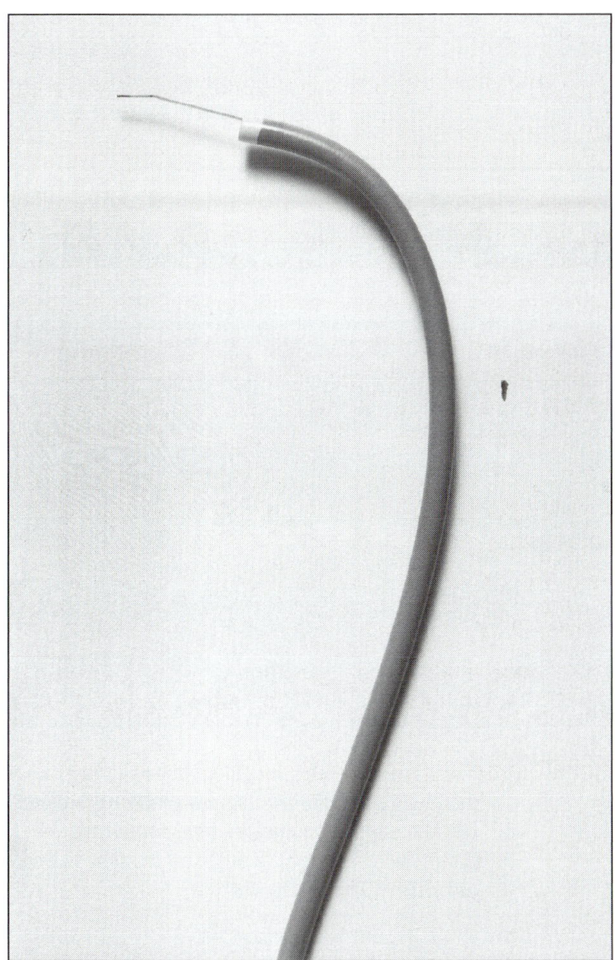

FIGURE 7.56 A guiding catheter.

if the balloon accidentally ruptures, no air will enter the arterial system.

On occasion when the balloon is inflated, the patient will experience similar, if not more, intense chest pain (angina) as compared to the initial incident before being admitted to the hospital. During PTCA, however, the patient experiences the angina under a controlled environment. Chest pain during PTCA does indicate to the physician that the correct artery has been selected and that the portion of the heart that is supplied by this artery still has viable muscle. Following two to three balloon inflations lasting 30 seconds to 5 minutes, the balloon is pulled back into the guide catheter leaving the wire across the lesion. An angiogram is performed at this time. If the physician is satisfied that the artery is sufficiently opened and there is minimal residual stenosis, the wire is removed. A final set of angiograms is performed (Figure 7.59).

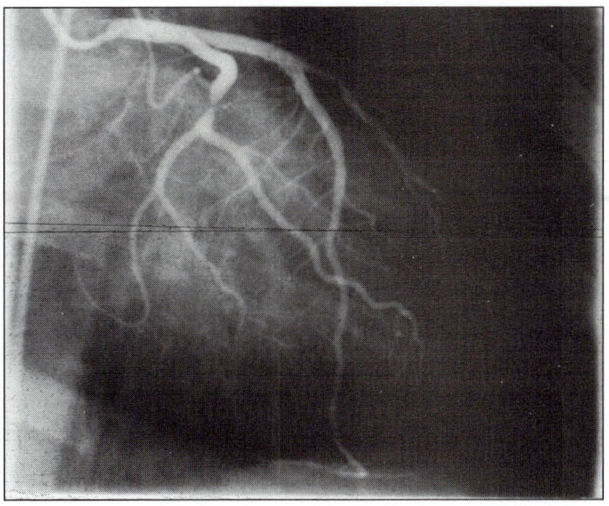

FIGURE 7.57 Stenotic circumflex artery.

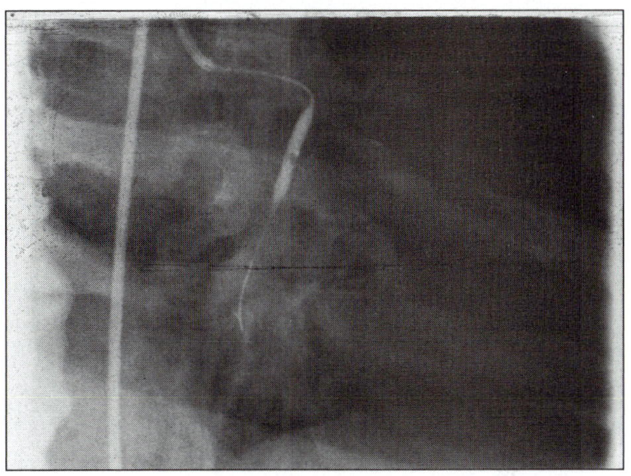

FIGURE 7.58 Inflated PTCA balloon in circumflex artery.

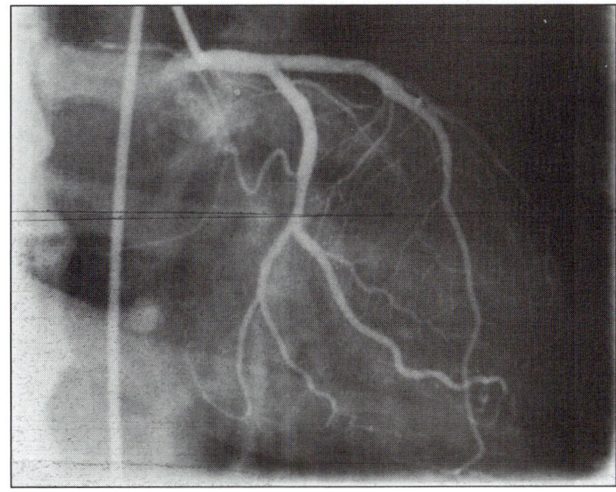

FIGURE 7.59 Angiogram after PTCA.

The catheter sheath remains in place and is sutured to prevent accidental removal. If the sheath is removed prematurely, bleeding at the puncture site is difficult to control. A patient having PTCA is given large doses of heparin, an anticoagulant. Following PTCA, the patient is hospitalized for 24 to 72 hours for observation.

A complete discussion of angioplasty can be found in Chapter 6, Angiographic Procedures and Equipment.

STENTS

Stents are wire scaffolds that provide structural support to arteries and thus prevent arteries from restenosing (Figure 7.60). Before stent deployment, an angioplasty is performed on the stenotic vessel. Stents are either of the self-expanding type or balloon-expanding type. The self-expanding type of stent does not require the use of a balloon catheter. When deployed, this type of stent becomes decompressed when released. The balloon-expanding stent is carefully mounted on a PTCA (intracoronary) or PTA (**intra-arterial**) balloon catheter for delivery. All balloon catheters have a radiopaque marker to locate the position of the balloon within the artery. Once the stent is centered at the lesion (as verified by placement of the radiopaque marker over the lesion), the balloon is then inflated and the stent deployed. Both pre- and poststent placement angiograms of the vessel are obtained (Figures 7.61 and 7.62).

Postprocedure care of stent placement differs from that of arteriography by administering anticoagulant therapy to the patient for 6 to 8 weeks following the procedure. Stents cannot be removed and are permanent. Stents and their placements are carefully documented and are registered with the company that manufactured the stent.

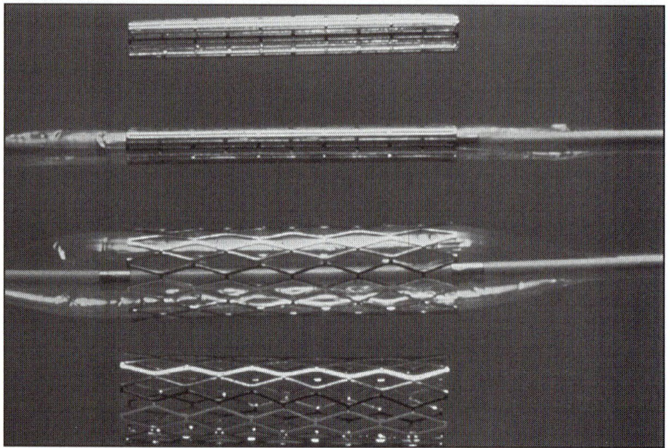

FIGURE 7.60 Four stages of stent placement (top to bottom): nondeployed stent, stent on delivery balloon, balloon inflated stent expanded, and expanded stent (Courtesy of Cordis®, a Johnson & Johnson Company, New Brunswick, NJ).

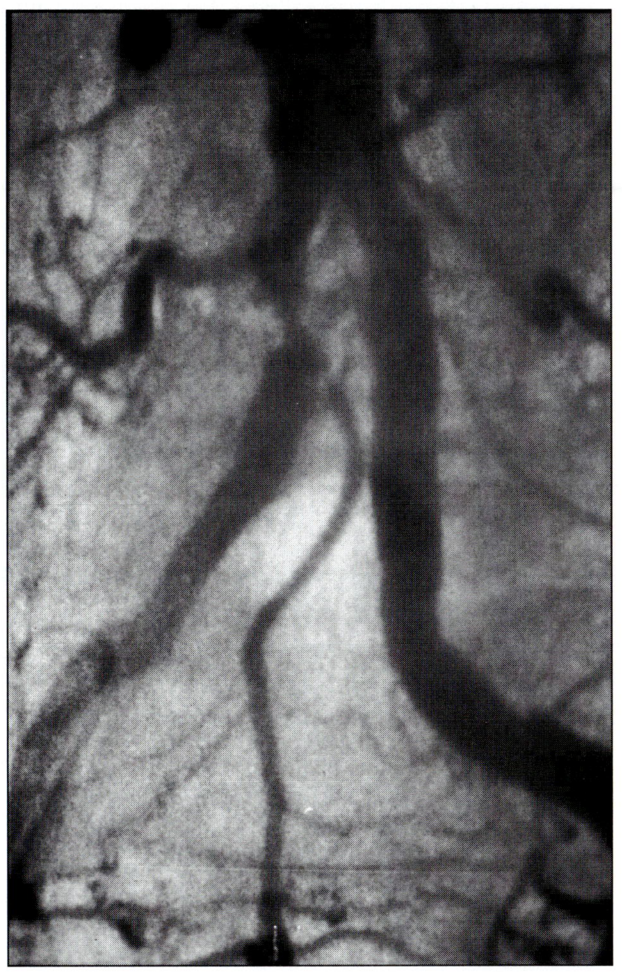

FIGURE 7.61 Stenosed iliac artery, prestent placement.

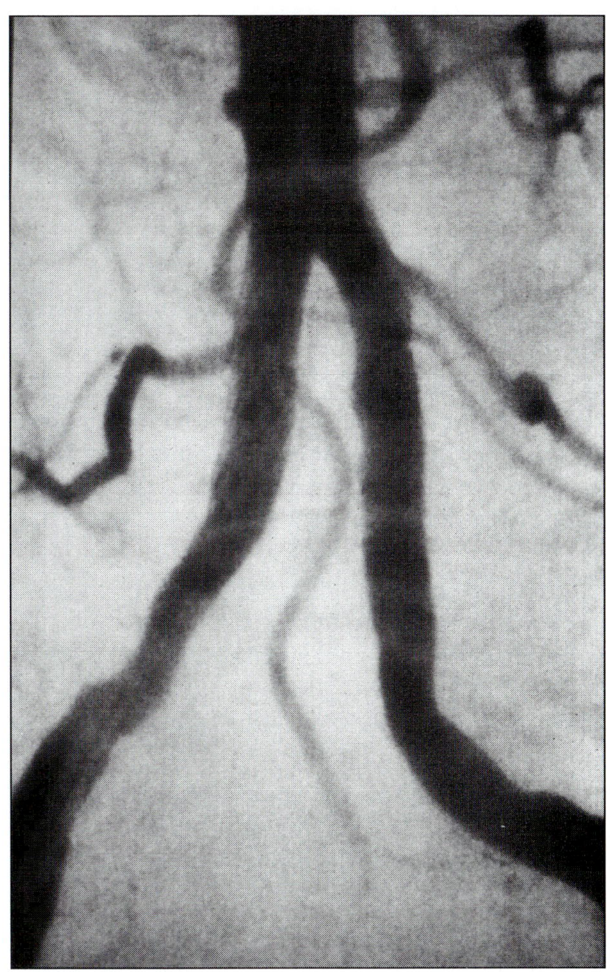

FIGURE 7.62 Iliac artery with stent.

EMBOLIZATION

Embolization is the use of mechanical, chemical, or particulate methods of stopping blood flow, either normal or abnormal. The procedure of embolization involves the (usually) superselective placement of a catheter at the site of a bleed. Through this catheter the liquid particulate or solid embolization material is deployed. Embolization may be performed either as a temporary or permanent intervention. Follow-up radiographs, usually DSA, are taken to assure the occlusion of the artery. Coronary arteries are not embolized.

A complete discussion of embolization can be found in Chapter 6, Angiographic Procedures and Equipment.

Review Questions

1. List the equipment needed for a heart catheterization procedure.

2. Identify radiation protection practices currently in use in the angiography suite.

3. Identify and differentiate between the structure and use of a pigtail catheter and a Judkin's catheter.

4. A "selective" angiogram refers to:
   a. a general type of angiogram
   b. a specific vessel angiogram other than aortic
   c. the use of fluoroscopy for an aortic angiogram
   d. the use of digital films for an angiogram

5. The pulmonary artery pumps ___________ to the lungs.
   a. oxygenated blood
   b. unoxygenated blood

6. The celiac axis consists of the ________________ arteries.
   a. left gastric, hepatic, and splenic
   b. right gastric, hepatic, and duodenal
   c. hepatic, splenic, and gastroduodenal
   d. mesenteric, hepatic, and splenic

7. Identify the pathways through which blood flows in and out of the heart.

8. The aortic valve is a tricuspid structure made up of:
   a. three cusps, left, right, and coronary
   b. three cusps, left, right and noncoronary
   c. two cusps, left and right
   d. two cusps, coronary and noncoronary

9. Identify one type of pathology for each of the following angiograms
   a. Peripheral arteriography ________________
   b. Abdominal aortogram ________________
      Renal ________________
      Superior mesenteric ________________
   c. Cardiac catheterization ________________
   d. Pulmonary arteriography ________________

CASE STUDY

A 45-year-old man presents at the emergency room with shoulder pain radiating down the left arm. The patient has a history of smoking; his father died of "heart problems" at 53 years of age. What angiographic studies and which alternate imaging modalities would support the diagnosis of this patient?

____

____

____

____

____

____

____

____

____

____

References and Recommended Reading

Ballinger, P. (1995). *Merrill's atlas of radiographic positions and radiologic procedures.* St. Louis: Mosby-Year Book.

Grossman, W. (1980). *Cardiac catheterization and angiography.* Philadelphia: Lea & Febiger.

Johnson, L., Moore, R., & Balter, S. (1992, March). Review of radiation safety in the cardiac catheterization laboratory. *Catheterization and Cardiovascular Diagnosis, 25,* 3.

Kern, M. (1995). *The cardiac catheterization handbook.* St. Louis: Mosby-Year Book.

Laudicina, P., & Wean, D. (1994). *Applied angiography for radiographers.* Philadelphia: Saunders.

Marcus, M., Schelbert, H., Skorton, D., & Wolf, G. (1991). *Cardiac imaging: A companion to Braunwald's heart disease.* Philadelphia: Saunders.

Meschan, I. (1978). *Radiographic positioning and related anatomy.* Philadelphia: Saunders.

Miller, B., & Keane, C. B. (1987). *Encyclopedia and dictionary of medicine, nursing, and allied health* (4th ed.). Philadelphia: Saunders.

Mosby's medical encyclopedia for health professionals. St. Louis: Mosby-Year Book.

Snopek, A. (1992). *Fundamentals of special radiographic procedures.* Philadelphia: Saunders.

Tortorici, M., & Apfel, P. (1995). *Advanced radiographic and angiographic procedures.* Philadelphia: Davis.

CHAPTER 8

Venous System

CYNTHIA COWLING, BSc, MEd, MRT(R), ACR

OBJECTIVES

At the completion of this chapter, the student should be able to:

1. Describe the main features of the venous system.
2. Describe the procedures used in the diagnostic study of the venous system.
3. List the major equipment used for each procedure.
4. List the major indications and contraindications for each study.
5. Describe and compare the different modalities used to image the venous system.
6. Apply knowledge of angiography to the studies described in this chapter.
7. Discuss safe practices used for each procedure.
8. Identify normal radiographic appearances.
9. Identify radiographically some simple pathologies as listed in this chapter.
10. List usual contrast used, if any, for each procedure.
11. Describe patient care principles used for each procedure.
12. Describe the interventional procedures used therapeutically on the venous system.
13. List the major reasons for performing each interventional procedure.

Introduction and Historical Overview

The first radiographs taken of the veins was in 1923 when Berberich and Hirsch injected strontium bromide intravenously. In 1929, lipiodil was used and in 1934 the first indirect venograms were performed after an arterial study. Although this seemed successful for demonstrating the major abdominal vessels, it was not very successful in demonstrating the leg vessels because of the amount of blood present in the veins and the consequential dilation of the contrast. Dos Santos first attempted ascending venography in 1938. The only problem with this study at the time was the inability to determine when exactly the contrast would be in the leg. Application of tourniquets slowed the process, but it was not until image intensification was able to visualize dynamically the rapid movement of the contrast that venography became an established procedure. It became the main technique for assessing for deep vein thrombosis until ultrasound developed the ability to demonstrate thrombotic vessels, in a simpler, noninvasive, and cost-effective way.

Anatomy

The venous system is extensive and can be divided into the deep and superficial systems. With one major exception, the venous system transports deoxygenated blood back to the heart. The exceptions to this are the pulmonary veins, which transport oxygenated blood from the lungs back to the heart. The superficial veins usually provide the injection site for entry into the venous and arterial systems (Figure 8.1).

All veins empty eventually into the superior vena cava, inferior vena cava, or into the coronary sinus from the heart.

VEINS OF THE UPPER EXTREMITY

The subclavian vein, which accompanies the subclavian artery, is the major vein that drains the upper extremity. It receives venous blood from the shoulder and upper extremity. Superficial drainage is by the basilic and cephalic veins. These drain into the brachial and axillary vein, respectively. The median cubital vein in the arm is the major injection site for entry into the blood supply (Figure 8.2).

VEINS OF THE LOWER EXTREMITY

The external iliac vein, the major vein of the lower extremity, lies next to the artery that bears the same name. The deep veins parallel the arteries and are so named. The major superficial veins are the short and long saphenous (sǎ-fē´nŭs) veins, which drain into the popliteal and femoral veins, respectively.

The major deep veins are the inferior and superior vena cava, into which all veins drain. The inferior vena cava lies slightly to the right of midline and receives drainage from the common iliac, renal, suprarenal, right gonadal, hepatic, and lumbar veins.

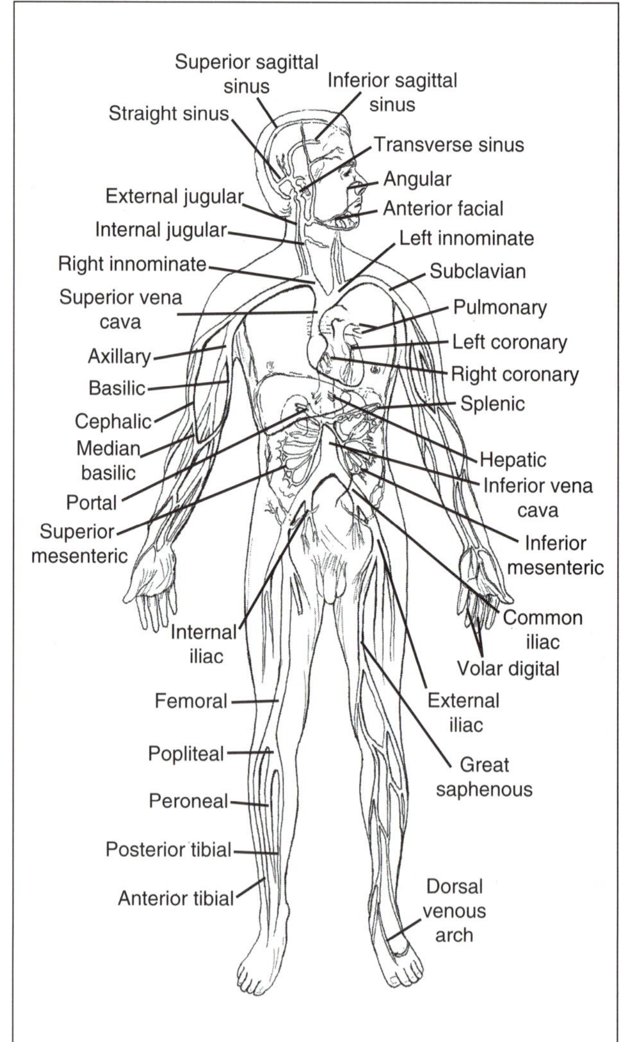

FIGURE 8.1 The venous system.

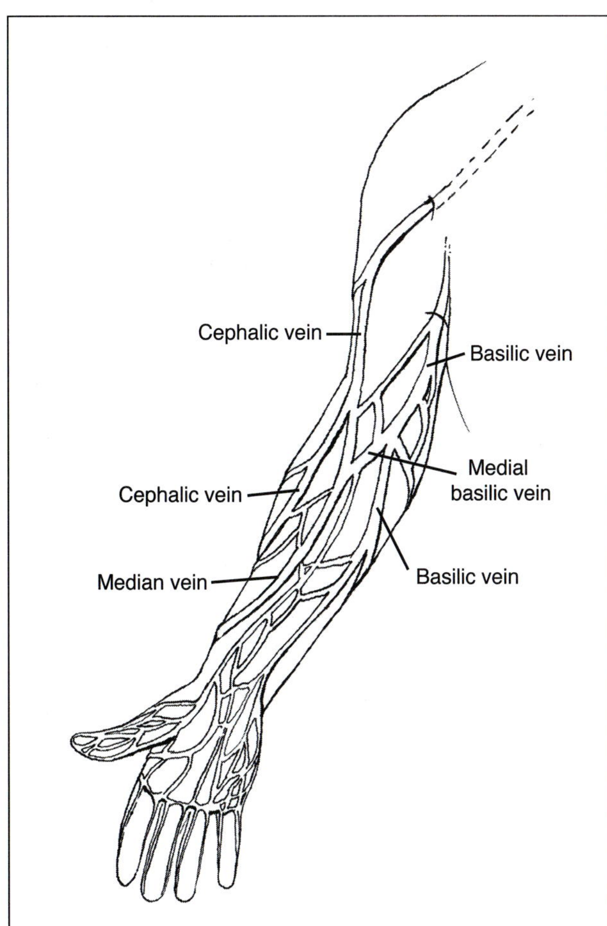

FIGURE 8.2 Superficial system of the upper extremity.

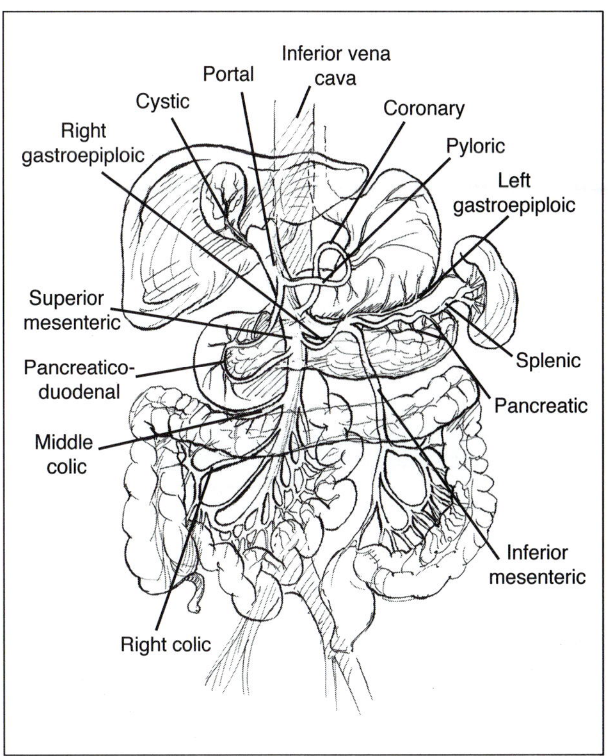

FIGURE 8.3 Portal system.

The hepatic portal venous system drains the digestive organs of the abdomen, excluding the stomach, pancreas, spleen, and small and large intestine. The ultimate site and drainage of these organs or structures is the portal vein formed by the **anastomosis** (ă-năs´´tō-mō´sĭs) of the splenic and superior mesenteric veins, which drain the spleen and small intestine, respectively. The portal vein enters the liver via the porta hepatis, where its venous contents enter the liver sinusoids (Figure 8.3). The ultimate drainage is into the inferior vena cava through the hepatic veins. The posterior thorax is drained by the hemiazygos (hĕm´´ē-ăz´ĭ-gŏs) veins, which empty ultimately into the superior vena cava.

About two-thirds of the body's blood supply sits within the venous system at any given time. The flow to the heart is controlled partially by gradient and partially by muscle contractions (particularly in the lower limb). Within most veins are valves, which prevent the retrograde movement of blood (Figure 8.4).

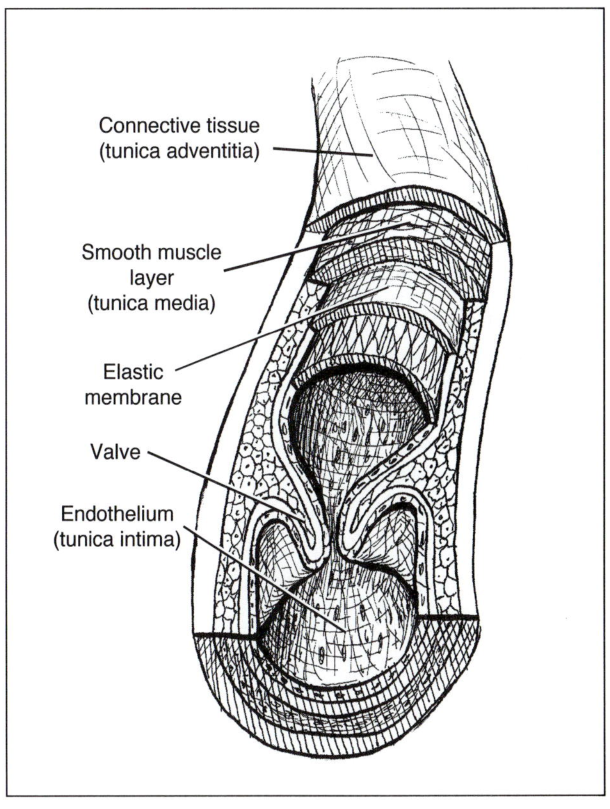

FIGURE 8.4 Valve system in veins.

Procedures

VENOGRAPHY

Venography can also be called venous angiography or phlebography and is the radiographic examination of the venous system by the introduction of contrast media into the venous system. The contrast can be introduced either directly via an injection or catheter into the venous system or indirectly following an arteriogram. Veins examined include abdominal and peripheral systems, but the number of peripheral examinations has decreased with the extensive use of Doppler ultrasound, a noninvasive, relatively inexpensive technique.

PERIPHERAL VENOGRAPHY

Venous studies of the extremities are usually referred to as peripheral venography.

LOWER LIMB VENOGRAPHY

This procedure examines the condition of superficial and deep veins of the leg. At one time it was a common procedure that did not necessitate the use of the angiographic suite. Today its use has been curtailed by the advances of ultrasound. The most common reason for this examination is suspected **deep vein thrombosis (DVT)**.

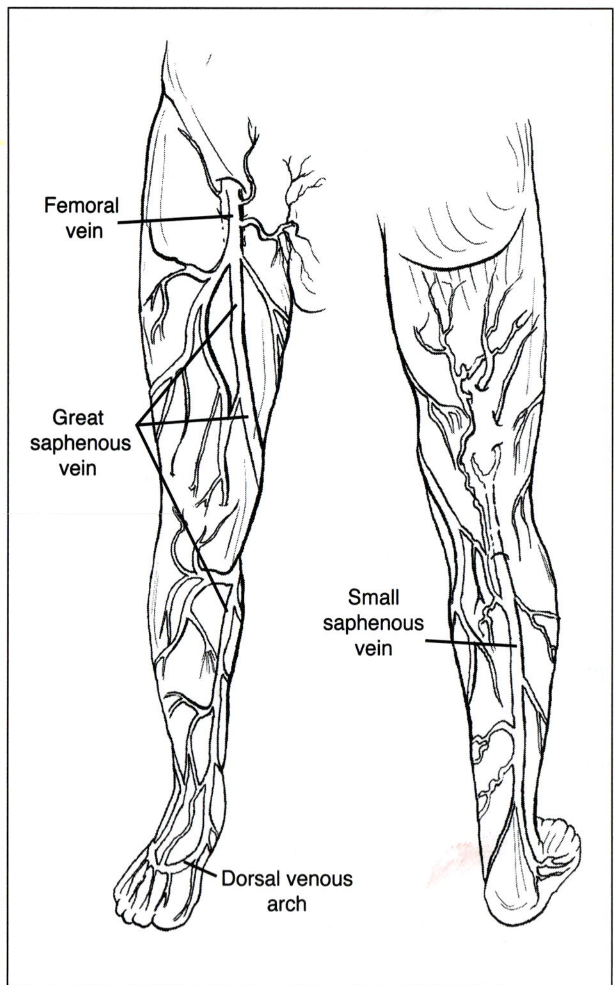

FIGURE 8.5 Superficial veins of the leg.

Applied Anatomy (Figures 8.5 and 8.6)

Indications

- DVT
- Venous obstruction due to tumor or other extrinsic factors
- Recurrent **varicose** (văr´ĭ-kōs) **veins**
- Swollen legs of unknown etiology
- **Varicose ulcers**
- Venous malformations

Contraindications

- Contrast allergy
- Local sepsis
- Significant compromising of the veins, which would inhibit their competence and contrast flow. Ultrasound should always be recommended for these conditions.

Equipment

- Fluoroscopy unit with spot film device
- Tilting table top
- Tourniquet
- 19-gauge butterfly needle
- 20- or 50-mL syringe
- Cleansing swabs

Contrast Media Iodine-based water-soluble contrast is used. Ideally a low-osmolarity contrast is preferable. This is better tolerated by the patient, reduces pain, and has a history of fewer complications or reactions. It is also more expensive.

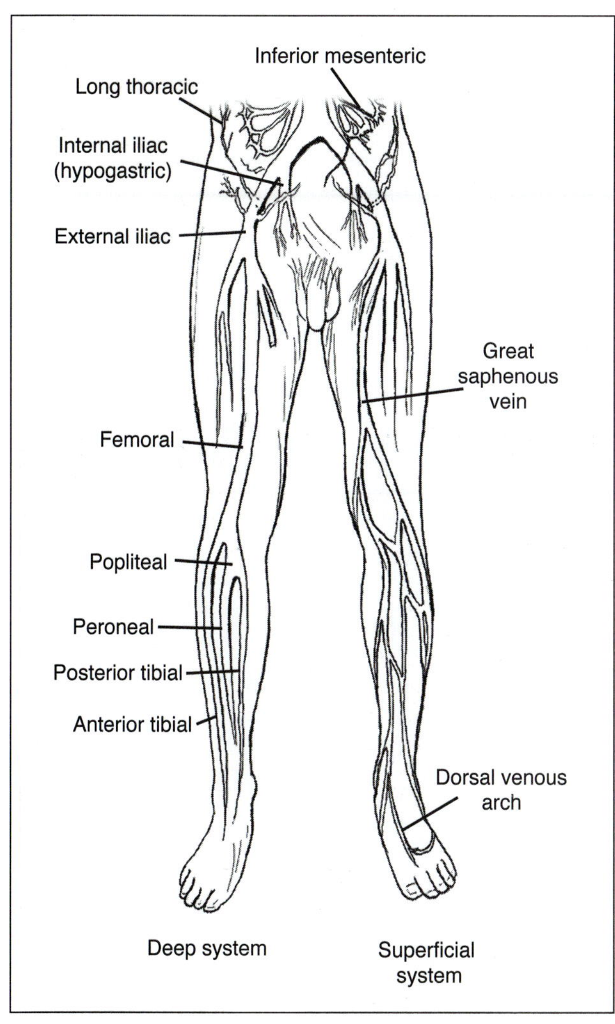

FIGURE 8.6 Deep and superficial veins of the leg.

Radiation Protection Fluoroscopy time kept to a minimum

Preliminary Radiographs

- AP projection of the area using an overhead tube or PA projection of the knee, calf, and ankle taken with the undercouch tube, before injection to check exposure factors.
- Doppler ultrasound is sometimes performed at this point to determine the condition of the veins.

Patient Preparation

- If there is severe swelling of the leg (**edema**), the leg should be elevated the previous night.
- The patient must be informed of the risks of the procedure and sign a consent form.

Procedure Sequence For ascending, IV venography:

- Patient is supine on the table with the head raised and body at about 40° (**Fowler's position**).
- Injection area is cleansed.
- A small butterfly needle (19 or 21 gauge) is inserted into a distal superficial vein on the dorsum of the foot.
- This foot should not be weight-bearing so that the calf muscles can remain relaxed to allow smooth movement of the contrast.
- If there is significant swelling of the foot, a small incision can be made, the vein exposed, and the needle inserted.
- A **tourniquet** or inflatable cuff is applied to affected limb. The pressure should occlude the superficial veins, but not the deep veins.
- Forty to 50 mL of contrast is injected by hand and the flow monitored by the fluoroscopy unit. This can take up to 30 seconds. Care should be taken to avoid **extravasation** (ěks-trăv´´ă-sā´shŭn) of contrast into the dorsum of the foot because this is painful and can cause **necrosis** (nĕ-krō´sĭs) in a foot that already has a compromised circulation.
- Spot films are taken as injection is given.
- With any additional injection, the patient is asked to perform the **Valsalva** (văl-săl-vă) **maneuver**, which slows down the movement of the contrast into the pelvic region.
- Just before removal of the needle, it should be flushed with 0.9% saline to prevent any risk of phlebitis due to the presence of contrast.
- Injection site can be covered with small dressing. No prolonged pressure should be needed.

> Very occasionally, because an ascending approach is not possible and an injection of contrast is definitely required, descending venography can be performed by puncturing the femoral vein and having the contrast moved down the leg by the patient being stood erect and performing the Valsalva maneuver. The radiographs taken remain the same as for the ascending technique.

Procedure Radiographs AP of the leg, using the spot film device, during the procedure, to include all vessels up to the common femoral and iliac veins. The leg should be slightly medially rotated to separate the tibia and fibula and the deep veins of the calf (Figure 8.7).

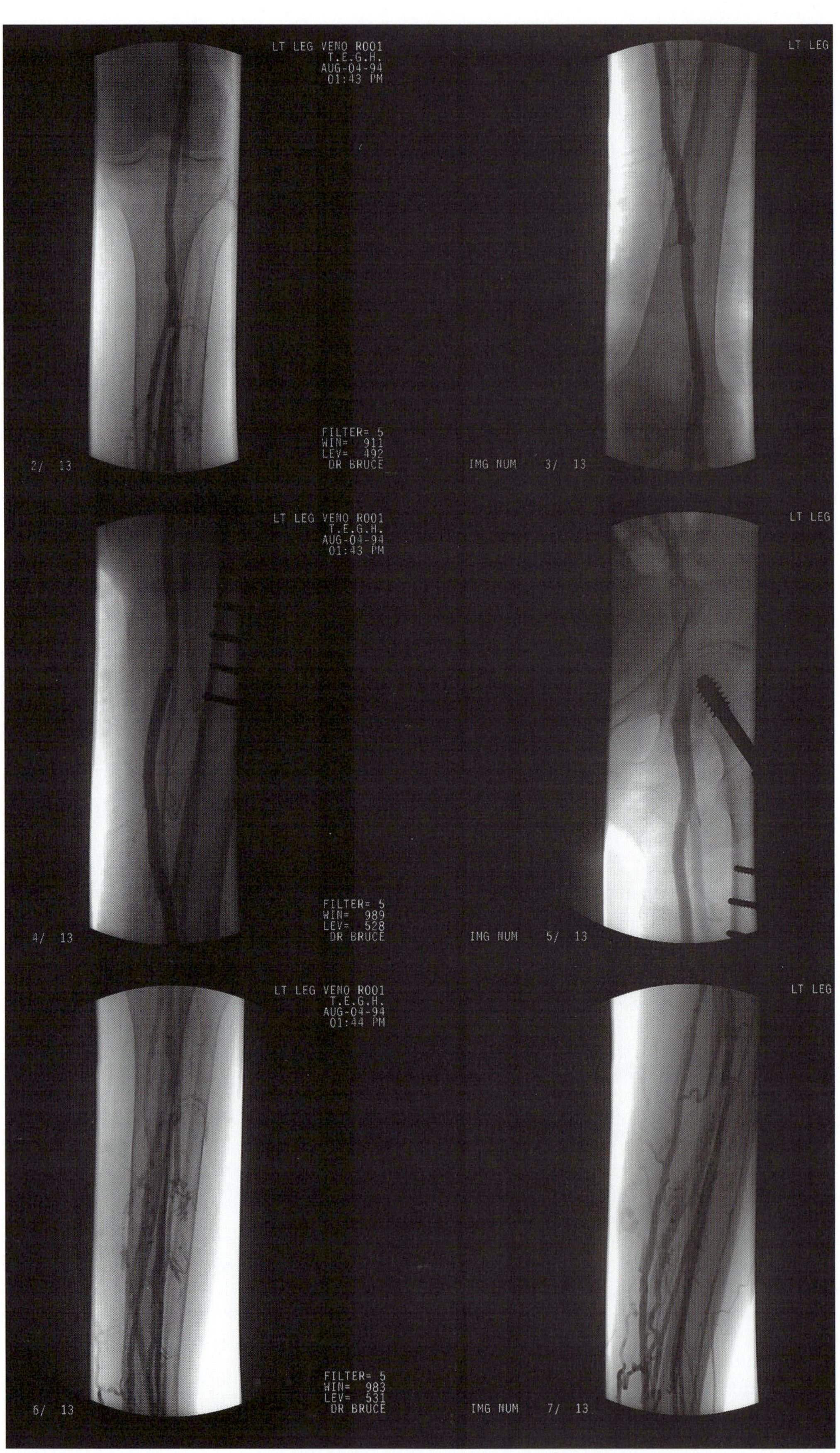

FIGURE 8.7
Serial view of leg.

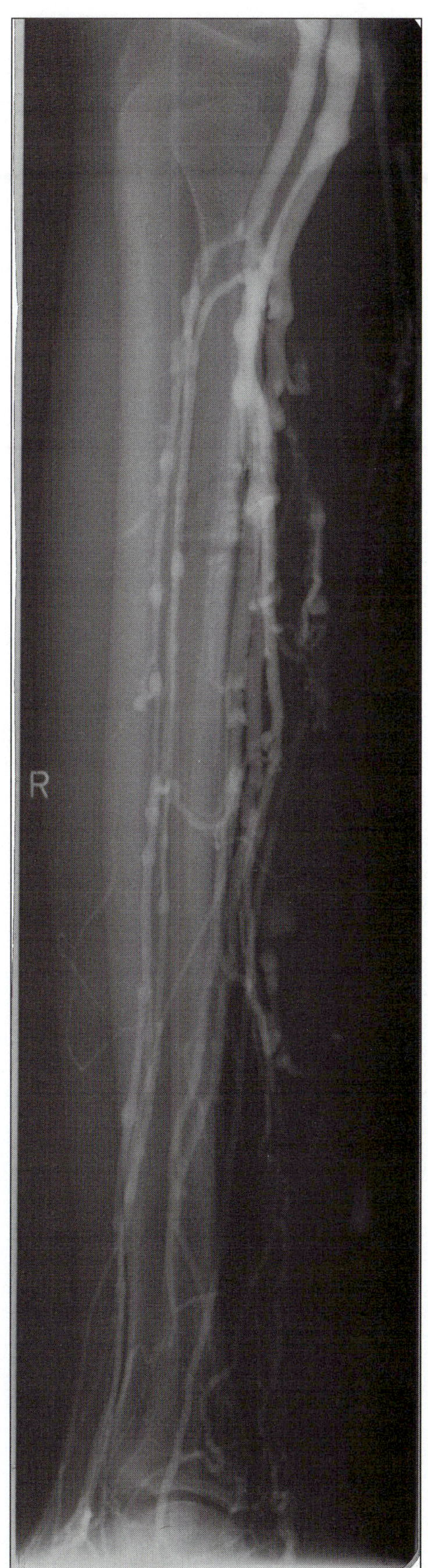

FIGURE 8.8 Lateral view of leg.

Alternative Radiographs Overhead radiographs, using long film cassettes (7 × 17 inch) can be taken of calf and thigh level immediately after the needle has been removed (Figure 8.8). Keeping the patient in the Fowler's position helps to keep the contrast in the peripheral veins.

Postprocedure Care

- The patient should be encouraged to exercise the limb.
- The injection site should be examined periodically to ensure there is no inflammation, infection, or necrosis.
- Any changes to the leg pain should be examined in the rare event of the presence of **thrombophlebitis**.
- There are no other conditions required. This is usually performed as an outpatient procedure.

Common Pathologies

- DVT (Figure 8.9)
- Acute thrombosis
- Recurrent varicose veins

Varicography

Occasionally, a study of the distribution of varicose veins is requested, and contrast is injected via a varicosed vein below the knee. By filling the venous system at this point, spot films are able to determine the extent of varicosed involvement. Sometimes, the leg has to be repunctured above the knee, if there are a large number of varicosed veins. This is an uncommon procedure.

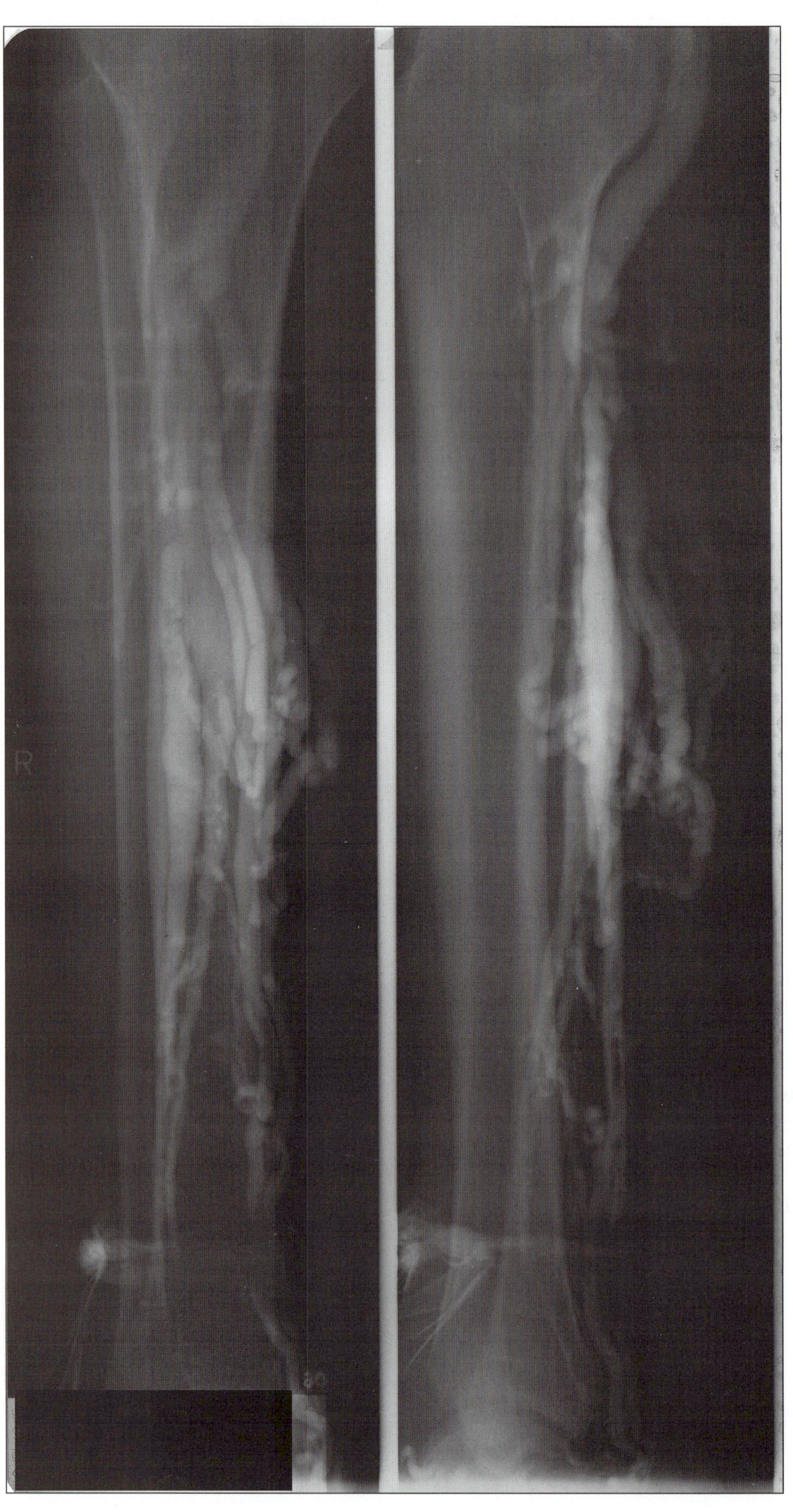

FIGURE 8.9
DVT 7 cm above ankle.

UPPER LIMB VENOGRAPHY

This procedure demonstrates the venous system of the arm. The upper arm is usually of more interest because there is a greater likelihood of **thrombus** in these vessels. Introduction of contrast is usually by direct injection.

Applied Anatomy It is important to note the vasculature of the arm. The medial cubital vein should be used for direct or indirect injections because contrast will flow through and, therefore, opacify the axillary vein. An injection into the median cephalic vein will bypass the axillary vein, which is the major venous vessel of the upper arm, and more significant if found to be thrombosed.

Indications

- Edema of the arm or hand
- Venous obstruction
- Suspected thrombosis

Contraindications Contrast allergy

Equipment

- Fluoroscopy unit with spot film device
- Butterfly needle, 18, 19, or 21 gauge
- Syringes
- Tourniquet

Contrast Media Water-soluble, iodine-based with low osmolarity

Radiation Protection

- Fluoroscopy time kept to a minimum
- Lead protection to the gonadal region

Preliminary Radiographs An AP or PA radiograph of affected site, usually the shoulder and upper arm, is obtained.

Patient Preparation Patient must be informed of the procedure and its risks and sign a consent form; otherwise, none.

Procedure Sequence

- Patient lies supine, the hand is supinated and abducted from the torso.
- Approximately 30 mL of contrast is injected under fluoroscopic control into the median cubital vein or more distal into the superficial system at the wrist or forearm.
- Tourniquet can be applied at the level of the elbow to force the contrast into the deep venous system.
- Radiographs are taken using spot film device.
- Before removal, the needle is flushed with 0.9% saline solution to prevent the occurrence of phlebitis.

Procedure Radiographs

- Spot films of the affected area.
- PA and obliques (to separate the vessels) can be taken with the overhead tube immediately after the insertion of the contrast (Figure 8.10).

Postprocedure Care Same as for lower limb. The same complications can occur, although these are very rare.

Common Pathologies Thrombosis

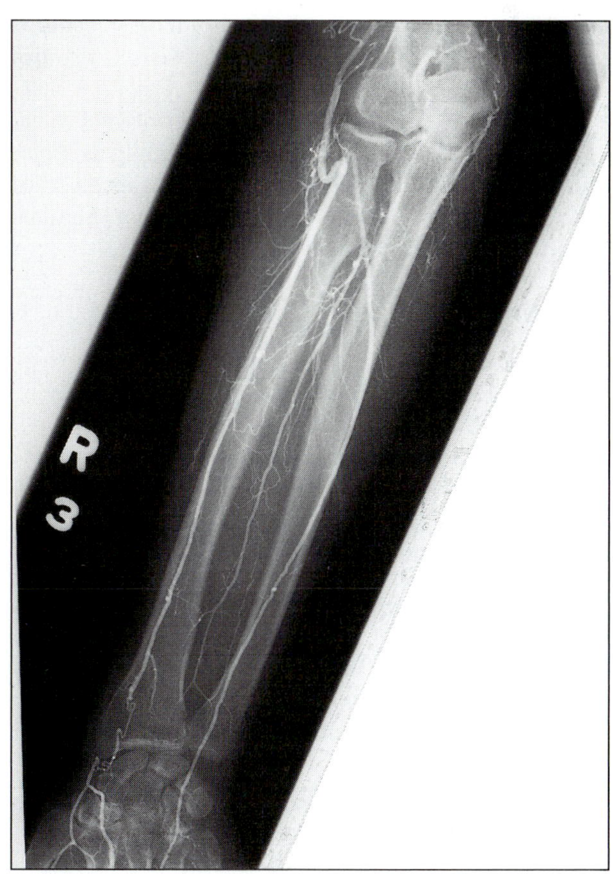

FIGURE 8.10 Upper limb venogram.

Vena Cava Venography

The two main vessels of the venous system are the superior and inferior vena cava. These are sometimes visualized as part of a peripheral examination (superior vena cava with upper limb venography; inferior vena cava with lower limb venography). However, they are usually better demonstrated by direct injection or indirectly by catheterization.

ABDOMINAL VENOGRAPHY

This procedure demonstrates the inferior vena cava and its branches, most particularly the iliac and renal veins. Contrast can be introduced either by direct injection through the femoral vein or indirectly by catheterization via the femoral vein or median cubital vein.

Applied Anatomy

- Pelvic and abdominal venous system (Refer back to Figure 8.1). It is important to note that the iliac veins and inferior vena cava do not have valves and therefore appear smooth and tubular on a radiograph.
- When there is a blockage in the inferior vena cava, collateral vessels move the venous supply and can become quite enlarged. The usual veins involved in the event of an obstruction are the azygos, hemiazygos, and lumbar veins.

Indications

- Venous obstruction, either extrinsic pressure or intrinsic such as a clot or tumor invasion
- Posttraumatic venous damage
- Pelvic varices
- Congenital abnormalities

Contraindications Contrast allergies

Equipment

- Rapid serial radiographic equipment (see Chapter 7, Heart and Arterial System). Single or biplane can be used depending on pathologies to be visualized.
- Pressure injector (if using indirect approach)
- Sterile tray to include:
  —16-gauge needles (for direct approach)
  —Seldinger-type needle (for indirect approach)
  —Syringes
  —Guidewires
- 5 French straight catheter with side holes

Contrast Media Nonionic, water-soluble contrast with low osmolarity

Radiation Protection Minimize fluoroscopy time

Preliminary Radiographs A scout radiograph of the area of interest is taken using overhead tube with serial changer to assess exposure factors. This will usually be an AP of lower abdominal region.

Patient Preparation

- NPO for 5 hours prior to procedure
- Patient is usually admitted for an overnight stay for observation.
- The patient must be informed of the procedure and its risks and then sign a consent form.

Procedure Sequence (Direct Approach)

- Patient lies supine on the angiographic table.
- The groin area is cleansed and prepared on both sides.
- A venous puncture is made into the femoral vein. Unless there is significant obstruction, needles can be inserted into each femoral vein at the same time, connected via a Y-connector and tubing and injected simultaneously.
- Thirty to 40 mL of contrast is injected as a single **bolus** (bō´lŭs) (usually takes 2–4 seconds).
- During injection, the patient is asked to perform the Valsalva maneuver. This helps keep the contrast in the abdominal area.
- Serial radiographs are taken. One exposure per second for 10 seconds.
- Needle(s) are removed and pressure applied for a short time at venipuncture site.

Procedure Sequence (Indirect Approach)

- Patient lies supine on angiographic table.
- Puncture and Seldinger procedure are carried out via the femoral vein (see Chapters 6 and 7).

- A 5 French catheter is inserted and passed 5 to 8 cm up the vein, under fluoroscopic guidance.
- Contrast (40 mL) injected using pressure injector.
- Serial radiographs taken, one per second for 10 seconds.
- Catheter is removed and pressure applied to venipuncture site.

> Occasionally, the median cubital approach is used when both femoral veins are known to be occluded or are extremely tortuous. A long catheter is inserted using the Seldinger technique and advanced via the superior vena cava to the inferior vena cava, and if necessary, into the external iliac vein.

Procedure Radiographs

- Single-plane serial radiography: AP of area of interest (Figure 8.11).
- Biplane serial radiography: AP and lateral of area of interest.

Postprocedure Care

- Observation of puncture sites for 2 hours
- Routine observation of vital signs for 2 hours

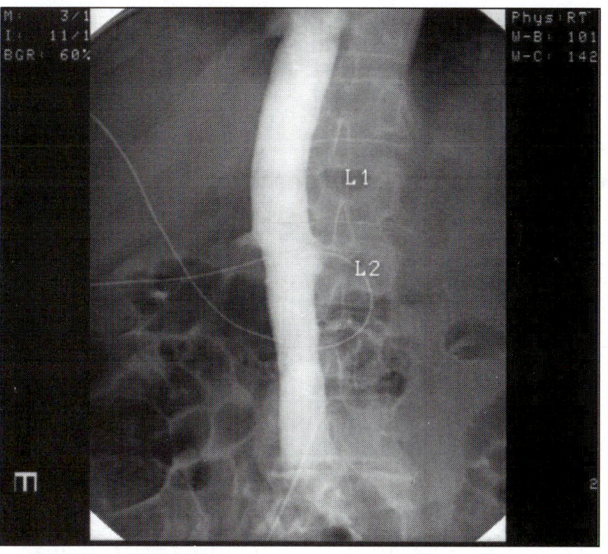

FIGURE 8.11 Abdominal venogram, inferior vena cava.

Common Pathologies

- Thrombosis
- Glandular and neoplastic masses
- Enlargement of **collateral circulation** (azygos, hemiazygos, and lumbar veins).

RENAL VENOGRAPHY

The renal veins can be demonstrated by selective catheterization using the Seldinger technique. Each vessel is selected separately using a fine catheter (maximum size 5 French) and 10 mL of contrast injected for each side. Serial AP radiographs taken of the area will be able to confirm the presence of a thrombosis. Although the contrast will move into the kidney, renal arteriography will provide a better examination of the renal vasculature.

SUPERIOR VENA CAVA VENOGRAPHY

As with the lower limb, the superior vena cava can be visualized by means of a direct injection via the median cubital vein, but better visualization of the superior vena cava is obtained using a catheter and a pressure injector. Rapid blood flow through a large vessel requires a large bolus of contrast administered quickly.

Applied Anatomy (Figure 8.12)

Indications

- Venous obstruction
- Congenital abnormalities, such as left-sided superior vena cava
- Thrombosis of vena cava branches, axillary, subclavian, or innominate veins

Contraindications Known allergy to contrast

Equipment

- Angiographic unit with rapid serial radiography and fluoroscopy. Usually single plane only is required, but biplane can be used if necessary.
- Sterile tray to include:
  —Seldinger type of needle
  —Syringes
  —Guidewires
- 5 French catheter with side holes

Contrast Media Nonionic, water-soluble contrast with low osmolarity

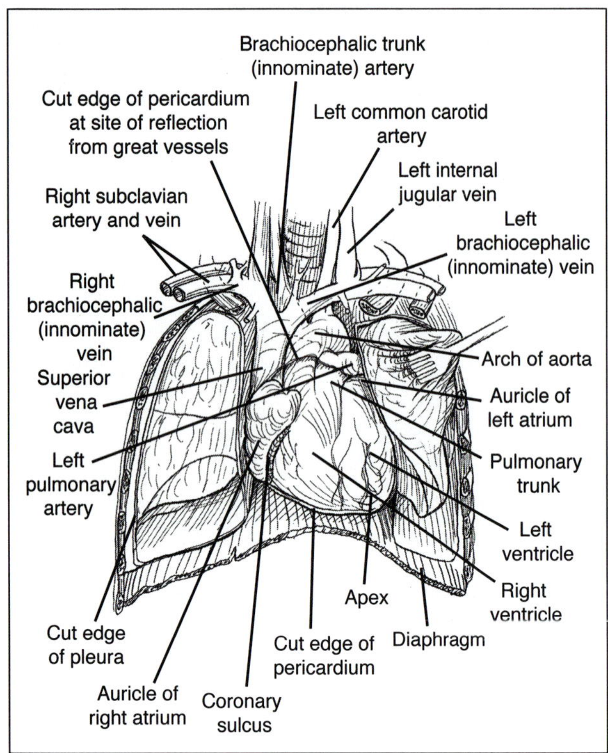

FIGURE 8.12 Superior vena cava and heart.

Radiation Protection Minimize fluoroscopy time

Preliminary Radiographs Scout AP or PA of area of interest, usually upper chest and lower neck, to assess radiographic technique using the angiographic equipment

Patient Preparation

- NPO for 5 hours prior to procedure
- The patient must be informed about the procedure and its risks and then sign a consent form.

Procedure Sequence

- Patient lies supine on the angiographic table with the arm supinated.
- The elbow region is prepared for injection by cleansing with an aseptic solution.
- The median cubital or median basilic vein is catheterized using the Seldinger technique.
- Occasionally a small incision is required to expose the correct vein.
- A 5 French catheter is advanced several centimeters up the arm, under fluoroscopic guidance.
- Contrast (30 mL) is injected, using a pressure injector, in a single bolus.
- Serial radiographs are taken at the rate of one or two films per second for 5 to 10 seconds.
- The catheter is removed and pressure exerted over the venipuncture site for a short period.

Procedure Radiographs

- AP serial radiographs of interested area
- Lateral serial radiographs if biplane is requested

Postprocedure Care Observation of the patient for vital signs and puncture site for 2 hours after the procedure.

Common Pathologies

- Extrinsic obstruction due to malignant neoplasm (usually of the lung)
- Congenital abnormality. Left-sided superior vena cava occurs quite frequently in association with congenital heart disease. With this condition, the vein drains into the coronary sinus.

Portal Venography

The venous pathway that drains into the liver from the abdominal contents is known as the portal system. The examination of this area will demonstrate the condition of the vessels and assess their involvement with a diagnosis of portal hypertension. **Cirrhosis** of the liver is the most usual pathology that involves the venous system, but this examination is also done to determine the patency of the portal vessels. Because these vessels do not directly branch from a major vessel it cannot be easily selected. There are several methods of approach:

Percutaneous splenic puncture
Transhepatic portal venography (usually performed on patients with cirrhosis for whom surgery is contraindicated)
Arteriovenography
Operative mesenteric venography (rarely performed today and will not be described)
Transjugular approach

Less invasive studies are often performed today and are mentioned later in this chapter. However, there are instances where only the following procedures provide the information needed in the diagnosis or treatment of a patient.

TRANSSPLENIC AND TRANSHEPATIC APPROACHES

Applied Anatomy The portal system carries nutrient-rich, deoxygenated blood to the liver to be detoxified before it is carried to the vena cava via the hepatic veins. The portal vein itself is formed by the union of the splenic and superior mesenteric vein. The gastric, pancreatic, and inferior mesenteric veins drain into the splenic vein before it becomes the portal vein (see Figure 8.13).

Indications

- Portal hypertension
- Ascites
- To check patency of a **portosystemic** anastomosis

Contraindications

- Allergy to contrast
- Certain approaches may not be possible due to specific condition of the patient. For example, a transhepatic approach may be more difficult for a patient with severe cirrhosis of the liver.

Equipment

- Rapid serial radiography unit with fluoroscopy; generally only single plane is used.
- Needles or catheters depending on approach (listed under procedure).
- This is a sterile procedure and must be carried out under aseptic conditions.

Contrast Media Nonionic, water-soluble, contrast with low osmolarity

Radiation Protection Minimize fluoroscopy and number of radiographs required

Preliminary Radiographs

- Previous AP abdomen radiographs.
- A scout radiograph of the area of interest taken on the angiographic table to assess radiographic technique and to determine the position of spleen and liver. Soft tissue technique should be used. The centering point used to include the complete portal system is about 2.5 cm to the right of the midline halfway between the xiphisternum and umbilicus.

Patient Preparation

- This procedure requires admission to hospital whatever the approach taken.
- All clotting factors should be carefully screened and medications checked and halted if necessary.
- NPO for 5 hours prior to the procedure
- The patient must be informed of the procedure and possible complications and sign a consent form.
- A sedative and analgesic can be prescribed if required.
- On the morning of the examination, the patient must be suitably attired in a gown, as for an aseptic procedure.

Procedure Sequence

Transsplenic Approach

- The patient lies supine on the angiographic table, and the position of the spleen is verified. The site of puncture is usually along the lateral border at the level of the tenth or eleventh intercostal space.
- The region is prepared and anesthetized using aseptic technique.

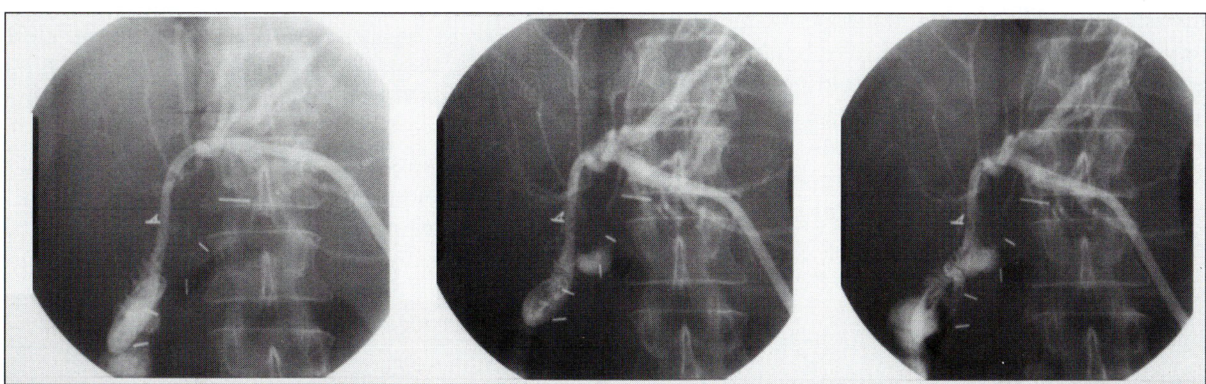

FIGURE 8.13 Portal system with contrast.

On inspiration a long 20-gauge needle with a stilette and malleable plastic outer cannula is inserted into the spleen by an upward and inward motion. The point of the needle can be felt puncturing the splenic capsule. Once in the splenic pulp, there will be a backflow of blood into the connecting tube attached to the needle.

- The needle and stilette are withdrawn and a test dose of contrast is administered under fluoroscopic control to check needle position.
- With the cannula in place, the patient is asked to breathe as shallowly as possible to prevent undue movement of the cannula.
- Portal pressure can be measured at this point by means of a manometer. A raised pressure will be indicated by a rapid reflux of blood during insertion of the needle and cannula.
- A manual injection of 20 to 50 mL of contrast is administered in about 5 seconds and at a point two-thirds through the injection, serial radiographs are taken at two per second for about 10 seconds.
- The cannula should be removed as soon as possible to minimize the risk of damage to the spleen.

Transhepatic Approach

- The patient lies supine on the angiographic table.
- The portal vein can be localized using real-time ultrasound and the appropriate entry points marked on the body.
- The region is prepared and anesthetized using aseptic technique.
- A long needle with stilette and cannula is inserted at the point determined by the ultrasound.
- After removal of the needle and stilette a syringe is attached to the cannula and gentle suction applied to the syringe as it is being withdrawn until a flow of blood occurs.
- A test injection of contrast is made under fluoroscopic control to determine which vessel has been selected.
- When it has been verified that the portal vein has been entered, a J guidewire with a movable core is advanced through to the splenic vein.
- When in the correct position, the catheter is threaded over the guidewire and the guidewire removed.
- Blood samples can be taken at this point along the length of the portal system, which are helpful in the localization of hormone-producing pancreatic tumors.
- An injection of 40 mL is given, using a pressure injector at the rate of 10 mL per second.
- Serial radiographs are taken at the rate of one per second for 8 seconds.
- On completion of the study, the cannula and catheter are removed.
- The patient is hospitalized overnight for observation.

> This approach can also be used to occlude **esophageal varices** (văr´ĭ-sēz), by the process of embolization. This has largely been replaced with direct endoscopic injection of esophageal varices.

ARTERIOVENOGRAPHY (LATE-PHASE ARTERIOGRAPHY)

Branches of the portal system can be opacified and demonstrated during the late phase of abdominal arteriograms. The superior mesenteric and portal veins will be visualized when the superior mesenteric artery is selectively catheterized. The celiac trunk and specifically the splenic artery should be catheterized to visualize the splenic vein. This is a useful approach, particularly if the arterial system is also required. It is, however, a lengthy and difficult procedure to catheterize the celiac branches. The transsplenic is a simpler and quicker study, providing better visualization of the vessels because of the direct injection.

Procedure Radiographs For all of these approaches, serial radiographs are taken in the AP position, using the rapid serial changer (Figure 8.13).

Postprocedure Care

- For patients undergoing direct injection into the spleen or liver, where pressure cannot be applied to prevent bleeding, the patient must be closely observed. Vital signs should be taken every 15 minutes for the first hour and then half hourly for 3 hours.
- These patients must be hospitalized overnight for continued observation.
- Patients having late-phase arteriovenography, the procedures used following a femoral arterial insertion should be followed (see Chapter 6, Angiographic Procedures and Equipment).

Use of Digital Imaging and Digital Subtraction Imaging in Venography

All venous studies can be enhanced by using digital imaging and digital subtraction because they allow better visualization with less contrast of a lower concentration. With the broader latitude afforded with digital fluoroscopic imaging, peripheral vessels can be better visualized. Digital subtraction angiography (DSA) is extremely useful for abdominal and superior vena cava venography as well as peripheral venography. (Figure 8.14). The technique is the same, with the reminder that there must be an initial scout film that has no contrast and that provides the subtracted image. Most pressure injectors and serial programmers can be adjusted to provide this.

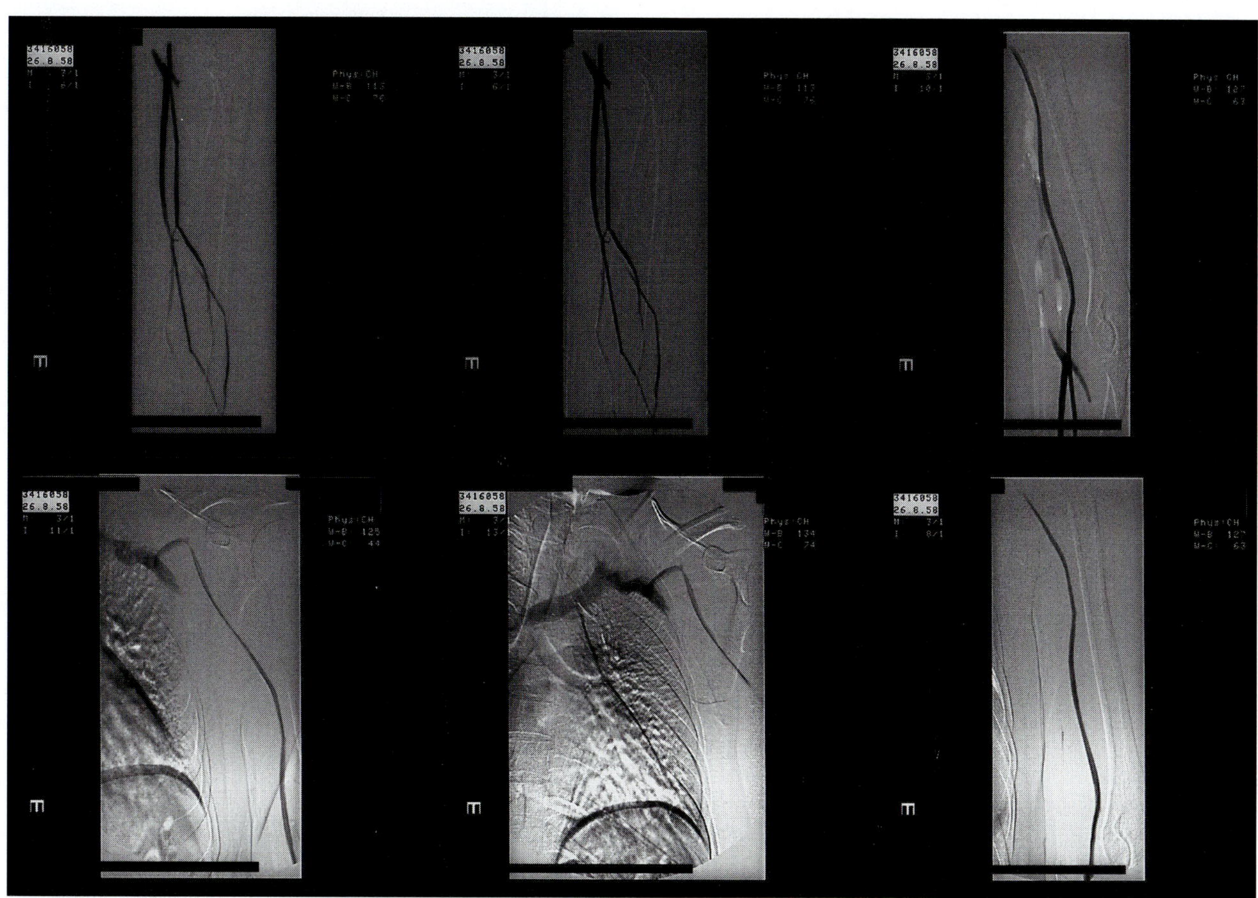

FIGURE 8.14 Use of DSA in upper limb venography.

Other Imaging Modalities

COMPUTED TOMOGRAPHY

Larger veins can be visualized using CT, and any significant involvement of the inferior vena cava or of the renal vein can be demonstrated (Figure 8.15). However, the vessels are only seen at their best with a contrast injection, which makes the procedure more costly and time-consuming. Contrast is usually given intravenously either as a drip infusion or a single injection using a pressure injector. Ultrasound is more cost efficient and MRI provides better visualization without the use of contrast.

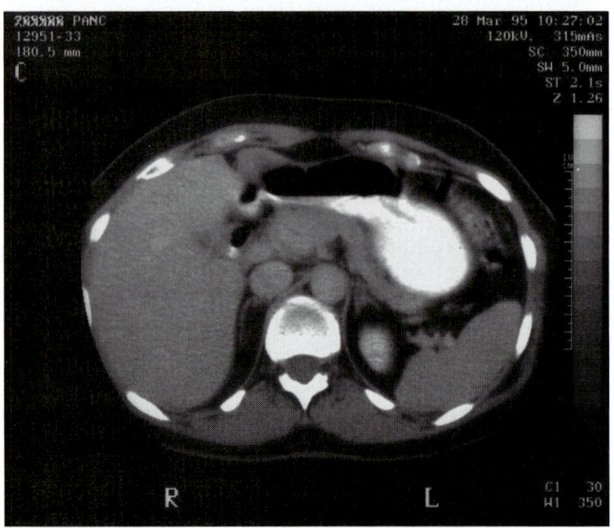

FIGURE 8.15 CT image of inferior vena cava.

MAGNETIC RESONANCE IMAGING

This is an excellent method of imaging the larger veins. Flowing blood, being a moving structure, contrasts with surrounding or nonmoving structures and provides a high contrast between the flowing blood and the lumen of the vessel. Absence of flow in the case of thrombus or clot can, therefore, be well demonstrated because it is contrasted with the moving blood. It is for this reason that it is advocated as a useful method of imaging some larger venous vessels, such as the inferior vena cava, because thrombus is the number one pathologic condition demonstrated by all forms of diagnostic imaging. Smaller branches are more difficult to define. With the technical advances of postprocessing into two- and three-dimensional display, and contrast enhanced angiography, MRI is being used more frequently. An advantage is its ability to demonstrate not only the morphology but also the function of the vessels. It also has the ability to distinguish between an acute or "new" and a chronic or "old" thrombus (Figure 8.16).

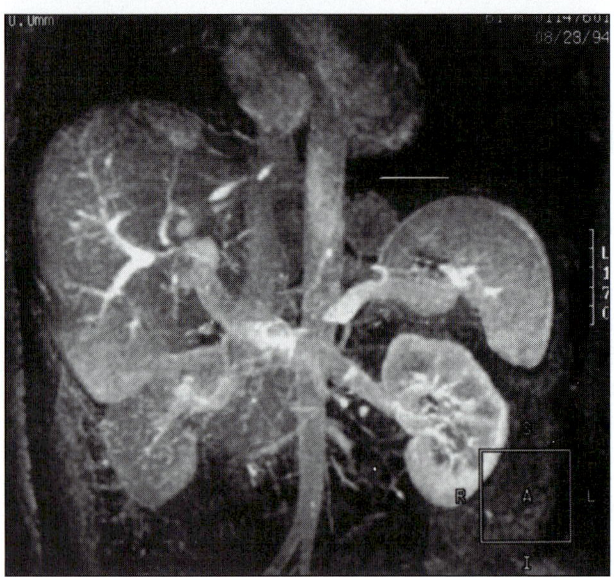

FIGURE 8.16 MRI of inferior vena cava and vessels of the abdomen.

The ability of MRI to image blood and the vessels is complex and beyond the scope of this chapter. Standard T1- and T2-weighted images will demonstrate vessels. Magnetic resonance angiographic techniques continue to improve visualization. The use of surface coils improves the imaging of peripheral veins, but even then, small vessels may not be adequately seen.

Because of the noninvasive and cost-efficient features of ultrasound and the gold standard capabilities of angiography, it is unlikely at this point that MRI will become the sole imaging modality for the vasculature.

ULTRASOUND

Ultrasound is used extensively to demonstrate certain conditions of the venous system, in particular DVT. A combination of continuous-wave, B-scan, pulsed Doppler and color Doppler will provide an accurate assessment of the condition of the veins and has replaced peripheral venography in some centers as the primary imaging modality of choice (Figure 8.17).

- Continuous-wave ultrasound only assesses movement and is useful only as a tool to scan the major vessels for significant involvement. It does not have a high sensitivity and should be used in conjunction with other methods.
- Duplex imaging is a combination of B-scan and pulsed Doppler. The flow signals from the femoral, popliteal, and posterior tibial veins can be assessed using this method. DVT can be determined if there is an interruption or change of signal, or when muscle contractions of the leg do not produce the expected elevation in blood flow. When a normal, healthy vein is compressed it should collapse. Those filled with thrombus will not. This examination is very operator dependent, with the more experienced individual providing a greater degree of accuracy.
- Color Doppler provides an even greater amount of detail. As well as assessing the presence of a clot, or thrombus, it is able to demonstrate the extent of blood flow around a clot.

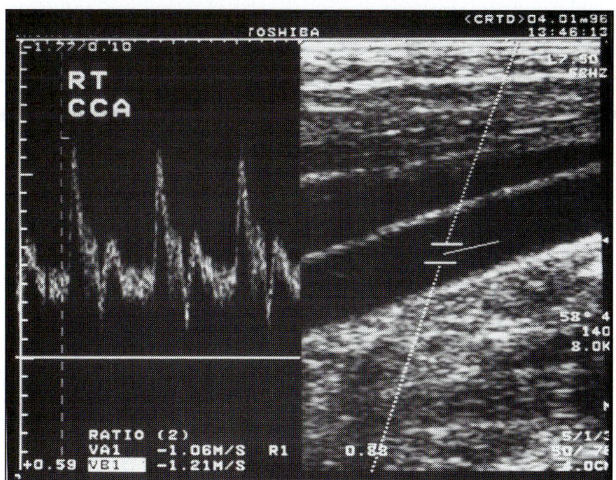

FIGURE 8.17 Doppler ultrasound.

Doppler and color Doppler are used extensively in the assessment of renal and liver transplants, checking the patency of the arterial and venous vasculature.

RADIONUCLIDE IMAGING

This modality has generally not been the primary imaging chosen to demonstrate the venous system. Fibrinogen I 125 has been used to diagnose DVT. It is injected into the venous system of the arm and is taken up by the developing thrombosis. It is accurate in determining large recent thrombi in the leg and is a useful procedure if the patient is high risk or has an allergy to contrast. Its main disadvantage is that the uptake can take from 24 to 48 hours, and false-positive results can occur if there has been recent injury leading to hematoma or inflammation.

Technetium 99m is also used to determine venous obstruction. It is injected into each foot simultaneously and then recorded as it passes along the system. Delay to one leg demonstrates an obstruction. This same nuclide can be followed through the renal system and any abnormalities to uptake will determine changes to blood flow and serves as a screen in the interpretation of renal hypertension. It is not the definitive study, but it does provide a noninvasive assessment. It is particularly useful when dealing with high-risk patients.

Interventional Procedures

THERAPEUTIC INTERRUPTION OF THE INFERIOR VENA CAVA

This technique is occasionally used to occlude the inferior vena cava when there has been a past history of pulmonary **embolus**, a major cause of death. After treatment or surgical removal of a pulmonary embolus, there is a 60% possibility that the embolus will return. Its most usual origin is the venous system of the legs. By occluding the inferior vena cava, it prohibits movement into the pulmonary artery.

- A preliminary venogram is necessary to ensure that there is collateral circulation and also to confirm the level of the renal veins.
- A transjugular approach is taken. Using the Seldinger technique, a guidewire is advanced into the venous system and into the inferior vena cava via the superior vena cava.
- An embolization device (usually a detachable balloon-Hunter) is then advanced under fluoroscopic control to just below the renal vein, and detached and stabilized.

There are now also filters that can be placed at the same level, consisting of steel wires, which prevent the emboli from moving up the system.

TRANSJUGULAR BIOPSY OF THE LIVER

Liver biopsies are generally performed percutaneously. However, there are some indications for a transvenous approach. These include:

- Bleeding problems (a disturbed clotting mechanism).
- Ascites
- Biopsy done during venography or pressure studies (Figure 8.18).

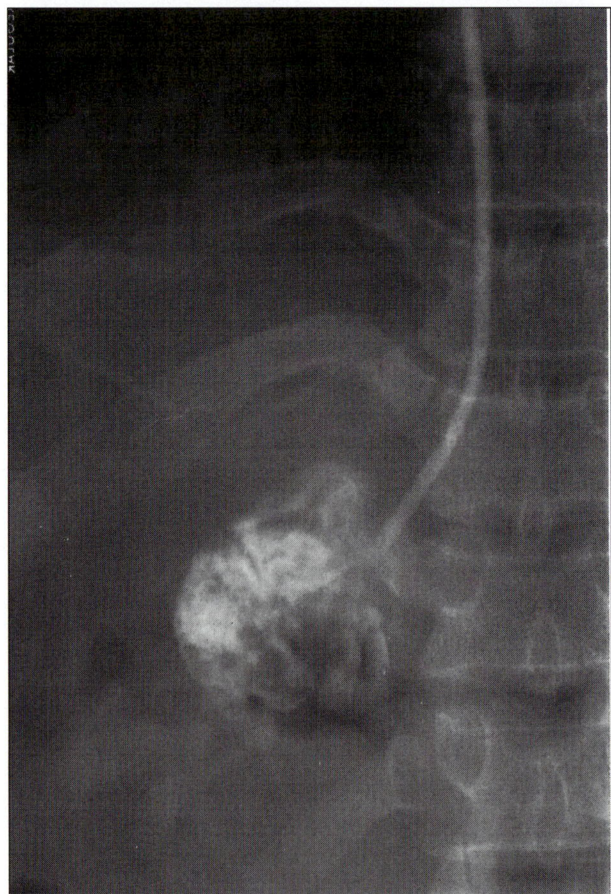

FIGURE 8.18 Transjugular biopsy.

EMBOLIZATION OF ESOPHAGEAL VARICES

In the past this has been performed in combination with transhepatic portal venography. However, these varices, which bleed into the lower esophagus, can be embolized directly via an endoscope or a transjugular catheterization.

TRANSJUGULAR INTRAHEPATIC PORTOSYSTEMIC SHUNT (TIPS)

A catheter is passed transhepatically to the portal vein and the gastric vein is embolized with Gelfoam. Using a transjugular approach, a second catheter is advanced into the portal vein, using a special rigid needle advanced over the guidewire. A balloon catheter is then advanced to this site, inflated and left in situ for about 12 hours. When deflated, the portal vein remains patent. A catheter is often left in place for a while to determine portal pressures.

DILATATION OF SYSTEMIC VENOUS OBSTRUCTIONS

Occasionally, stenosis of the pulmonary veins can occur, either congenitally or postoperatively. Surgery has not been successful and balloon dilatation therapy has been attempted. A balloon 2 1/2 times the width of the stenosis is placed at the affected site and inflated. This is still an experimental procedure, showing short-term success, but lack of improvement in the long term.

THROMBOLYTIC THERAPY

This last procedure is an example of the numerous ways in which therapeutic interventions are being carried out and assessed. Some are more successful than others, but all are attempting an alternative method of treatment that is less invasive and safer than surgery. Other procedures that are being assessed include thrombolytic therapy, which is introduction of a thrombus-reducing chemical directly to the thrombus itself. **Streptokinase** (strĕp´´tō-kī´nās) has been used in varying amounts with varying success and reaction rates. Also, methods of performing a mechanical thrombectomy are being studied experimentally at present.

RENAL VEIN SAMPLING

The presence of an elevated **renin** ratio in blood draining from the kidney is one indicator of hypertension. Samples of this venous blood can be obtained from a catheter introduced into the vein as described above. Venous blood samples are also taken from the arm so that a comparison can be made between the two sites. A ratio between the two greater than 1.5:1 is significant and indicates that any hypertension may be renovascular in origin. Although a rather invasive study that necessitates a femoral venipuncture and catheterization, it does provide information unattainable in any other form.

Review Questions

1. Compare the structure and function of the arterial and venous systems and suggest how the variance between the two affects the procedures carried out on them.

2. Discuss the difference between examinations of the deep and superficial systems of the venous system.

3. Compression in the form of a tourniquet can be useful in:
   a. splenoportography
   b. ascending lower limb venography
   c. vena cava venography
   d. superficial upper limb venography

4. Which of the following is the initial imaging modality of choice for deep vein thrombosis?
   a. radionuclide imaging
   b. MRI
   c. ascending venography
   d. ultrasound

5. Which of the following reduces the probability of pulmonary emboli?
   a. pulmonary arteriography
   b. vena caval shunt
   c. venal caval filter
   d. streptokinase injection

6. The portal system:
   a. is part of the arterial and venous system of the liver
   b. can be imaged indirectly by injection into the inferior mesenteric artery
   c. cannot be imaged by direct injection
   d. can be visualized by injecting into the splenic artery

CASE STUDY

A patient has been diagnosed with thrombophlebitis. Discuss the various methods of imaging that can be used to visualize this problem. The patient has a history of "throwing an embolus." Suggest what other procedures could be performed within the vascular imaging department.

References and Recommended Reading

Abrams, H. L. (1983). *Abrams' angiography: Vascular and interventional radiology* (3rd ed.). Boston: Little, Brown.

Ballinger, P. W. (1991). *Merrill's atlas of radiographic positions and radiologic procedures* (7th ed.). St. Louis: Mosby -Year Book.

Castaneda-Zuniga, W. R., & Tadavarthy, S. T. (1992). *Interventional radiology.* Baltimore: Williams & Wilkins.

Chapman, S., & Nakielny, R. (1993). *A guide to radiological procedures* (3rd ed.) London: Bailliere Tindall.

Colapinto, R. F. (1985). Transjugular biopsy of the liver. *Clinics in Gastroenterology, 14*(2) 451–467.

Colapinto, R. F., Stronell, R. D., et. al. (1982). Creation of an intrahepatic portosystemic shunt with a Gruntzig balloon catheter. *Canadian Medical Association Journal, 126*(3), 267–268.

Cope, C., Burke, D., & Meranze, S. (1990). *Atlas of interventional radiology.* Philadelphia: Lippincott.

Cope, C. (1990). *Interventional arterial catheterization techniques* (Cook Inc.). New York: Gower Medical Publishers.

Cullinan, A., & Cullinan, J. (1994). *Producing quality radiographs.* Philadelphia: Lippincott.

Curry, T. S., Dowdey, J. E., & Murray, R.C. (1990). *Christensen's physics of diagnostic radiology* (4th ed.). Philadelphia: Lea & Febiger.

Dowd, S.B., & Wilson, B.G. (1995). *Encyclopedia of radiographic positioning.* Philadelphia: Saunders.

Doyle, T., Hare, W., Thomson K., & Tress, B. (1989). *Procedures in diagnostic radiology.* London: Churchill Livingstone.

Eisenberg, R.L. (1992). *Radiology, an illustrated history.* St. Louis: Mosby-Year Book.

Gilbertson, J. J., et. al. (1992). A blinded comparison of angiography, angioscopy and duplex scanning in the intraoperative evaluation of in-situ saphenous vein bypass grafts. *Journal of Vascular Surgery, 15*(1), 121–127.

Greene, R. E., & Oestmann, J-W. (1992). *Computed digital radiography in clinical practice.* New York: Thieme.

Rodgers, P. M., et. al. (1994). Dynamic contrast-enhanced MR imaging of the portal venous system. Comparison with x-ray angiography. *Radiology, 191*(3), 741–745.

Snopek, A. M. (1992). *Fundamentals of special radiographic procedures* (3rd ed.) Philadelphia: Saunders.

Sutton, D. A. (1993). *Textbook of radiology and imaging* (5th ed.). Edinburgh: Churchill Livingstone.

Taber's cyclopedic medical dictionary (1989) (17th ed.). Philadelphia: F. A. Davis.

Tortorici, M. R., & Apfel, P. J. (1995). *Advanced radiographic and angiographic procedures.* Philadelphia: Davis.

CHAPTER 9

Head and Neck Vessels, Arterial and Venous

CYNTHIA COWLING, BSc, MEd, MRT(R), ACR

OBJECTIVES

At the completion of this chapter, the student should be able to:

1. Describe the main features of the vascular system of the head and neck.
2. List the major procedures used to demonstrate the cerebral vascular system.
3. Describe the procedure sequence for each examination.
4. Identify the main indications and contraindications for each procedure.
5. Apply safe practice to all procedures performed.
6. Discuss the use of digital subtraction angiography in vascular studies of the head and neck.
7. List the main equipment used in the special procedures suite.
8. List the contrast media used for each examination.
9. Compare the various imaging modalities and their usefulness in cerebral vasculature examinations.
10. List the main indications for interventional embolization of the cerebral circulation.
11. Describe the embolization procedure.

Introduction and Historical Overview

The first angiogram on head vessels was performed in 1927. Moniz had been working on a method to image the brain radiographically with positive contrast and experimented with dogs and rabbits to find the best, least toxic substance to inject into the cerebral vessels. The first human injections were unsuccessful (the contrast did not appear in the vessels). So Moniz cut down to the carotid artery and injected directly. This became a successful procedure, but left an unpleasant scar, particularly if both sides of the brain were surgically exposed. In 1936, the first percutaneous carotid artery puncture was performed. The contrast first used by Moniz was a sodium iodide, but in 1929, he switched to thorium dioxide, which produced excellent films with low toxicity. However, the repercussions of using a radioactive substance such as thorium was only realized years later, when tumors appeared in the endothelial-reticular system 20 to 30 years after the use of thorium dioxide.

Since then, huge strides have been made in contrast and technique in the examination of cerebral vessels. Until the 1970s, cerebral angiography was recognized as the foremost method of demonstrating neurologic, vascular conditions. With the advent of CT and then MRI, diagnostic imaging of the cerebral vasculature profoundly changed, and angiography plays a smaller role today. The use of interventional techniques in this area has increased dramatically and angiography is often performed in association with interventional procedures. Techniques such as digital subtraction angiography (DSA) and magnification are often used in these studies to improve visualization.

Anatomy

The arterial supply of the brain is derived from the right and left internal carotid arteries and the right and left vertebral arteries. Each internal carotid artery arises from its respective common carotid artery at the level of the upper border of the thyroid cartilage. It courses upward posterolateral to the pharynx to enter the carotid canal at the base of the skull.

Within this carotid canal the internal carotid passes medially and slightly forward in the petrous portion of the temporal bone for an inch. From here each artery enters the side of the foramen lacerum, where it turns superiority to enter the cranial cavity. The internal carotid passes forward, lateral to the body of the sphenoid bone as far as the anterior clinoid process where it turns sharply upward to enter the subarachnoid space. The internal carotid ends by dividing into the anterior cerebral, middle cerebral, and posterior communicating arteries (Figure 9.1).

The bilateral vertebral arteries arise from the subclavian arteries and ascend the neck through the transverse foramina of the cervical vertebrae, from the sixth to the first, to enter the cranial cavity at the foramen magnum (Figure 9.2). Each vertebral artery runs forward and medially on the side of the medulla to end at the lower border of the pons and joins the opposite vertebral artery to form the basilar artery. The basilar artery ends at the upper border of the pons by bifurcating into the posterior cerebral arteries.

Arterial branches that supply the brain and upper end of the spinal cord arise from the internal carotid, vertebral, and basilar arteries.

The internal carotids are joined by the anterior communicating artery while the posterior communicating arteries communicate with the posterior cerebral arteries to complete the circle of Willis, which is found within the subarachnoid space (Figure 9.3).

In general, the venous drainage of the head and neck collect into three large veins, the internal jugular, the external jugular, and the vertebral veins. The external jugular veins drain into the internal jugular veins and the subclavian veins join the internal jugular to form the right and left brachiocephalic veins (Figure 9.4). The brachiocephalic veins, in turn, join to form the superior vena cava. This latter vein empties into the right atrium of the heart.

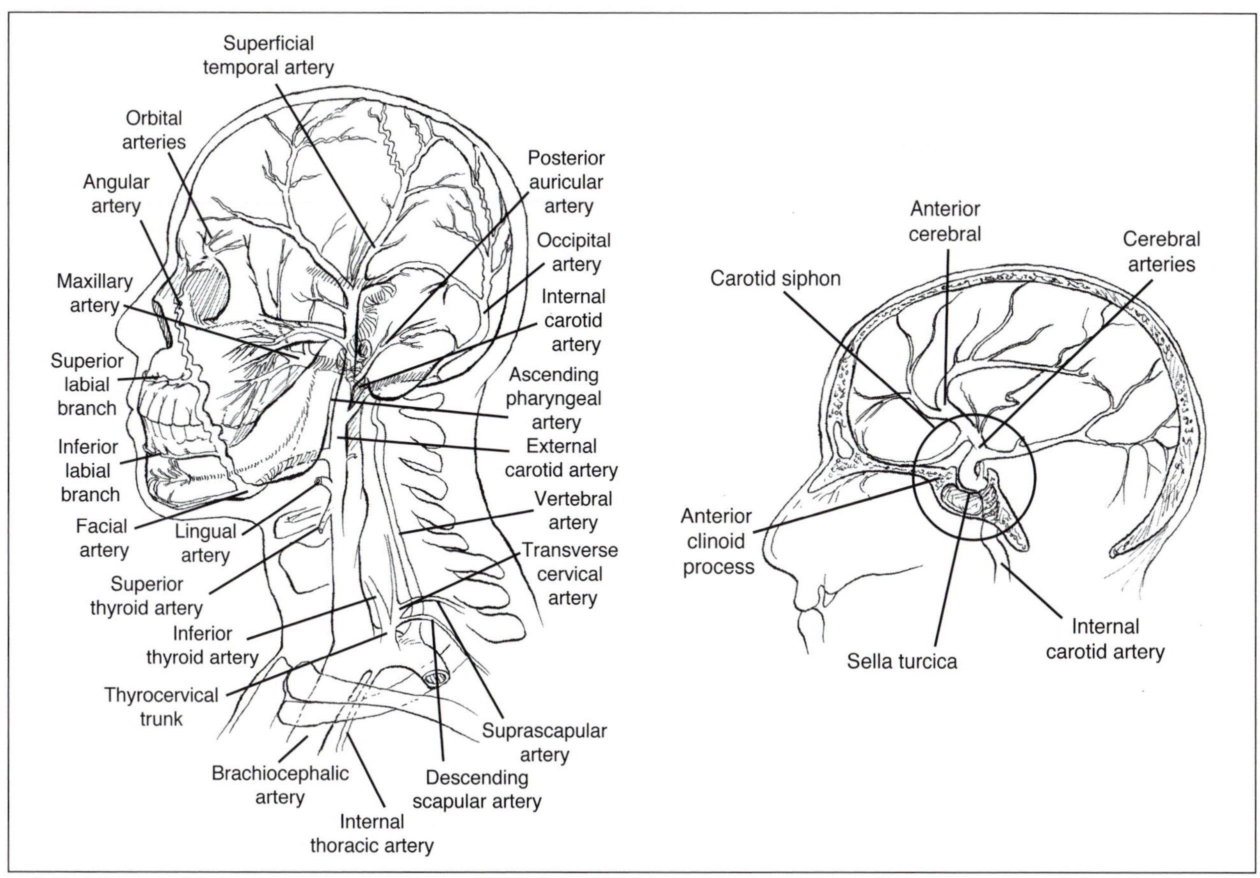

FIGURE 9.1 Arterial supply to head and neck.

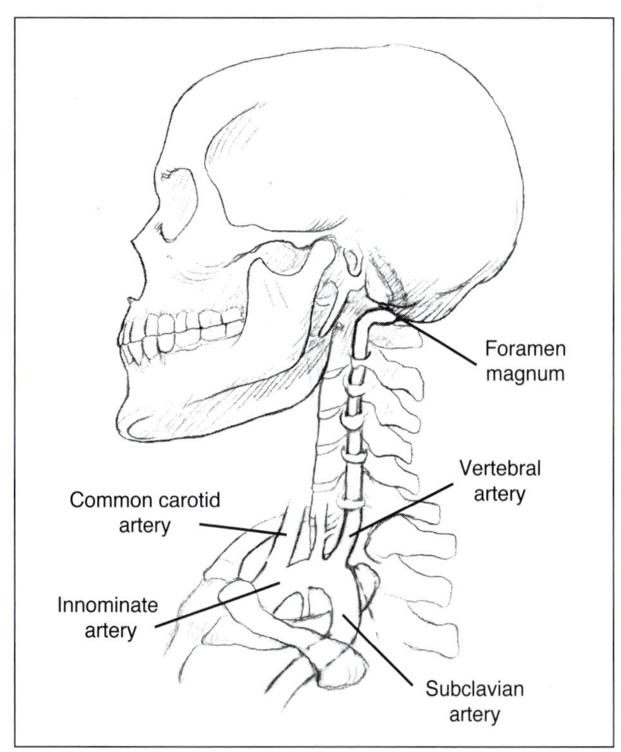

FIGURE 9.2
Position of vertebral arteries.

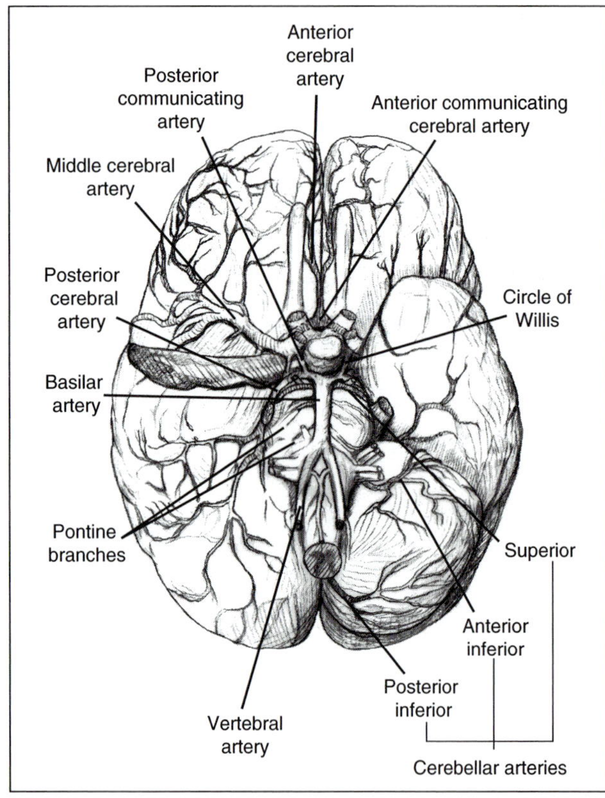

FIGURE 9.3 Arteries at base of brain.

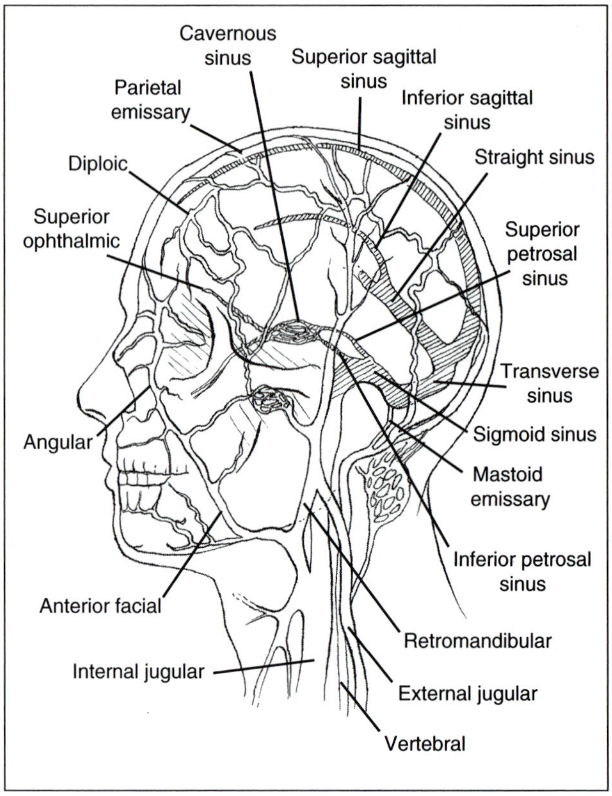

FIGURE 9.4 Venous supply to head and neck.

Procedures

CEREBRAL ANGIOGRAPHY

This is a general term that refers to the examination of the vascular system of the head and major vessels feeding the brain and draining from the brain. The arterial, capillary, and venous supplies are usually done in a single procedure, when demonstrating the intracerebral vasculature. At one time contrast was often administered via a direct injection into the carotid artery. Today, the carotid and cerebral vessels are generally catheterized using the Seldinger technique, with the femoral artery, occasionally the brachial artery, as the entry point. Although direct injection is occasionally performed if catheterization is not possible, it is rarely done. Other techniques are also providing information on these areas, such as MRI and carotid Doppler ultrasound. For this reason, the direct injection is not discussed in this chapter.

Risks and complications arising from these procedures are the same as for all angiography. There are, however, additional concerns of which all radiologic staff should be aware. When direct injection to the carotid and vertebral arteries was performed, there was a risk of local trauma to the vessels, leading to dissection of the vessel wall, or thrombosis. With the prevalence of catheter use, there has been a raised incidence of a clot embolus, which can give rise to cerebral **infarction**, **hemiplegia** (hĕm-ē-plē´jē-ă), or even death in extreme cases. Although rare, it is important that the staff be fully aware of these risks and perform the examination in the safest and most expedient manner.

ARCH OF AORTA ANGIOGRAM (ARCHOGRAM)

Occlusion or partial occlusion of the origins or branches of the four major vessels feeding the brain can be the cause of abnormal neurologic conditions. This examination enables the visualization of these vessels. It may also be the preliminary procedure to a selective study to demonstrate the intracranial circulation, or as part of an interventional procedure. Congenital anomalies in this area are common with variants in placement of arterial origins found in about 25% of the population.

Applied Anatomy (Figure 9.5)

Indications

- Vascular disease
  —Atherosclerosis
- Aneurysms
- Congenital anomalies
- Aortic stenosis

Contraindications Allergy to contrast

Equipment

- Biplane radiographic unit with fluoroscopy. Biplane is useful for this examination and should be the 35 × 35 cm (14 × 14 in.) size. They must have the ability to be off-set (see procedure). DSA capability is an asset. In some instances this can replace the series radiographs.
- Pressure injector
- Sterile tray setup for Seldinger puncture
- Guidewires
- Catheters (pigtail catheter for aortic contrast injection)

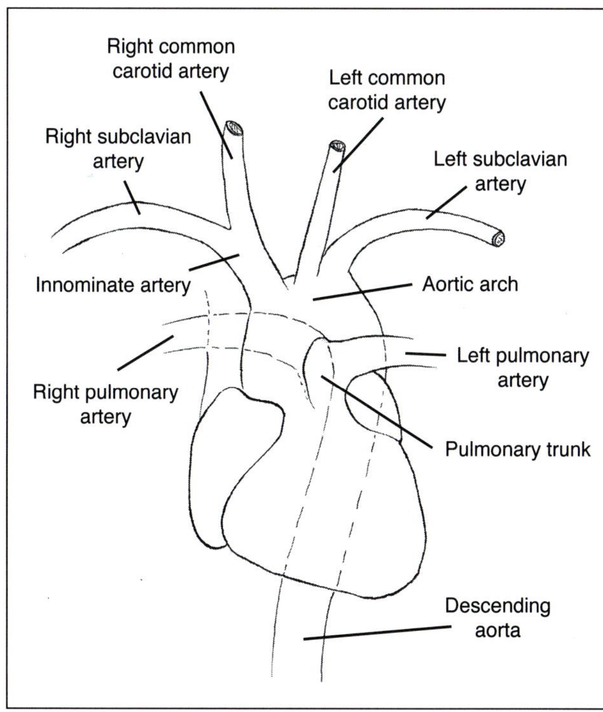

FIGURE 9.5 Vessels arising from the aortic arch.

Contrast Media Nonionic, water-soluble contrast media with low osmolarity

Radiation Protection

- Protection to the gonadal region
- Fluoroscopy kept to a minimum
- Repeat series avoided

Preliminary Radiographs Scout radiographs are taken of the area of interest. The patient is generally positioned RPO on the angiographic table. This will open up the aortic arch and allow the origins of the four main vessels to be well visualized. A rotating table such as that used in cardiac catheterization makes positioning simple without the need to move the patient. However, careful preliminary positioning and radiographs are a satisfactory technique.

Patient Preparation

- Patients are usually hospitalized for this procedure. The use of very small catheters (<5 French) will require a very small puncture and these patients can be admitted as day surgery patients.
- The patient is prepared as for a femoral puncture.
- Clotting factors should be assessed.
- The patient must be informed of the procedure and its risks and sign a consent form before any premedication is administered.
- The puncture site is prepared and shaved if necessary.

Procedure Sequence

- The patient lies supine on the table. The radiographs are taken in an oblique position and the patient can either be set up in this position at the onset of the procedure or immediately before the series radiographs are to be taken. This latter approach is more comfortable for the patient but raises the likelihood that the catheter placement may be affected.

- The femoral artery area is prepared, and a catheter introduced using the Seldinger procedure.
- The catheter should be long (145 cm) and be a pigtail design. This is because the catheter will sit in the large lumen of the aorta and will tend to flail during the large bolus injection. The pigtail catheter design will help to prevent recoil.
- The catheter is advanced under fluoroscopic control until the tip sits in the arch of the aorta.
- The patient is carefully placed and supported in the oblique position, rotated about 45° to the right and with the head lateral. The head and neck must also be supported to avoid superimposition of the mandible over the neck vessels. Because the patient may be in this position for quite some time, it is important that he or she be made as comfortable as possible and reassured at every opportunity.
- Forty to 60 mL of contrast is injected as a single bolus (40 mL in 2 seconds) using a pressure injector.
- Series radiographs are taken.
- When these are satisfactory, the examination is completed and the catheter removed. If there is a need to visualize the branches more clearly, selective catheterization of the individual vessels can be performed.
- Each vessel can be selected by following the procedure for catheter changing. A guidewire is inserted into the pigtail catheter. (This straightens the pigtail for its removal and serves as a guide for the replacement catheter.) The type of catheter is based on observations made by the radiologist using the arch aortogram just performed. The two usual types used for this procedure are the headhunter and sidewinder type (size 5 French). The selection of the vessels can be a delicate and even time-consuming task particularly if the vessels are atypical, tortuous, or partially occluded. Great care must be taken by the radiologist to ensure that there is no trauma caused to these vessels because any dislodging of thrombus can have devastating effects in the head.
- Selective radiographic series can then be performed on each individual vessel if required. It is important that there be the minimum of catheter changes and manipulation with no repeat examinations required.

DSA is a useful tool in this particular examination. An IV injection can provide a satisfactory overview of the condition of the arch and its four branches. It is useful when a patient's condition contraindicates the use of catheters. There are disadvantages. Large quantities of contrast and often multiple injections are required for the IV study. DSA can be performed using a direct arterial injection, using contrast that has been diluted by 50% and reduced in amount to less than 50%. Using DSA in conjunction with the angiogram is now common. This allows for just one contrast injection to be made and for postprocessing manipulation to achieve the visualization and information required (Figure 9.6). In some sites film has been completely replaced by the computerized image.

Procedure Radiographs

Using Biplane Equipment:

- RPO view, centered to the upper chest, using the AP changer. This opens up the arch and frees the vessel origins from superimposition.
- LPO view centered to the neck (usually about 15 cm higher) using the lateral changer. This demonstrates the vessels in the neck.

Selective Catheterization:

- Series or video images are taken in the AP position or at an angle determined by the radiologist.
- It is important to create scout images if using DSA, and not to move the patient until the contrast-filled images are complete.

Alternative Radiographs Use of DSA, as mentioned

Postprocedure Care

- As for any percutaneous femoral catheterization
- Observation for any neurologic signs, facial movements, and upper limb muscle movement

Common pathologies

- Stenosis of vessel origins
- Congenital abnormality of the arch

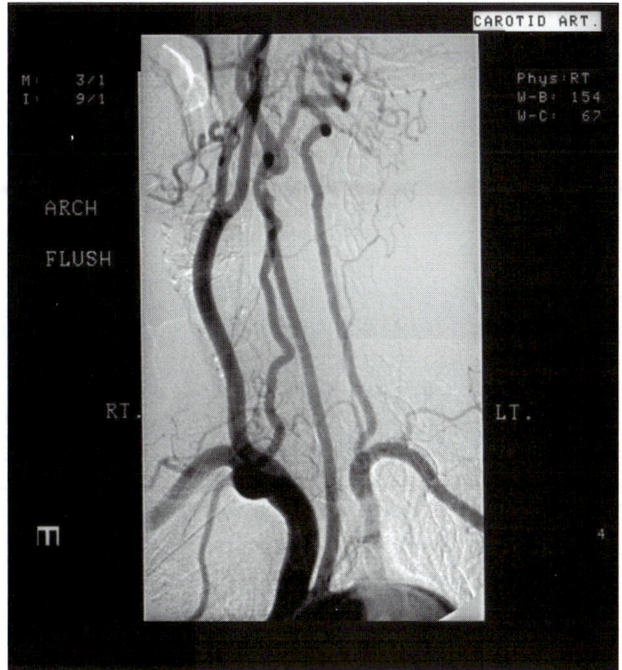

FIGURE 9.6
DSA image of neck vessels.

Carotid Angiography

This examination can be classified under two main headings, extracerebral and intracerebral and the intracerebral is subdivided into the internal and external carotid angiogram. The extracerebral carotid consists of the common carotid and its bifurcation into the internal and external carotid vessels. This is usually demonstrated on an archogram. By demonstrating the vasculature of the head, the angiographer aims to identify either an aberrant or abnormal blood supply or a displacement of vessels due to the presence of pathology.

INTERNAL CAROTID ANGIOGRAPHY

This is the more commonly performed carotid angiogram because it demonstrates a significant portion of the vasculature of each hemisphere. The normal method of approach is transfemorally with selective catheterization of the internal branch of the common carotid artery. The angiogram can be divided into three sections: arterial, capillary, and venous.

Contrast takes approximately 4 to 7 seconds to circulate through these three areas. Sometimes a late-phase venous radiograph is taken to demonstrate the deep venous system. A carotid angiogram will only demonstrate one hemispheric circulation, so that if both sides need to be demonstrated, the examination with have to be repeated on the contralateral side. Using catheterization techniques and a patient in a suitable condition, both sides can be done from a single percutaneous femoral puncture by selecting the internal carotids in turn. Careful record must be kept of the amount of contrast administered if multiple series are attempted during one procedure because a critical toxic level may be reached.

Applied Anatomy (see Figure 9.1)

Indications

- **Transient ischemic attack** (TIA)
- Additional information on tumors (CT and MRI are usually the primary method of imaging) to provide preoperative information
- As a preliminary for interventional procedures such as embolization
- **Subarachnoid hemorrhage**
- Arteriovenous (AV) malformation

Contraindications

- All contraindications related to angiography apply for carotid angiography.
- Allergy to contrast
- Severe arteriosclerosis
- Severe arachnoid or intracerebral hemorrhaging

Equipment

- Angiographic suite with biplane serial film changers and fluoroscopy unit
- Pressure injector
- Sterile tray equipment for Seldinger technique
- Guidewires
- Catheters for selecting the internal carotid artery
- Immobilization device for the head (usually a binder)

Contrast Media Nonionic, water-soluble contrast with low osmolarity

Radiation Protection

- Fluoroscopic time kept to a minimum
- Repeat exposures/series avoided

Preliminary Radiographs If a complete set of skull radiographs has not been taken before the examination, AP projection and lateral views should be done before contrast is injected. Any previous CT or MRI scans should also accompany the patient.

Patient Preparation

- As for angiography
- The patient must be made aware that the procedure requires the head to be very still during the sensation of a warm flush through the head and that an immobilization device like a bucky band across the forehead may be required.

Procedure Sequence

- The patient is placed supine on the angiographic table.
- The groin area is prepared for a percutaneous puncture.
- The Seldinger procedure is performed.
- If there are no previous studies of the extracerebral carotid artery, the catheter is placed in the common carotid and a flush injection made under fluoroscopy to determine the condition and patency of the common carotid, the bifurcation, and the internal and external carotids. Occasionally a short series of radiographs may be required, preferably in the lateral position to obtain a hard copy of the neck vessels.
- The internal carotid is then **superselected** using guidewire catheters designed to follow the curve. The (5 French) headhunter is the usual type, although there are even smaller catheters now available, 3 and 4 French.
- The catheter tip is advanced 3 to 4 cm beyond the bifurcation so that during the injection no major reflux occurs into the other vessels.
- The head is positioned ready for the radiographic series. Biplane should be used wherever possible to reduce the number of injections and exposures.
- The head is placed in the true AP position (orbitomeatal line perpendicular to the table) with an angle of about 15° caudad on the tube. The head must be carefully positioned and a binder or band used to inhibit movement.
- The central ray should pass through the frontal bone and external auditory meatus and care should be taken to ensure that the resultant image of the entire head falls within the film and collimation field.
- Collimation must be precise and as effective as possible to reduce secondary scatter and exposure.
- For the lateral view, the horizontal ray should pass 2.5 cm anterior and superior to the external auditory meatus. The biplane equipment allows positioning of the head to meet both AP and lateral requirements at the same time.
- An injection is made using a pressure injector. Because all three phases of the circulation are to be demonstrated, the injector has to be carefully programmed. The average circulation time is about 4.5 seconds, from carotid to jugular vein, and films are required at differing intervals during this time. An average program would be:

  One mask exposure made for subtraction purposes, before contrast.

Arterial phase:	3 exposures per second for 2 seconds.
Capillary phase:	1 exposure per second for 2 seconds.
Venous phase:	1 exposure per 2 seconds for 3 or 4 seconds (one film every other second).

- The program is decided by the radiologist and may vary from the normal because of certain pathologic conditions. An AV malformation may shorten the transit time; raised intracranial pressure may lengthen it. The program should be customized so that it best demonstrates the suspected pathology.

- Additional series may be taken in oblique positions if required (see alternative radiographs that follow).
- With the series satisfactorily completed, the catheter is removed and pressure exerted on the puncture site, or a guidewire is inserted into the catheter and a further neck vessel is selected provided the patient's condition is stable.

Procedure Radiographs AP series: central ray 15° caudad will demonstrate:

- Arterial phase—anterior, middle cerebral arteries (only about one-third of carotid angiograms show the posterior cerebral) (Figure 9.7).
- Capillary/venous phases—superficial veins vary with every patient and are not of major consequence in diagnosis. However, the deep veins are more consistent and important to demonstrate. They include the internal cerebral veins and the vein of Galen, which passes into the inferior sagittal sinus to form the straight sinus.

Lateral series: patient supine, central ray horizontal:

- Arterial phase—lateral view of anterior and middle carotid and the carotid syphon (Figure 9.8)
- Capillary/venous phase—superficial and deep veins of that hemisphere

Alternative Radiographs

- Posterior oblique view:
  —The head is rotated away from the injected side between 30° and 60° depending on need. This opens up the anterior communicating artery, a fairly common site for aneurysms.
  —The central ray is angled 15° to 20° caudad and centered over the raised side about 2.5 cm above the orbital margin.
- **Tangential** views are occasionally required to demonstrate a subdural hematoma.
- Transorbital views can be taken to demonstrate the first section of the middle cerebral artery, another common site for aneurysms. The head is rotated about 10° toward the affected side and the central ray passes through the raised orbit at an angle of about 5° cephalad.
- DSA can be used to provide an overall demonstration of the intracerebral vasculature.
- Macroradiography can be used to demonstrate developing aneurysms or aberrant vasculature (Figure 9.9).

Postprocedure Care

- As for angiogram with femoral puncture
- There must be close observation of neurologic signs as discussed with arch aortograms.

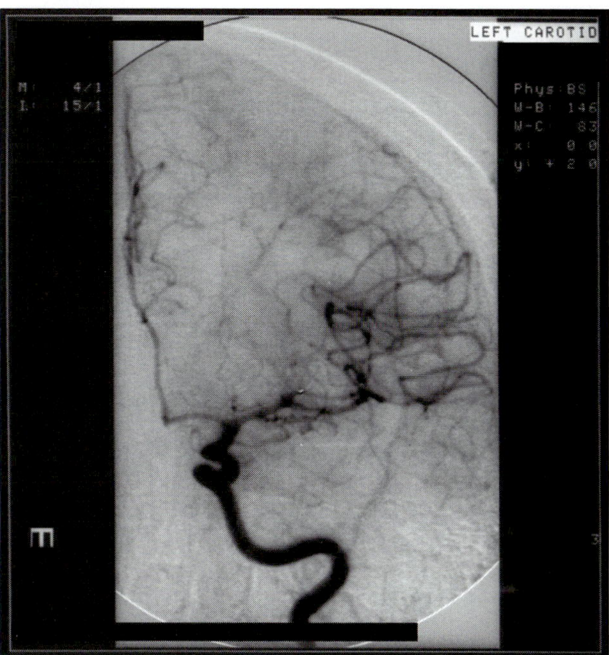

FIGURE 9.7 Cerebral arterial flow.

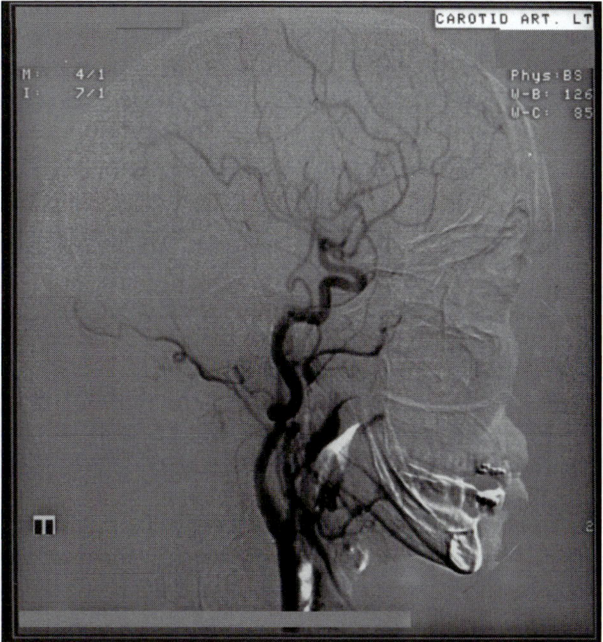

FIGURE 9.8 Lateral flow.

Common Pathologies

- Aneurysm
- AV malformation

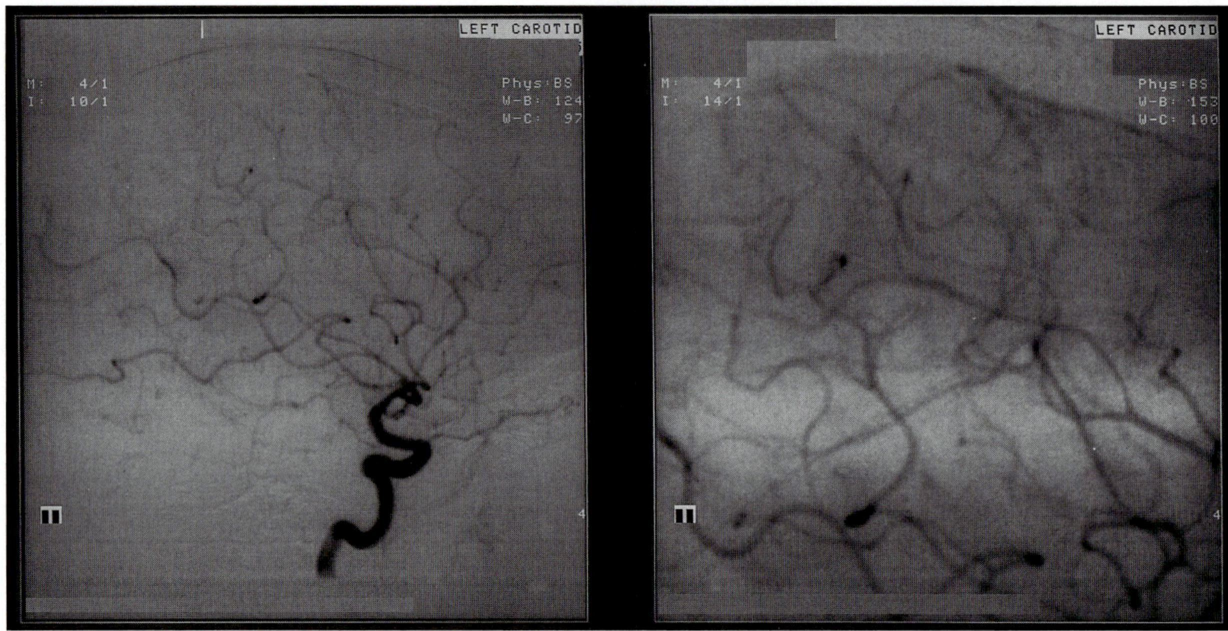

FIGURE 9.9 **Postprocessing macroradiography.**

EXTERNAL CAROTID ANGIOGRAPHY

The method of selecting and demonstrating the external carotid and its branches is the same as for the internal carotid. This procedure is becoming more common as embolizing techniques are more frequently used to assist in the treatment of tumors of the face and tongue.

The head position during exposure should be in the true AP position, but centering points and central ray angulation may vary according to the area to be demonstrated.

VERTEBRAL ANGIOGRAPHY

Unlike the carotid angiogram, one vertebral injection will demonstrate both hemispheres of the posterior brain vasculature. This is due to the circle of Willis. The vertebral artery is more difficult to select because it arises from the subclavian arteries and not directly from the aortic arch. Congenital anomalies are fairly common. The left vertebral artery actually arises from the arch itself in over 50% of the population. It is important to have the flush aortogram to determine the position of the vessels before proceeding with the vertebral selection (or any of the branches).

Applied Anatomy (Figure 9.10)

Indications

- Basilar thrombosis
- Basilar artery aneurysm
- Posterior fossa tumors

Contraindications As for carotid angiography

Equipment Biplane angiographic unit with fluoroscopy

Contrast Media Water-soluble, nonionic contrast with low osmolarity

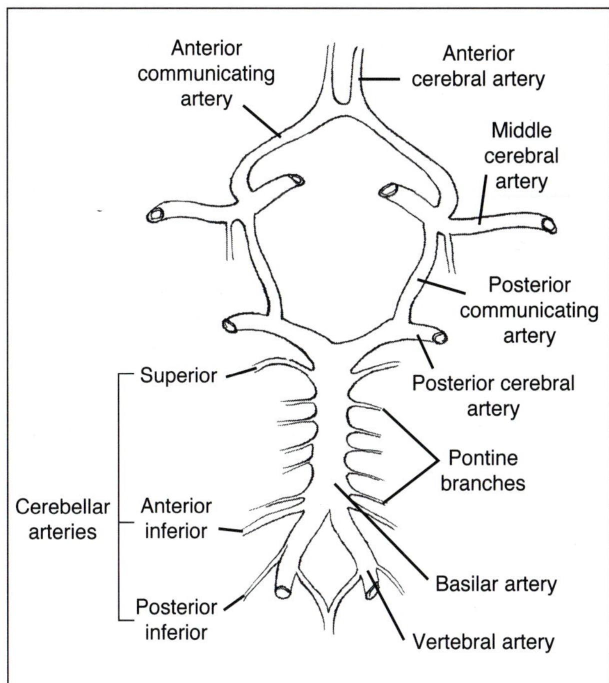

FIGURE 9.10 Circle of Willis.

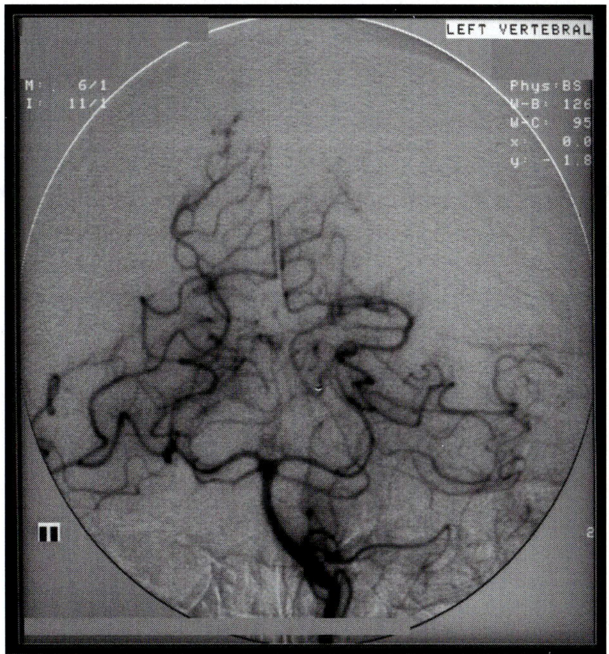

FIGURE 9.11 Left vertebral angiogram.

Radiation Protection Fluoroscopy time and radiographic series are kept to the minimum.

Preliminary Radiographs

- Set of skull radiographs
- Flush study of the aortic arch to determine placement of catheter (may not always require a hard copy)

Procedure Sequence

- The procedure for performing the vertebral is the same as for the carotid. A femoral puncture is performed and the vertebral artery selected by a catheter.
- The left vertebral artery is most often catheterized because it is generally easier to select.
- Eight to 10 mL of contrast usually provides adequate visualization.

Procedure Radiographs

- Head position is the same as for the carotid angiogram. However, a central ray caudad angulation of 25° is recommended for the AP radiographic series and centered to the midline to demonstrate both sides simultaneously (Figure 9.11).
- The lateral central point is 2.5 cm superior and 2.5 cm *posterior* to the external auditory meatus.

Alternative Radiographs

- DSA can provide a satisfactory overall demonstration of the vertebral circulation.
- Macroradiography can be used to demonstrate small areas of interest such as a small, developing aneurysm or an abnormal blood supply indicating a lesion.

Postprocedure Care As for carotid angiography

Common Pathologies Basilar aneurysm

Other Imaging Modalities

COMPUTED TOMOGRAPHY

There are several pathologies for which CT has become the primary imaging modality. (In some sites, most of the pathologies mentioned are now imaged primarily by MRI, including all lesions and the presence of metastases.) Intracranial lesions are well demonstrated in some situations, dispelling the need for plain radiographs of the skull (see Chapter 14, Brain).

Applied Anatomy (Figure 9.12)

Indications

- Congenital lesions
- Inflammatory lesions
- Trauma
- Neoplasms
- Metastases

Contraindications

- No specific contraindications
- Allergy to contrast if enhancement is being considered
- In the case of a suspected intracranial bleed, contrast use is contraindicated.

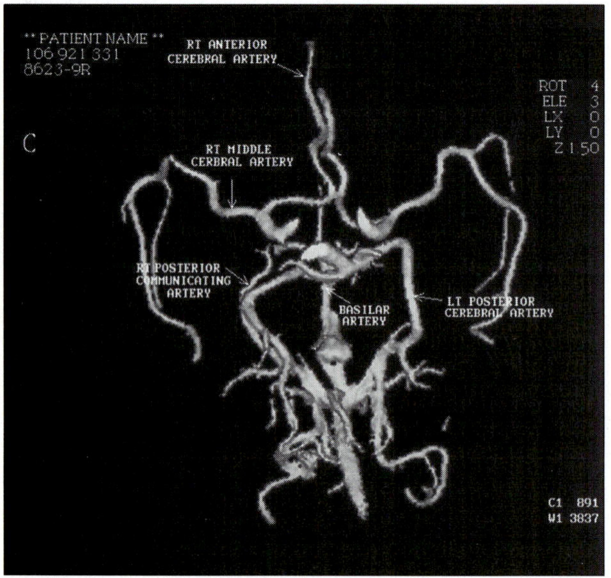

FIGURE 9.12 CT three-dimensional reconstruction of head vessels.

Equipment CT scanner with tilting gantry

Contrast Media

- Abnormal tissue in the brain accepts water-soluble iodinated contrast in a different way than normal tissue because of a breakdown in the blood–brain barrier and because the presence of abnormal vasculature will attract more contrast. Gray matter is better defined than white matter because of its higher levels of blood.
- Vascular abnormalities are best defined immediately after a bolus injection.
- The enhancement of lesions via the blood-brain barrier takes about 30 minutes to achieve the best concentration of contrast.

Radiation Protection

- Radiation exposure is high (although not as high as a complete angiogram), so care must be taken to avoid repeat examinations.
- A slight angling of the gantry to the orbits will decrease the amount of direct radiation to the sensitive lens of the eye.

Procedure Sequence

- Nonenhanced scans are made initially and then protocols are determined that will best demonstrate the suspected pathology.
- Coronal sections are usually performed with the patient in the AP position and the gantry at 10° to 25° caudad to Reid's baseline (Figure 9.13).
- Sagittal sections are obtained by having the patient turn on the side. However, three-dimensional reconstruction can provide this information and with the advent of MRI patients requiring this particular section would probably be referred to that modality.

Procedure Radiographs (Figure 9.14).

Postprocedure Care No significant care is needed.

Common Pathologies

- AV malformation
- Malignant vascular tumor

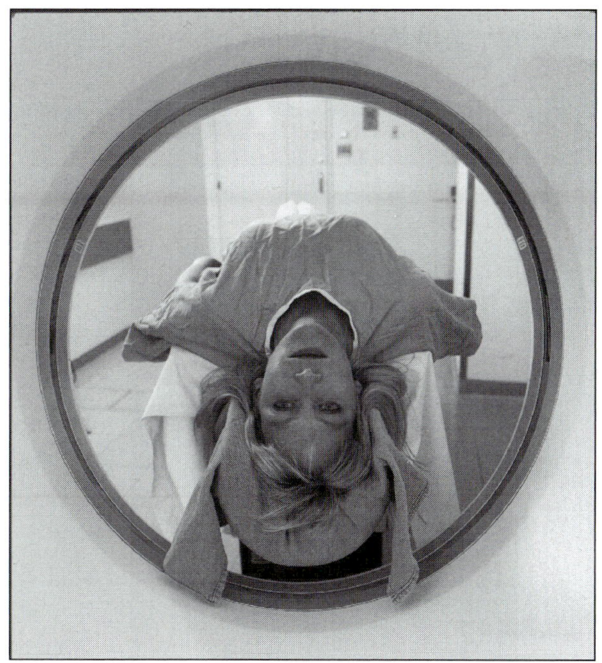

FIGURE 9.13
Patient position for head CT.

MAGNETIC RESONANCE IMAGING

Although CT continues to be the main brain imaging source, MRI has made huge gains and is considered the primary imaging modality of choice for many conditions. Its availability and cost do have implications, but its noninvasive character and ability to image in any plane required have made it a preferred source of diagnostic information. The addition of contrast enhancement with gadolinium and the advances of magnetic resonance angiography will doubtless expand the usefulness of this modality (Figures 9.14 and 9.15).

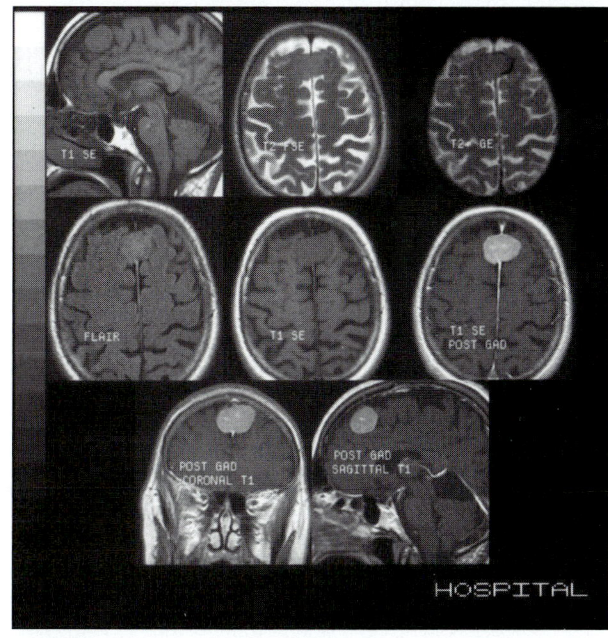

FIGURE 9.14 MRI studies to demonstrate meningioma.

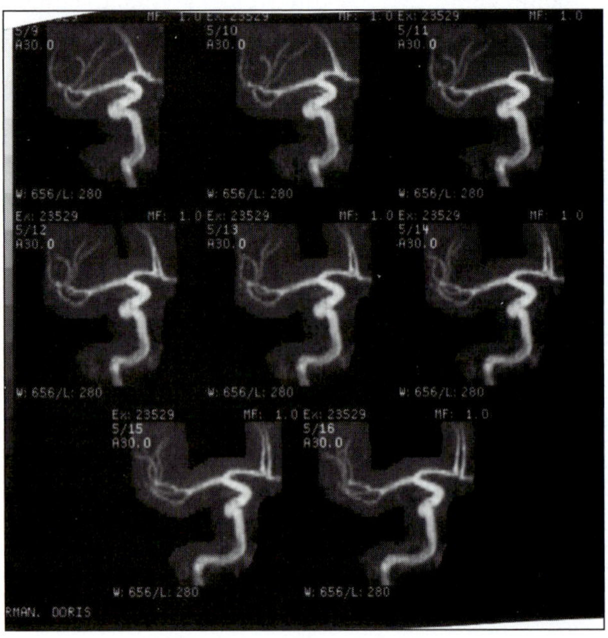

FIGURE 9.15 MRI angiogram demonstrating vertebral vessels.

The use of angiography in determining the type and presence of tumors has virtually disappeared with the advance of CT and MRI. Avascular tumors in angiography were demonstrated as a displacement (and therefore an indirect visualization) and the vascular tumors were shown with their abnormal blood supply.

CT and MRI have advantages and disadvantages for the demonstration of tumors. Early tumors are well demonstrated using MRI because the changes are better shown using resonance rather than x-ray attenuation. However, older lesions are not as well shown with MRI because of the inability to image calcification. (Enhancement with gadolinium has helped this problem.)

ULTRASOUND

Ultrasound does not play a part in the imaging of the adult intracranial circulation. However, two important developments are currently in use.

- Ultrasound of the neonate brain (neurosonography). Specialized equipment allows the cranial contents to be visualized via the anterior fontanelle. It is possible to image this way until about the sixth month when the fontanelle becomes too small to provide an effective accoustic window. Hydrocephalus and hemorrhage are the most common pathologies for which this examination is requested.
- Carotid Doppler. This examination of the blood flow within the carotid arteries has become extremely useful in the diagnosis of TIAs and strokes, and has certainly replaced angiography in this particular area as an initial form of imaging (Figure 9.16).

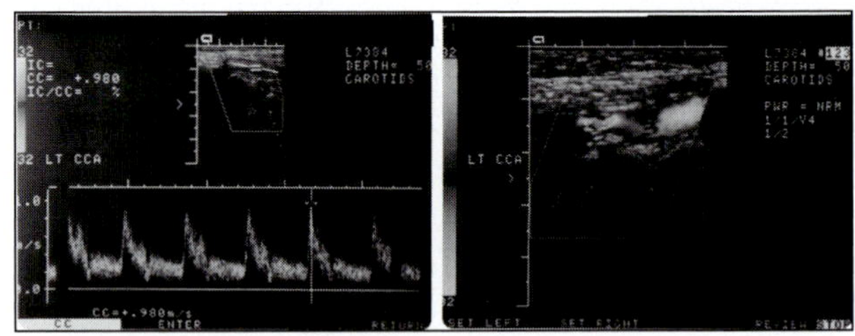

FIGURE 9.16 Carotid Doppler study.

RADIONUCLIDE IMAGING

The use of radionuclides in the determination of lesions has decreased, but **positron emission tomography (PET)** does have some useful qualities by being able to assess differing metabolic rates within the brain. However, it continues to be an extremely expensive procedure.

Flow studies of the brain can be done, in the absence of CT and as a less invasive technique than angiography. Comparisons of takeup time between hemispheres will demonstrate the presence of an infarction, but cannot accurately determine its position (Figure 9.17).

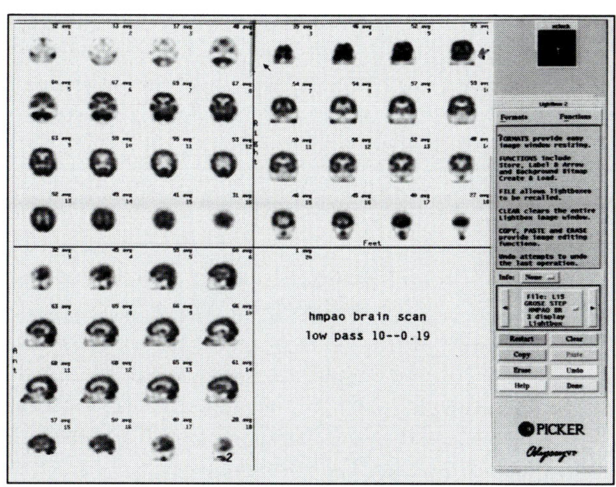

FIGURE 9.17 Nuclear medicine brain scan.

Some highly vascular tumors can be demonstrated (e.g., meningiomas), but in several others activity during the radionuclide scan does not differ appreciably from the surrounding tissue (e.g., gliomas).

Imaging with PET can provide qualitative information on the cerebral blood flow. By using a lipid-soluble blood–brain barrier-penetrating agent, PET provides a rough picture of the cerebral circulation. This is definitely less invasive than angiography, but has the drawback that the agent described is not always readily available because it must be produced in a **cyclotron**.

Interventional Procedures

The use of interventional techniques as an alternative to vascular surgery has increased rapidly in the last 20 years. The use of techniques such as angioplasty has evolved more slowly with cranial blood vessels because of the serious consequences of a failed attempt or the resultant effects from a dislodged plaque. These procedures are always performed with the assistance of angiography and, preferably, the addition of DSA, which can provide rapid information on the circulatory pathways and accurate site of a lesion. The most common type of intervention in this area is embolotherapy (see Chapter 6).

EMBOLIZATION

Embolization may be used as a method of treatment, that is, to starve a tumor by inhibiting its blood supply or as a complement to surgery or radiation therapy (see also Chapter 6).

Indications

- Occlusion of AV fistulae
- Before radiation therapy, to reduce circulation and thus increase effectiveness of the therapy
- Before surgery to decrease vascularity
- Inoperable tumors
- Unmanageable **epistaxis**

Contraindications Specific to the condition of the patient. The decision to embolize is made only after careful scrutiny of all aspects of the patient's physical condition and anatomy. As with all procedures that carry with them the element of risk, the risk versus benefit must be carefully analyzed.

Equipment

- Cerebral embolizations will be carried out in an angiographic suite with fluoroscopy, video playback and DSA available.
- Sterile tray for percutaneous puncture and Seldinger technique
- Catheters
- Appropriate embolizing agent. This will depend on the pathology being treated as well as physician preference. The list below, although not definitive, offers suggestions on the type of embolizing materials that could be used:
  —AV fistulae and aneurysms—a permanent detachable balloon. The balloon is delivered via a coaxial catheter and detachment occurs either by gentle traction or manipulation after the balloon has been inflated and is firmly in place.
  —Hemorrhage, preoperative procedure—particulates such as Ivalon or Gelfoam, which are reabsorbed over several days, are made radiopaque by being

suspended in contrast. Gelfoam is prepared by cutting into strips or small 1- to 2-mm particles and can be introduced either as a single piece or strip or as a suspension in contrast through the catheter.
—AV malformations—liquid embolics that can be used to systematically reduce blood flow to a large inoperable AV malformation. One such is an acrylic or polymerizing agent that hardens on contact with the body and is injected through the catheter behind a bolus of 5% glucose. (At the time of writing this mechanism had not met with full federal approval.)

Contrast Media A water-soluble, nonionic contrast with low osmolarity is used to determine placement only.

Radiation Protection

- Usually significant fluoroscopy is required during the placement of the embolus.
- Care should be taken that all the operators are well protected with gloves where possible, as well as the patient.
- Fluoroscopy should be kept to the minimum by using a pulse signal and video freeze frame wherever possible.

Preliminary Radiographs All prospective embolizing candidates must have had an angiogram to provide a good map of the cerebral vasculature, particularly the vessels to be embolized and the pathway to be selected to get to the site.

Patient Preparation

- As for an angiogram
- Prescribed drugs depending on the condition of the patient

Procedure Sequence

- Vessels are selected and catheterized so that the end of the catheter sits exactly in the correct spot for embolizing. This procedure alone necessitates great skill on the part of the physician because placement is critical. If the embolus is positioned too far from the specific site to be occluded, it will mean the vessel will not become fully occluded. If the catheter tip is too close, there is the risk of recoil of the embolizing agent. Embolizing should always be in the direction of the blood flow. Sometimes an AV malformation produces an abnormal flow, and it is somewhat difficult to determine the flow direction.
- Contrast flush injections during placement are essential to determine flow as well as vessel position.
- Injections of particulates or liquid are made slowly and steadily to reduce the risk of an aberrant embolus. The risk is particularly high in the brain where serious complications can occur.
- The embolization can take a considerable amount of time, particularly where there are a number of vessels to occlude. If the patient is tiring or showing a deteriorating condition, it is more advisable to stop before all the vessels are occluded and proceed again at a later date.

Postprocedure Care

- As for an angiogram and embolization (see Chapter 6, Angiographic Procedures and Equipment)
- Special observations must be made of neurologic signs to ensure that the embolization has been successful and that the embolizing agent has not become dislodged and moved elsewhere. For this reason, the pulmonary area must be closely observed for any sign of a pulmonary embolus.

> This area of brain imaging is rapidly evolving and it is beyond the scope of this text to incorporate all the latest developments. New products are constantly surfacing and experiments being performed. Sometimes procedures that showed initial promise of effective treatment fall out of favor when long-term studies show a return to the previous state. It is a fascinating area, full of challenge for the radiographer willing to learn more about the therapeutic capabilities of imaging in the brain.

Review Questions

1. Compare and contrast the imaging modalities used in the demonstration of the vascular system to the brain.

2. Develop a chart that identifies which modality best demonstrates which pathology and why.

3. Pigtail catheters are useful because they:
   a. are small (less than 4 French)
   b. can be easily withdrawn
   c. have a higher tensile strength
   d. prevent recoil during injection

4. Which of the following is used most often in conjunction with angiography?
   a. SPECT
   b. ultrasound
   c. DSA
   d. MRI

5. TIAs most often occur because this vessel is occluded?
   a. common carotid artery
   b. internal carotid artery
   c. basilar artery
   d. jugular vein

CASE STUDY

A child is admitted with a suspected AV malformation. Describe the different studies/procedures that may be performed within the imaging department.

References and Recommended Reading

Abrams, H. L. (1983). *Abrams angiography: Vascular and interventional radiology* (3rd ed.). Boston: Little, Brown.

Castaneda-Zuniga, W. R., & Tadavarthy, S. M. (1992). *Interventional radiology* (2nd ed.). Baltimore: Williams & Wilkins.

Chapman, S., & Nakielny, R. (1993). *A guide to radiological procedures* (3rd ed.). London: Bailliere & Tindall.

Dowd, S. B., & Wilson, B. G. (1995). *Encyclopedia of radiographic positioning.* Philadelphia: Saunders.

Doyle, T., Hare W., Thomson K., & Tress B. (1989). *Procedures in diagnostic radiology.* London: Churchill Livingstone.

Eisenberg, R. L. (1992). *Radiology, an illustrated history.* St. Louis: Mosby-Year Book.

Greene, R. E., & Oestmann, J-W. (1992). *Computed digital radiography in clinical practice.* New York: Thieme.

Potchen, E. J., Haacke, E. M., Siebert, J. E., & Gottschalk, A. (1993). *Magnetic resonance angiography, concepts and applications.* St. Louis: Mosby-Year Book.

Prayer, L. M., et al. (1993). MRI, a non invasive tool for evaluating therapeutic embolization of cerebral arteriovenous malformations. *European Radiology, 1.*

Schweitzer, J. S., Chang, B. S., et al. (1993). Pathology of arteriovenous malformations of the brain treated by embolotherapy. *Neuroradiology, 35*(6), 468–474.

Snopek, A. M. (1992). *Fundamentals of special radiographic procedures* (3rd ed.). Philadelphia: Saunders.

Sutton, D. A. (1993). *Textbook of radiology and imaging* (5th ed.). Edinburgh: Churchill Livingstone.

Taber's Cyclopedic medical dictionary (17th ed.). (1989). Philadelphia: Davis.

Tortorici, M. R., & Apfel, P. J. (1995). *Advanced radiographic and angiographic procedures.* Philadelphia: Davis.

Warach, S., et al. (1992) Acute cerebral ischemia; evaluation with dynamic contrast-enhanced MR imaging and MR angiography. *Radiology, 182*(1), 41–47.

CHAPTER 10

Lymphatic System

CYNTHIA COWLING, BSc, MEd, MRT(R), ACR

OBJECTIVES

At the completion of this chapter, the student should be able to:

1. Describe the main features of the lymph system.
2. List the major procedures used to demonstrate the lymph system.
3. Identify the main indications and contraindications for each procedure.
4. Describe the procedure for lymphangiography.
5. Discuss the application of diagnostic procedures to radiation and chemotherapeutic procedures.
6. Compare the different imaging modalities used to demonstrate the lymph system.
7. Apply safe practice to each procedure.
8. Apply good patient care techniques.
9. Describe interventional techniques used to assist in the treatment of lymph pathology.

Introduction and Historical Overview

The earliest radiographs depicting the lymph system were achieved in 1930 by injecting Thorotrast into cadavers. Because the lymph vessels are small and much more difficult to inject directly, it was not until the 1950s that the procedure used today was first performed. In the 1930s, scientists at the Rockefeller Institute had outlined the lymphatic system of the extremities by injecting a blue dye, but it was not until 1952 that this method was used to visualize lymph vessels to allow an injection of contrast that would pass throughout the system. A minor cut-down procedure exposed the dyed vessel on the dorsum of the foot and the injection made with a fine needle and catheter. The use of an oily contrast enhanced the visualization of lymph nodes, lymph channels, and the thoracic duct.

With the advent of CT scanning, ultrasound, and radionuclide imaging, this method of imaging the lymph system has fallen into disfavor. The necessity to perform a surgical procedure and the sometimes frail nature of the lymph vessels can make this a frustrating and time-consuming exercise. Successfully performed, it does, however, produce excellent images of the lymph system and is particularly useful in the diagnosis and staging of **Hodgkin's disease**.

Anatomy

The lymphatic system is part of the circulatory system although it can also be considered part of the immune system because it contributes lymphocytes to the circulatory system.

The fluid moving within lymphatic vessels is called lymph and is derived from the blood and it returns to the blood. Lymph resembles blood plasma but it contains fewer proteins and salts than does blood.

The lymphatic system returns fluid lost in capillary interstitial spaces, fills the blood and debris at the lymph nodes, adds lymphocytes to the general circulation, and transports fats from the small intestine to the circulation. On its return to the general circulation, lymph passes through filtering systems called lymph nodes. These are placed in strategic locations such as the inguinal, iliac, paraorta, and axillary areas. There is no pump to propel the lymph through the lymphatic vessels. The driving force depends on muscle massage and the pulsating accompanying arteries (Figure 10.1).

The two major lymph vessels are the thoracic duct and the right lymphatic duct. The thoracic duct (left lymphatic duct) originates anterior to the second lumbar vertebra. It passes up the posterior thorax to the root of the neck. It receives lymph from the left side of the head, neck, thorax, abdomen, pelvis, left upper extremity, and lower extremities. All lymph from the thoracic duct empties into the venous system at the junction of the left internal jugular and subclavian veins. The short right lymphatic duct lies anterior to the anterior scloneus muscle. It drains the right side of the head, neck thorax, and right upper extremity. The right lymphatic duct empties into the venous system at the junction of the right internal jugular and subclavian veins (Figure 10.2).

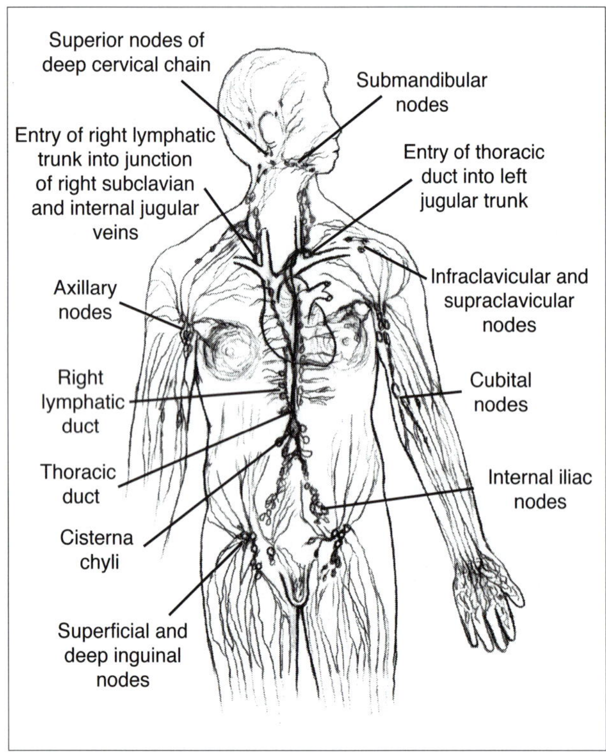

FIGURE 10.1 Lymphatic system.

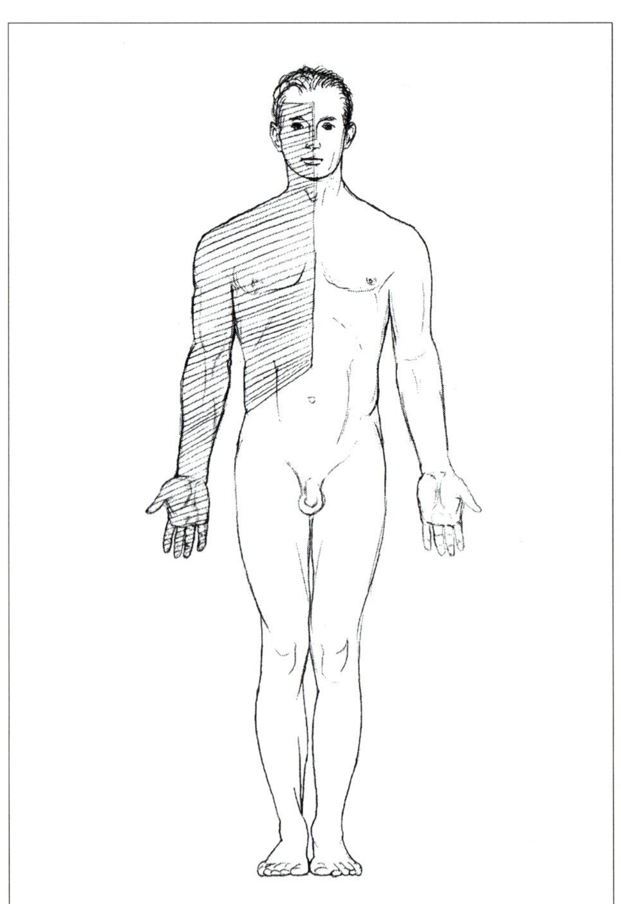

FIGURE 10.2 Outline of lymphatic drainage system.

Procedures

LYMPHOGRAPHY

This term describes the examination of the lymph system by using a contrast medium injected into the vessels. It can be subdivided into:

- **Lymphangiography** (lĭm-făn´´jē-ŏg´ră-fē)—the study of the vessels
- **Lymphadenography** (lĭm-făd´´ĕ-nŏg´ră-fē)—The study of the lymph nodes

Lymphadenography is generally achieved after a lymphangiogram because the nodes are best seen at least 24 hours after injection of contrast media.

LYMPHANGIOGRAPHY

Applied Anatomy The lymph system is a transport and drainage system that returns certain fats, proteins, and tissue fluids to the general circulation. It does not circulate in the same way as the blood supply. Instead, capillaries arise from intercellular spaces in soft tissue areas. These enlarge to form the drainage vessels that culminate and drain into the main lymphatic trunks, the right lymphatic trunk, and the thoracic duct. The origin of the thoracic duct is the cisterna chyli, a dilated sac found in the lumbar region and into which drains lymph from the intestinal and lumbar area (Figure 10.3).

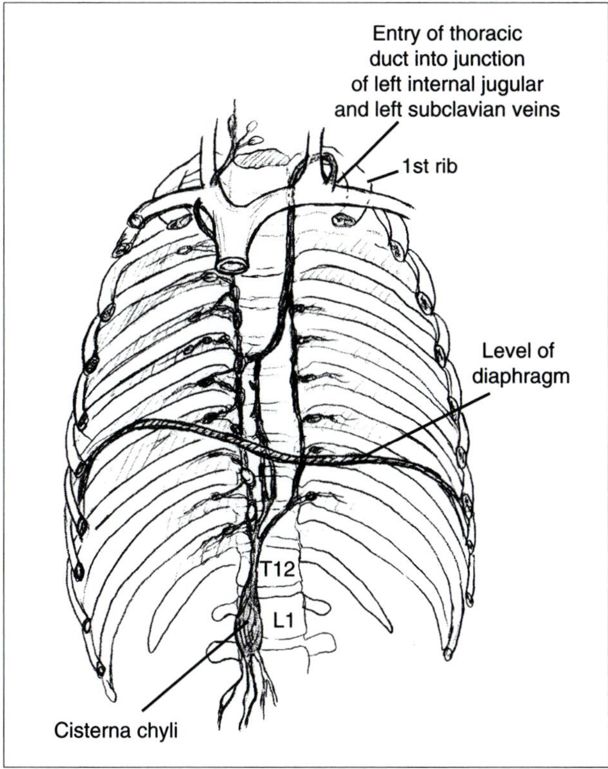

FIGURE 10.3 Central lymph system showing the cisterna chyli.

Lymph nodes (or glands) are oval-shaped structures enclosed within a fibrous capsule that serves as a filter at various points along the vessel transport system. They are found in clumps in specific areas of the body—the floor of the mouth, the neck, the axilla, and the groin area (Figure 10.4).

Indications

- Hodgkin's disease
- Prostatic carcinoma
- Other carcinomas of unknown origin
- Swellings of the extremities
- Assessment of posttreatment changes in nodes
- Negative CT scan in a patient with a suspected **lymphoma**

Contraindications

- Allergy to contrast (specifically iodine)
- Serious tremors of the extremities
- Within 3 weeks of radiation therapy, which can destroy parts of the system and increase the risk of

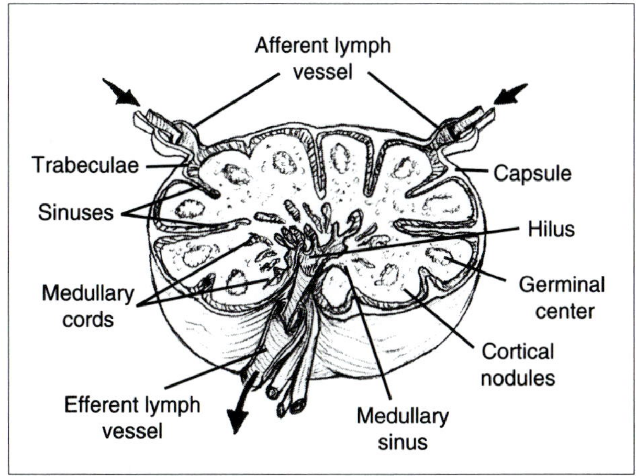

FIGURE 10.4 Lymph node.

oily contrast getting into the systemic circulation or the lungs and producing oil emboli. (Radiation should not be administered for at least a week after this procedure, for the same reason.)

- Thrombophlebitis
- Respiratory disease that may have led to tissue destruction

Equipment

- A regular x-ray table with overhead tube
- A slow-speed pressure injector
- Sterile tray to include syringes, needles, and sponges
- Lymphangiography set with cannula for contrast injection
- Good lighting to the cut-down and injection site

Contrast Media

- Contrast for vessel visualization. A blue dye is injected subcutaneously that drains initially into the peripheral and superficial lymph vessels. Two common types are:
  —Direct blue (Chicago Blue 6B)
  —Alphazurine 2G (Patent Blue)
- Contrast for radiographic visualization of lymphatic system. Oil-based iodine compounds are usually used (Lipiodil ultrafluid). Water-soluble medium is occasionally used, but it does not opacify the lymph nodes and can be irritating to the lymph vessels.

Radiation Protection Radiographs for this procedure are normal overhead tube studies and normal precautions must be taken.

Preliminary Radiographs

- PA chest—will demonstrate enlargement of mediastinal nodes and hilar lymph nodes. (This can sometimes negate the need for the procedure.) It will also show evidence of serious respiratory conditions.
- AP abdomen—less useful, but very enlarged nodes can sometimes be seen.

Patient Preparation

- This procedure can be performed on an outpatient basis, but the patient will be required to return on day 2 for delay radiographs.
- The patient must be made aware of the procedure, including the fact that there will be a cut-down procedure requiring postprocedure sutures on the dorsum of the foot, which may be painful for a few days.
- The patient should also be aware that the blue dye may stain the whole foot for several days.
- If the leg is **edematous**, (ĕ-dĕm´ăt-ŭs) it should be elevated for 24 hours before the procedure.
- The area to be incised should be shaved.
- The patient should void the bladder immediately before the procedure.

Procedure Sequence (for Lower Extremity Injection)

- The patient lies comfortably supine on the radiographic table. This is a long procedure so every care should be taken to make the patient as comfortable as possible.
- A small dose of 1% lignocaine is mixed with 2 mL of blue dye and injected subcutaneously between the first and second toes. Both feet can be injected. This allows a choice of injection points in case one side is better visualized. Some examiners do both sides automatically.
- The dye will reach the lymph capillaries in about 15 minutes. Some recommend exercising to encourage movement of the dye. The dye will eventually arrive in the systemic circulation so it is important not to exercise too vigorously or wait too long because the venous system could obscure the lymph vessels.
- The dorsum of the foot is prepared using sterile technique.
- An incision of 2 to 3 cm is made on the dorsum of the foot where a lymph vessel has been visualized with the dye, and the vessel is exposed and dissected.
- Using either the prepackaged lymphangiogram setup or a piece of card, the lymph vessel is lifted from the fascia to enable ease of cannulation.
- Massaging of the foot distal to the incision sometimes enlarges the vessel.
- Suture thread can be placed on either side of the exposed vessel and tightened as required to increase dilation of the vessel.
- The vessel is cannulated using a 27-gauge needle and the cannula secured with the silk ties.
- The pressure injector, which has been prepared with saline along its connector with air excluded, is attached to the cannula.
- A small amount of saline is injected to confirm that the cannula is in place in the lymph system and not the venous system and that there is no leakage.
- Approximately 7 mL of oily contrast is injected slowly over a period of about 45 minutes. (If this

procedure were being performed on the upper extremity half of that amount would be required.)

- Radiographs are taken at various intervals during the injection. These will determine the level that the contrast has reached. Fluoroscopy can replace these radiographs if preferred.
- The injection is terminated as soon as the nodes at the lumbar level have been opacified, even if the full amount has not yet been injected.
- When the injection is complete, the cannula is removed and the incision sutured.

Procedure Radiographs

- Radiographs are taken at 10-minute intervals along the length of the leg to confirm the position of the contrast and to ensure that the contrast is in the lymph system.
- A 30-minute AP radiograph of the pelvis
- A 40-minute AP radiograph of the abdomen
- Radiographs every 15 minutes thereafter until the contrast has reached L3 or until the injection is complete
- At 2 hours postinjection
  —AP abdomen
  —PA chest
  —AP pelvis and upper femora (Figure 10.5)
- At 24 hours postinjection (This procedure is known as lymphadenography.)
  —AP abdomen
  —PA chest
  —AP upper femora and pelvis

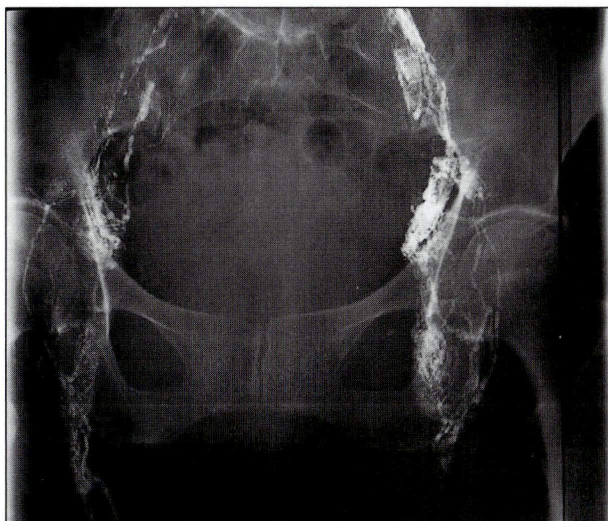

FIGURE 10.5 Pelvic area with contrast.

Alternative Radiographs

- A 45° AP oblique of either side of pelvic area to separate nodes
- Lateral view of lumbar area to demonstrate the cisterna chyli

Postprocedure Care

- The incision(s) must be carefully observed for infection and bleeding and some investigators prefer to admit their patients overnight.
- No radiation or chemotherapy is to be given for a week after the procedure to reduce the likelihood of oil embolus.
- Patients occasionally experience a low fever after this examination.
- Stitches can be removed after 10 days.

Common Pathologies

- Hodgkin's disease
- Metastatic disease

Advantages of lymphography:

- The ability to determine a lesion within a normal-sized node or gland and to assess whether the gland is diseased or reacting as part of its normal function
- Retaining of contrast within a node for several weeks allows for ongoing evaluation of those nodes.

Disadvantages of lymphography:

- Does not image the abdominal lymph nodes
- Requires a cut-down procedure, can be time-consuming and painful for the patient at injection site

Advantages of CT

- Easier procedure for the patient
- Simpler procedure to perform
- Abdominal nodes well visualized
- Provides accurate assessment for treatment planning for radiation therapy

Disadvantages of CT

- Does not visualize the internal structure of the lymph nodes and glands

Ultrasound, radionuclide imaging, and MRI are all used to visualize the lymph system to a lesser degree.

Other Imaging Modalities

COMPUTED TOMOGRAPHY

This has become the primary imaging modality for the visualization of several conditions related to the lymph system. It is particularly effective in the demonstration of normal and abnormal lymph nodes, indicators of direct lymphomas such as Hodgkin's or indirect indicators of malignant and metastatic disease. Scanning of the lymph system is usually divided into those areas where nodes are most evident—thorax, abdomen, and head and neck.

Applied Anatomy In CT nodes are seen in cross section and assessed for size and shape. Nodes affected by Hodgkin's differ in their irregular shape more than non-Hodgkin's lymphomas and CT can demonstrate these differences well.

Indications

- Hodgkin's disease
- **Lymphedema**
- Metastatic changes—staging of disease; very useful for treatment planning for radiation therapy

Contraindications

- Early metastatic changes
- Lymph drainage problems
- Presence of oily contrast in nodes (sometimes produces a reactive enlargement and creates a very high contrast area, degrading the CT image)
- Known allergy to contrast

Equipment CT scanner with fast scan times

Contrast Media

- Water-soluble, nonionic contrast
- Enhancement is beneficial for only some areas and will be administered intravenously.

Radiation Protection Minimize scans and repeats.

Preliminary Radiographs Chest and abdomen radiographs are usually taken although they only demonstrate very enlarged nodes.

Patient Preparation None specific

Procedure Sequence

For Thorax

- Patient lies supine.
- IV contrast is established; 100 mL should be injected over a period of 1 to 2 minutes while the scan is being performed. Contrast is helpful in the thoracic region because it is not taken up by the lungs and therefore does not obscure the mediastinal structures.
- Contiguous sections are made through the area of interest at 1-cm intervals. Scans should be made on inspiration and be as short as possible to avoid movement.
- Wide window setting

For Abdomen

- Patient is supine.
- An oral contrast is administered to outline the bowel.
- Sections are taken at 1.5-cm intervals from the pelvic region to the liver and spleen. Spleen and liver can be affected by lymphoma, but these are difficult to detect with CT.

For Neck and Head

- Patient lies supine with head supported in the AP position.
- IV infusion of contrast is established.
- Scans taken at 3 to 6 mm contiguously, depending on the initial investigation. Nodes in this area are often palpable so that size can be estimated.
- The hilar region may be included, using scans at 5 to 10-mm intervals.

Procedure Radiographs For all areas, scans will depict the nodes in cross-section demonstrating any nodular enlargement (Figure 10.6).

Postprocedure Care None specific

Common Pathologies

- Hodgkin's disease
- Non-Hodgkin's lymphoma

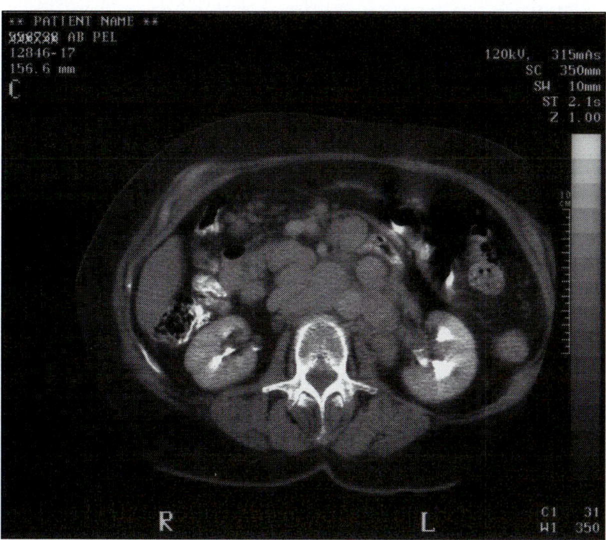

FIGURE 10.6 CT showing lymphoma.

As well as demonstrating abnormal lymph nodes, the sections through the abdomen and chest will also demonstrate any spread of metastatic disease. This information together with the determination of the type of lymphatic disease has made CT an essential part of treatment planning in radiation therapy. MRI, while holding the potential for demonstrating soft tissue admirably, is a more expensive method and has not yet replaced CT in this important area.

MAGNETIC RESONANCE IMAGING

An MRI scan can be used in the thoracic and abdominal areas to determine the presence of abnormal lymph nodes.

MRI has several advantages over CT:

- There is no need for contrast.
- It is easier to distinguish between vascular and soft tissue structures.
- The areas can be imaged along any plane.
- T1-weighted images allow for discrimination between fat and the lymph nodes.

Disadvantages to MRI include:

- High cost
- Inability to distinguish calcification of nodes
- Poorer spatial resolution, making it more difficult to determine the difference between a single large node and several smaller ones
- In the abdomen, bowel contents can sometimes prevent optimum imaging of the lymphatic areas.

ULTRASOUND

Lymphadenopathy can be visualized using ultrasound, but a very skilled operator is needed to locate the abdominal nodes by means of a sonographic silhouette. Bowel gas can adversely affect the success of this procedure.

RADIONUCLIDE IMAGING

Radionuclides are used extensively to study the lymph system. Lymphoscintography is an examination where a **colloid** is injected subcutaneously adjacent to the area of interest. It is taken up by the lymph nodes and images are recorded using a gamma camera at 15, 30, 60 minutes, and 3 hours. This can continue until the liver is demonstrated, which indicates some patency of the lymphatic system.

A number of different radiopharmaceuticals can be administered intravenously. Some attach to **leukocytes** and some to **granulocytes** and increased uptake is seen at sites of infection or inflammation. Images can be taken with the gamma camera at the suspected area as well as a total body scan to rule out problems elsewhere. The actual timing of the images varies according to the radiopharmaceutical used, but delay scans at 24 or 48 hours are often requested to visualize the liver.

Gallium imaging uses ^{67}Ga gallium citrate injected intravenously to demonstrate lymphomas and to assess and predict their response to therapy. Delay films are taken at 48 and 72 hours, including whole body scans, and if possible, single photon emission CT images.

Interventional Procedures

LYMPH NODE BIOPSY

A percutaneous biopsy will enable diagnosis of the cause of abnormally sized lymph nodes. This is not a common procedure because results of the biopsy are not always definitive. The biopsy needle can be guided using:

- Fluoroscopy following opacification of the lymph nodes by lymphangiography
- CT guidance
- Ultrasound guidance

Review Questions

1. Discuss the advantages and disadvantages of using lymphangiography as a diagnostic tool as compared to CT.

2. Describe how radiation therapy can affect the success of lymphangiography and indicate its effects if administered shortly after this examination.

3. Radiographs taken after contrast injection usually stop after:
   a. contrast is seen at the level of L3
   b. 2 hours postinjection
   c. 24 hours postinjection
   d. when contrast is visualized at the mediastinal level

4. The study of lymph nodes is known as:
   a. lymphadenography
   b. lymphography
   c. lymphangiography
   d. lymphoscintography

5. Iodine contrast for a lymphangiogram is injected:
   a. as a single bolus
   b. to determine position of superficial lymph vessels
   c. slowly over 45 minutes
   d. at 15-minute intervals until 2 hours

CASE STUDY

A teenager, who appears asymptomatic but with suspected Hodgkin's disease, is admitted. Describe the main features of this disease and discuss the various diagnostic procedures she might undergo.

References and Recommended Reading

Berland, L. L. (1987). *Practical CT technology and techniques.* New York: Raven Press.

Brant, W. E., & Helms, C. A. (1994). *Fundamentals of diagnostic radiology.* Baltimore: Williams & Wilkins.

Castenada-Zuniga, W., & Tadavarthy, S. M., (1992). *Interventional radiology (Vol. 2).* Baltimore: Williams & Wilkins.

Chapman, S., & Nakielny, R. (1993). *A guide to radiological procedures* (3rd ed.). London: Bailliere Tindall.

Dowd, S. B., & Wilson, B. G. (1995). *Encyclopedia of radiographic positioning.* Philadelphia: Saunders.

Doyle, T., Hare, W., Thomson, K., & Tress, B. (1989). *Procedures in diagnostic radiology.* London: Churchill Livingstone.

Eisenberg, R. L. (1992). *Radiology, an illustrated history.* St. Louis: Mosby-Year Book.

Greene, R. E., & Oestmann, J-W. (1992). *Computed digital radiography in clinical practice.* New York: Thieme.

Pond, G. D., & Castellino, R. A., et al. (1989). Non-Hodgkin lymphoma: Influence of lymphography, CT and bone marrow biopsy on staging and management. *Radiology, 170*(1), 159–164.

Selby, P., & McElwain, T. J. (Eds.). (1987). *Hodgkin's Disease.* Oxford: Blackwell Scientific.

Snopek, A.M. (1992). *Fundamentals of special radiographic procedures* (3rd. ed.). Philadelphia: Saunders.

Sutton, D.A. (1992). *Textbook of radiology and imaging* (5th ed.). Edinburgh: Churchill Livingstone.

Taber's Cyclopedic Medical Dictionary (17th ed.). (1989). Philadelphia: F. A. Davis.

Tortorici, M.R., & Apfel, P. (1995). *Advanced radiographic and angiographic procedures.* Philadelphia: Davis.

SECTION V

URINARY SYSTEM

CHAPTER 11

Urinary System

PETER LLOYD, DCR, ARMIT, Grad Dip, FEd

OBJECTIVES

At the completion of this chapter, the student should be able to:

1. Describe the procedures used in the studies of the urinary system.
2. Describe the applied anatomy of all relevant areas of study.
3. List the major indications and contraindications for each procedure.
4. Identify the equipment used.
5. List contrast media types.
6. Identify radiation protection methods used.
7. List radiographs/images for each procedure.
8. Describe patient preparation for the procedures.
9. Describe procedure sequences.
10. List alternative radiographs/images.
11. Describe postprocedure care.
12. List common pathologies.
13. Identify other imaging modalities used for the urinary system.
14. Describe basic concepts of alternative imaging routines.
15. Describe interventional procedures used for the urinary system.

Introduction and Historical Overview

Imaging of the urinary system has advanced greatly since early plain film radiography. The development of a satisfactory cystoscope allowed the introduction of catheters into the ureters and the first attempt to outline the ureters was by Tuffier in 1897, using a radiopaque catheter. In 1903, Wittek was able to demonstrate a stone in a bladder by filling it with air. By 1905, the same examination was performed using an early form of contrast media.

The development of contrast agents opened up a whole new range of radiologic examinations. IV urography became possible when nontoxic iodinated substances were discovered that provided a safe study (1929). Cystography and retrograde pyelography soon used this type of contrast, and angiography of the renal system followed. The use of radioisotopes (now called radiopharmaceuticals) further developed diagnostic procedures. In more recent years CT, diagnostic ultrasound, MRI, and digital radiography have played a key part in urologic imaging. **Interventional** radiologic techniques first pioneered in the early 1900s have further expanded the field and are now used widely. Many surgical procedures have become obsolete having been replaced by the more simple and less traumatic interventional procedures.

Anatomy

The urinary system consists of two kidneys that form and excrete urine at the rate of approximately 1 ml/min, bilateral ureters that transport the urine by peristalsis (pĕr-ĭ-stăl´sĭs) to a muscular bladder, and a urethra, which conveys urine from the bladder.

Each kidney is retroperitoneal, paravertebral, and subdiaphragmatic and extends from T11 to L3. The right kidney is approximately 2.5 cm lower than the left because of the liver above (Figure 11.1).

An abundance of adipose tissue surrounds each kidney with an outer layer of tissue, the renal fascia. This fascia, along with surrounding organs and renal vessels, maintains the kidney in somewhat of a stable position.

The kidneys are generally perfused with about 600 mL of blood per minute, representing about 20% to 25% of cardiac output during that time. From the abdominal aorta, the renal artery enters the hilum (hī´lŭm) of the kidney and divides into major branches directed toward the superior, middle, and inferior segments of the kidney.

The interlobar arteries arise from the branches of the renal artery that lie on the renal columns between adjacent pyramids. On the bases of the pyramids, each interlobar artery arches over the pyramid base to become the arcuate artery. All interlobar arteries arising from the arcuate arteries extend into the cortex to give rise to the afferent arterioles that supply the microscopic glomeruli (glō-mĕr´ū-lī) (Figures 11.2 and 11.3).

The bilateral ureters, muscular tubes that convey the urine to the bladder, have both an abdominal part and a pelvic component. The abdominal part lies on the psoas (sō-´ăs) major muscle; the pelvic portion is against the pelvic wall. Each empties into the bladder at the ureteropelvic junction.

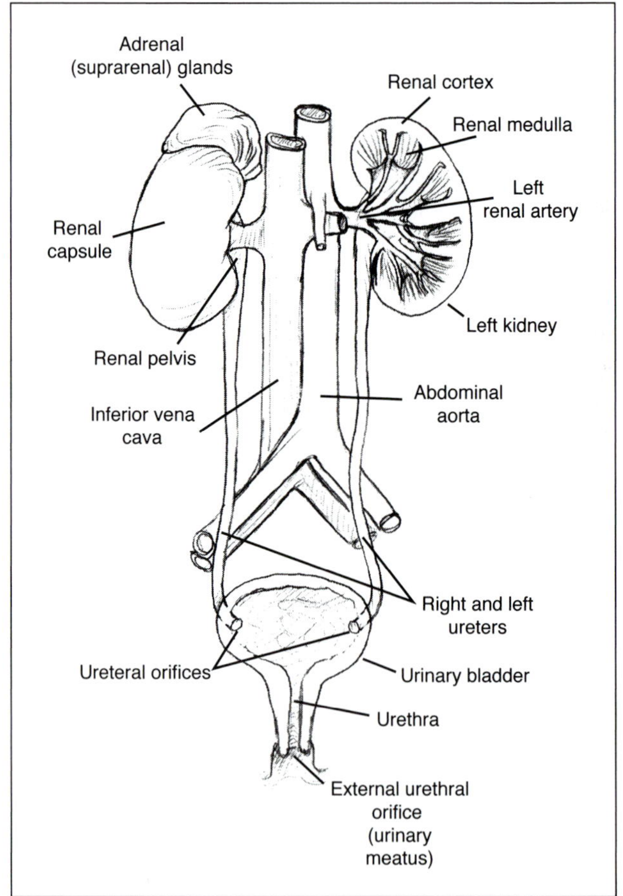

FIGURE 11.1 Anatomy of urinary system.

The muscular urinary bladder, situated in the pelvic cavity, is anterior to the rectum in the male and anterior to the vagina and neck of the uterus in the female (Figure 11.4).

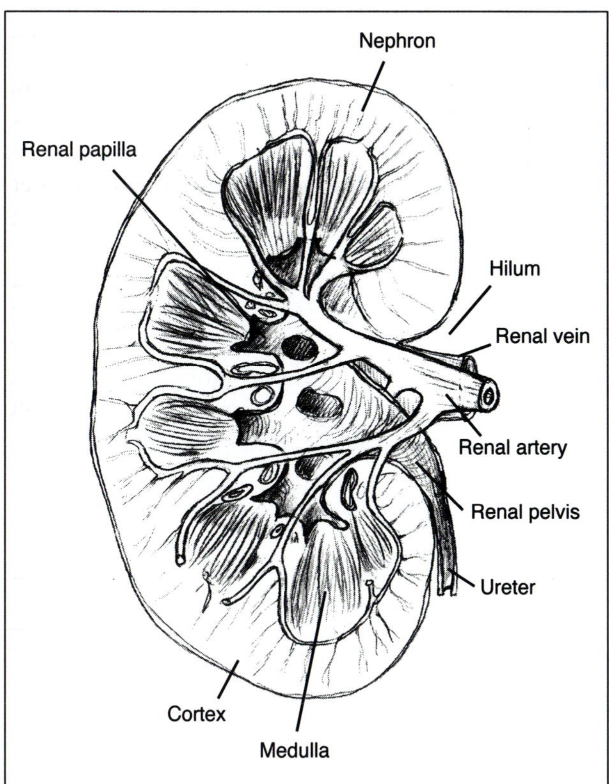

FIGURE 11.2 Internal structures of the kidney.

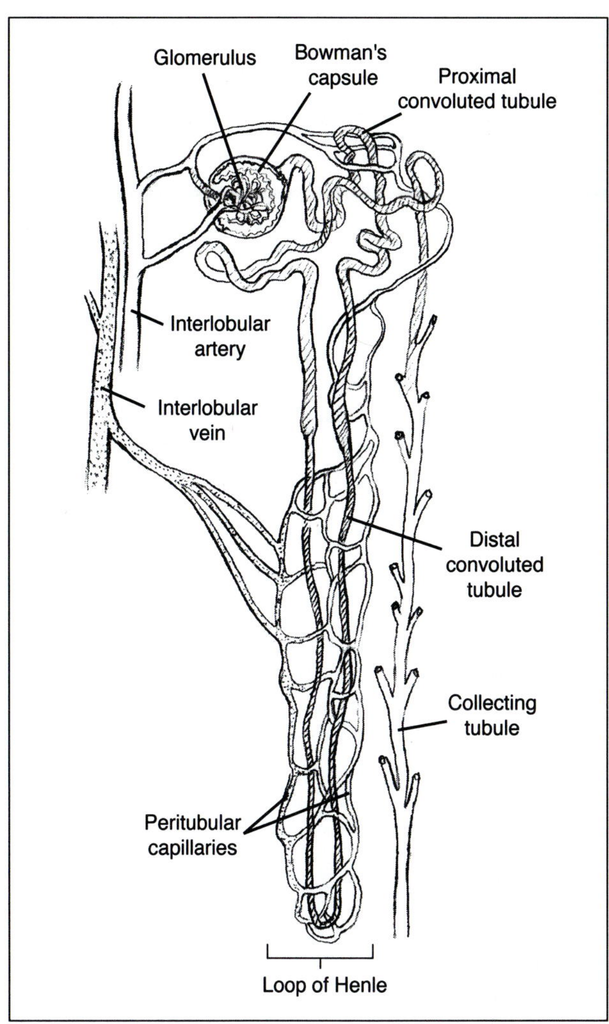

FIGURE 11.3 Blood supply of the kidney.

The urethra carries the urine from the bladder. In the male it is divided into prostatic, membranous, and spongy components. The female urethra is approximately 4 cm in length and is closely applied to the anterior wall of the vagina.

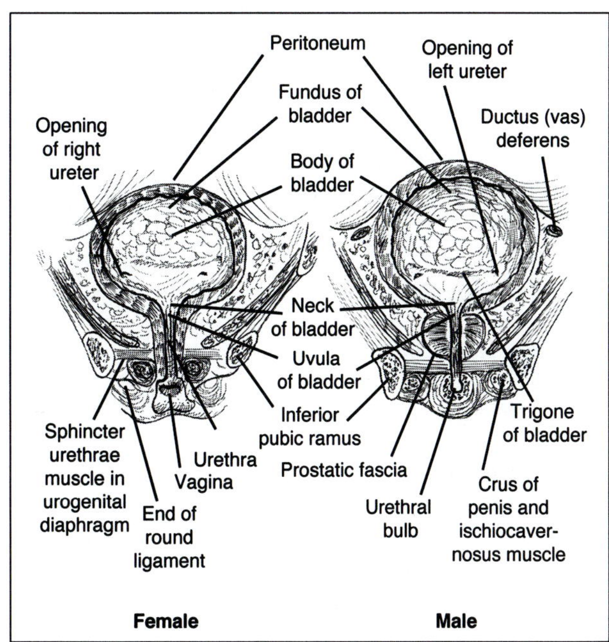

FIGURE 11.4 Female and male bladder.

Procedures

RETROGRADE PYELOGRAPHY

Retrograde pyelography (pī´´ĕ-lŏg´ră-fē) is a radiologic examination of the kidney and ureter using a contrast medium that is introduced by inserting a catheter into the ureter, via the bladder using a cystoscope. This examination has specific but limited use because it only determines structure and not function of the urinary system. The procedure is carried out under aseptic conditions in a specially adapted x-ray room or operating theater. It can be performed under sedation, although general anesthesia is more common.

Applied Anatomy The retrograde pyelogram shows only the structure of the urinary system (Figure 11.5).

Indications

- Unsatisfactory or inconclusive IV urogram
- Patient unable to receive IV contrast
- More accurate demonstration of ureteral fistula required
- Presence of **calculi** (kăl´kū-lī)
- Filling defect demonstrated on an IV urogram

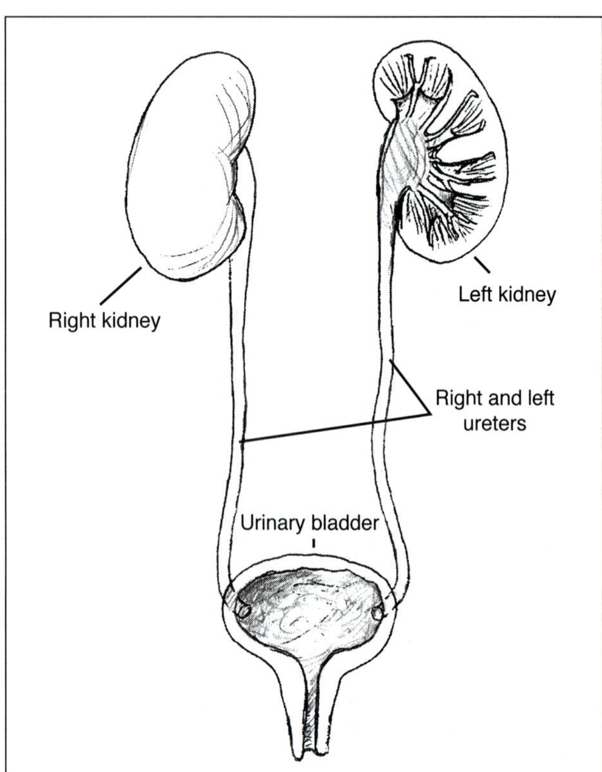

FIGURE 11.5 Kidneys, ureters, and bladder (KUB).

Contraindications Contrast reactions are possible but rare.

Equipment

- Conventional fluoroscopy x-ray unit with spot film device or
- Fluoroscopy unit in conjunction with cystoscopy table or
- Conventional general purpose x-ray unit or
- General purpose x-ray tube and gantry in conjunction with cystoscopy table
- Leg stirrups should always be available.
- Sterile tray containing cystoscope, catheters, syringe, cleansing equipment
- Gloves and sterile clothing available

Contrast Media

- Water-soluble, nonionic medium is preferred, but due to its expense and the fact that the contrast will remain only within the urinary system, thus reducing the likelihood of reaction, water-soluble, ionic media may be used.
- Three to 5 mL per normal-sized adult kidney
- Syringe injection or infusion. The syringe injection is more popular because it allows for control of the contrast by the administrator.

Radiation Protection

- Adequate collimation
- Minimal fluoroscopy time
- Minimal number of radiographic exposures (gonadal protection not possible)

Preliminary Radiographs An AP projection covering whole of renal tract (including the bladder) is taken with the catheter in place.

Patient Preparation Sedation or premedication appropriate to general anesthesia

Procedure Sequence

- Patient is placed supine on appropriate table, with the knees flexed over stirrups.
- The patient is draped appropriately (Figure 11.6).
- A radiopaque catheter is inserted into the ureter via cystoscope, usually a 4 to 7 French (Figure 11.7).
- The position of the catheter is checked by fluoroscopy or preliminary radiograph.

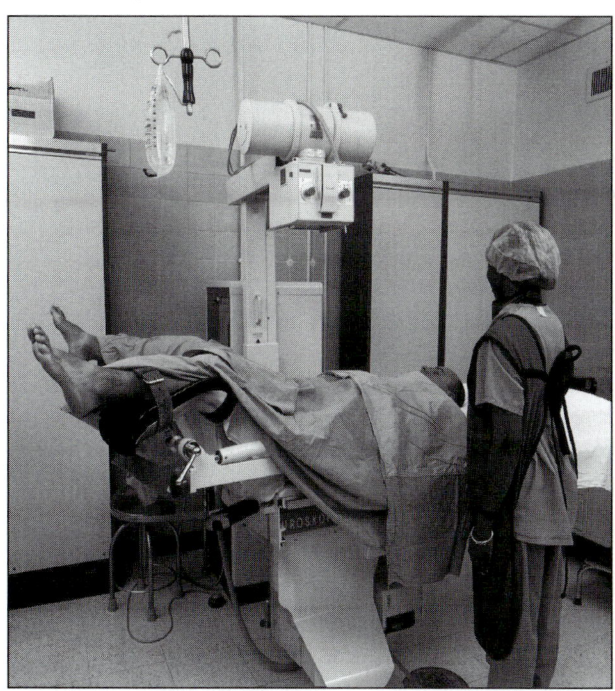

FIGURE 11.6 Patient draped and prepared for retrograde pyelogram.

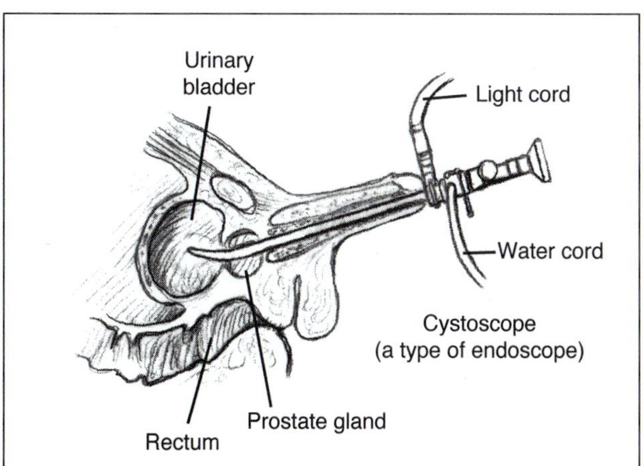

FIGURE 11.7 Catheter introduced via cystoscope.

- Three to 5 mL of contrast is injected. Fluoroscopic control may be used to visualize the pathway of the contrast media.
- Radiographs are taken on arrested respiration.

Procedure Radiographs Depending on the type of equipment used, radiographs will be AP for over-couch tube (or PA for under-couch tube)

- AP projection of kidneys and ureters with maximum filling (Figure 11.8)

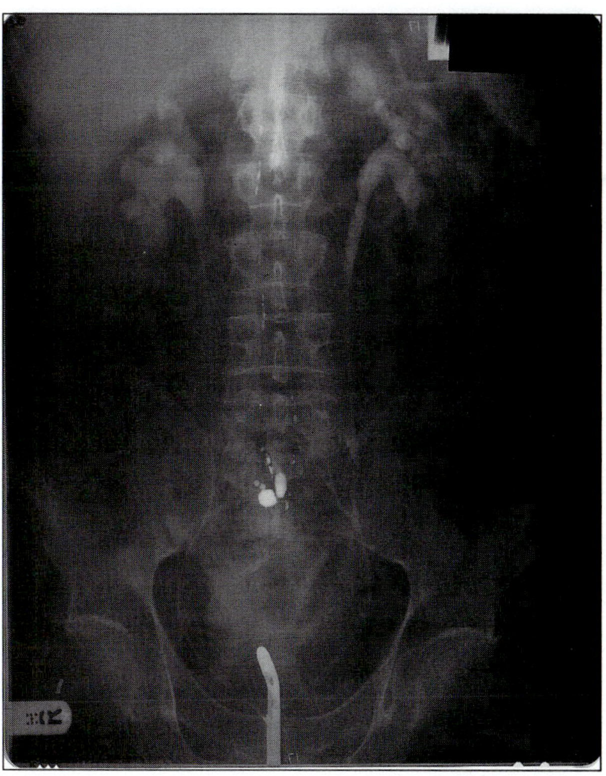

FIGURE 11.8 Abdomen (kidneys, ureter, bladder) with catheter.

- AP projection of kidneys and ureters immediately following removal of catheter (Figure 11.9). A further injection of contrast is required, with the catheter withdrawn during the latter part of the injection. This enables the ureters to be filled with contrast before draining.

NOTE: Sometimes the catheter is left in place to drain an obstruction and withdrawal radiographs are not possible.

Alternative Radiographs

- 35° posterior oblique views of each kidney and ureter (Figure 11.10)
- Lateral view of kidney or ureters
- AP projection of kidneys and ureters 5 to 15 minutes after removal of catheter

NOTE: All radiographs should be numbered sequentially to identify them.

Postprocedure Care

- Normal postanesthetic care as required
- Observe for blood in urine (**hematuria**) (hē´´mă-tū´rē-ă).

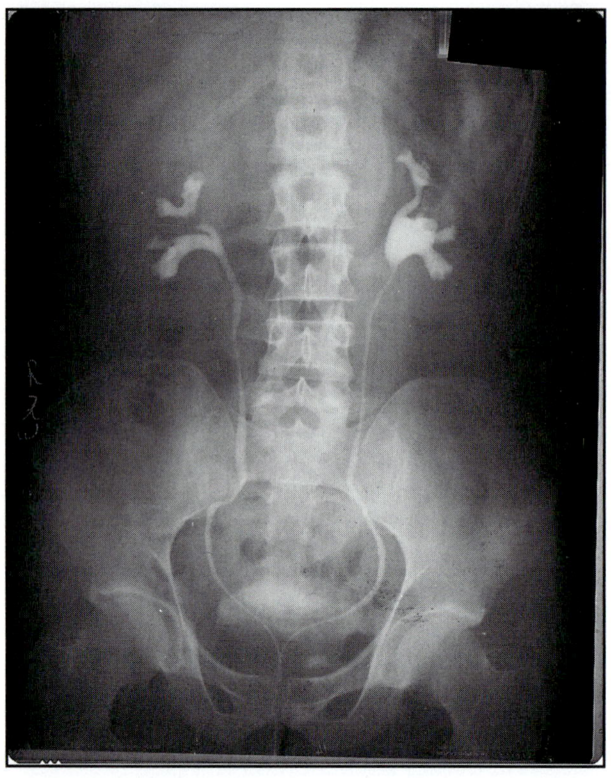

FIGURE 11.9 AP projection of abdomen (KUB) without catheter.

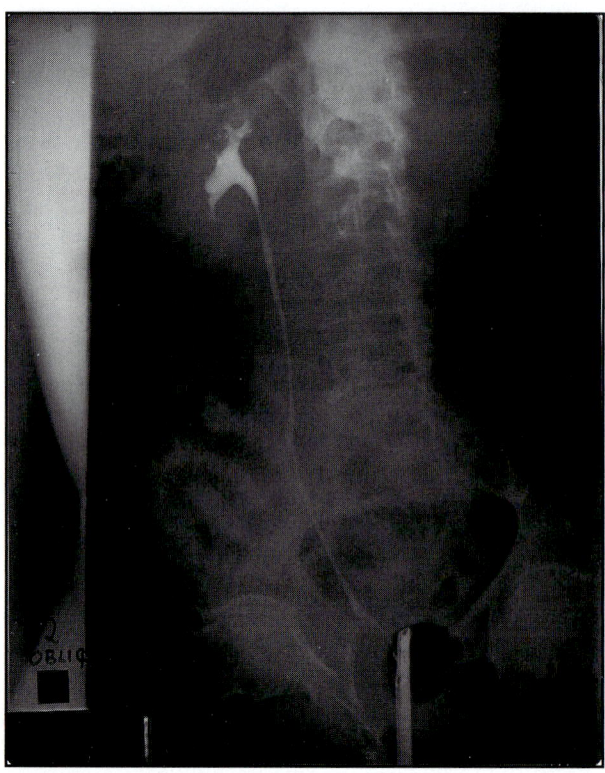

FIGURE 11.10 35° oblique posterior view of ureter.

- Hydrate. Intake and output should be monitored for 24 hours to ensure that the kidney is functioning appropriately.

Common Pathologies

- Presence of stones (Figure 11.11)
- **Hydronephrosis** (hī′drō-nĕf-rō′sĭs) (Figure 11.12)

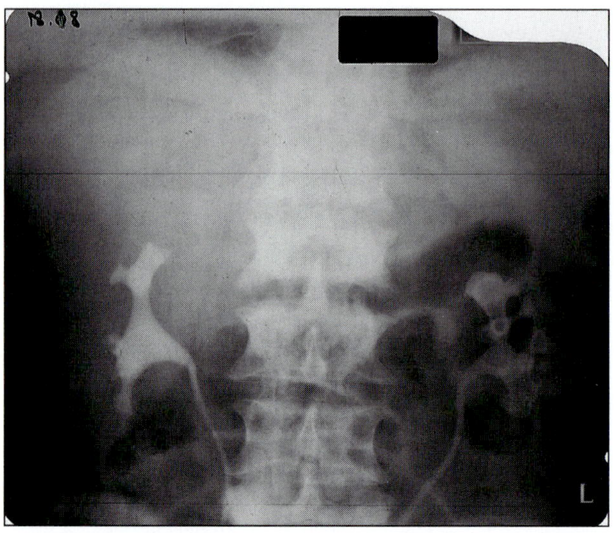

FIGURE 11.11 Presence of stones.

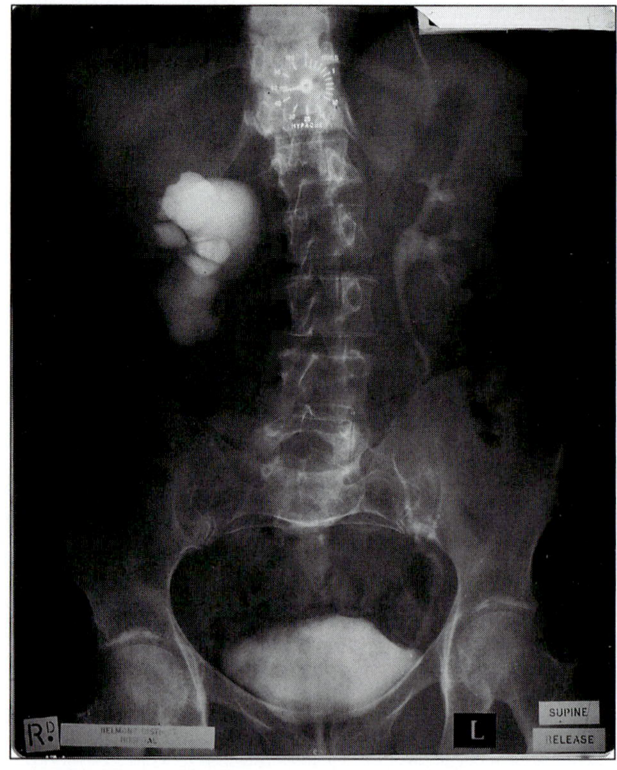

FIGURE 11.12 Hydronephrosis.

ASCENDING URETHROGRAPHY

Ascending (or retrograde) urethrography is a contrast examination of the male urethra. In most cases the voiding (micturating) cystourethrogram adequately visualizes the urethra (see Chapter 18, Urinary System, in Volume I). In some cases a retrograde urethrogram is necessary to adequately demonstrate strictures or anterior urethral disease.

Indications

- Stricture
- Anterior urethral disease
- Trauma

Contraindications None

Equipment

- Conventional fluoroscopy x-ray unit with spot film device
- Sterile gloves available

Contrast Media

- Water-soluble, ionic media may be used. Because this examination has little likelihood of reaction, the less expensive ionic rather than the nonionic media can be used.
- Hand injection via catheter
- Inject under fluoroscopic control

Radiation Protection

- Adequate collimation
- Minimize fluoroscopy time
- Minimize number of radiographic exposures

Preliminary Radiograph

- Patient lies in a 45° posterior oblique position
- Lower limb flexed at hip and knee
- Penis lies on flexed thigh.
- Film coverage to include bladder and whole urethra

Patient Preparation Empty bladder if possible

Procedure Sequence

- Patient lies in a 45° posterior oblique position as for preliminary radiograph.
- A small Foley catheter is inserted into distal end of urethra and positioned so that the balloon of the catheter is placed in the fossa navicularis of the penis.
- The balloon is distended with 1 to 2 mL saline to close off the urethral opening and to help maintain the catheter in position.
- Contrast is injected via catheter under fluoroscopic control.
- Contrast should be seen to enter bladder to ensure complete filling of urethra.

NOTE: Various forms of clamps have been used in the past, to maintain position of the catheter, but the balloon catheter is the preferred method in current use.

Procedure Radiographs

- 45° posterior oblique view of whole urethra and bladder on completion of injection (Figure 11.13)
- Postdrainage film in same position after the catheter has been removed

Alternative Radiographs

- Opposite oblique view
- Lateral view

Postprocedure Care There is usually no routine care required but specialized care relevant to the pathology being investigated may be appropriate.

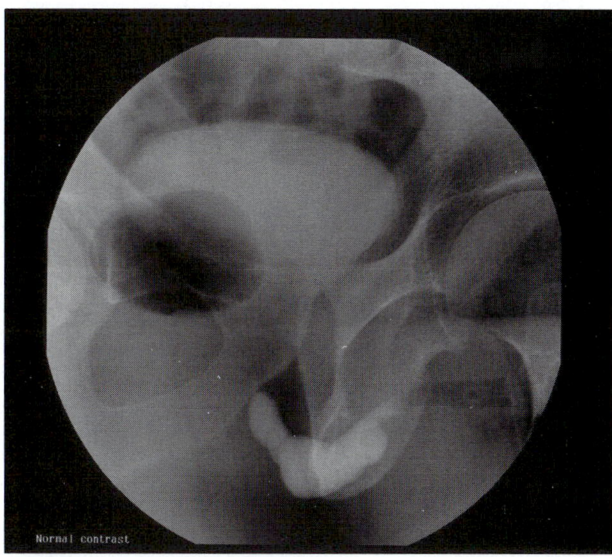

FIGURE 11.13 45° posterior oblique.

Common Pathologies

- Strictures (Figure 11.14)
- Anterior urethral disease
- Trauma

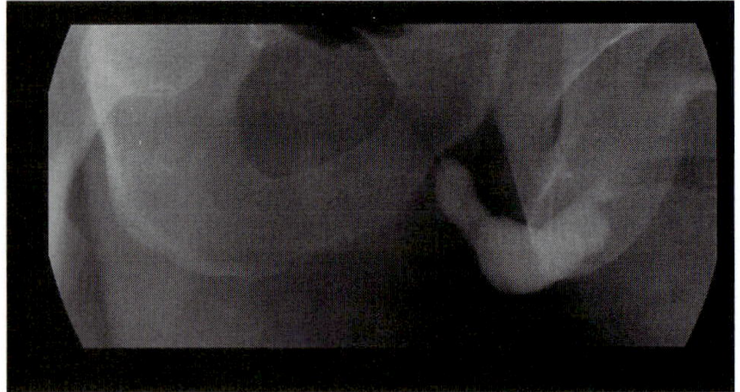

FIGURE 11.14 Demonstration of urethral stricture.

Other Imaging Modalities

COMPUTED TOMOGRAPHY

Computed tomography has a limited but positive role in the investigation of the urinary tract and is usually used in a follow-up role to IV urography and diagnostic ultrasound. CT demonstrates upper urinary tract and surrounding structures in good detail particularly when used in conjunction with an IV contrast medium. Dynamic scanning in conjunction with the use of a contrast medium demonstrates vascular anatomy well and this technique has greatly reduced the use of angiography for lesions of the kidney.

Applied Anatomy (Figure 11.15)

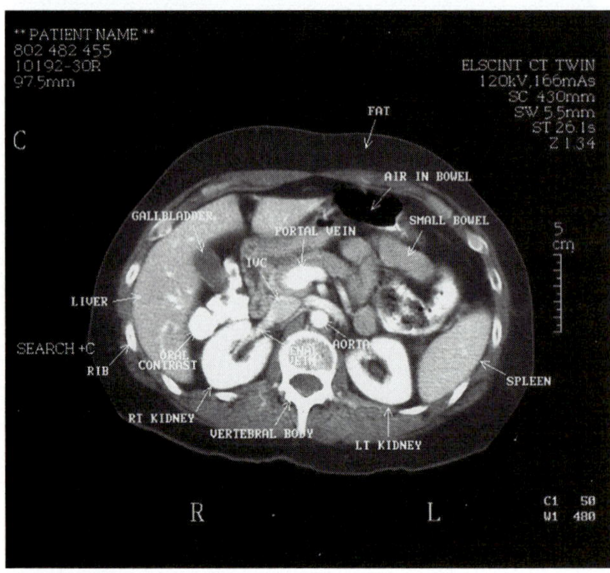

FIGURE 11.15 CT of renal system.

Indications

- Trauma
- Stone
- Tumor
- Hematuria
- Unexplained abdominal pain
- Infection (pus in urine, pyuria)
- Kidney present or not
- Transplant workup

Contraindications Contrast allergy. This can usually be overcome by steroid cover. An IV injection of 4 to 8 mg dexamethasone administered 12 hours before and then again on the day of the examination reduces the risk of an allergic reaction.

Equipment CT scanner

Contrast Media

- Water-soluble, nonionic when injected—approximately 100 mL (see above for steroid cover).
- A 2.5% barium sulfate solution may also be used, PO, to outline alimentary tract.

Radiation Protection Minimize number of exposures.

Preliminary Radiographs Scout of area to be scanned. This will be a planar view of the abdomen to ascertain the level of the kidneys.

Patient Preparation

- Steroid cover if contrast allergy (see above)
- Fluids only for 4 hours before procedure
- 500 mL oral contrast 1 hour before scan

Procedure Sequence

- Patient is supine.
- Position markers are set.
- Scout (AP of abdomen)
- Kidney—pre- and postcontrast scans; 10 mm every 10-mm slice throughout entire kidney.
- Contrast is administered either by IV infusion or bolus injection.
- Scans taken of renal tract (to demonstrate stones)—10-mm slices from top of kidney to base of bladder (precontrast slices 5 mm or 2 mm can be taken).
- Scans to demonstrate condition of bladder (i.e., for presence of a tumor)—10-mm slices every 20 mm, postcontrast, from top of liver to top of bladder, then 5 mm every 5 mm from top of bladder to symphysis pubis.
- Each scan is taken on arrested respiration.

Procedure Radiographs

- High-detail images are preferred because it is sometimes difficult to interpret and differentiate cystic from solid lesions. (Ultrasound does this better.)
- At 60-second postcontrast injection, the cortex is shown with greater attenuation than the medulla (Figure 11.16).

Postprocedure Care

None

Common Pathologies

- Tumor
- Hydronephrosis (Figure 11.17)
- Perirenal pathology
- Renal calculi
- Cysts
- Trauma

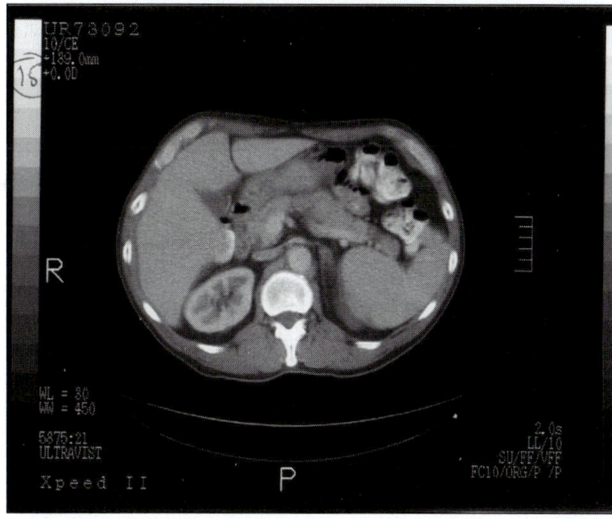

FIGURE 11.16 CT of right kidney.

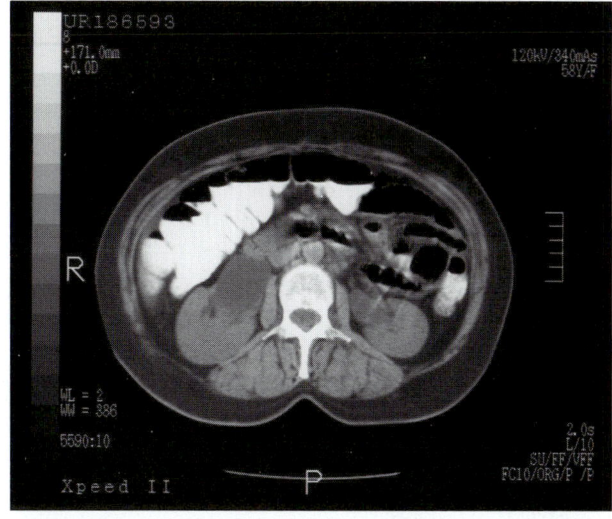

FIGURE 11.17 Hydronephrosis (right kidney).

MAGNETIC RESONANCE IMAGING

Only gradually has MRI evolved as a tool to investigate the urinary tract. Unlike some anatomic areas (e.g., knees) where MRI quickly became the imaging modality of choice, MRI still has only certain advantages over IV pyelograms (IVPs), ultrasound, radionuclide imaging, and CT.

It does have some advantages over CT, including higher intraorgan contrast without the need to inject contrast media. However, the paramagnetic agent, gadolinium, is now being used occasionally to enhance the medulla of the kidney, the ureters, and bladder.

Disadvantages of MRI include the inability to detect small calcifications (new hybrid sequences under investigation may change this); the inability to distinguish between benign and malignant tumors in tissue identification; long image sequences, making movement more likely (although recent developments are making image acquisition faster); and artifacts.

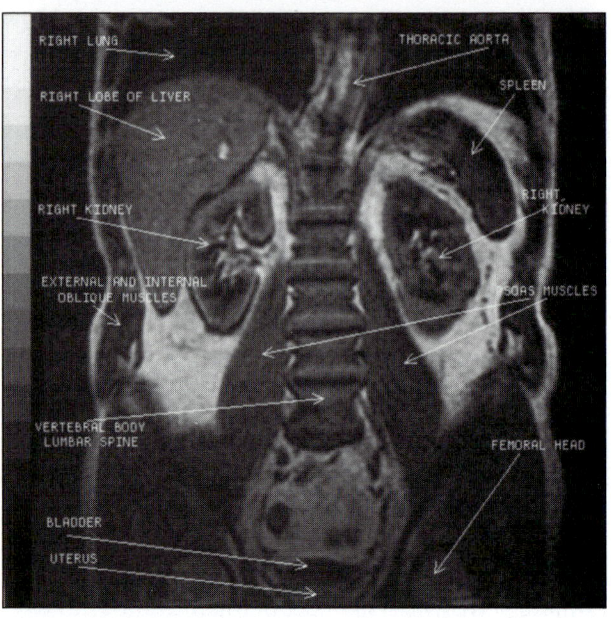

FIGURE 11.19 MRI coronal view of abdomen.

Applied Anatomy (Figures 11.18 and 11.19)

Indications

- Evaluation of mass lesions
- Staging of renal carcinoma for therapy management
- Localization and evaluation of perirenal fluid collections

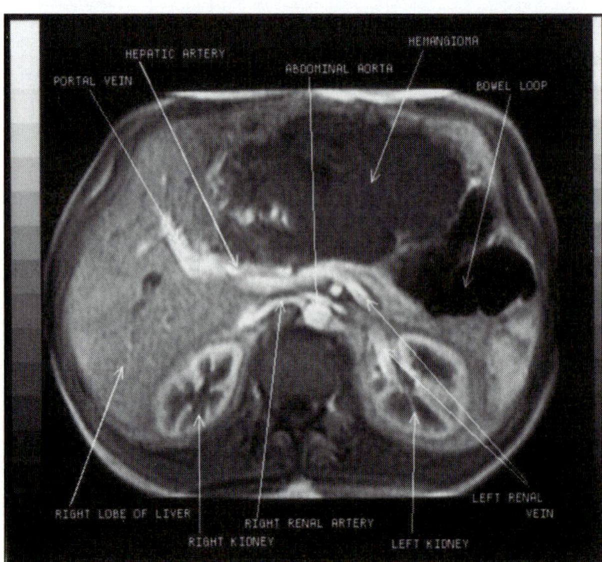

FIGURE 11.18 MRI axial view of abdomen.

Contraindications

- Cardiac pacemaker and other implanted electromechanical devices (i.e., cochlear implants)
- Inability of patient to remain still
- Ferromagnetic objects unable to be removed (especially in strategic locations)
- Intraocular metallic foreign bodies
- Inability to fit into unit (although recent designs will eliminate this contraindication)

Equipment MRI scanner

Contrast Media

- None usually
- Gadolinium occasionally used (a paramagnetic contrast media)

Radiation Protection Not applicable

Patient Preparation

- Remove all ferromagnetic objects where possible (screen patients by means of a questionnaire).
- Sedation may be necessary.

Procedure Sequence

- Patient supine. The patient is scanned using various protocols, which are generally defined according to the patient condition and pathology. T1- and T2-weighted images are acquired.
- T1 contrast displays the best anatomy and cortex medulla differentiation (Figure 11.20).
- T2 images allow characterization of fluids and distinction between hemorrhage and cystic transudate.

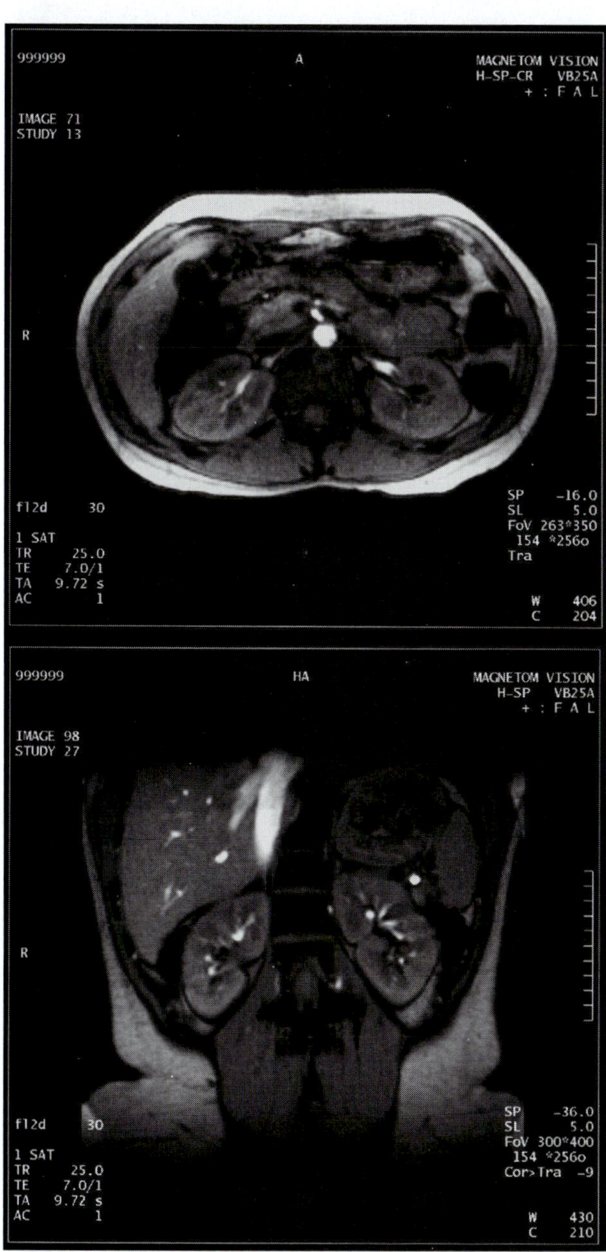

FIGURE 11.20 MRI T1 scan.

> The reconstructional ability of MRI and the development of magnetic resonance angiography has enabled blood vessels to be demonstrated at the same time as the renal structures (Figure 11.21).

Postprocedure Care None

Common Pathologies

- Renal mass lesion
- Simple and complex cysts
- Renal cell carcinoma and other primary solid masses
- Obstructed hydronephrosis

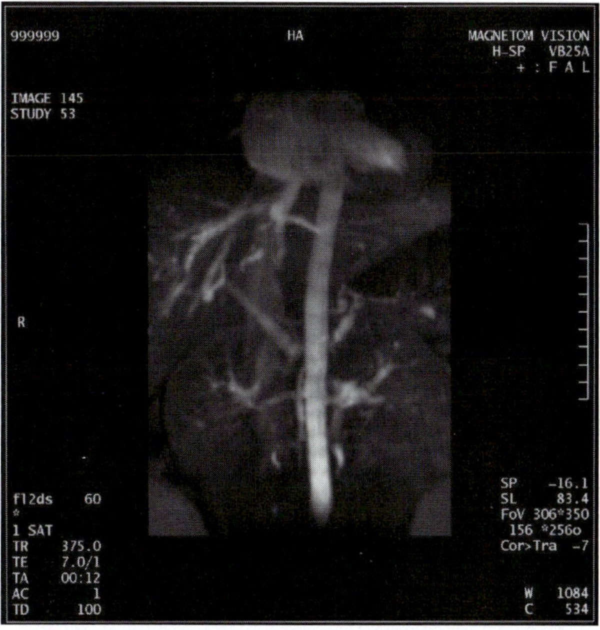

FIGURE 11.21 MRI demonstrating blood supply to kidney.

ULTRASOUND

Ultrasound plays a leading role in renal imaging because it is often the first imaging modality of choice when determining the condition of the kidney. It has no known adverse side effects and does not require contrast medium. Ultrasound can provide sectional images in any plane and real-time images. The only disadvantage acknowledged is its dependency on the operator. As with all ultrasound examinations, false-negative and false-positive results can be created unless the technologist or physician is an experienced and trained ultrasonographer.

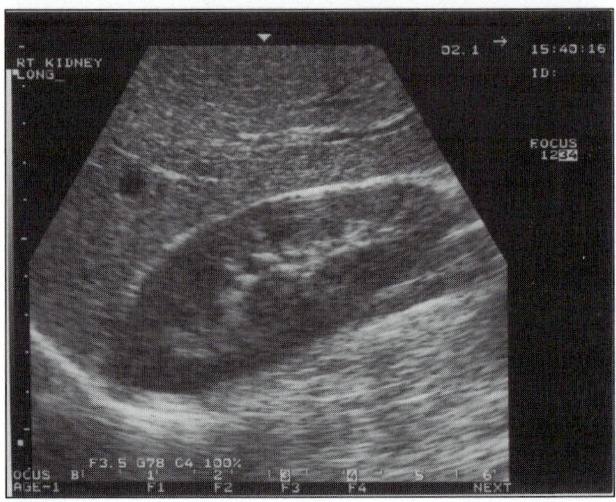

FIGURE 11.22 Ultrasound of right kidney—longitudinal scan.

Indications

- Hydronephrosis
- Adult polycystic kidneys
- Renal mass lesions
- Renal calculi

Contraindications None

Equipment

- Real-time ultrasound unit
- .5-3.5-MHz transducers

Contrast Media None

Radiation Protection Not applicable

Patient Preparation

- May require full bladder, but only if the bladder is the area of interest.
- Contact gel on skin. Gel should be warmed to body heat.

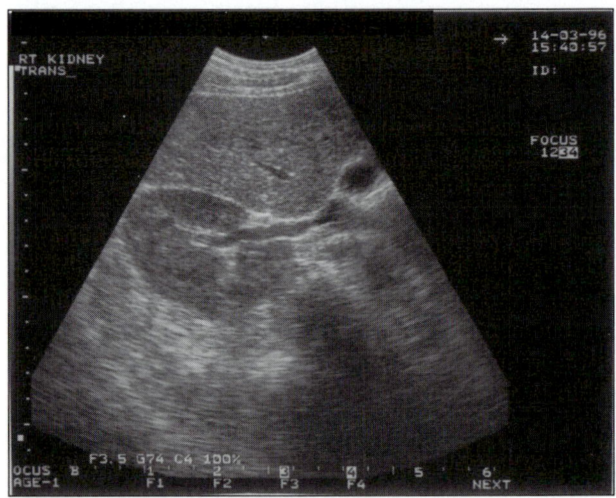

FIGURE 11.23 Ultrasound of right kidney—transverse scan.

Procedure Sequence

- Right kidney—supine longitudinal and transverse (coronal) scans (Figures 11.22 and 11.23)
- Left kidney—decubitus longitudinal (coronal) and transverse scans

Postprocedure Care Empty bladder if appropriate.

Common Pathologies

- Hydronephrosis
- Adult polycystic kidney
- Renal mass lesion
- Renal calculi

RADIONUCLIDE IMAGING

Radionuclide imaging of the renal tract has developed into one of the primary diagnostic tools. As in most studies, it requires an injection of a radiopharmaceutical and relies on organ uptake of a radiopharmaceutical. Emitted radiation patterns are detected and data acquisition methods are used to display the uptake. Copy information is also available. Radionuclide imaging can demonstrate blood supply to and function of kidneys and drainage of urine from kidneys by the ureters into the bladder.

Indications

- Determination of relative renal function
- Determination of glomerular filtration rate
- Ureteral obstruction
- Hydronephrosis
- Renal masses
- Evaluation of hypertension
- Evaluation of renal transplant

Patient Preparation

- Patient is hydrated by drinking 1 to 2 glasses of water.
- Patient is asked to void the bladder.

Procedure Sequence

- Patient is placed over a scintillation gamma camera and a radiopharmaceutical injected. The type depends on the particular study being undertaken.
- Data are acquired at 3-second intervals up to 40 seconds after injection. One minute perfusion for 5 minutes then at 15 and 30 minutes. Other routines can be used depending on specialist need.

Common Pathologies

- Renal function
- Hydronephrosis
- Ureteral reflux
- Renovascular hypertension
- Renal transplant
- Pyelonephritis
- Residual urine
- Urinary tract obstruction
- Renal artery stenosis
- Pelvic ureteric junction obstruction

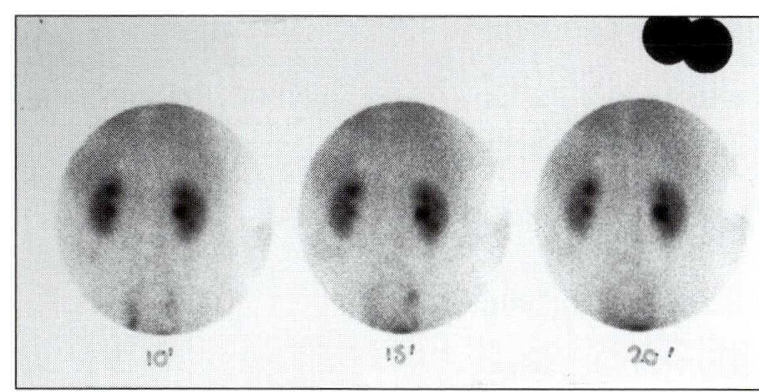

FIGURE 11.24 Nuclear medicine scans of kidney.

Interventional Procedures

Interventional procedures of the renal system are mainly carried out by means of percutaneous injection or insertion. They are procedures that can be diagnostic or therapeutic or both. Aseptic technique is used to perform these procedures, which are usually carried out under fluoroscopic control, preferably using a C-arm x-ray system. Sedation and local anesthetic are generally used.

Indications

- Acute hydronephrosis
- Obstruction, intra- or extraureteral
- Tumor
- Acute renal failure

Contraindications Abnormal bleeding parameters

Equipment

- Fluoroscopic C-arm unit preferred
- Other biplane or single plane fluoroscopic units can be used.
- Sterile tray containing percutaneous equipment, catheters, stents, and so on
- Gloves and gown for aseptic technique

Contrast Media Water-soluble, nonionic

Radiation Protection

- Adequate collimation
- Minimize fluoroscopy time.
- Minimize number of radiographic exposures.
- Gonad shielding if possible

Preliminary Radiograph A plain film of the area may be required.

Patient Preparation Conventional **neurolept sedation** is preferred.

ANTEGRADE PYELOGRAPHY

Antegrade pyelography involves a percutaneous needle puncture of the kidney collecting system. It is a diagnostic examination used independently or as the initial part of other interventional procedures. It involves the direct injection of a contrast medium into the kidney.

Indications Failed routine methods, IV urogram and retrograde pyelogram.

Contraindications Abnormal bleeding parameters

Procedure Sequence

- Patient prone (position may vary depending on personal preference, condition of the patient and type of equipment used).
- An IV injection of contrast may be administered before start of the pyelogram to aid renal visualization.
- Ultrasound can also be used to locate the kidney.
- Local anesthetic is injected subcutaneously at the site of entry.
- A 22- to 23-gauge needle is inserted percutaneously directly into the kidney collecting system (Figure 11.25).
- The injection site is posterior and subcostal, although intercostal injection sites may be necessary.
- The needle is vertical.
- Opinion differs on the question of arrested respiration or not, although arrested respiration appears to be the more common procedure.
- Anesthetizing the entire needle track is optional.
- Aspiration of urine confirms that the needle tip is correctly sited.
- Contrast medium is injected.

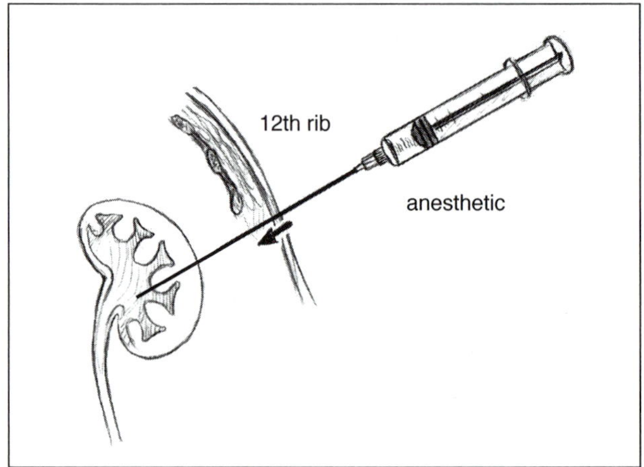

FIGURE 11.25 Needle entering kidney.

Procedure Radiographs Spot films may be taken as required.

Postprocedure Care

- Standard postsedation observations
- Fluids given
- Puncture site checked

Common Pathologies

- Acute hydronephrosis
- Obstructions
- Tumor

PERCUTANEOUS NEPHROSTOMY

Percutaneous **nephrostomy** is the insertion of a percutaneous access tube directly into the kidney using the Seldinger technique to facilitate remedial procedures. A contrast medium is often used. This aseptic procedure is commonly performed under sedation and local anesthesia.

Indications

- Obstruction
- Functional assessment
- Collecting system access
  - Stricture dilatation
  - **Stent** placement
  - Calculus therapy
  - Biopsy
  - Nephroscopy
  - Internal surgery

Contraindications

- Abnormal bleeding parameters
- Untreated urinary tract infection
- Surgical mass lesion
- Dermatologic reasons
- Anatomic abnormalities

Procedure Sequence

- Patient prone (position may vary depending on personal preference, condition of the patient and type of equipment used).
- Local anesthetic is injected subcutaneously at the site of entry.
- An antegrade pyelogram is carried out first.
- A 22- to 23-gauge needle is inserted percutaneously directly into a kidney calyx.
- The injection site is posterolateral and subcostal, although intercostal injection sites may be necessary.
- A needle angle of 30° lateromedially is required to ensure that the kidney is punctured and the needle enters the kidney at its lateral aspect.
- Opinion differs on the question of arrested respiration or not.
- Anesthetizing the entire needle track is optional.
- Aspiration of urine confirms that the needle tip is correctly sited.
- Contrast media and fluoroscopy may be used to confirm correct location and aid visualization of the system (Figure 11.26).
- A guidewire is inserted through the needle and advanced to the bladder if possible. It is felt by some that a small coil of wire in the pelvis of the kidney is sufficient.

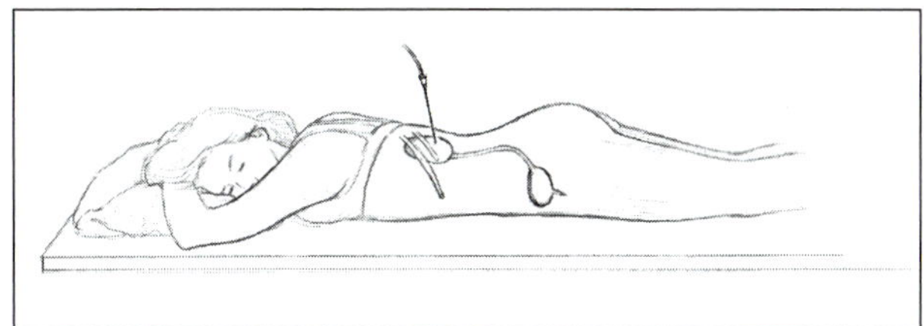

FIGURE 11.26 Patient in position for percutaneous nephrostomy.

- The needle is removed and a 5 French catheter is threaded over the guidewire until its tip lies within the kidney pelvis (Figure 11.27). (A cobra catheter is sometimes preferred.)
- The fine guidewire may be replaced by one of more rigid structure.
- The 5 French catheter is then replaced by progressively larger dilators, which are advanced over the guidewire.
- Fluoroscopic visualization is essential.
- When the track is sufficiently dilated a multihole pigtail drainage tube of 7 to 11 French is advanced over the guidewire.
- Once the drainage tube is in place the guidewire is removed. (It may be left in place if further procedures are likely.)
- The tube must be fixed securely to the skin surface. Several devices are available for this purpose.
- Stone removal, stricture dilation, drainage, or stent placement may be carried out via this tube.
- A drainage bag may be connected.

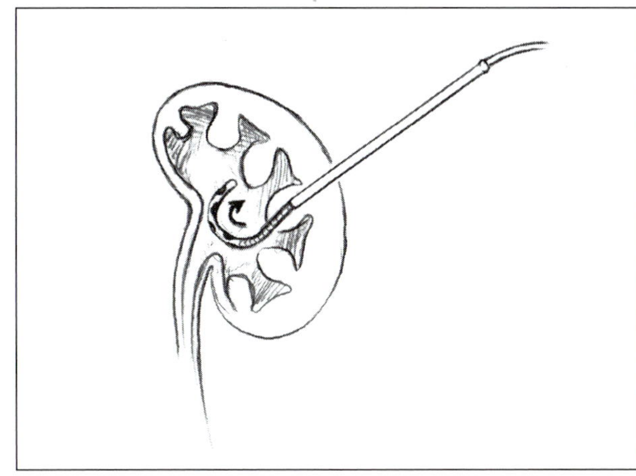

FIGURE 11.27 Catheter inserted through dilator.

Procedure Radiographs Spot films may be taken as required (Figures 11.28 and 11.29).

Postprocedure Care

- Standard postsedation observations.
- Check puncture site.
- Give fluids.
- Check tube fixation.
- Check tube draining if appropriate.

Common Pathologies

- Obstruction
- Stones
- Trauma

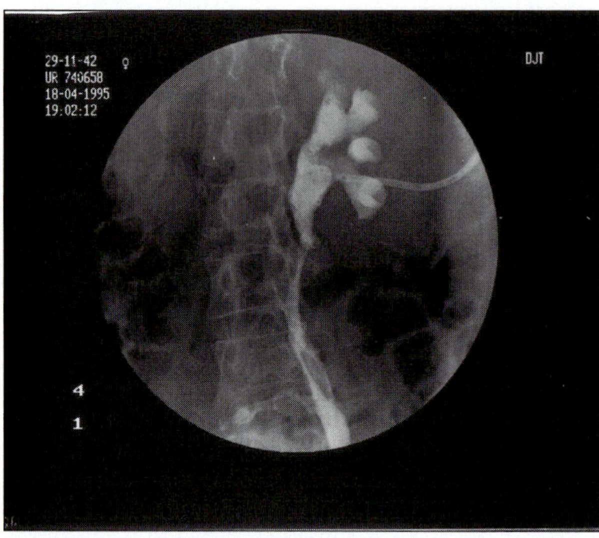

FIGURE 11.28 Injection into kidney.

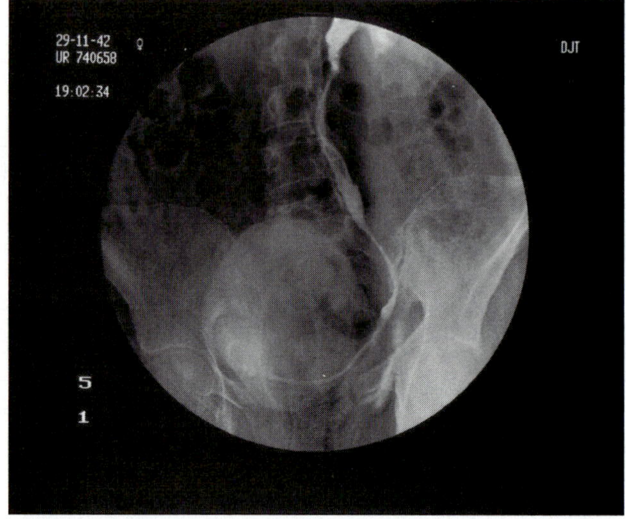

FIGURE 11.29 Catheter fed through to bladder.

PERCUTANEOUS REMOVAL OF URINARY CALCULI

This is carried out via a percutaneous drainage tube. The procedure is similar to that described for percutaneous nephrostomy. General anesthesia is usually required.

Indications Renal calculi

Contraindications

- Abnormal bleeding parameters
- Untreated urinary tract infection
- Surgical mass lesion
- Dermatologic reasons
- Anatomic abnormalities

Procedure Sequence

- The procedure up to the insertion of the drainage tube is the same as for percutaneous nephrostomy.
- The drainage tube used would be of larger size, 14 to 15 French.
- A conventional cystoscope or nephroscope may be used in conjunction with any one of the many stone removal devices (Figure 11.30).

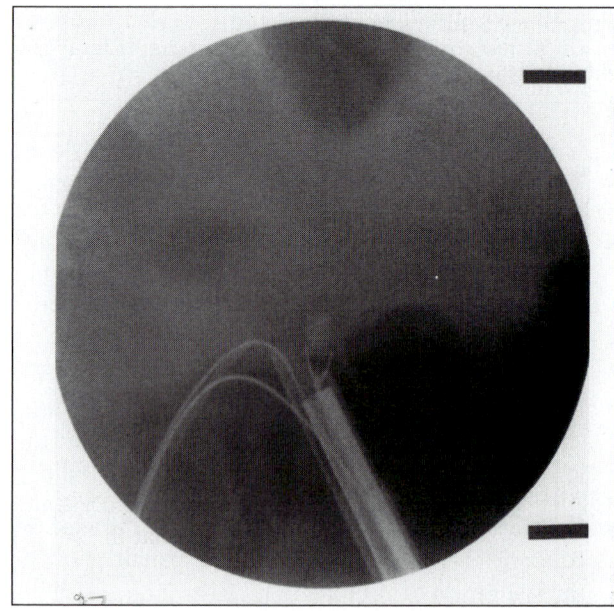

FIGURE 11.30 Percutaneous stone removal.

- For large stones an ultrasonic lithotripsy unit may be used to break them up before removal.
- Some stones may be completely shattered and flushed out.
- More modern ultrasonic lithotripsy units are capable of completely disintegrating calculi from outside the patient, eliminating the need for percutaneous procedures.

Postprocedure Care

- Standard postsedation observations
- Check puncture site.
- Give fluids.
- Check tube fixation and drainage.

Common Pathologies

- Obstruction
- Stones
- Trauma

PLACEMENT OF URETERIC STENTS

This insertion of a catheter inside a ureter is performed following percutaneous nephrostomy. A retrograde method can be used if necessary.

Indications

- Obstructions (ureteric or extrinsic)
- Fistula
- Stenosis
- Trauma

Contraindications

- Untreated urinary tract infection
- Bladder abnormality
- Untreated bleeding disorder
- Wire unable to pass stricture

Procedure Sequence

Antegrade Approach

- The procedure is carried out following percutaneous nephrostomy.
- Fluoroscopic control is used throughout the procedure.
- Several types of stents are available but a double pigtail radiopaque catheter (one at each end) is popular (Figure 11.31).
- A guidewire is introduced via the nephrostomy tube until its tip reaches the bladder.
- The stent is advanced over the guidewire until the tip of the catheter almost reaches the tip of the guidewire.
- A pushing device may be used to advance the stent.
- The guidewire is then withdrawn so that the pigtail the ends of the catheter (stent) remain curled in the bladder and kidney pelvis.
- The nephrostomy tube is often left in place for 24 hours to ensure good drainage.

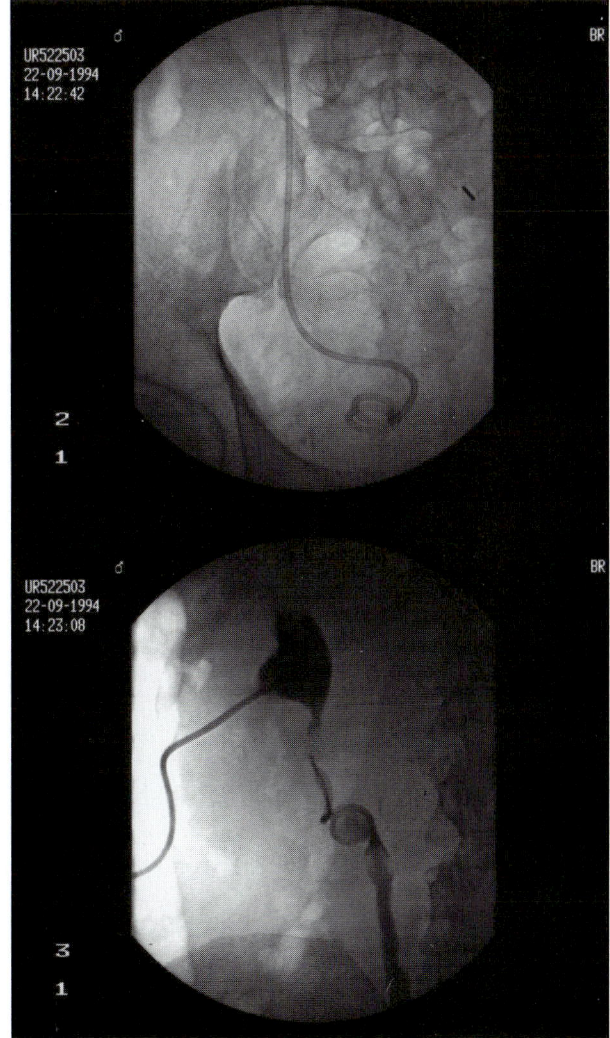

FIGURE 11.31 Stents in place.

Retrograde Approach This technique is similar to the insertion of retrograde catheters, but a pigtail stent and guidewire advanced via the urethra using a cystoscope.

Postprocedure Care

- Standard postsedation observations
- Check puncture site.
- Give fluids.
- Check tube fixation and drainage.

Common Pathologies Ureteric stenosis

PLACEMENT OF DILATION BALLOONS

A balloon catheter inserted into a stricture of the urethra or ureter will, when blown up, dilate the stricture. Ureteral dilations can be carried out by an antegrade or retrograde method. A range of balloon catheters is available.

Indications Stricture of urethra or ureter

Contraindications

- Retrograde—no real contraindications.
- Antegrade—similar to those of a percutaneous nephrostomy

Procedure Sequence

Antegrade Ureter

- This is carried out following the procedure for a percutaneous nephrostomy.
- The guidewire is introduced via the nephrostomy until the tip is well past the ureter stricture.
- A catheter with a 4 to 6mm balloon is advanced over the guidewire until the balloon covers the area of the stricture.
- The balloon is blown up and kept in position for a short while.
- The balloon is then deflated and the catheter removed.
- The wire remains in place temporarily in case further dilation is required.
- A stent may be inserted on a temporary basis.

Retrograde Ureter

- A guidewire is inserted into the ureter via the urethra using a cystoscope.
- A catheter with a 4 to 6mm balloon is advanced up the guidewire until the balloon is within the stricture.
- The balloon is blown up and kept in position for a short while.
- The balloon is then deflated and the catheter removed.
- The wire remains in place temporarily in case further dilation is required.
- A stent may be inserted on a temporary basis.

Retrograde Urethra

- A guidewire is inserted into the urethra until the tip enters the bladder.
- A catheter with a 4 to 6mm balloon is advanced over the guidewire until the balloon is within the stricture.
- The balloon is blown up and kept in position for a short while.
- The balloon is then deflated and the catheter removed.
- The wire remains in place temporarily in case further dilation is required.
- A stent is then placed in the urethra for a period of approximately 24 hours.

Postprocedure Care

- Standard postsedation observations
- Check puncture site if appropriate.
- Give fluids.
- Check stent for drainage.

Common Pathologies Stricture

LITHOTRIPSY

Extracorporeal Shock Wave Lithotripsy (ESWL)

Lithotripsy involves the disintegration of urinary calculi using sound waves. It does not require any invasive procedures because the shock waves are applied through the tissues. The procedure is performed under x-ray fluoroscopy control.

Indications Renal, ureteral, or bladder stones

Contraindications

- Pregnancy
- Hemophilia
- Receiving blood thinning drugs
- Weight more than 380 lb (172.4 kg)
- Stone not seen on x-ray
- Obstruction distal to stone

Equipment Extracorporeal shock wave lithotriptor with C-arm or biplane x-ray fluoroscopy and water-coupling cushion (Figure 11.32) (A gel-coated water cushion ensures efficient passage of shock waves.)

Contrast Media None

Radiation Protection

- Adequate collimation
- Minimize fluoroscopy time.

Preliminary Radiographs None

Patient Preparation

- NPO for 8 hours before treatment
- Blood pressure and vital signs taken
- Neurolept sedation in approximately 60% to 70% of patients
- General anesthetic preparation if required

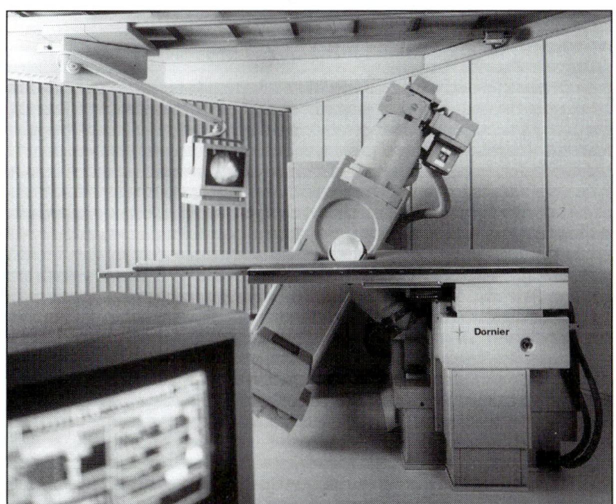

FIGURE 11.32 Lithotriptor (Courtesy of Dornier Medical Systems, Inc.).

Procedure Sequence

- Patient lies supine on the lithotriptor table with relevant area in contact with the gel-coated water cushion.
- Blood pressure cuff is placed on the arm and ECG electrodes are attached to chest.
- The fluoroscopy unit is positioned over the area of interest.
- The stone is localized using the fluoroscopy unit and computerized localizing system.
- The patient's position is automatically adjusted to place the stone in the exact shock wave field (Figure 11.33).
- Shock wave treatment is carried out based on the rhythm of the heartbeat or respiration.
- The disintegration of the stone is monitored throughout.
- Treatment is continued until the stone is reduced to particles small enough to be flushed out in the normal way.
- Treatment may last from 30 to 45 minutes.

Postprocedure Care

- Vital signs monitored for a short while
- Clinical examination
- Plain x-ray may be taken.
- Patient is advised of possible minor pain as stone particles are passed.
- Patient should drink at least 2 liters of fluid a day for 2 or 3 days.

Common Pathologies Urinary stones

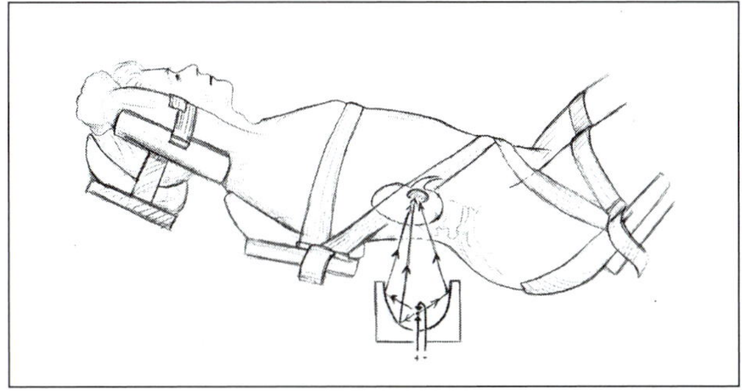

FIGURE 11.33 Patient position for lithotripsy.

Intracorporeal Shock Wave Lithotripsy

This is disintegration of urinary calculi using shock waves and requires direct contact between the tip of the probe and stone. It does not generate heat and there is no limit to number of pulses applied. The probe is introduced using an endoscope via percutaneous nephrostomy or cystoscopy and done under x-ray fluoroscopy control.

Indications Renal, ureteral, or bladder stones not retrieved by other methods

Contraindications Only those associated with percutaneous nephrostomy or cystoscopy.

Equipment

- Intracorporeal shock wave lithotriptor with probes ranging from 0.8 to 2.0 mm in diameter and pulse wave variation (Figures 11.34, 11.35, and 11.36).

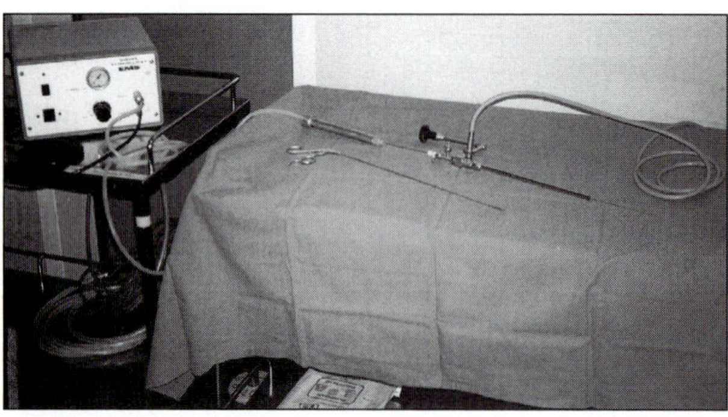

FIGURE 11.34 Intracorporeal lithotriptor.

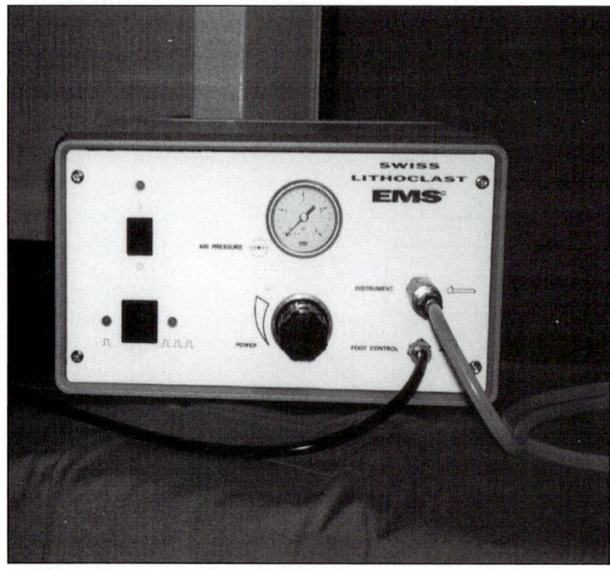

FIGURE 11.35 Lithoclast machine.

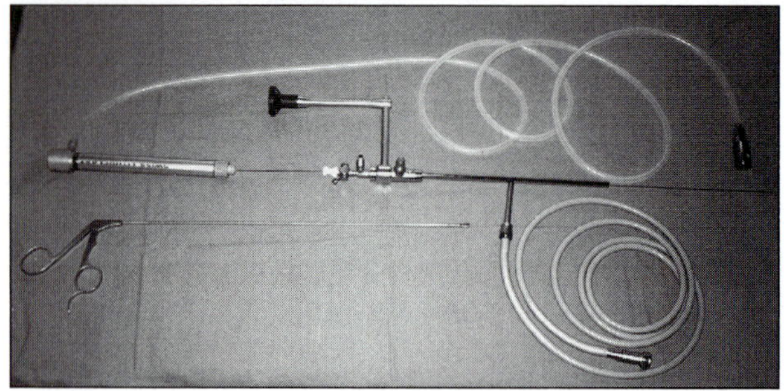

FIGURE 11.36 Lithotriptor equipment—forceps in foreground for grasping stone fragments.

- Endoscope
- X-ray fluoroscopy unit, C-arm or biplane

Contrast Media None

Radiation Protection

- Adequate collimation
- Minimize fluoroscopy time.

Preliminary Radiographs Any radiographs associated with percutaneous nephrostomy

Patient Preparation Preparation associated with percutaneous nephrostomy or cystoscopy

Procedure Sequence

- A percutaneous nephrostomy or cystoscopy is first performed.
- The stone is localized.
- The probe is introduced via an endoscope.
- The probe tip should exceed the tip of the endoscope by 10 to 20 mm, but no more.
- The endoscope is advanced until the tip of the probe is in contact with the stone.
- Single pulse on half power is used initially, but may be increased depending on the size and fragility of the stone.
- Shock waves are continued until stone has been fragmented to a size that will allow easy passage.
- Movable stones, especially in the bladder, may need to be held against the bladder wall by slightly dilating the bladder with fluid.
- Ureteral stones may require holding with a dormia basket or balloon catheter.
- Fragments are finally flushed out.
- Larger fragments may be individually retrieved.

Postprocedure Care Care only related to percutaneous nephrostomy or cystoscopy

Common Pathologies Urinary stones

Review Questions

1. For a percutaneous nephrostomy, identify the type of x-ray unit preferred. Explain what advantages this unit has over other types.

2. What does ESWL stand for? Explain the principles involved.

3. Identify any complications likely to arise from a percutaneous nephrostomy.

4. Discuss the role of diagnostic ultrasound in renal imaging. Identify its advantages and disadvantages.

5. Which of the following pathologies would contraindicate the placement of a stent?
   a. fistula
   b. bladder abnormality
   c. ureteric stenosis
   d. obstruction

6. Contrast media in CT imaging of the renal system:
   a. is a paramagnetic agent
   b. is always administered as a single bolus
   c. is sometimes a barium sulfate compound
   d. enhances the cortex at 60 seconds

7. "Opinion differs on the question of arrested respiration or not" with regard to percutaneous punctures of the kidney. Discuss this statement.

8. What is neurolept sedation and what does it achieve?

9. Outline the radiographer's role during a retrograde pyelogram. What film sequence would be used? Identify likely problems and explain how you would overcome them.

CASE STUDY

A patient is admitted into the emergency department complaining of acute pain in the right kidney region, symptomatic of a renal stone. Describe the imaging modalities used to determine this diagnosis and any imaging therapeutic procedures that might help this patient.

References and Recommended Reading

Alazraki, N., & Mishkin, F. S. (1991). *Fundamentals of nuclear medicine* (2nd ed.). New York: The Society of Nuclear Medicine.

Ballinger, P. W. (1991). *Merrill's atlas of radiographic positions and radiologic procedures* (Vols. 1, 2 and 3, 7th ed.). St. Louis: Mosby-Year Book.

Bentrager, P. W. (1987). *Textbook of radiographic positions and radiologic procedures* (7th ed.). St. Louis: Mosby.

Bernier, D. R., Christian, P. E., & Langan, J. K. (1994) *Nuclear medicine technology and techniques* (3rd ed.). St. Louis: Mosby-Year Book.

Chapman, S., & Nakielny, R. (1988). *A guide to radiological procedures* (2nd ed.). London: Bailliere Tindall.

Cass, A. (Ed.). (1992). *Imaging of urologic disorders.* Mt. Kisco, NY: Futura.

Datz, F. L. (1993). *Handbooks in radiology: Nuclear medicine* (2nd ed.). St. Louis: Mosby-Year Book.

Dixon, D. L., & Dugdale, L. M. (1988). *An introduction to clinical imaging.* New York: Churchill Livingstone.

Dondellinger, R. F., et al. (1990). *Interventional radiology,* New York: Thieme.

Dorland's illustrated medical dictionary. (1994). (28th ed.). Philadelphia: Saunders.

Early, P. J., & Sodee, D. B. (1995). *Principles and practice of nuclear medicine* (2nd ed.). St. Louis: Mosby-Year Book.

Eisenberg, R. L. (1992). *Radiology, An illustrated history.* St. Louis: Mosby-Year Book.

Federle, M. P., et al. (1993). *Year book of diagnostic radiology 1993.* St. Louis: Mosby -Year Book.

Fleischer, A. C., & James, A.E. (1989). *Diagnostic sonography—Principles and clinical applications.* Philadelphia: Saunders.

Gaylord, G. M., Davis, L. P., & Baker, S. R. (1989). *Diagnostic and interventional radiology. A clinical manual.* Philadelphia: Saunders.

Goldman, S., & Fishman, E. (1991). Upper urinary tract infection: The current role of CT, Ultrasound and MRI. *Seminars in ultrasound, CT and MR, 12* (4), 335–360.

Griffith, H. J. (1990). *Radiology of renal failure* (2nd ed.). Philadelphia: Saunders.

Kreel, L., & Thornton, A. (1992). *Outline of medical imaging.* Oxford: Butterworth Heinemann.

Lau, L. S. (1993). *Imaging guidelines* (2nd ed.). Royal Australasian College of Radiologists and Victorian Medical Postgraduate Foundation.

Mettler, F. A., & Guiberteu, M. J. (1991). *Essentials of nuclear medicine imaging* (3rd ed.) Philadelphia: Saunders.

Pellack, H. M., et al. (1990). *Clinical urography* (Vols. 1, 2, and 3) Philadelphia: Saunders.

Posniak, M., Kelcz, F., & Dodd, G., III. (1991). *Renal transplant ultrasound imaging and Doppler. Seminars in Ultrasound, CT and MR, 12*(4), 319–334.

Rominger, M. B., Kenney, P. J., Morgan, D. E., Bernrenker, W. K., & Listinsky, J. J. (1992). Gadolinium-enhanced MR imaging of renal masses. *Radiographics, 12*(6), 1047–1116.

Rumack, C. M., Wilson, S. R., & Charbeneau, J. W. (1991). *Diagnostic ultrasound* (Vols. 1 and 2). St. Louis: Mosby-Year Book.

Sanders, R. C. (1991). *Clinical sonography. A practical guide* (2nd ed.). Boston: Little, Brown.

Sarti, D. A., & Sample, W. F. (1987). *Diagnostic ultrasound text and cases* (2nd ed.). Chicago: Year Book Medical Publishers.

Sharp, P. F., Gemmell, H. G., & Smith, F. W. (1989). *Practical nuclear medicine.* IRL: Press at Oxford University Press.

Snopek, A. M. (1992). *Fundamentals of special radiographic procedures* (3rd ed.). Philadelphia: Saunders.

Stark, D. D., & Bradley, W. G. (1988). *Magnetic resonance imaging.* St. Louis: Mosby.

Swallow, R. A., & Naylor, E. (1986). *Clark's positioning in radiography* (11th ed.). Oxford: William Heinemann Medical Books.

Weir, J., & Abrahms, P. (1986). *An atlas of radiological anatomy* (2nd ed.). New York: Churchill Livingstone.

Wojtowycz, M. (1993). *Interventional radiology and angiography. Handbooks in Radiology.* St. Louis: Mosby-Year Book.

SECTION VI

REPRODUCTIVE SYSTEM

CHAPTER 12

Reproductive Organs

CYNTHIA COWLING, BSc, MEd, MRT(R), ACR

OBJECTIVES

At the completion of this chapter, the student should be able to:

1. Describe the procedures used in the diagnostic studies of the male and nongravid female reproductive system as listed.
2. Describe the imaging studies used to assess and diagnose the gravid female.
3. Describe the anatomy of all relevant areas of study.
4. Describe the similarities and differences between gynecologic and obstetric imaging.
5. List the major indications and reasons for performing the studies listed.
6. Compare the resultant images provided in the various imaging modalities used in each study.
7. Identify radiographs indicated for each procedure.
8. Discuss safe practice procedures for each examination.
9. Identify common radiographic appearances of resultant images for each procedure.
10. List usual contrast media used, if any, for each procedure.
11. Identify appropriate patient care practices for each examination.
12. Discuss the importance of ultrasound as the imaging modality of choice in this area.
13. Discuss and explain the changes in imaging procedures in this area.

Introduction and Historical Overview

This chapter describes the imaging of the male and female reproductive systems and includes **obstetric** and **gynecologic** imaging. These areas have been superseded almost entirely by ultrasound and this chapter will deal only with radiographic procedures still performed on a regular basis.

In today's environment of an acute awareness of the risks of radiation, the history of the radiography of the female reproductive system has a fearsome ring. As early as 1896, physicians were attempting to image the fetus in utero, using exposure times of over an hour. The physicians correctly assumed that it would be useful to know the position and condition of the fetus before delivery, but, of course, at that time had no inkling of the long-term damage that could be incurred. In fact, Dr. Edward Parker Davis was quoted as saying, "There has not been the slightest evidence that the passage of the rays through the uterus has affected either mother or child."

Pelvimetry (pĕl-vĭm´ĕ-trē), the measurement of pelvic proportions to assess the delivery of the fetus, became common practice. The mechanism for measuring the bony pelvic landmarks became much more accurate with the introduction of the Colcher-Sussman ruler method in 1944, which enabled the reader to eliminate distortion by having a metal ruler with holes at regular intervals, placed at the same level and angle as the pelvis itself. Although ultrasound has replaced this procedure to a large degree, specifically because of its nonionizing nature, on occasion having the accuracy and clarity of radiographs is an advantage.

Other studies such as placentography (plă´´sĕn-tŏg´ră-fē) and the study of the in utero fetus have been replaced by ultrasound entirely. Ian Donald at the University of Glasgow was the first to examine the fetus in this way in the 1950s amid fears that the ultrasound could have some kind of toxic affect. MRI can demonstrate certain conditions of the female pelvis extremely well and without the hazards of radiation that has been inherent with the use of CT in this area. MRI has proven to be most effective in the localization and staging of ovarian and **endometrial** (ĕn´´dō-mē´trē-ăl) carcinomas.

Studies of the reproductive organs themselves (or gynecologic radiography) were carried out in the early 1900s. By 1919, physicians were experimenting with gas as a form of contrast, inserting it into the peritoneal cavity. The dangers of a gas emboli were thought to be reduced by using carbon dioxide or nitrous oxide, which were quickly absorbable. In 1914, Dr. Walter Rindfleisch injected bismuth salts into the uterine cavity and thus began the hysterosalpingogram (hĭs´´tĕr-ō-săl´´pĭng´ō-grăm). A long evolution of changing contrast agents has resulted in today's study that uses less toxic materials, which are safer and less painful for the patient.

On plain radiography, uterine tumors can be distinguished from a full bladder by a thin fat line between the two. Ovarian dermoid cysts, fibromas, and uterine fibroids can often be determined. Plain films are sometimes obtained to determine the position of an **interuterine device (IUD)**, although ultrasound is the first modality of choice.

The examination of the male reproductive system has become the almost exclusive domain of ultrasound. The prostate gland is imaged via the rectum and the seminal ducts can be visualized transrectally by filling the bladder with an ultrasound gel. Testicles can be imaged to check for masses or metastases. Vesiculography provides an accurate assessment of the seminal vesicles, seminal ducts, and epididymis but requires incisions to be made and radiation administered directly to the reproductive sites. MRI provides an opportunity to study the prostate for staging of neoplasms. CT can also supply this information, but MRI has the added advantage of no ionizing radiation.

Plain radiographs can be useful when identifying a mass. Sometimes radiography of other areas will help to determine the presence of a mass. For instance, a study of the ureters and bladder (usually forming part of an intravenous pyelogram or IVP) can show a mass if these organs are displaced.

Sometimes barium enemas can help identify the spread of carcinomas from the reproductive organs.

Anatomy

FEMALE GENITAL SYSTEM

The female reproductive system is composed of the following principal structures:

1. Right and left ovaries and the ligaments of the ovaries
2. Right and left uterine or fallopian tubes
3. Uterus and the broad and round ligaments
4. Vagina

The ovaries lie in contact with the peritoneum against the lateral walls of the pelvis at the level of the origins of the internal iliac arteries. Each is suspended from the posterior surface of the broad ligament by a fold of peritoneum, the mesovarium (mĕs′′ō-vā′rē-ŭm). The uterine tubes are on the free edge of the broad ligament and open laterally into the peritoneal cavity. Medially, each tube opens into the uterus, between the fundus and body of that structure.

The uterus is positioned with its long axis directed downward and backward. It is maintained in the anteflexed position by the round ligament, which extends from the upper outer angle of the uterus to fuse with the labia majora of the external genitalia.

The cervix of the uterus is inserted into the anterior aspect of the upper part of the vagina. As the cervix projects into the vagina the vaginal wall is deflected onto the external aspect of the cervix. The cavity created between the cervix and the vagina is divided into the anterior, posterior, and lateral fornices (for′nĭ-sēz).

The vagina is directed downward and forward to lie at right angles to the long axis of the uterus. It passes through the perineal membrane to end in the vestibule of the vagina.

The broad ligament of the uterus is comprised of two folds of peritoneum and lies across the middle of the pelvis. The broad ligament encloses all the genital structures except the ovaries, vagina, and cervix of the uterus (Figure 12.1).

MALE GENITAL SYSTEM

The reproductive system of the male consists of the following parts:

1. Testes
2. Efferent ducts of the testes
3. Epididymies
4. Vas deferens (seminal ducts)
5. Seminal vesicles
6. Ejaculatory ducts
7. Prostate glands

The scrotum contains the testes and each is surrounded by a double-walled sac called the tunica vaginalis. Internally, the testis consists of a number of tubes, the seminiferous tubules, which are the sites of sperm formation. These tubules communicate by a network of tubes at the hilum of the testis, which become the efferent ductules, which in turn empty into the epididymis.

The epididymis, a long twisting tube, ends in the vas deferens, which leads from the scrotum through the inguinal canal to enter the abdomen. The vas deferens crosses the external iliac vessels and the ureter to reach the base of the bladder. At this point it is joined by the seminal vesicles to become the ejaculating duct, which passes though the posterior aspect of the prostate gland to enter the prostatic urethra. This then passes through the main body of the prostate gland, which lies against the neck of the bladder and contributes to the seminal fluids (Figure 12.2).

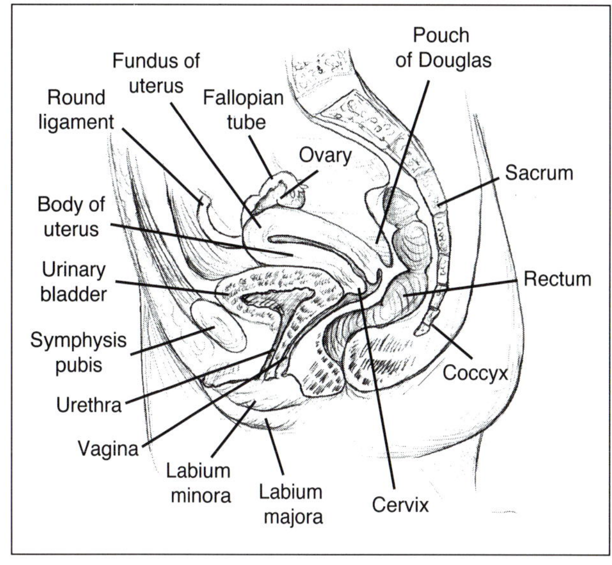

FIGURE 12.1 Female reproductive system.

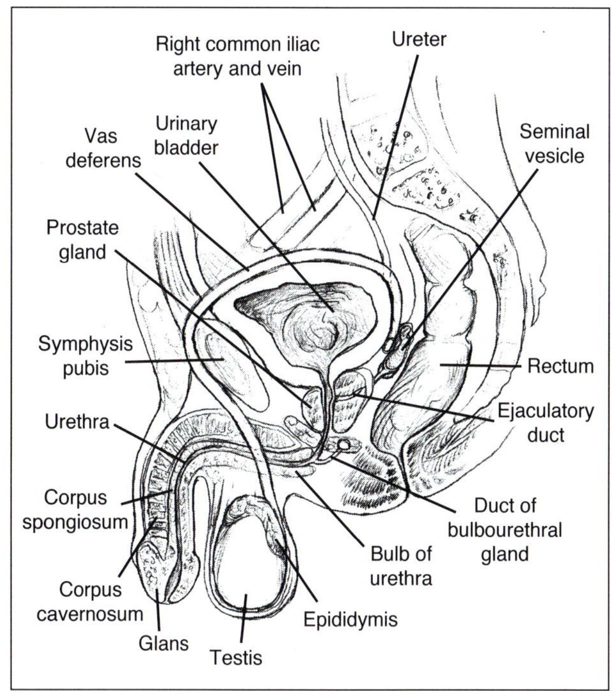

FIGURE 12.2 Male reproductive system.

Procedures for Gynecologic Imaging

This covers the examinations and procedures of the nongravid female pelvis.

HYSTEROSALPINGOGRAPHY

Applied Anatomy This study outlines the fallopian tubes and uterus (Figure 12.3).

Indications

- Infertility
- Recurrent miscarriages
- Following tubal surgery

Contraindications

- Pregnancy
- Purulent discharge
- Recent dilatation and curettage or abortion

Equipment

- Fluoroscopy unit with spot film device
- **Vaginal speculum** and uterine cannula (Figure 12.4).

Contrast Media

- Oily or water-soluble contrast media
- Advantages—oily media
  - —Very opaque (highly viscous)
  - —Remains within cavities for up to 24 hours to give good indication of patency
  - —Low incidence of pain
- Advantages—water-soluble media
  - —Quickly absorbed and does not leave any residue
  - —Remains primarily in a cavity, therefore, little need for nonionic compounds

Patient Preparation

- Patient should be guaranteed as not pregnant.
- The examination can be scheduled between the fourth and tenth day following the commencement of menstruation.

Procedure Sequence

- Patient lies supine on the table with knees flexed, and legs abducted (or **lithotomy** (lĭth-ŏt′ō-mē) **position** with the ankles in stirrups).
- Using aseptic technique, the operator inserts a speculum and cleanses the vagina.
- A cannula is inserted into the cervical canal.
- A syringe containing contrast material (and no bubbles) is attached and the contrast slowly injected under fluoroscopic control.

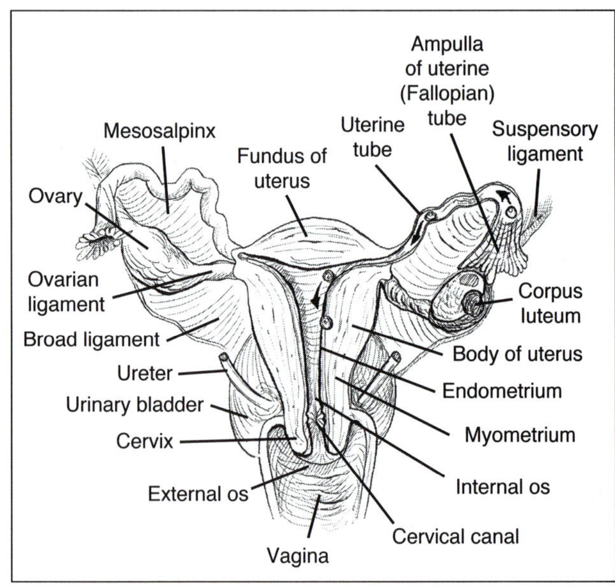

FIGURE 12.3 Fallopian tubes and uterus.

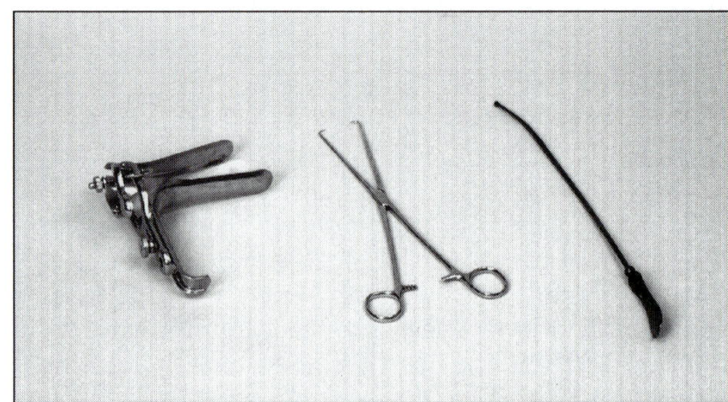

FIGURE 12.4 Speculum, forceps, and cannula.

Procedure Radiographs

- Under fluoroscopic control, radiographs are taken as the fallopian tubes fill, and contrast is injected until it is seen to be spilling into the peritoneum. The sign demonstrates a clear pathway and therefore **patent** fallopian tubes (Figure 12.5).
- A single PA projection of the pelvic area is sometimes taken.
- If an oily contrast medium is used, a 24-hour delay radiograph of the area is taken to check for spilled contrast medium in the peritoneum.

Complications

- Allergies
- Pain (more so with water-soluble contrast medium)
- Bleeding
- Transient nausea
- Infection
- Spontaneous abortion

This procedure can have a therapeutic affect. The force of the contrast medium passing through the fallopian tube can make it patent, allowing for movement of the ovum to the uterus.

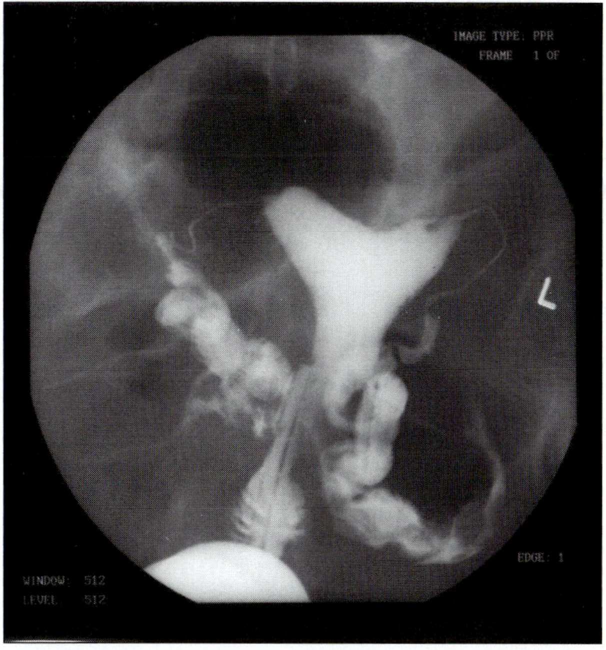

FIGURE 12.5 Hysterogram with spill.

Other Imaging Modalities

COMPUTED TOMOGRAPHY

A CT scan of the female pelvis is generally obtained only for gynecologic problems when the patient is obese, has had recent surgery, or has major bladder problems. It is also able to stage gynecologic tumors.

To determine structures, it is useful to insert a tampon, since this outlines the vaginal wall and defines the position of the cervix.

MAGNETIC RESONANCE IMAGING

An MRI is important in the evaluation of pelvic pathology because it is able to discern small variations in soft tissue. It is also considered noninvasive. It is, however, expensive, particularly compared to ultrasound and so would not be used on a regular basis. It is the modality of choice, if available, for the staging of pelvic malignancies. The use of IV gadolinium (DPTA) assists in the discrimination of normal and abnormal endometrial tissue, as well as the various tissue layers of the cervix.

An MRI can demonstrate the uterus, cervix, and vagina very clearly as well as changes to the uterine walls, the presence of tumor material, or ovarian masses. CT is more sensitive to mesenteric and serosal metastases and is therefore used for the detection of ovarian cancer.

Where possible, examinations of the **gravid** and nongravid individual are performed using a noninvasive method, the most common being ultrasound.

ULTRASOUND

Ultrasound of the female pelvic cavity works on the principle that sound passes easiest through a structure that is homogenous. Therefore, for gynecologic ultrasound, the patient is asked to fill her bladder, so that the pulse can pass through without bouncing off irregular contents (Figure 12.6).

Indications

- Management of IUD
- **Ectopic** (ĕk-tŏp´ik) **pregnancy**
- Endometriosis (ĕn´´dō-mē´´trē-ō´sĭs) and pelvic inflammatory disease (PID)
- Pelvic abscess
- Tuberculosis (in fallopian tubes)
- Neoplasms
- Ovarian masses

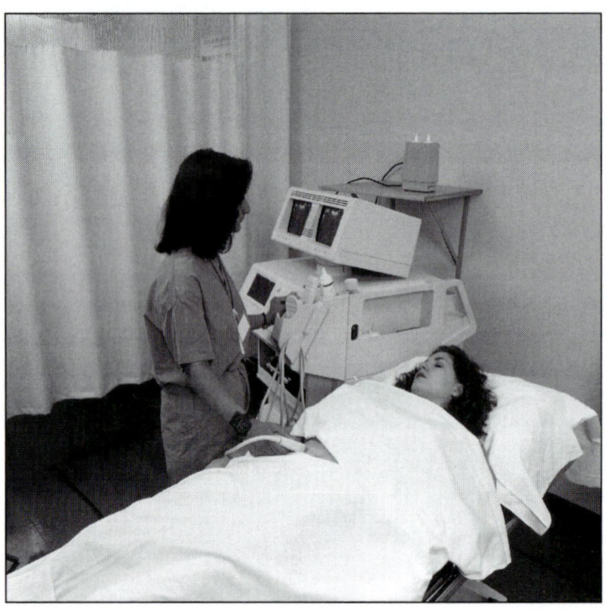

FIGURE 12.6 Patient having ultrasound.

The differential diagnosis is based on the accoustic characteristics of the pelvic structures such as the uterine wall, and great skill is required by the operator to determine the likely diagnosis.

Ultrasound is also able to recognize the variation in size of the follicles that grow during a normal menstrual cycle, and when it erupts (ovulation). Ultrasound scanning has become a regular screening part of subfertility studies.

Transvaginal Ultrasound

Rather than scan through a full bladder, a probe can be used that has a small transducer at its end. It is inserted into the vagina, often resulting in better detail of the pelvic contents.

Transrectal scanning is sometimes used for elderly patients. Using transvaginal probes, images can be obtained of the cervix, uterus, and ovaries.

The intrauterine device

Ultrasound of the pelvic region is the usual method used to determine placement of the device and to diagnose conditions that may be associated with the device, such as uterine perforation, inflammatory disease, or bleeding. If the IUD is "missing" (i.e., the nylon thread no longer visible in the vagina), a plain abdominal radiograph is taken to ensure that it has not migrated to the abdominal cavity (a rare occurrence). If it is necessary to demonstrate the extent of a perforation, it may be necessary to perform a hysterosalpingogram.

Procedures for Male Reproductive Imaging

VESICULOGRAPHY

Applied Anatomy (Figure 12.7)

Vesiculography is a rarely used study where a cut-down technique is used to place a needle in the vas deferens, so that contrast can be injected to determine the patency of the tubes and the condition of the seminal vesicles. Studies of the male reproductive system are most usually performed by ultrasound.

Ultrasound of the scrotum is performed to visualize testicular tumor, hydrocele (hī´drō-sēl), suspected variocele, or scrotal trauma, in the case of boys, acute torsion.

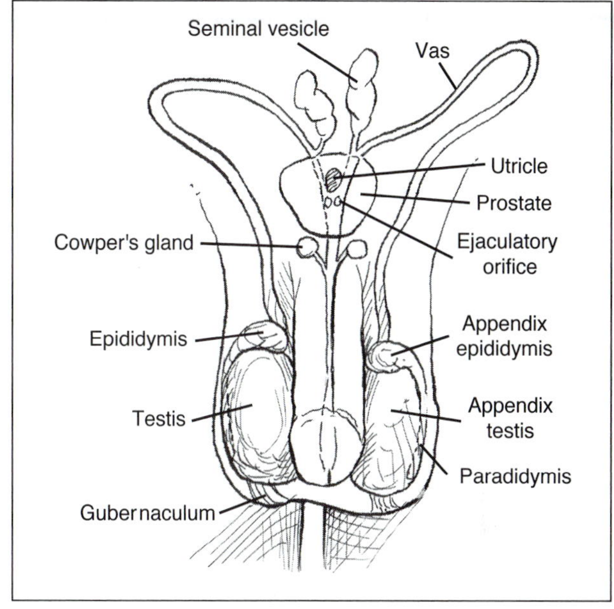

FIGURE 12.7 Anatomy of male duct system.

Other Imaging Modalities

RADIONUCLIDE IMAGING

This is occasionally performed to visualize acute scrotal disease.

ULTRASOUND PROSTATE IMAGING

Prostate cancer is the sixth most common tumor, which can be visualized by ultrasound either by scanning through the bladder or via transrectal scanner. Screening programs are available to enable men to determine the condition of their prostate, just as mammography screening offers the same opportunity for women and their breasts.

COMPUTED TOMOGRAPHY AND MAGNETIC RESONANCE IMAGING

A CT scan is rarely used to image the male system, but MRI is able to determine small changes in tissue composition. It is expensive but because of its noninvasive character and the fact that no preparation is required, it is recommended in certain situations (e.g., with small children).

Currently, there is little difference in success rates of the **staging** of prostatic cancer between ultrasound and MRI. However, changes in MRI technology may give it a higher prediction of accuracy.

Procedures for Obstetric Imaging

Radiography has been minimized to a great extent today because of its potential hazard to the unborn fetus, and ultrasound has become the imaging modality of choice. There have also been changes to clinical practice:

- Increased cesarian sections
- Fewer forceps deliveries
- More accurate biophysical diagnosis (usually via ultrasound)
- Improved biochemical diagnosis

The only procedure carried out radiographically is the Colcher-Sussman pelvimetry used during difficult obstetric delivery. It enables accurate measurements to be taken of the maternal pelvis and fetal skull. This procedure is used most frequently when the fetal head is partially engaged, so that ultrasound is unable to differentiate bony structures. In many centers even this procedure has been superseded by CT, which, although using potentially more radiation, allows for a rapid determination of measurements.

MODIFIED COLCHER-SUSSMAN PELVIMETRY

Because radiation during this examination poses a hazard to the fetus, only one radiograph is generally taken.

Applied Anatomy The lateral pelvimetry is taken to determine the bony landmarks of the pelvis in relation to the fetal head (Figure 12.8).

Indications

- Persistent **breech delivery**
- Prolonged labor
- Pelvic deformity
- Unusually large fetus

Contraindications Additional radiation dose to fetus

Equipment

- Normal radiographic table and x-ray source
- Steel ruler with holes at 1 cm distance (Figure 12.9)

Contrast Media None

Radiation Protection

- It is essential to keep radiation to the minimum. Therefore extreme care must be taken to avoid repeats.
- Very careful collimation must be used so that all the bony landmarks required are visualized but additional scatter is avoided.

Preliminary Radiographs None

Patient Preparation

- The patient is always anxious and often in active labor during this examination.
- The patient must be reassured and calmed as much as possible because this will help to reduce movement of the fetus as well as the mother.

Procedure Sequence

- The patient is asked to lie on her side on the radiographic table, with her back to the technologist.
- A perforated steel ruler is placed between the patient's legs at thigh level or between the buttocks, so that the ruler is at the midpoint of the patient, parallel to the table top. A sandbag will

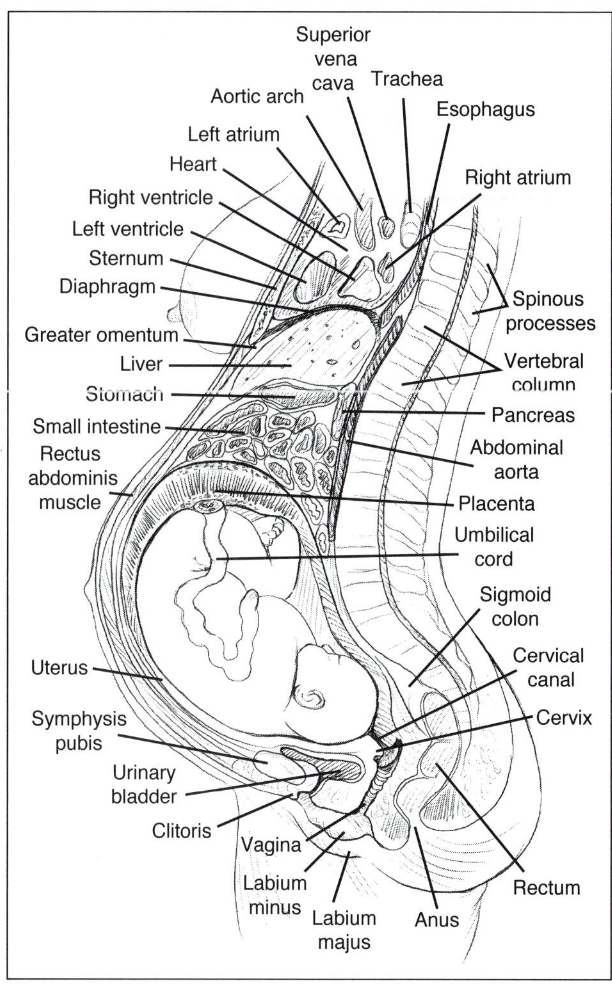

FIGURE 12.8 Lateral view of full-term pregnancy.

ensure stability of the ruler. The shadow produced by this ruler will therefore equate with the midpoint measurements of the maternal pelvis and fetal head.

- The patient is positioned in the true lateral position with legs partially flexed.
- Supports can be given between the knees and under the spine at waist level to ensure that the body is maintained in the lateral position.
- In the case of a very large abdomen, support can also be provided.
- A single exposure is taken, with the centering point at the level of the superimposed greater trochanters, using a 14 × 17 or 14 × 14 inch film and cassette size.

Procedure Radiographs

- A true lateral view of the pelvis, centered on the greater trochanters

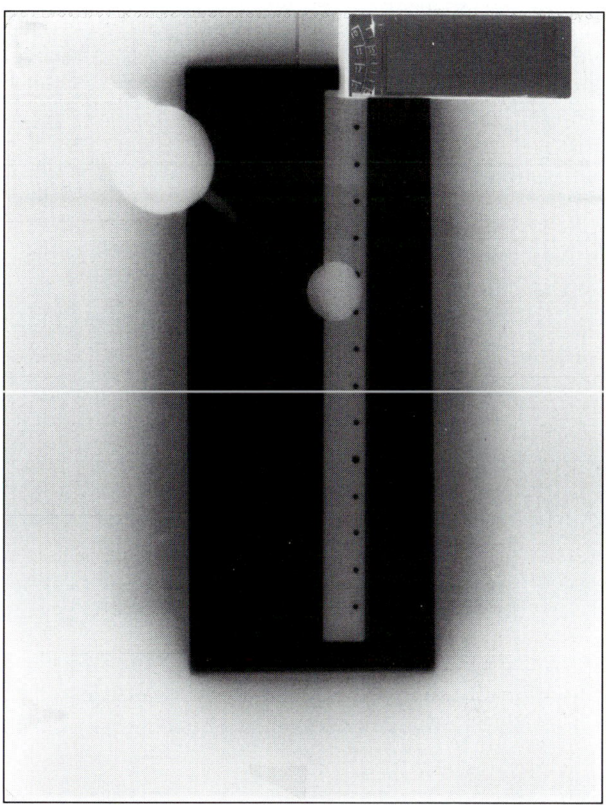

FIGURE 12.9 Ruler used in pelvimetry.

- Sacrum, coccyx, symphysis pubis, and ischial spines must all be visible (Figure 12.10).
- Exposure technique must be great enough to penetrate the pelvis to be able to demonstrate the bony landmarks.

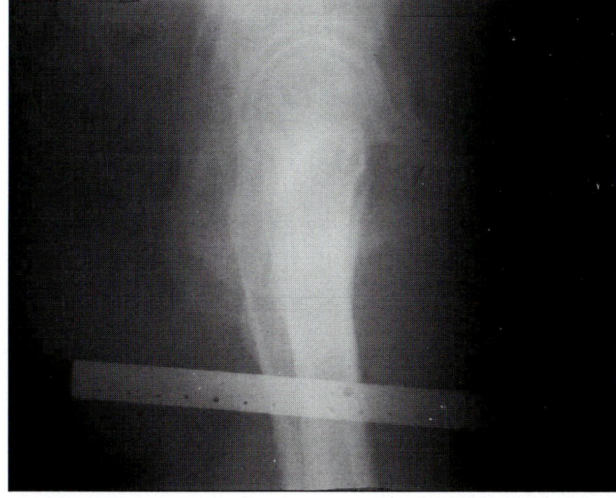

FIGURE 12.10 Lateral pelvimetry of breech delivery.

Alternative Radiographs An AP projection of the pelvic area has been taken in the past. This is now usually only done after delivery to assess the pelvic condition for future pregnancies.

Common Pathologies

- Deformed pelvis
- Enlarged fetal head
- Difficult breech delivery
- Those pathologies that make vaginal delivery more difficult.

> Fetal age and fetal death in the past have been undertaken using conventional radiography. A plain PA projection of the abdomen would determine size, position, and approximate age of the fetus. Condition of the bones such as overlapping of the cranial sutures would determine fetal death. This has been replaced by ultrasound studies. Late fetal age has been determined by a collimated radiograph of the fetal knee (usually a PA oblique projection) to assess epiphyseal development, but again, this has been mainly superseded by ultrasound.

Other Imaging Modalities

COMPUTED TOMOGRAPHY PELVIMETRY

A procedure has been developed that minimizes radiation dose to the patient. A single AP scan is taken to determine position and then a single 8- or 10-mm slice is taken at the level of the ischial spines. A low mAs factor is chosen. This allows for rapid and accurate assessment of the pelvic landmarks.

ULTRASOUND

Ultrasound has essentially taken over obstetric imaging, being considered significantly less harmful than ionizing radiation. There still exists some controversy regarding its use. Some countries and some physicians recommend ultrasound as a screening tool for pregnant women and advocate at least one scan per pregnancy. Others prefer to err on the side of caution and use ultrasound only when deemed clinically necessary. In both cases there is no doubt that ultrasound has revolutionized obstetric imaging, not only replacing existing radiographic studies but also allowing for many other diagnostic studies.

Normal ultrasound studies are usually divided into the three **trimesters**.

First trimester (usually performed at 8–9 weeks):

- Location of gestational sac
- Presence or absence of fetal life
- Fetal number
- Examination of uterus and **adnexal** structures

Second and third trimesters (Figure 12.11):

- Fetal life, age, and number
- Amount of **amniotic fluid**
- Placental location
- **Gestational** age (**biophysical profile**)
- Evaluation of uterine condition
- Demonstration of various parts of fetal anatomy: spine, ventricles, stomach, bladder, heart, kidneys, occasionally face

Equipment

- Sector transducers (for first trimester)
- Linear array transducers (for all obstetric applications)
- Transvaginal transducers (for detection of early pregnancy and ectopic pregnancy)
- Doppler ultrasound (for assessment of fetal well-being and umbilical arterial and venous flow)

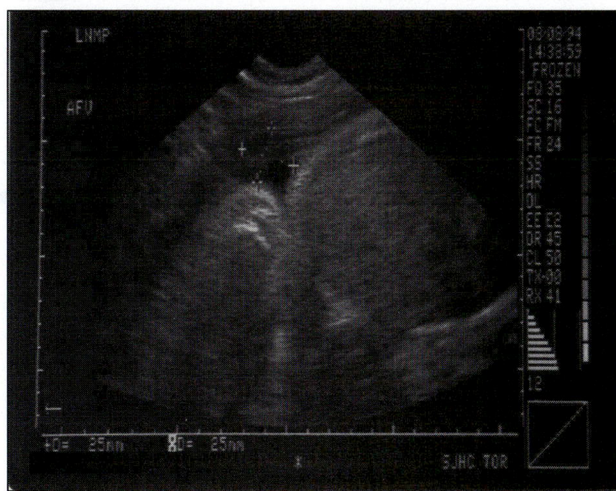

FIGURE 12.11 Full-term ultrasound of breech delivery.

Many abnormal or pathologic conditions as well as normal development seen with ultrasound are beyond the scope of this text. These procedures constitute a major portion of the ultrasound modality, which requires significant study to operate and interpret.

Genetic Screening

Ultrasound sound plays an important role in the assessment and diagnosis of genetic conditions. As well as specific examinations, ultrasound is used to guide tools required for extraction of fluids.

- Amniocentesis (ăm´nē-ō-sĕn-tē´sĭs). A needle is placed in the amniotic sac under ultrasound control. Amniotic fluid is withdrawn for testing. This is usually performed at 16 weeks' gestation, sometimes earlier.
- Chorionic villous sampling. Ultrasound is used to guide the catheter, which is introduced transcervically or transabdominally. Chorionic villous cells are aspirated from the trophoblast at about 9 to 11 weeks' gestation.
- Fetal blood sampling. Blood is removed under ultrasound guidance.
- Maternal serum α-fetoprotein screening. This is performed at 15 to 20 weeks' gestation and diagnoses 90% of all fetal neural tube defects.

Review Questions

1. Compare and contrast the ionizing and nonionizing studies used in obstetric imaging.

2. Imaging of the male and female reproductive organs has changed significantly in the last 25 years. Discuss this statement.

3. A missing IUD is best "found" by:
   a. ultrasound
   b. lateral pelvimetry
   c. plain radiograph
   d. single CT scan

4. When water-soluble contrast medium is used for hysterosalpingography, the most likely side effects are:
   a. cramping pain
   b. bleeding
   c. infection
   d. spontaneous abortion

5. In a lateral pelvimetry radiograph, which landmark must be seen to determine pelvic size?
   a. greater trochanters
   b. ischial spines
   c. fetal head
   d. iliac crest

CASE STUDY

A 36-year-old woman has recently determined that she is pregnant. Her first pregnancy was 10 years ago and was a difficult forceps delivery due to small pelvic proportions. There also appears to be some history of genetically inherited conditions in the family. Suggest all the types of imaging tests this woman may undergo during her pregnancy. Discuss how safety considerations to mother and fetus can be applied.

References and Recommended Readings

Ballinger, P. W. (1995). *Merrill's atlas of radiographic positioning and radiologic procedures* (8th ed.). St. Louis: Mosby-Year Book.

Barnes, P. D., Brody, J. D., Jaranmillo, D., Akbar, J. U., and Emans, J. B. (1993). Atypical ideopathic scoliosis, MR imaging evaluation. *Radiology, 186*(1), 247–253.

Berland, L. L. (1987). *Practical CT technology and techniques.* New York: Raven Press.

Chapman, S., & Nakielny, R. (1993). *A guide to radiological Procedures* (3rd ed.). London: Bailliere and Tindall.

Coleman, B. G. (Ed). (1992). The Female Pelvis. *Radiology, Clinics of North America, 30*(4).

Davis, E. P. (1986). The application of the Rontgen rays. III The study of the infant's body and of the pregnant womb by the Rontgen rays. *American Journal of Medical Science, 3,* 263–269.

Doyle, T., Hare, W., Thomson, K., & Tress, B. (1989). *Procedures in diagnostic radiology.* London: Churchill Livingstone.

Eisenberg, R., & Dennis, C. (1990). *Comprehensive radiographic pathology.* St. Louis: Mosby-Year Book.

Eisenberg, R. L. (1992). *Radiology, an illustrated history.* St. Louis: Mosby-Year Book.

Federle, M. P., et al. (1982). Pelvimetry by digital radiography: A low-dose examination. *Radiology, 143*(3), 733–735.

Fowler, R. (1990). Imaging the testis and scrotal structures [Review]. *Clinical Radiology, 41,* 81–85.

Green, R. E., & Oestmann, J. W. (1992). *Computed digital radiography in clinical practice.* New York: Thieme.

Grossman, L., Ellis, D., & Brigham, S. (1993). *The clinician's guides to diagnostic imaging.* New York: Raven Press.

Janus, C. (1991). Gynecologic magnetic resonance imaging. *Urologic Radiology, 13,* 29–40.

Kreel, L., & Thornton, A. (1992). *Outline of medical imaging.* Oxford: Butterworth, Heineman.

Miller, B. F., & Keane, C. B. (1987). *Encyclopedia and dictionary of medicine, nursing and allied health* (4th ed.). Philadelphia: Saunders.

Rumack, C. M., Wilson, S. R., & Charbeneau, J. W. (1991). *Diagnostic ultrasound* (Vols. 1 and 2). St. Louis: Mosby-Year Book.

Sanders, R. C. (1991). *Clinical sonography. A practical guide* (2nd ed.). Boston: Little, Brown.

Saxton, H. M., & Strickland, B. (1972). *Practical procedures in diagnostic radiology.* New York: Grune and Stratton.

Seeram, E. (1994). *Computed tomography. Physical properties. Clinical applications and quality control.* Philadelphia: Saunders.

Snopek, A. M. (1992). *Fundamentals of special radiographic procedures* (3rd ed.). Philadelphia: Saunders.

Sutton, D. A. (1993). *Textbook of radiology and imaging.* Edinburgh: Churchill Livingstone.

Wojtowycz, M. (1993). *Interventional radiology and angiography.* Handbooks in Radiology. St. Louis: Mosby-Year Book.

CHAPTER 13

Breast

BRONWYN CHAPPLE, MIR

OBJECTIVES

At the completion of this chapter, the student should be able to:

1. Describe the procedures used in the studies of the breast as listed.
2. Describe the anatomy and physiology of the breast.
3. Describe patient preparation and care for each procedure.
4. List the major indications and reasons for performing the studies listed.
5. Identify the relevant equipment used.
6. List the relevant radiographs/images indicated for each procedure.
7. Discuss safe practice procedures for each examination.
8. List contrast media used, if any, for each procedure.
9. Describe relevant postprocedure care.
10. List common pathologies.
11. Identify other relevant imaging modalities.
12. Describe relevant interventional procedures.

Introduction and Historical Overview

Breast cancer is a long-standing disease of women. References to treatment of the disease were made by the Romans as early as the 1st century A.D. Over the centuries many advances have been made in surgical treatment and management but the beginning of the 20th century brought no improvement in survival rates. Patients continued to present with advanced disease. The importance of early detection was recognized, and attention was focused on techniques for imaging the soft tissues of the breast as a means of detecting malignancies before they presented as clinical symptoms. In the 1960s, Robert Egan, MD, radiologist at the Anderson Hospital, in Houston, Texas investigated methods of improving the technical quality of breast roentgenology. His efforts resulted in the development of the low-kVp, high-mAs technique, which he named mammography (măm-ŏg´ră-fē). To obtain the contrast and detail required, the technique involved the use of a conventional diagnostic x-ray unit with a tungsten tube target, and nonscreen industrial film that required manual processing. The breast was not compressed and exposure times were long, resulting in some geometric unsharpness. Despite these shortcomings, contrast and detail were sufficient to demonstrate nonpalpable breast cancers and this breakthrough was hailed as a new era of mammographic imaging.

Further advances followed. In the 1970s the Xerox 125 process was developed with blue and white paper images. The attractions of xerography (zē-rŏg´ră-fē) over film methods were its lower x-ray dose and its ability to demonstrate more detail in the dense breast (especially **microcalcifications**). It was performed on a conventional x-ray unit but required special processing facilities.

The next 15 years saw huge improvements in mammographic imaging with film and equipment manufacturers taking up the challenge to produce better imaging systems. The introduction of appropriate screen/film combinations and x-ray tubes especially dedicated to mammography resulted in a lower radiation dose and images comparable to xerography, except in the dense breast. Compression of the breast during the examination and the introduction of a moving grid with carbon interspacers further improved the detail and contrast of the screen/film system, and xerography systems gradually disappeared.

Randomized trials were implemented to demonstrate the viability of population-based mammographic screening as a method of early breast cancer detection. The Health Insurance Plan in New York State (1963–1969) and W-E Study in Sweden (1977–1984) demonstrated a reduction in breast cancer mortality rates through mammographic screening, and film/screen mammography was adopted as the tool for breast cancer screening programs worldwide.

Advances in technology continue, and it is possible that the end of the century may see the replacement of film/screen mammography by digital mammography. In recent years ultrasound, CT, MRI, transillumination, and positron emission tomography (PET) scanning have been used as adjuncts in the diagnosis of breast abnormalities. Surgical procedures have altered due to the availability of simpler and less traumatic interventional techniques such as stereotactic and ultrasound-guided fine needle **aspiration** and core **biopsy**.

Anatomy

The breast is a modified sweat gland situated between the anterior and posterior layers of the superficial skin fascia. It lies anterior to the fascia of the pectoralis major muscle on the chest wall (Figure 13.1).

The internal structure consists of varying amounts of glandular and **adipose** (fatty) **tissue**, and blood and lymphatic vessels (Figures 13.2 and 13.3). The glandular tissue or **parenchyma** (păr-ĕn´kĭ-mă) extends radially from behind the nipple into the fatty tissue, and consists of 15 to 20 **lobes** made up of ductal structures and connective and supportive **stroma**. Each lobe consists of a collecting duct from the nipple orifice, a **lactiferous** sinus, and several ductule branchings that terminate in **lobules**. There are many lobule groupings in each lobe. A single lobule contains an extralobular terminal duct that divides into many intralobular terminal ducts and then ends bluntly at the terminal ductule and the **acinus** (ăs´ĭ-nŭs). Each of these structures, termed terminal duct lobular units (TDLUs), is loosely supported by connective tissue (Figure 13.4). The TDLU is the site of most breast pathology. Cooper's ligaments anchor the parenchyma to the anterior and posterior fascia and make up the supportive structure of the breast (Figure 13.5).

The breast, unlike other organs of the body, is continually changing. The total amount of glandular tissue will alter according to cyclical fluctuations, hormone therapy regimes, pregnancy, **lactation**, and the normal **involution** process that occurs during a woman's lifetime. The mammographic appearance will reflect these changes (Figures 13.6, 13.7, and 13.8).

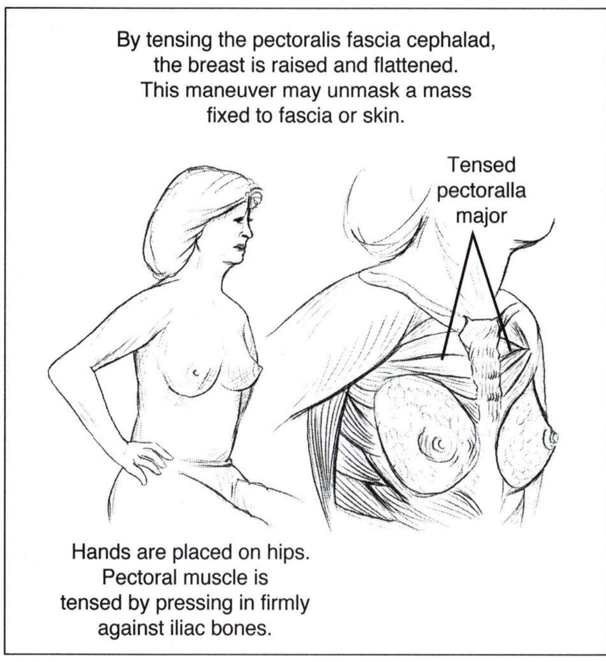

FIGURE 13.1 Anatomic location of the breast.

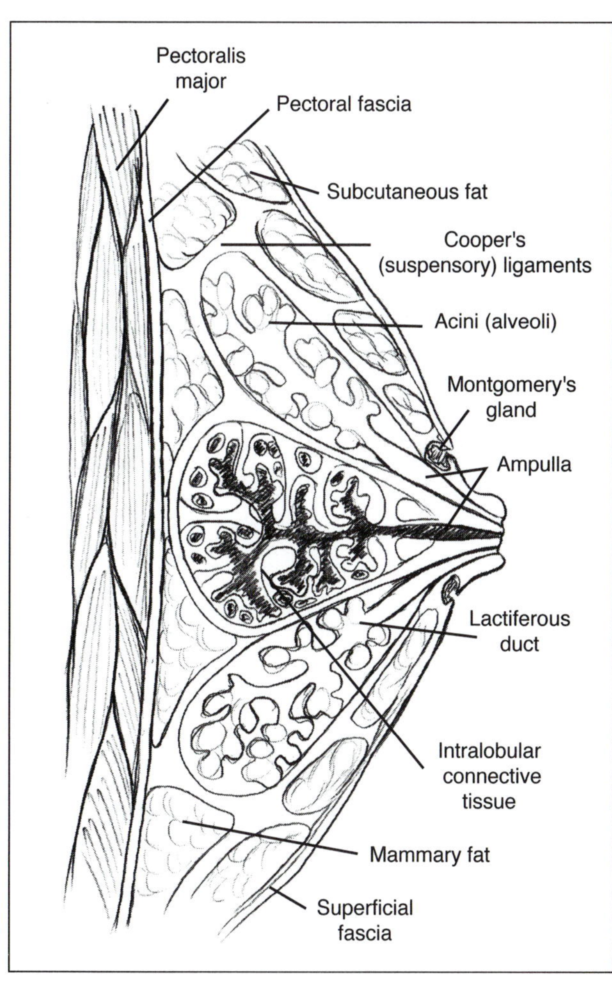

FIGURE 13.2 Internal breast composition.

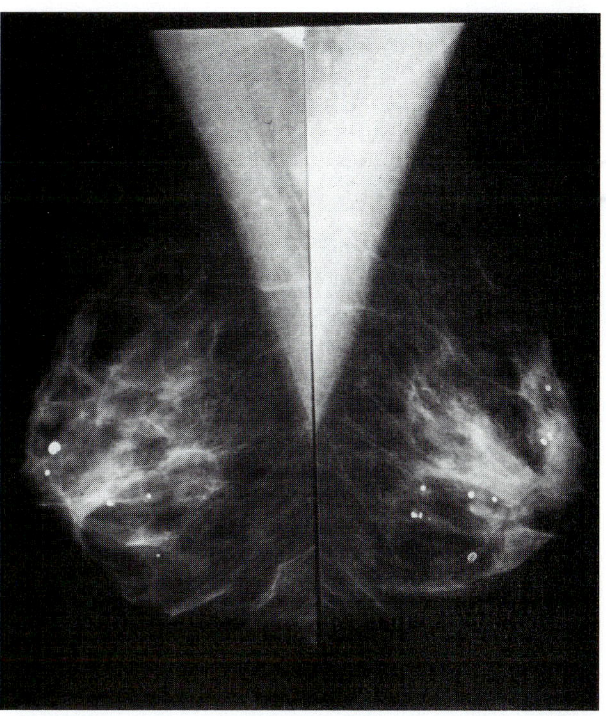

FIGURE 13.3 Mediolateral oblique (MLO) internal structures.

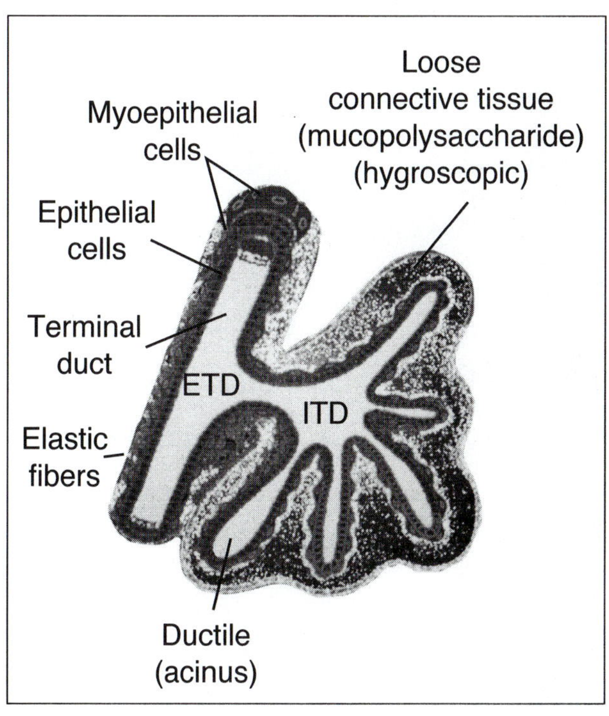

FIGURE 13.4 Terminal duct lobular units (TDLU) composition.

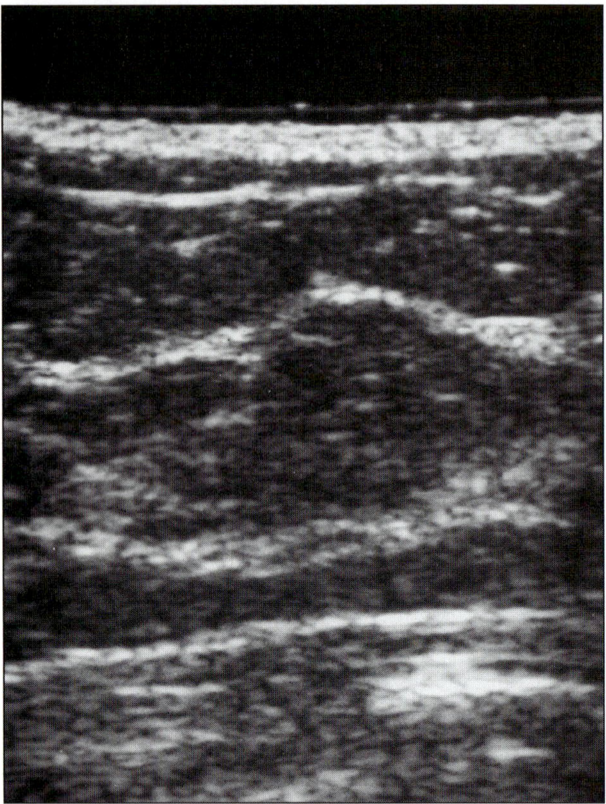

FIGURE 13.5 Ultrasound demonstrating Cooper's ligaments.

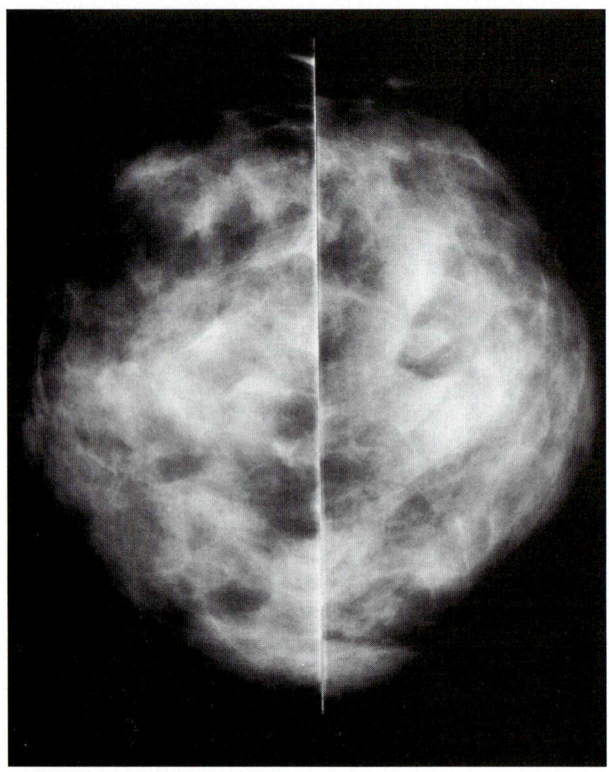

FIGURE 13.6 Glandular breast.

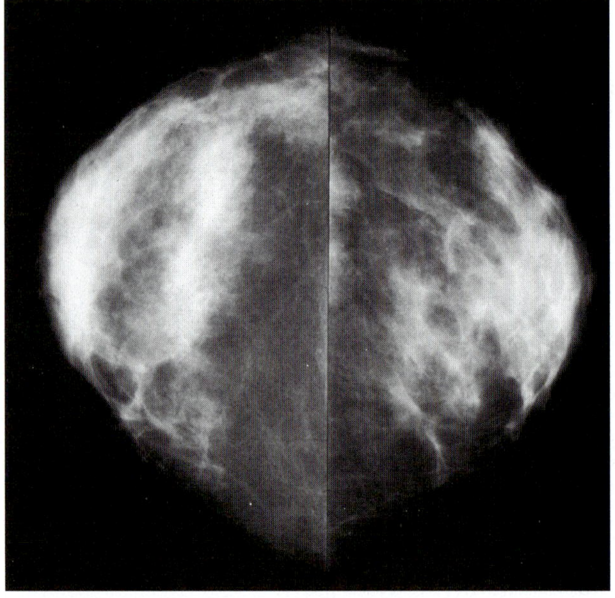

FIGURE 13.7 50/50 fatty/glandular breast.

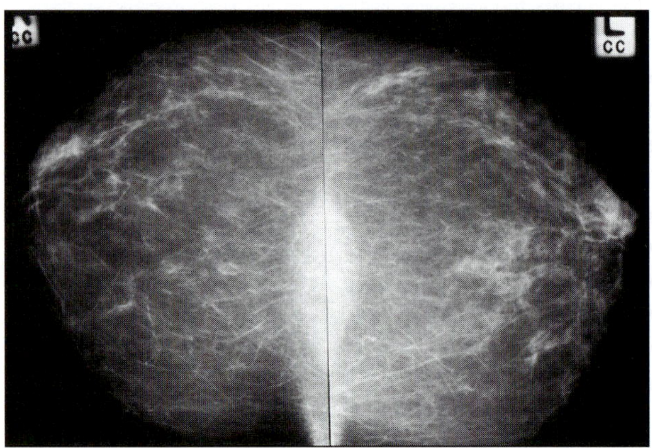

FIGURE 13.8 Fatty breast.

Procedures

MAMMOGRAPHY

Mammography is the radiologic examination of the breast using a dedicated x-ray unit that has the ability to produce consistently high-contrast images at an acceptable radiation dose (0.3 rads). The use of relatively fast screen/film combinations allows lower kVp selection (22–30) for better contrast and spatial resolution of the image. A small focal spot (0.3 mm), and a SID of 60 to 65 cm reduces geometric unsharpness.

Because the mA values are fixed on most mammography units, the radiologic technologist must choose the optimal kVp for image contrast, while limiting the exposure time to take best advantage of the reciprocity law failure for image density. A grid is used for most examinations to improve contrast.

The breast is compressed firmly during the examination by means of a thin plastic (Lexan) plate to reduce motion and geometric unsharpness, spread the tissue for more even density and increased contrast, and reduce scatter radiation. The compression device must be straight at the chest wall edge and remain parallel to the film holder during compression for best results.

A comprehensive quality assurance program is essential to maximize specificity and sensitivity in this demanding area of imaging. Quality control procedures for the monitoring of positioning techniques, technologist motivation and dedication, and the consistency of x-ray and processing equipment should be strictly adhered to.

Applied Anatomy

- Routine mammography is performed to:
  - —Detect clinically occult breast cancer (screening examination)
  - —Investigate clinical signs or symptoms in the breast (diagnostic examination)
- An understanding of the anatomy and physiology of the breast will allow the technologist to appreciate the necessity for quality mammographic images.

Indications

- Preventive health check for well women (screening)
- Inconclusive clinical findings (diagnostic)
- Family history of breast cancer
- Previous breast cancer
- Baseline study before commencement of hormone replacement therapy

Contraindications

- Dense glandular breast composition
- Due to the laws of physics relating to thickness of soft tissues and x-radiation, mammography is of limited value in the dense breast. Ultrasound is often used as an alternative method of evaluation in the young dense breast and is considered especially appropriate for examination of pregnant and adolescent females.

Equipment Dedicated mammography unit (Figure 13.9) with:

- High-frequency generator
- Molybdenum or rhodium tube target with a small focal spot (0.3 mm)

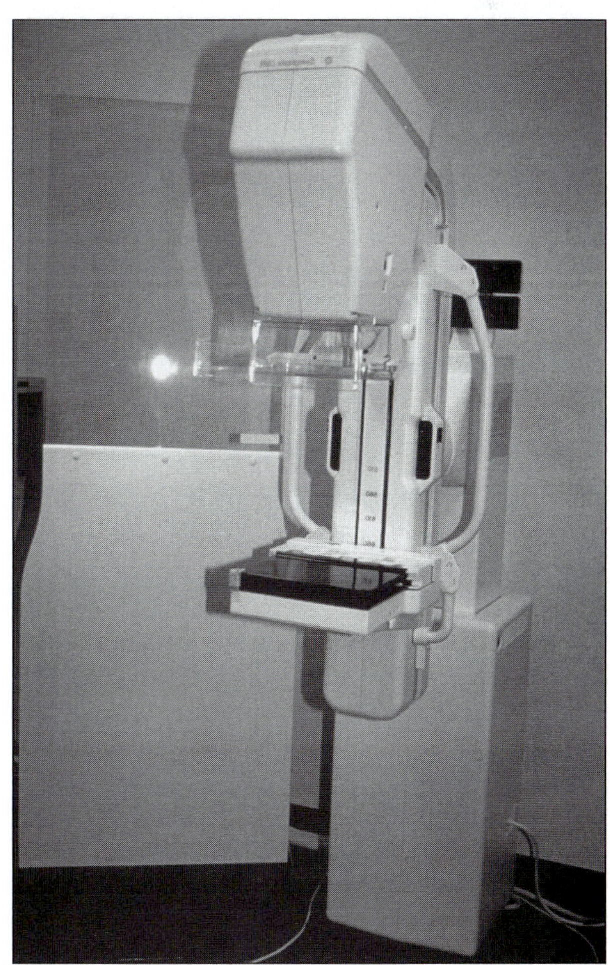

FIGURE 13.9 Mammography unit.

- Beryllium window with additional filtration of 0.03 mm of molybdenum or rhodium
- Automatic exposure control (AEC) device (Figure 13.10)
- Moving grid with carbon interspacers for low absorption of soft x-rays (Figure 13.11)
- Fixed source to image receptor distance (SID)
- Half-value layer (HVL) equal to 0.3 mm Al at 30 kVp
- Transparent plastic compression device with motorized operation (Figure 13.12)
- Scale in centimeters

Contrast Media Not applicable

Radiation Protection

- Collimation to film size, either by metal diaphragm or adjustable shutters
- Units must incorporate an automatic exposure cut-out when a diaphragm is not in place.

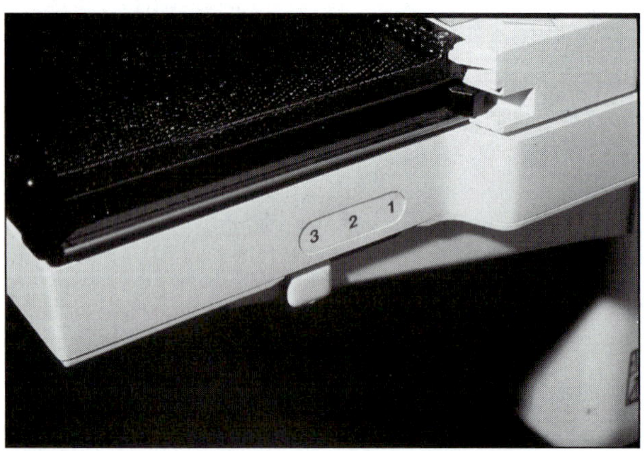

FIGURE 13.10 Automatic exposure control (AEC) unit.

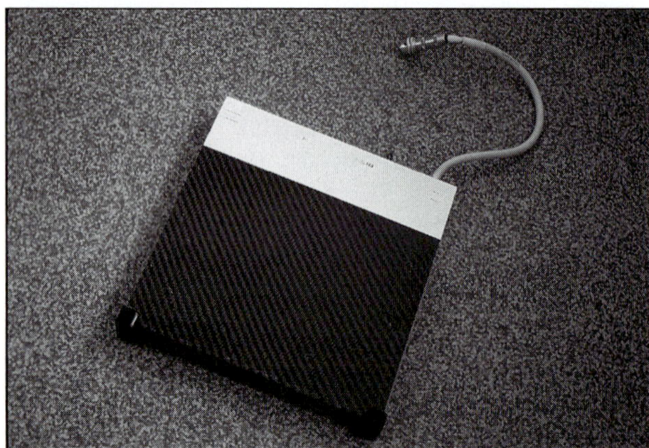

FIGURE 13.11 Grid assembly.

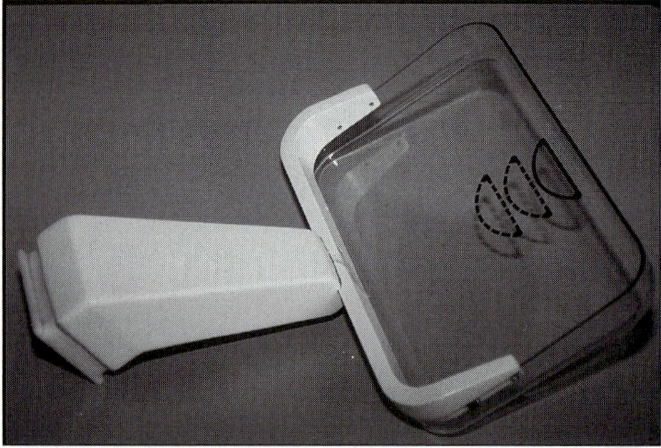

FIGURE 13.12 Compression device.

- Correct alignment of light and x-ray field especially at chest wall edge of film holder to ensure that no radiation extends beyond this border
- Gonad protection for the patient who may be pregnant

Preliminary Radiographs Not applicable

Patient Preparation

- The patient should be instructed not to use talc or deodorant on the day of the examination. Magnesium silicate may be imaged on the highly sensitive mammographic film, mimicking microcalcifications (Figure 13.13).
- The patient may be requested to reduce her intake of caffeine before the examination in an attempt to alleviate breast tenderness.
- The procedure should be explained fully to the patient before the examination, emphasizing the reasons for compressing the breast tissue.
- The patient's medical history is important to assist the radiologist. Scars from previous surgery, skin moles, and dimpling or nipple discharge (especially unilateral) should be recorded.

Procedure Sequence

- If possible, the examination should be performed with the patient standing.
- Correct positioning is important to ensure that all the breast tissue is visualized, and to ensure that imaging standards are maintained to allow reproduction of comparable images for subsequent studies.
- Despite the fact that symptoms may be unilateral, bilateral mammography is usually performed. This is for one of two reasons:

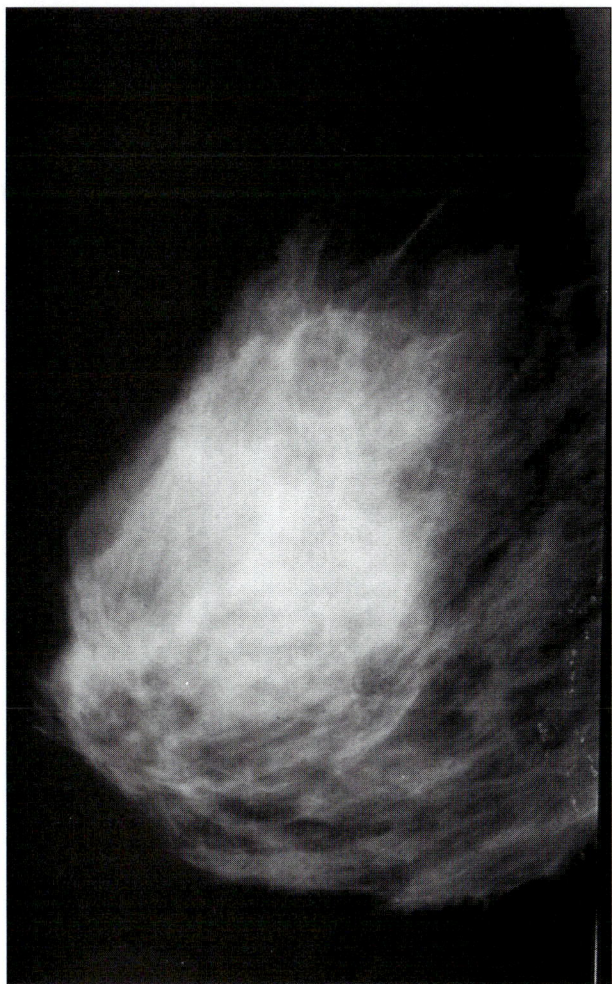

FIGURE 13.13 Talcum powder mimicking microcalcifications.

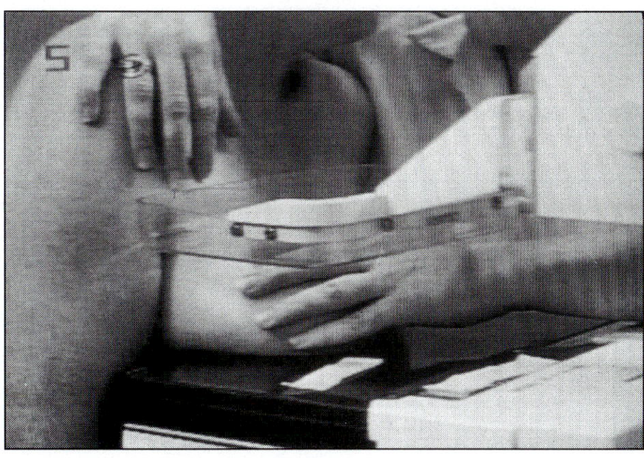

FIGURE 13.14 Craniocaudad (CC) procedure.

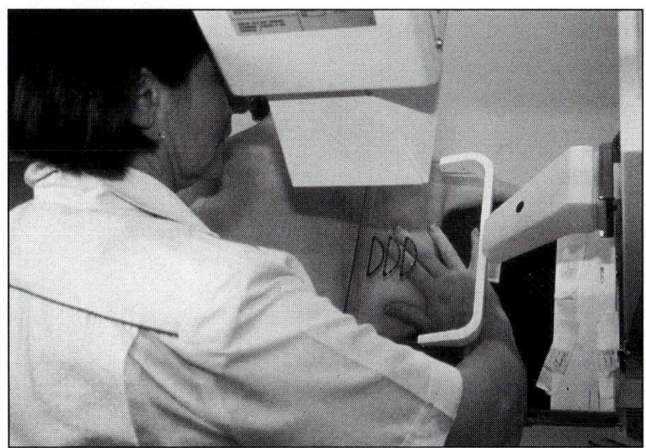

FIGURE 13.15 Mediolateral (MLO) procedure.

1. The tissue pattern of one breast is a mirror image of the other and marked asymmetry may be an early sign of a malignant process.
2. Malignancy may be bilateral because there is a lymphatic connection between the breasts.

- Two routine projections are performed on each breast: the craniocaudad (CC) projection (Figure 13.14) and the mediolateral oblique (MLO) projection (Figure 13.15).
- The CC projection is not able to demonstrate all the breast tissue (Figure 13.16). It is important to include as much as possible of the medial aspect of the breast on this view while not sacrificing the lateral aspect.
- The MLO projection, if performed correctly, demonstrates all the breast tissue (Figure 13.17). It has replaced the lateral projection in the routine series because it images more of the **axillary** tail and posterior portion of the breast than the lateral, and therefore complements the CC projection.
- An 18 × 24 cm (8 × 10 inch) film format is usual for mammography although a 24 × 30 cm (10 × 12 inch) format may be used for the larger breast. Image contrast can be affected by the inability to compress evenly with the larger compression paddle. An alternative is to perform two or three "jigsaw," 18 × 24 cm (8 × 10 inch) images of each breast to ensure adequate image contrast.
- Radiographs should be taken in arrested respiration.

Procedure Radiographs

- CC projection (Figure 13.18)
- MLO projection (Figure 13.19)

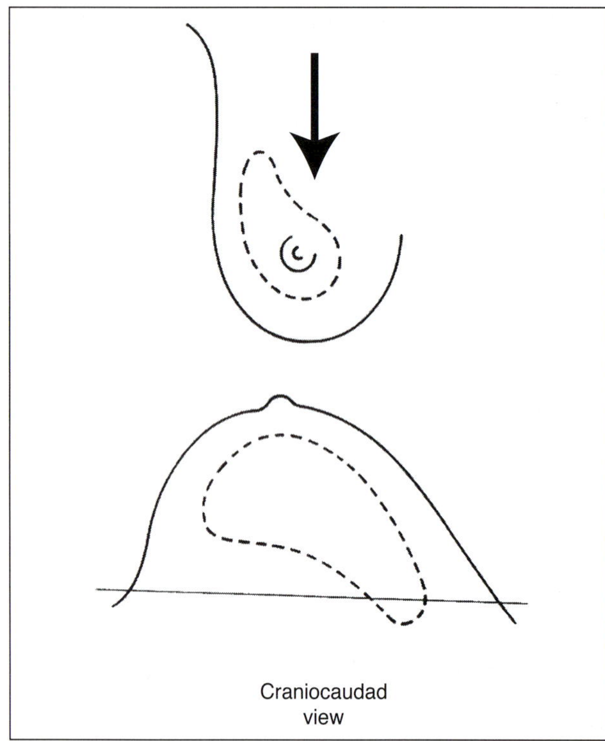

FIGURE 13.16 CC projection limitations.

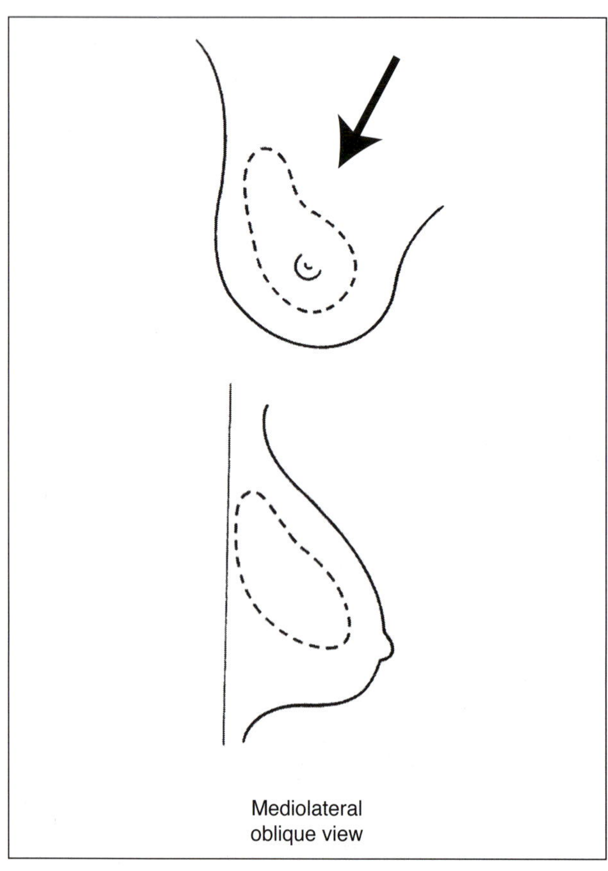

FIGURE 13.17 MLO projection limitations.

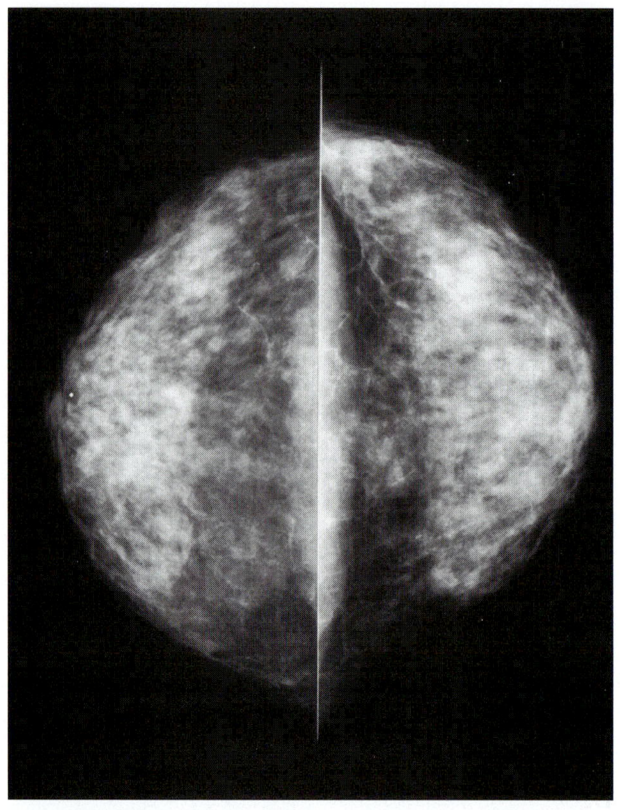

FIGURE 13.18 CC projections.

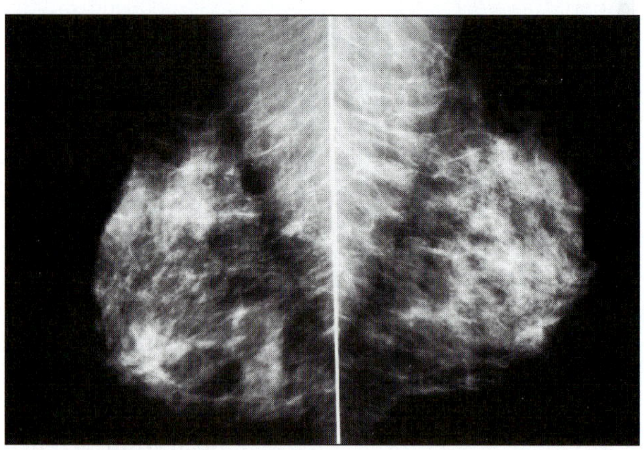

FIGURE 13.19 MLO projections.

Alternative Radiographs Specialized views may be used to:

- Visualize tissue not fully demonstrated in the routine views
- Allow for special positioning problems
- Further categorize the mammographic lesion

There are at least 15 "extra" views that can be used for specific problem-solving.

1. Extended CC View
   - May be done with lateral or medial bias
   - More commonly used to visualize extreme lateral breast tissue especially that which wraps around the lateral and posterior aspect of the pectoral muscle (Figures 13.20 and 13.21).

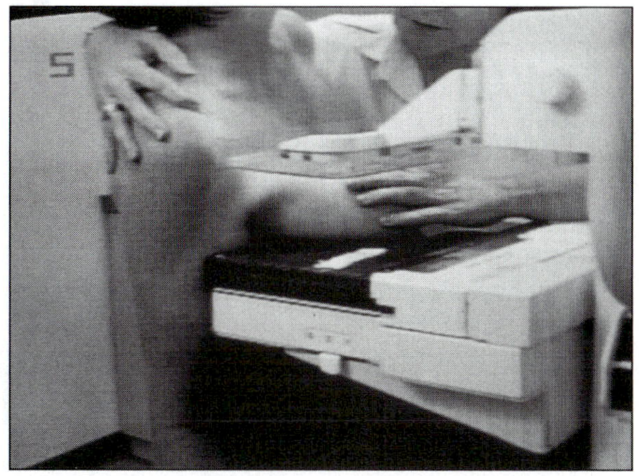

FIGURE 13.20 Positioning for extended CC view.

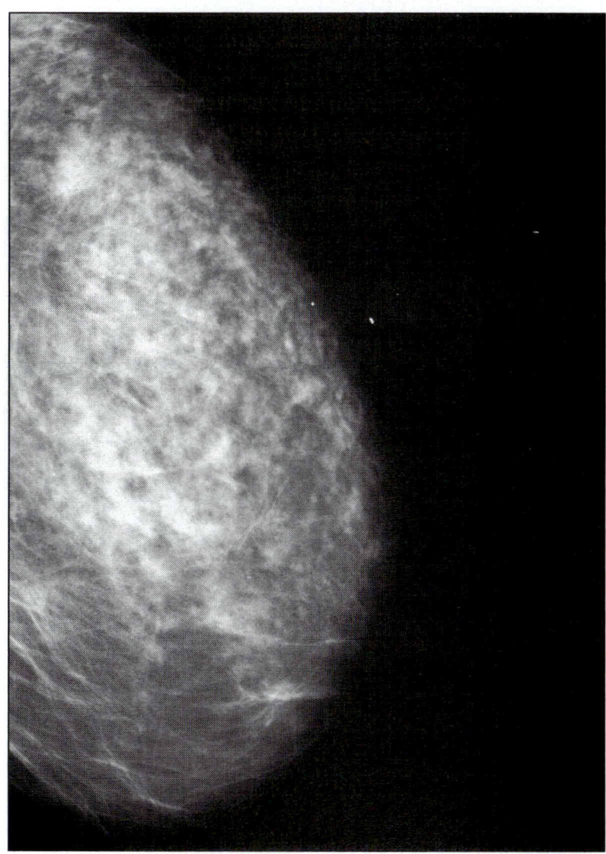

FIGURE 13.21 Extended CC radiograph.

2. 90° Lateral View (Mediolateral or Lateromedial)
   - The lateromedial projection complements the MLO view in that it demonstrates medial tissue and is the more frequently performed lateral (Figure 13.22).
   - The mediolateral projection is performed to better demonstrate an area of asymmetry laterally.
   - Both are used to demonstrate fluid or air levels.
   - Often performed as an orthogonal view before needle localization
   - Demonstrate "layering" of calcifications for **benign** versus malignant considerations (Figure 13.23)
   - Useful extra view for visualization of lower breast tissue in "difficult-to-position" women (e.g., depressed sternum)

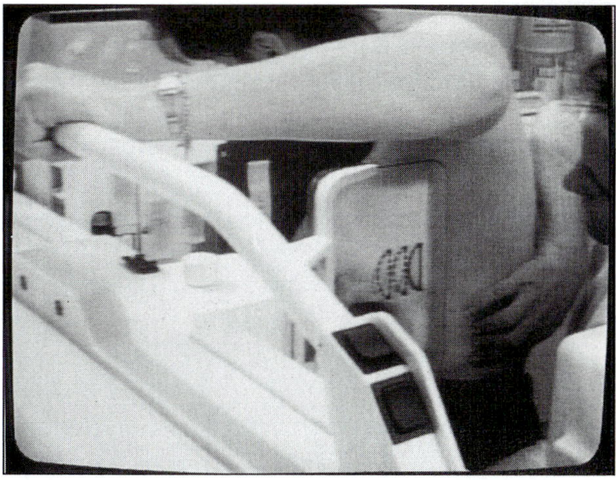

FIGURE 13.22 Positioning for lateromedial view.

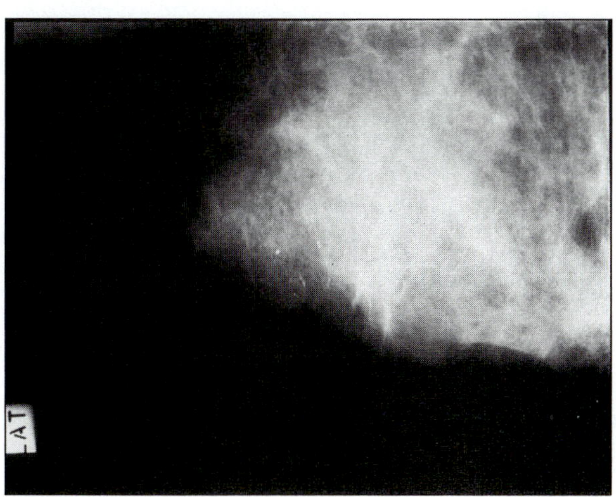

FIGURE 13.23 Layering of calcifications.

3. Cleopatra View
   - Used to visualize the axillary tail (Figures 13.24 and 13.25)
   - Provides local compression of lateral-most aspect of the breast close to the pectoral muscle

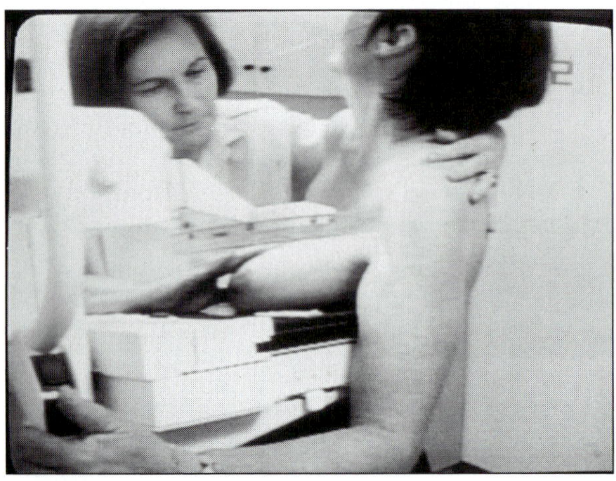

FIGURE 13.24 Positioning for Cleopatra view.

   - Client can lean sideways or more easily, the film holder can be rotated 10° to 15° so that it is parallel to the angle of axillary tail.
4. Cleavage View
   - Used to better visualize lesions deep in the medial aspect of the breast (Figure 13.26)
   - A manual exposure may be needed if the AEC is centered over the cleavage.
   - May be difficult on thin women
   - Some tissue posterior to the cleavage should be visible if correctly positioned (Figure 13.27)
5. Coned Compression View
   - May be taken in any projection
   - Allows better compression over a small area (Figure 13.28)
   - Allows separation of overlying structures and enhances image detail (Figure 13.29)
   - Useful for posterior lesions
   - Often combined with magnification
6. Magnification View
   - Especially useful to better define microcalcifications (Figure 13.30)

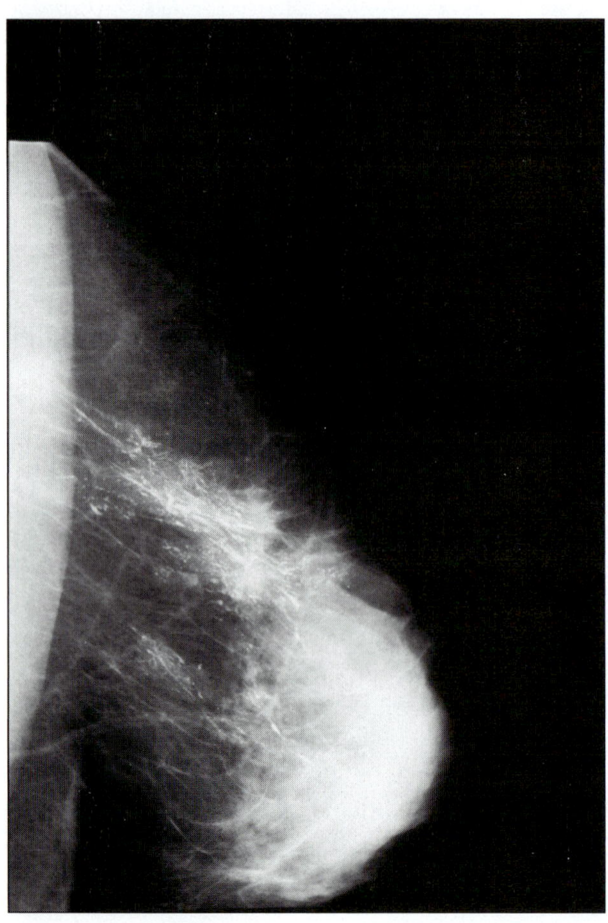

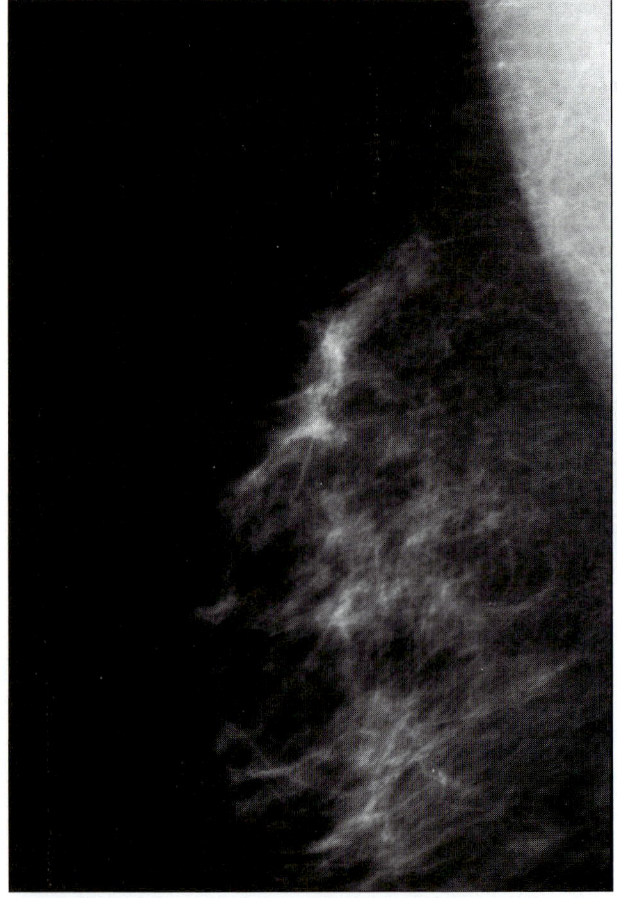

FIGURE 13.25 Cleopatra view radiographs.

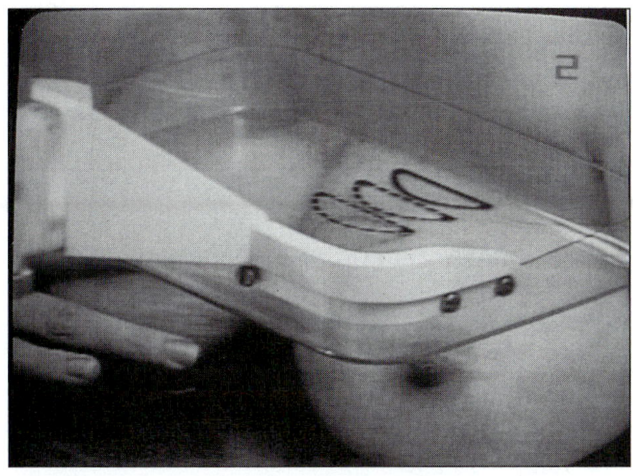

FIGURE 13.26 Positioning for cleavage view.

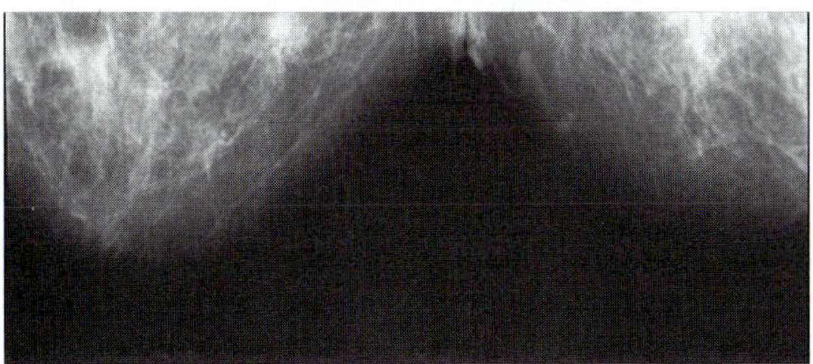

FIGURE 13.27 Cleavage view radiographs.

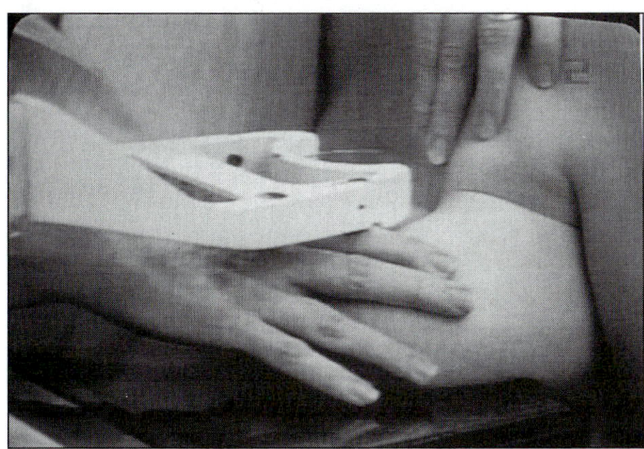

FIGURE 13.28 Positioning for coned compression view.

- Provides sharper, more defined image.
- No bucky is required because air gap is sufficient to reduce scatter radiation (Figure 13.31).
- Faster screens help reduce exposure time.
- Magnification is usually 1.5 to 2 times.
- "Spot" or "full" compression paddle may be used.
- Fine focus (0.1 mm) is required.

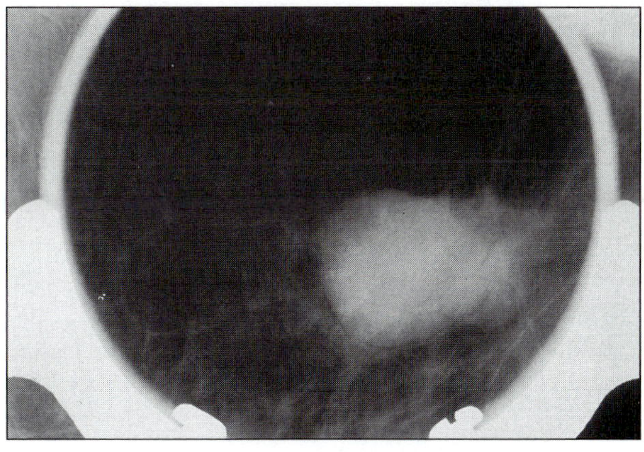

FIGURE 13.29 Coned compression view to demonstrate a cyst.

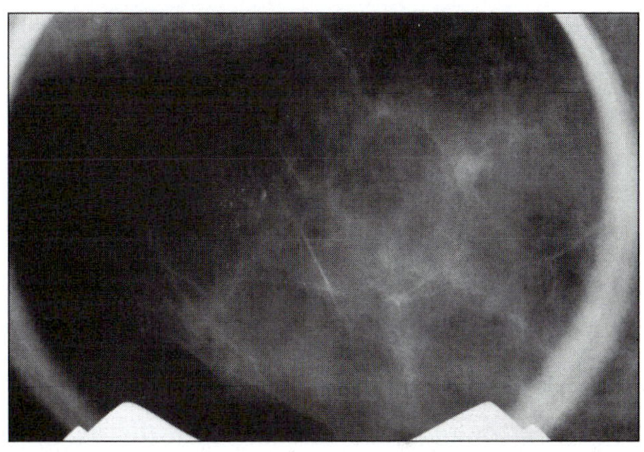

FIGURE 13.30 Coned magnification view to demonstrate calcification.

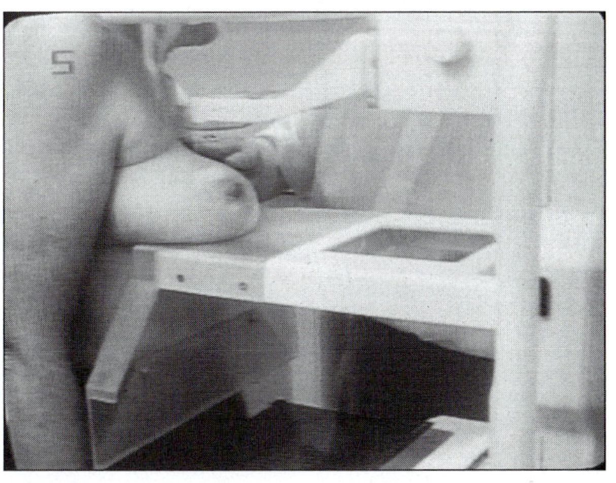

FIGURE 13.31 Positioning for magnification view.

7. Sponge View
   - A modified CC view
   - By placing a 15° triangular foam pad under the breast, more of the inferior tissue can be brought forward over the film holder (Figures 13.32 and 13.33).
   - Useful for imaging posterior medial lesions deep in the inferior area of the breast (Figure 13.34)
   - The breast is pulled up and away from the chest wall as the breast is compressed.
   - Geometric unsharpness may be increased due to the increased Object Image Receptor Distance (OID).
8. Uncompressed CC View
   - Useful to demonstrate posterior medial lesions in the most superior part of the breast
   - These lesions may be so close to the chest wall that they are "squeezed" out of view by the compression paddle in the routine CC.
   - Requires greater exposure (approximately double the mAs)
   - If the lesion is palpable, it can be rolled out and partial compression applied if possible (Figure 13.35).
   - The remainder of the breast will be poorly demonstrated.
   - Dense lesions will be demonstrated in relief against tissue at the chest wall.
9. "Pinch" Views for Augmented Breasts
   - Implants may inhibit breast compression, but every effort should be made to obtain the best mammographic images possible. There will always be some compromise when imaging the **augmented** breast.
   - Subpectoral or intramammary implants may obscure some breast tissue.

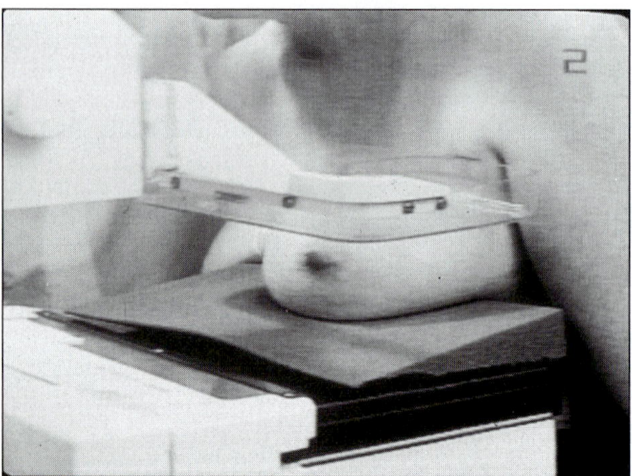

FIGURE 13.32 Positioning for sponge view.

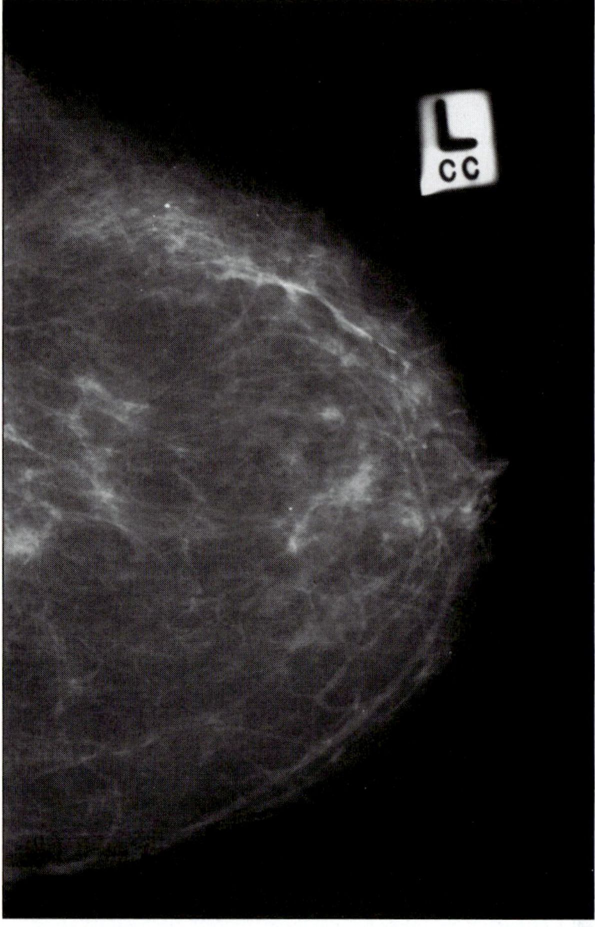

FIGURE 13.33 CC sponge views.

   - Mammography of the augmented breast involves an additional lateromedial view if the implant cannot be displaced.
   - Manual exposures are required.
   - For the implant that can be displaced, the routine views should be taken with the implant in place, and the implant displaced (four views/breast).
   - Modified compression technique (as described by Eklund, 1988) (Figure 13.36) enables significantly improved imaging of the breast tissue, free of the implant (Figures 13.37 and 13.38).
   - Even if the implant is fixed, the tissue can still be pulled over and in front of the implant.
10. Tangential View
   - To visualize superficial lesions close to the skin with the least amount of overlying tissue to allow better margin differentiation
   - The area of concern may be a palpable mass, a focal tenderness, skin dimpling, or calcifications (Figure 13.39).

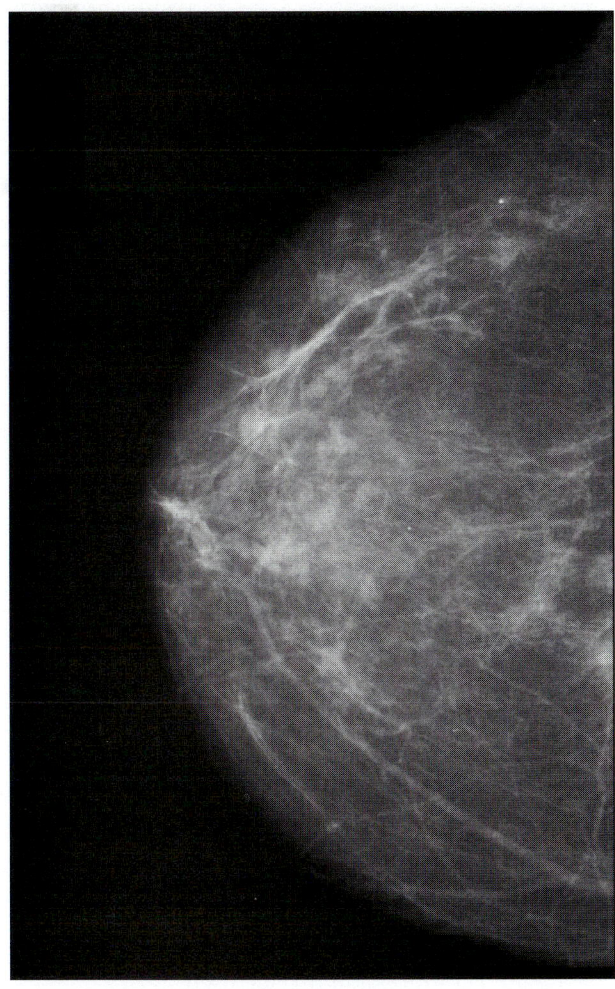

FIGURE 13.34 Deep lesion demonstrated by CC sponge view.

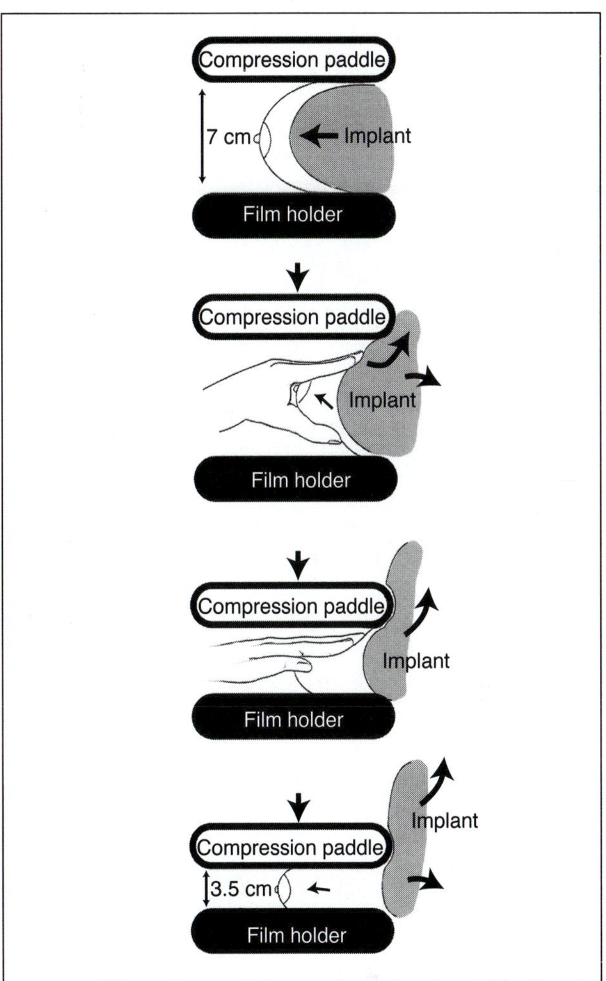

FIGURE 13.36 "Pinch" technique.

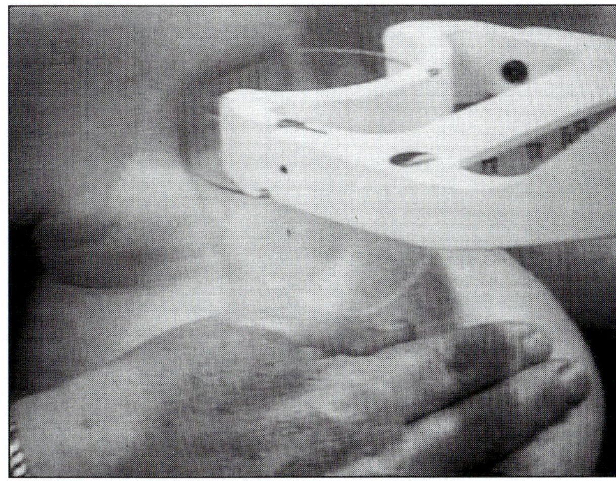

FIGURE 13.35 Positioning for uncompressed CC projection.

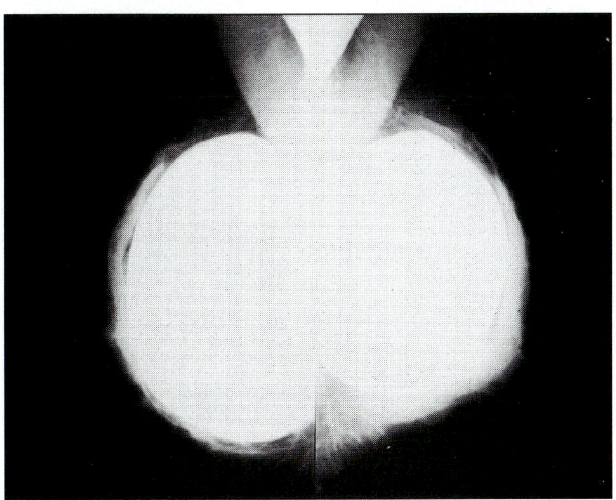

FIGURE 13.37 Implant in place.

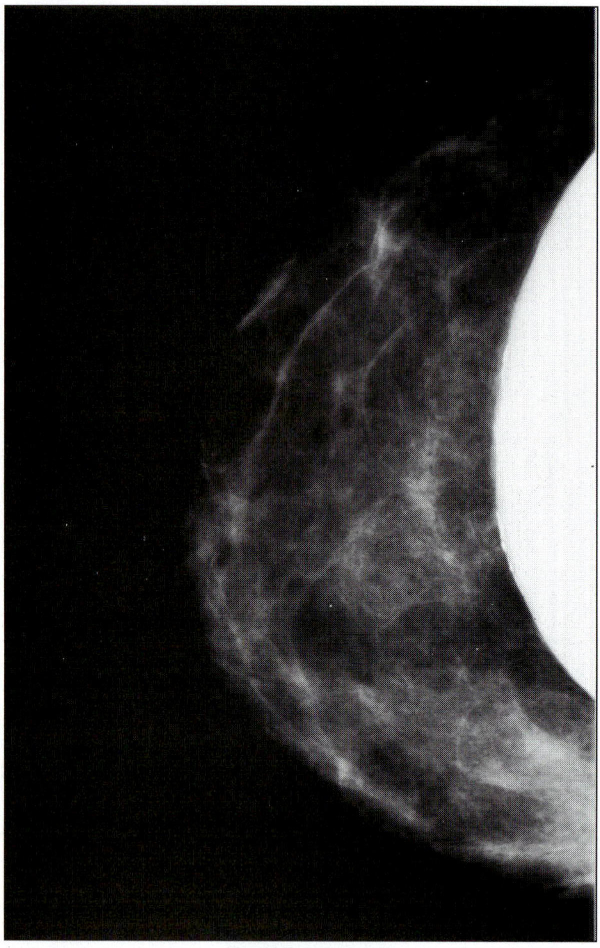

FIGURE 13.38 Implant "pushed" back.

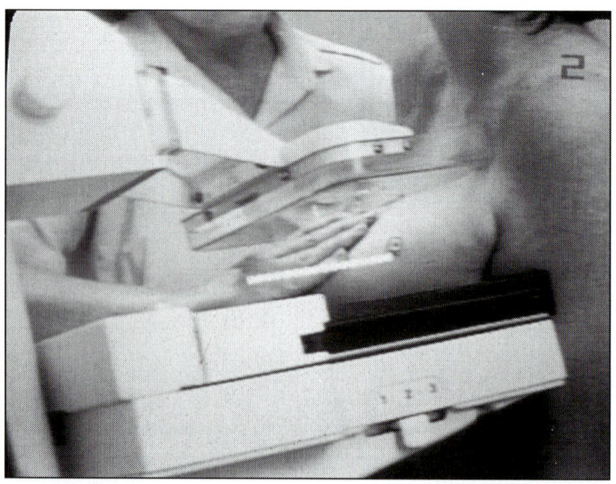

FIGURE 13.39 Positioning for tangential view.

- Reduce the mAs by approximately 20%.
- Manual exposure may be necessary.
- Use a spot compression paddle. The area can be magnified (Figure 13.40).

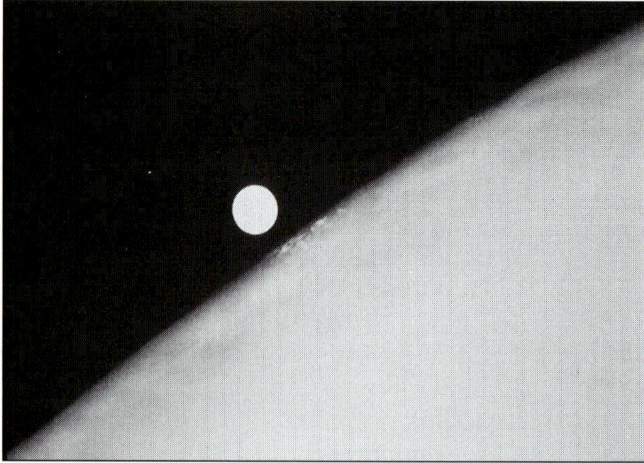

FIGURE 13.40 Magnified tangential view demonstrating calcifications.

11. Rotational View
    - Helpful in clarifying lesions obscured by overlying dense breast tissue
    - The angle of the x-ray beam as related to a particular point in the breast can be changed by rotating the film holder 10° to 20° (Figure 13.41) or by rotating the breast after 20°.
    - Useful to gain an understanding of the spatial relationship of lesions seen in only one view
    - Can be performed in either MLO or CC projection
    - Coned compression may be used.
    - Disappearance of the "lesion" indicates that it was probably a summation effect.
12. Postmastectomy View
    - After **mastectomy** (măs-tĕk´tŏ-mē) a portion of the axillary tail remains and this is a possible site for carcinoma recurrence (Figures 13.42).
    - A routine MLO projection of the mastectomy site may be obtained.
    - A manual exposure will be necessary.
    - An additional lateromedial view of the remaining breast should be included in the routine series on the premise that there is an increased risk of these women developing a further breast carcinoma.
    - Coned compression views of areas of clinical concern may be useful.
13. Axillary View
    - The axillary area can be imaged effectively by using a higher kVp (38–42 kVp with an aluminum filter).
    - Useful for visualizing axillary soft tissue or rib detail depending on mAs setting.

- The film holder is rotated 70° to 90° and placed behind the scapula (Figure 13.43).
- The breast tissue will be overpenetrated.

14. Caudocranial View
    - Useful for positioning women with kyphosis, pacemakers, limited head movement, or very small breasts
    - Produces better visualization of superior tissue especially high, superior lesion
    - The film holder is rotated 180° (Figure 13.44).
15. Lateromedial Oblique View (Reverse Oblique)
    - Can be used wherever MLO cannot be obtained (Figure 13.45)
    - Ideal for women with disabilities (e.g., in a wheelchair), a prominent sternum, a prominent pacemaker, recent open heart surgery, or a prominent pectoral muscle
    - Can be used to better demonstrate a posterior medial lesion (Figures 13.46 and 13.47)

Postprocedure Care

- On completion of the examination, it should be explained to patients that mammography is not 100% accurate in detecting breast cancer.
- Patients should be encouraged to continue carrying out breast self-examination on a regular basis and to consult their doctor if any symptoms present.

Common Pathologies

The pathologic lesions occurring in the breast can be grouped into four major categories according to their mammographic appearance.

1. Circumscribed tumors
2. **Stellate** lesions
3. **Calcifications**
4. Skin changes

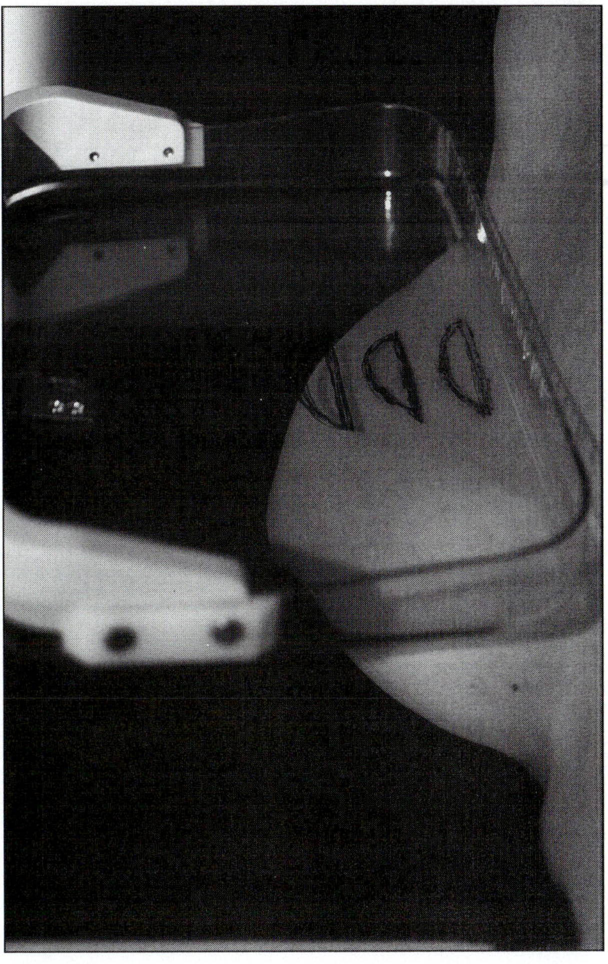

FIGURE 13.41 Positioning for rolled CC view.

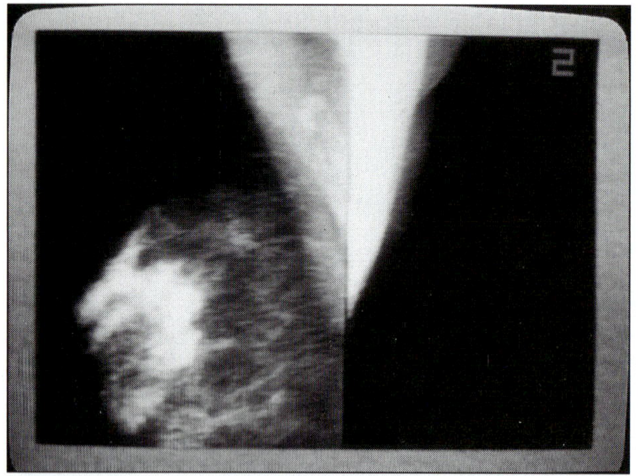

FIGURE 13.42 Postmastectomy radiograph.

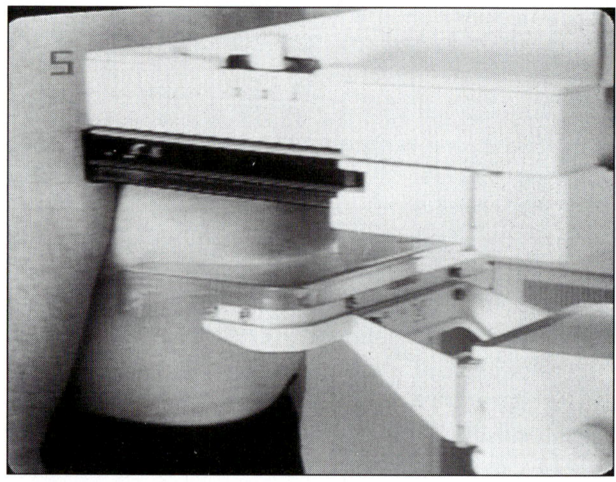

FIGURE 13.44 Positioning for caudocranial view.

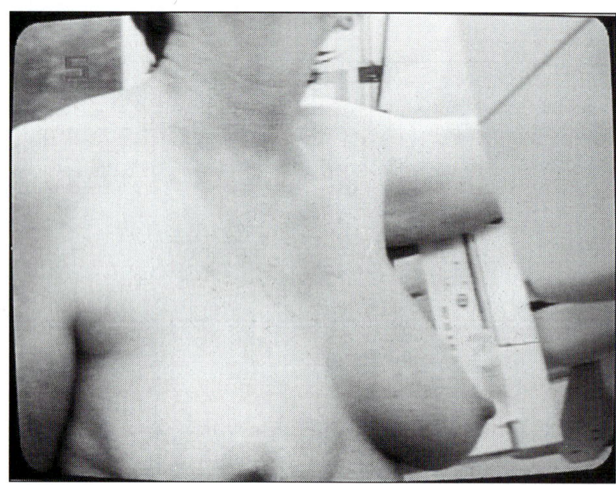

FIGURE 13.43 Positioning for axillary view.

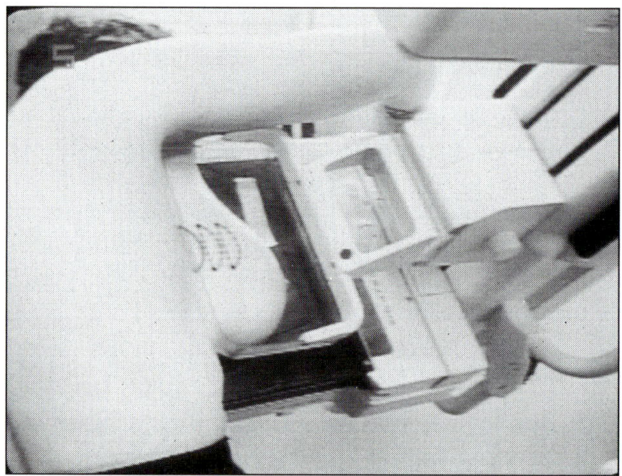

FIGURE 13.45 Positioning for reverse oblique view.

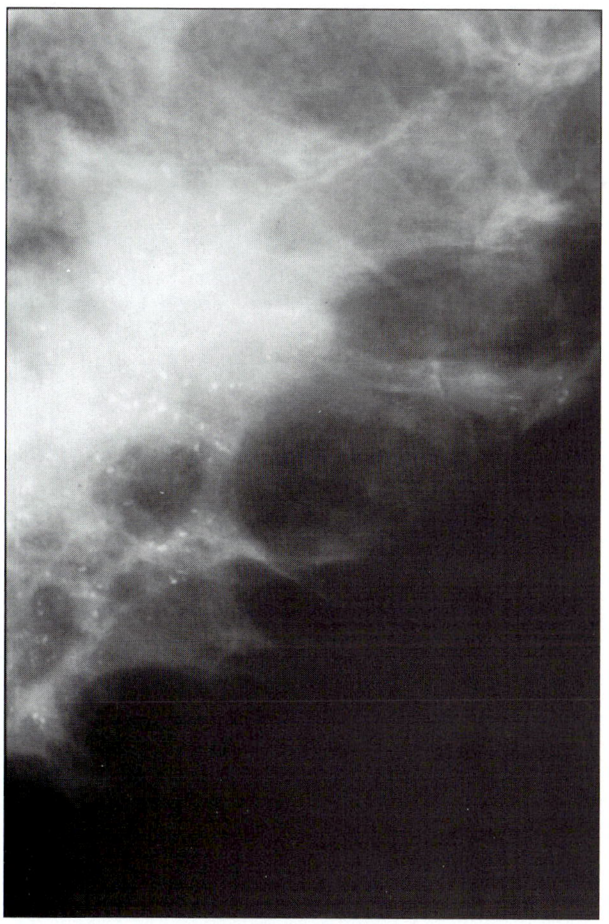

FIGURE 13.46 Calcifications demonstrated on medio-lateral oblique view.

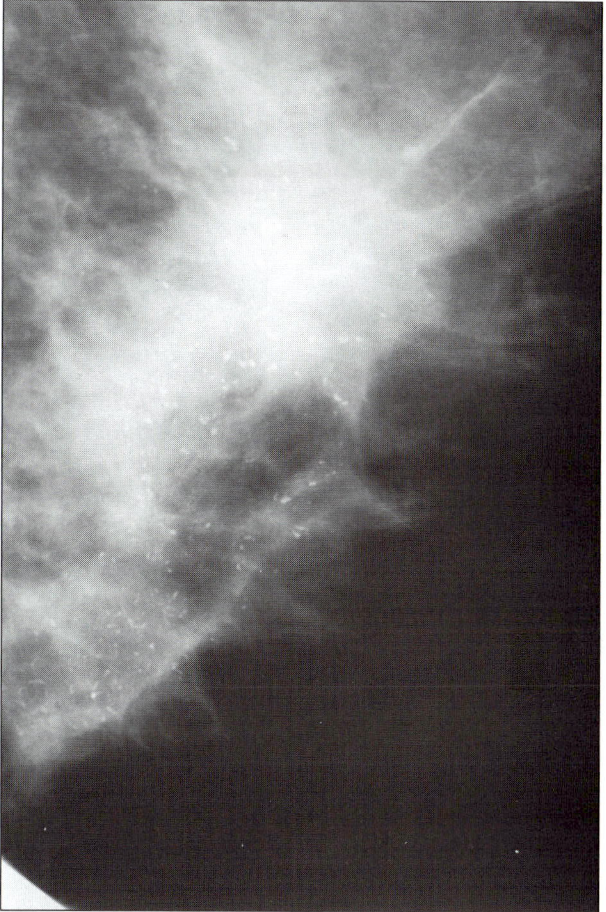

FIGURE 13.47 Calcifications demonstrated on reverse oblique view.

Circumscribed Tumors

Contour Analysis

- Important in the evaluation of circumscribed **tumors**.
- Benign breast tumors are sharply outlined in contour characteristically having a "halo" sign or capsule.
- Malignant tumors have an indistinct contour sometimes with short spicules or a comet tail.

Density Analysis

- Radiopaque—low density, usually benign; high density, usually cancer
- Radiolucent—mostly benign, containing oil or fat
- Radiopaque and radiolucent, mixed density—usually benign

Examples in this category include:

BENIGN

- **Cyst** (Figure 13.48)
- **Fibroadenoma** (fī´´brō-ăd´´ĕ-nō´mă) (Figure 13.49)

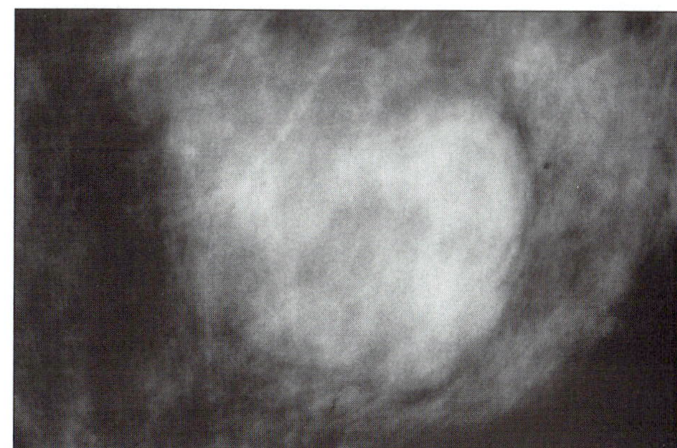

FIGURE 13.48 Benign cyst.

- **Fibroadenolipoma** (Figure 13.50)
- **Lipoma** (Figure 13.51)
- Oil cyst (Figure 13.52)
- **Abscess** (Figure 13.53)

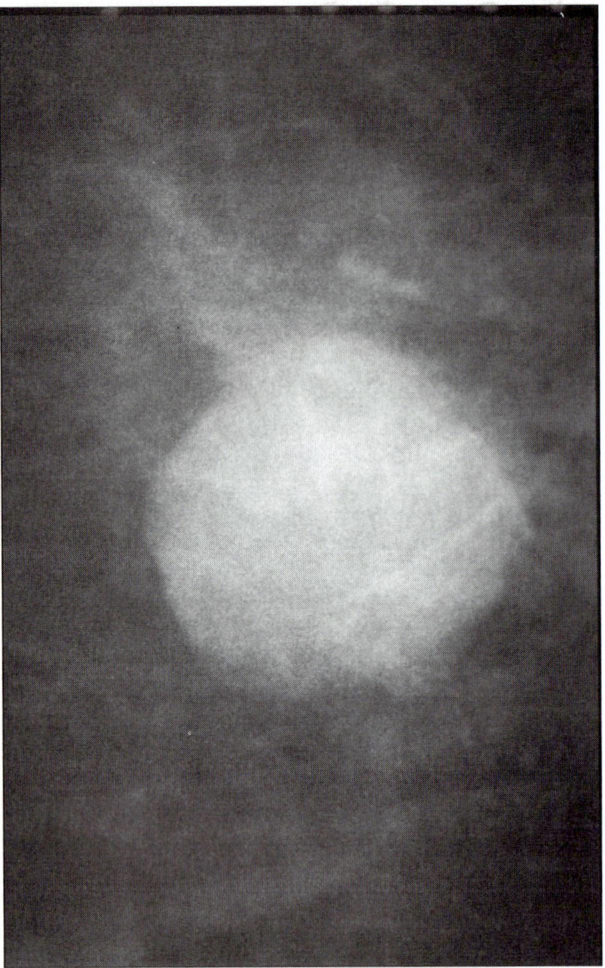

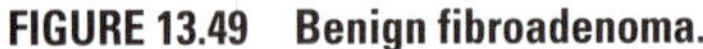
FIGURE 13.49 Benign fibroadenoma.

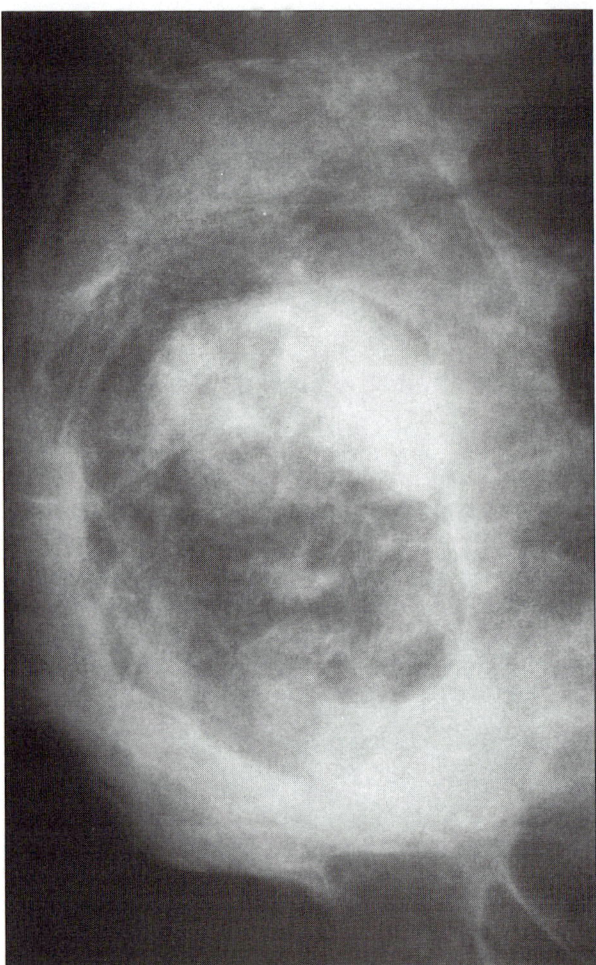

FIGURE 13.50 Fibroadenolipoma.

- **Cystosarcoma phyllodes** (Figure 13.54); can be malignant
- **Lymphoma** (Figure 13.55)
- **Papilloma** (Figure 13.56)
- **Lymph node** (Figure 13.57)

MALIGNANT

- Colloid carcinoma (Figure 13.58)
- **Medullary carcinoma** (Figure 13.59)
- **Sarcoma** (Figure 13.60)
- Melanoma
- Intracystic papillary carcinoma (Figure 13.61)

Stellate Lesions Most breast cancers present as stellate lesions. The characteristics most often seen on the mammogram are an area of increased density, irregular spiculated contour or margin with or without calcification. The exact type of tumor can be determined only by a histologic diagnosis.

Examples in this category are:

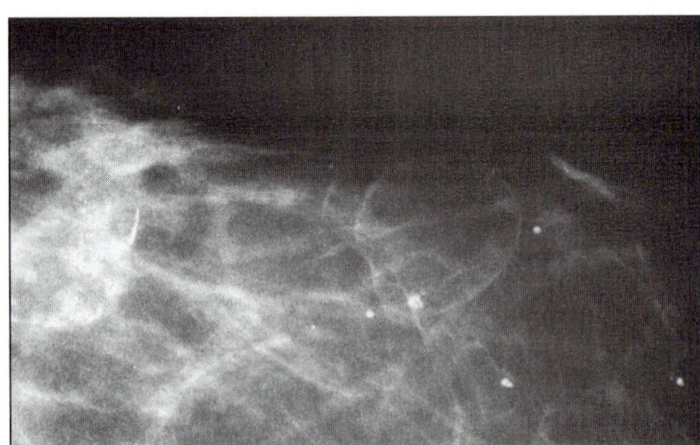

FIGURE 13.51 Lipoma.

BENIGN

- **Sclerosing** ductal **hyperplasia** (radial scar) (Figure 13.62)
- Traumatic **fat necrosis** (Figure 13.63)

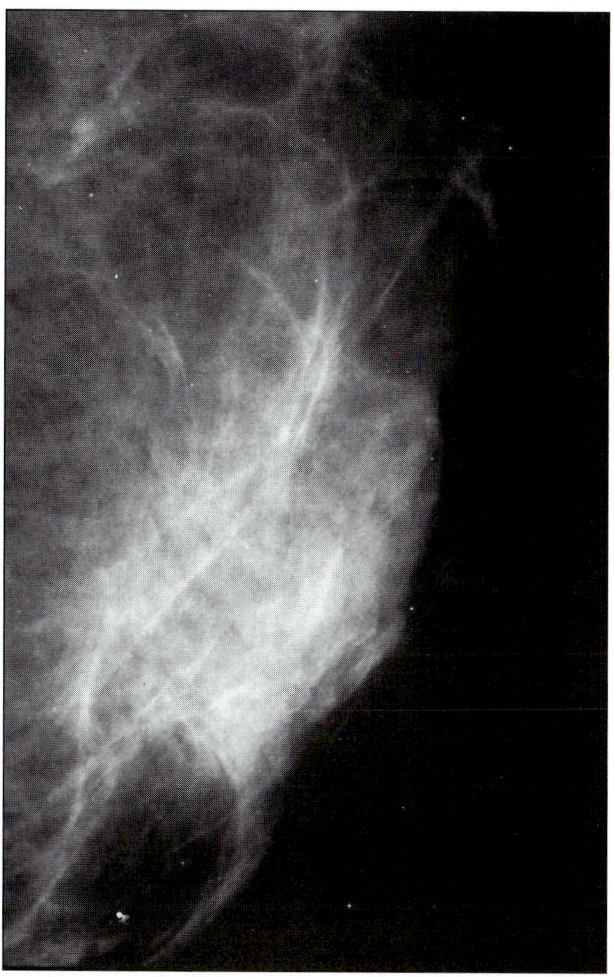

FIGURE 13.52 Oil cyst.

MALIGNANT

- Infiltrating ductal carcinoma (**scirrhous**)
- Tubular carcinoma (Figure 13.64)

Calcifications Calcifications can occur in both benign and malignant changes and must be analyzed according to their form, density, size, and distribution to define them as ductal, lobular, or miscellaneous. The ductal type of calcification occurs in breast cancer in two forms: **granular** or **casting**. The lobular type arises through the calcification of fluid within the lobules and is seen in benign processes. Miscellaneous calcification includes benign conditions such as calcified fibroadenoma, calcified papilloma, calcified traumatic fat necrosis, calcified **sebaceous** glands, and calcified arteries.

Examples in this category are:

BENIGN

- Calcified fibroadenoma (Figure 13.65)
- **Duct ectasia** (ĕk-tā´sē-ă)

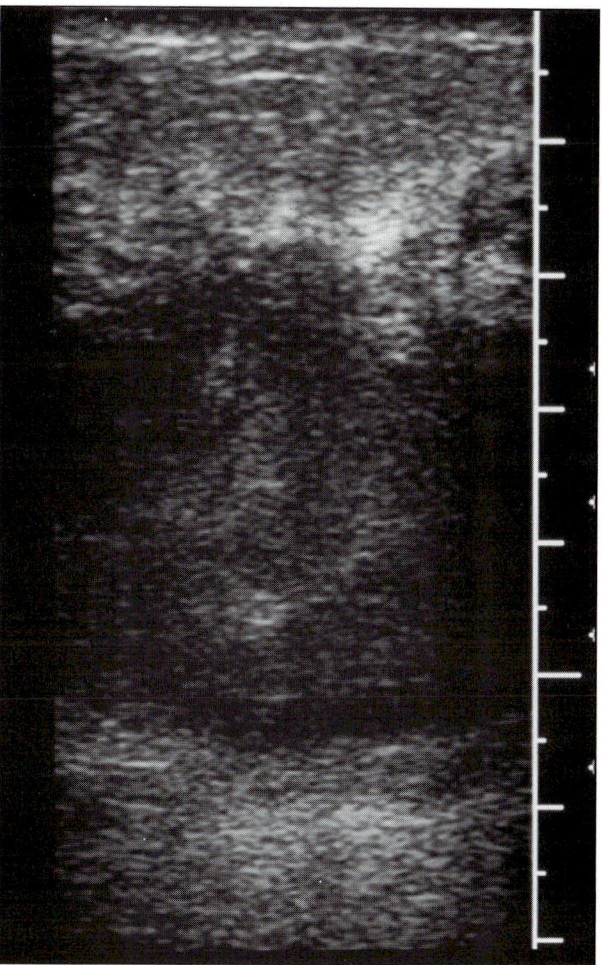

FIGURE 13.53 Abscess demonstrated with ultrasound.

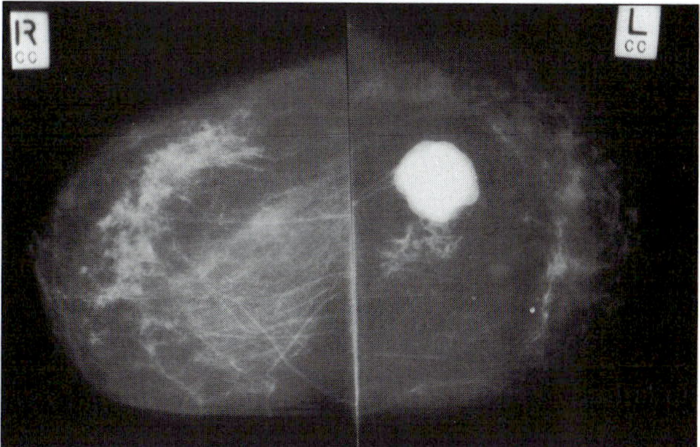

FIGURE 13.54 Cystosarcoma phyllodes (can be malignant).

- Calcified arteries (Figure 13.66)
- Milk of calcium
- Calcified sebaceous gland (Figure 13.67)
- **Intradermal calcifications**
- Calcified fat necrosis (Figure 13.68)

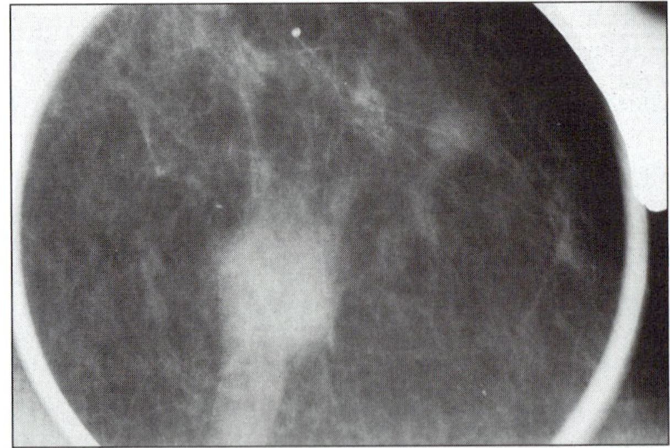

FIGURE 13.55 Lymphoma.

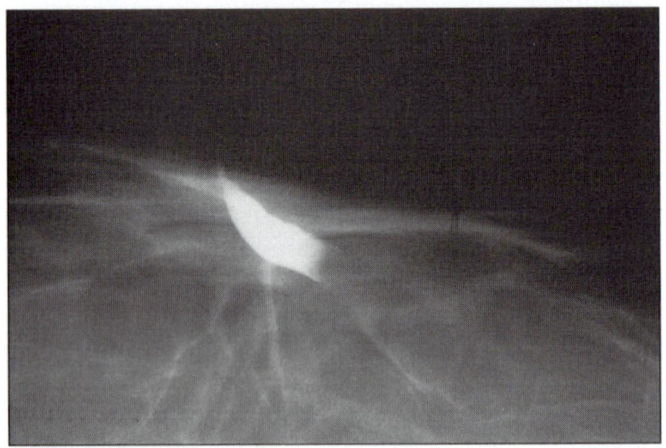

FIGURE 13.56 Papilloma.

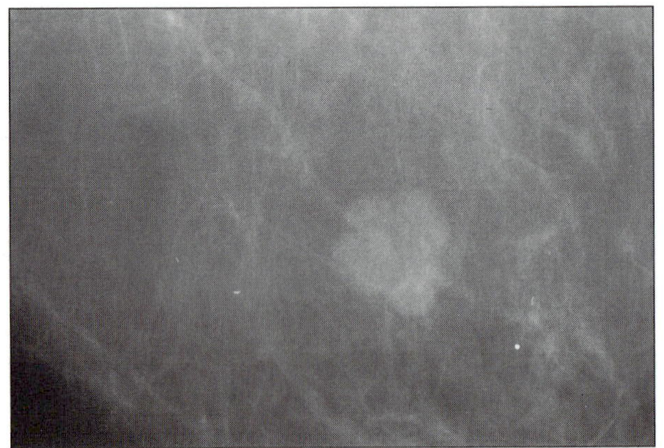

FIGURE 13.57 Intramammary lymph node.

MALIGNANT

- Comedo carcinoma (Figure 13.69)
- **Ductal carcinoma in situ**
- Invasive lobular carcinoma

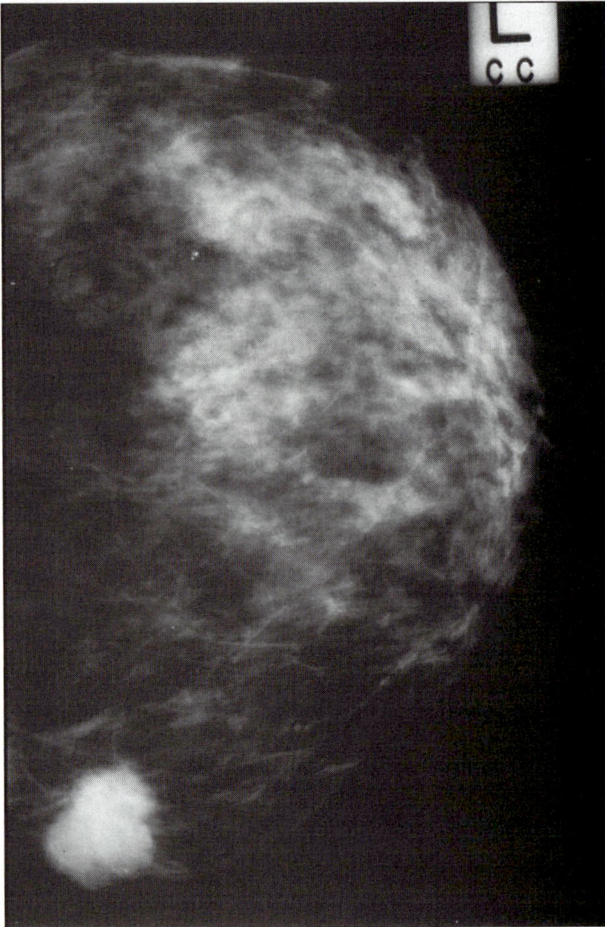

FIGURE 13.58 Colloid carcinoma.

Skin Changes Skin changes should be noted clinically and mammographically because they may represent a secondary sign of malignancy. Usually these are signs of lymphedema, which arises from blockage of the lymph drainage. Clinically the skin has a "peau d'orange" appearance (Figure 13.70) and mammographically there may be evidence of skin thickening especially in the dependent portion of the breast (Figure 13.71). The challenge is to find the primary cause. **Paget's** (păj′ĕt) **disease** (Figure 13.72) is the most common in this category, often associated with an underlying ductal carcinoma. Inflammatory carcinoma presents a similar clinical picture.

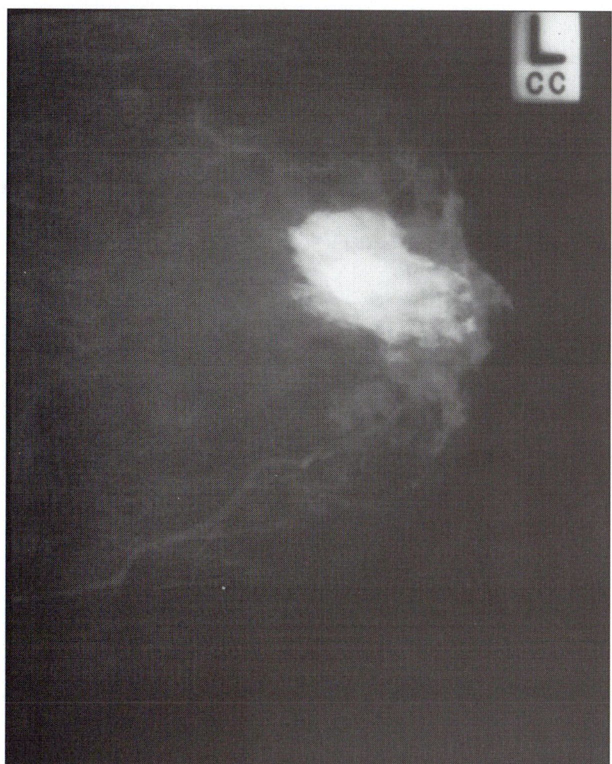

FIGURE 13.59 Medullary carcinoma.

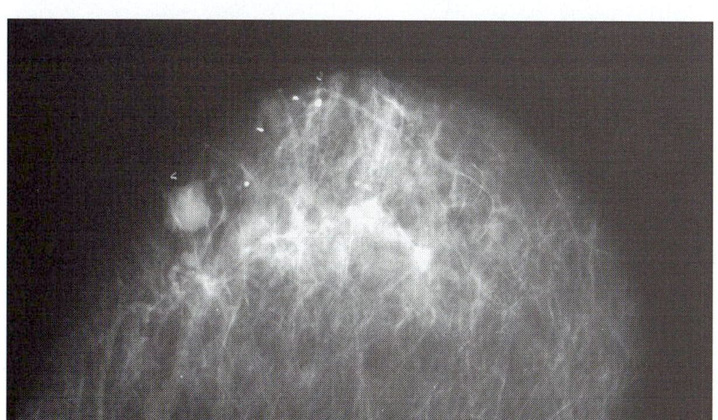

FIGURE 13.60 Sarcoma.

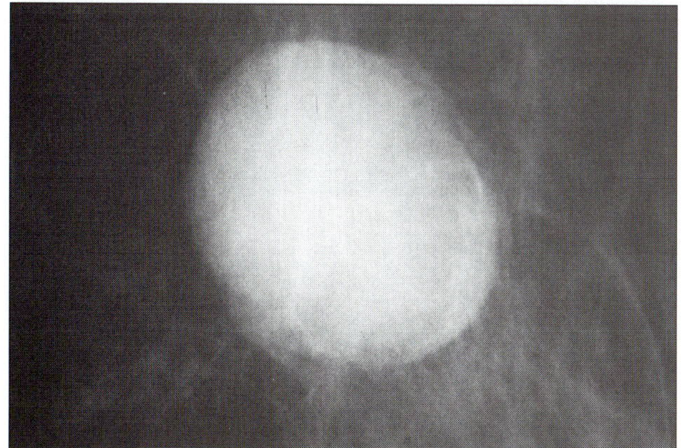

FIGURE 13.61 Papillary sarcoma.

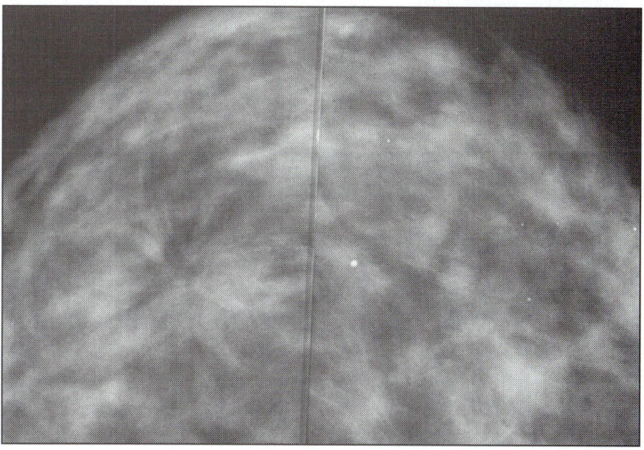

FIGURE 13.62 Radial scar.

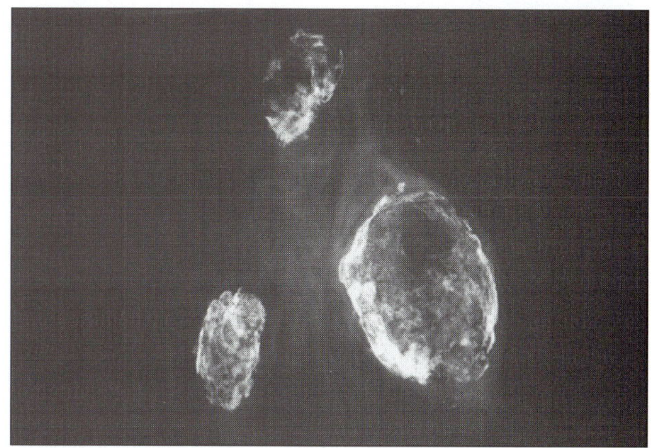

FIGURE 13.63 Fat necrosis.

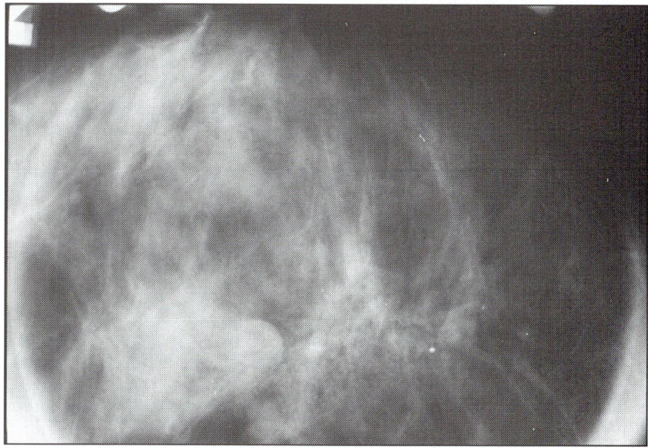

FIGURE 13.64 Tubular carcinoma.

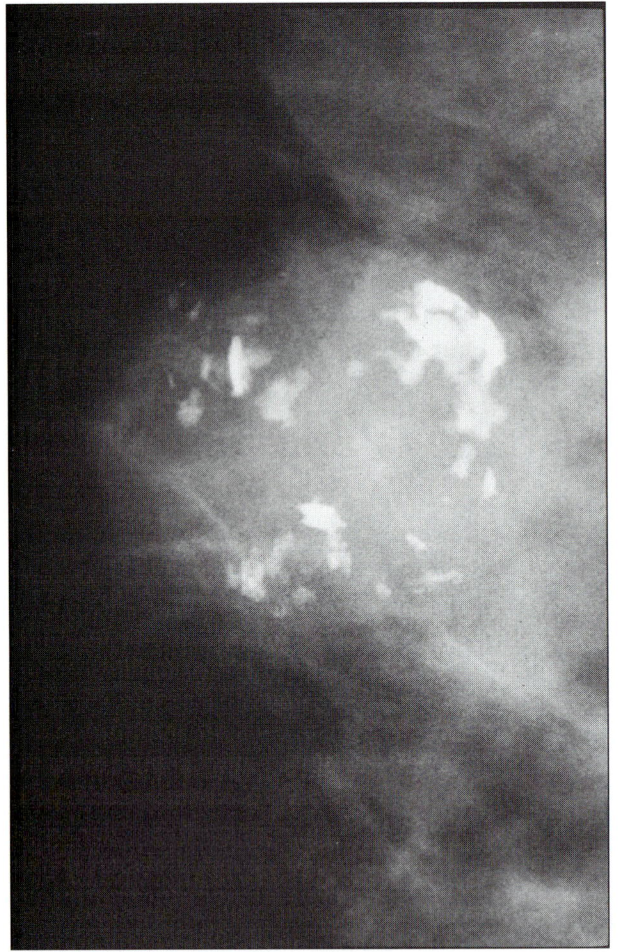

FIGURE 13.65 Calcified fibroadenoma.

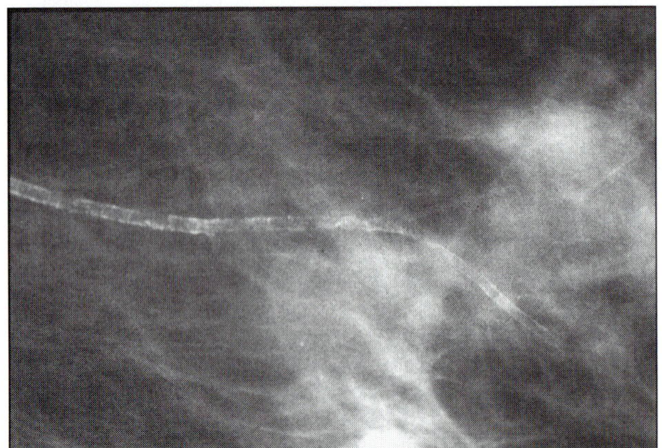

FIGURE 13.66 Calcified artery.

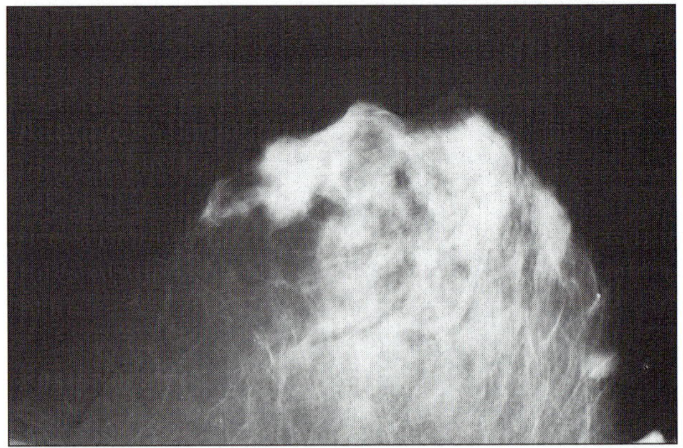

FIGURE 13.67 Calcified sebaceous cyst.

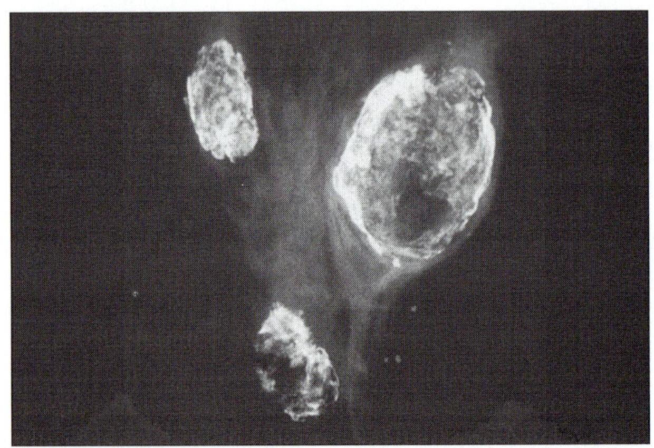

FIGURE 13.68 Calcified fat necrosis.

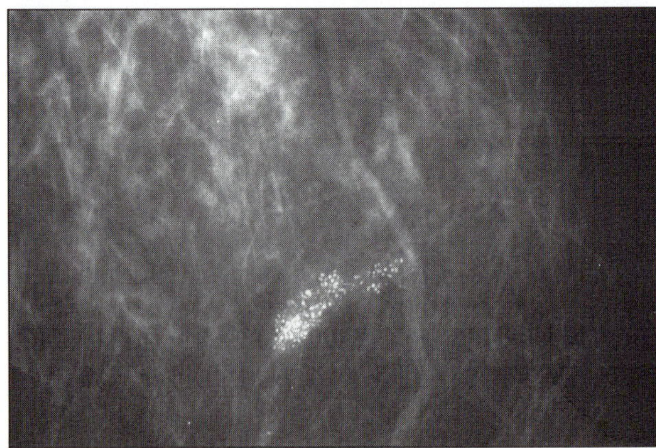

FIGURE 13.69 Comedo carcinoma.

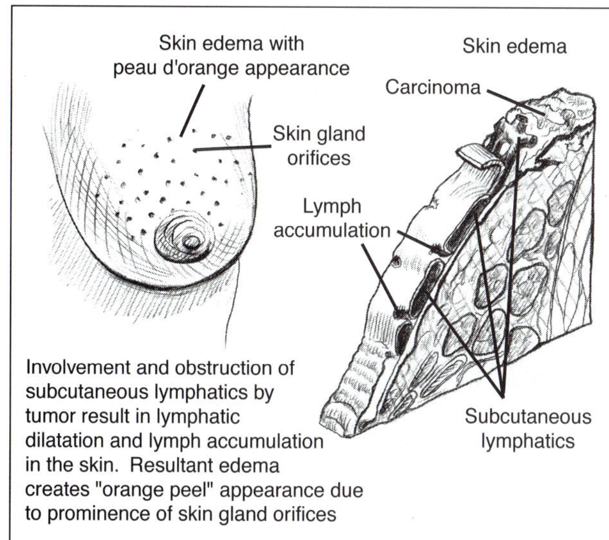

FIGURE 13.70 Peau d'orange.

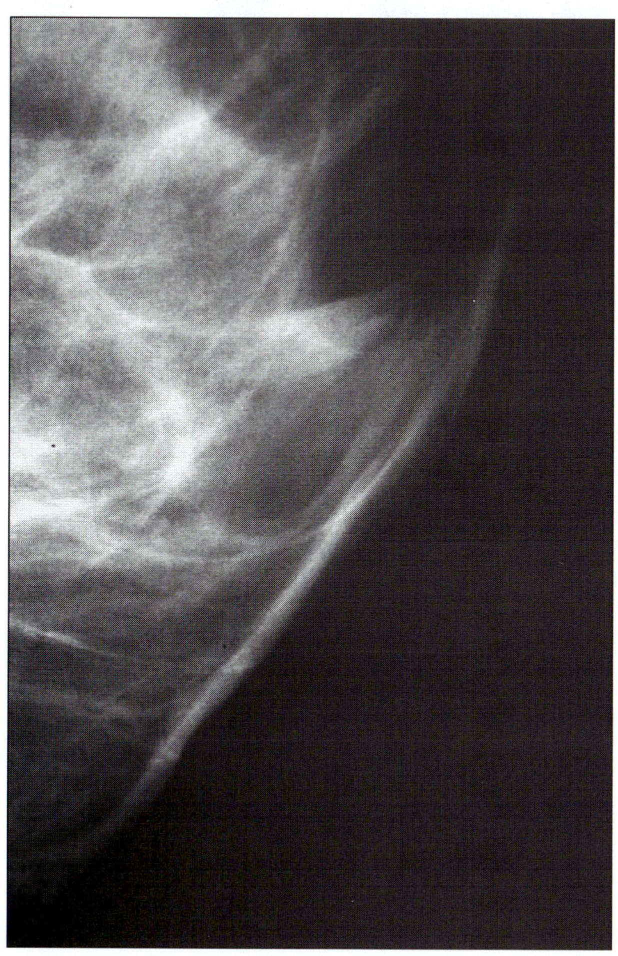

FIGURE 13.71 Skin thickening.

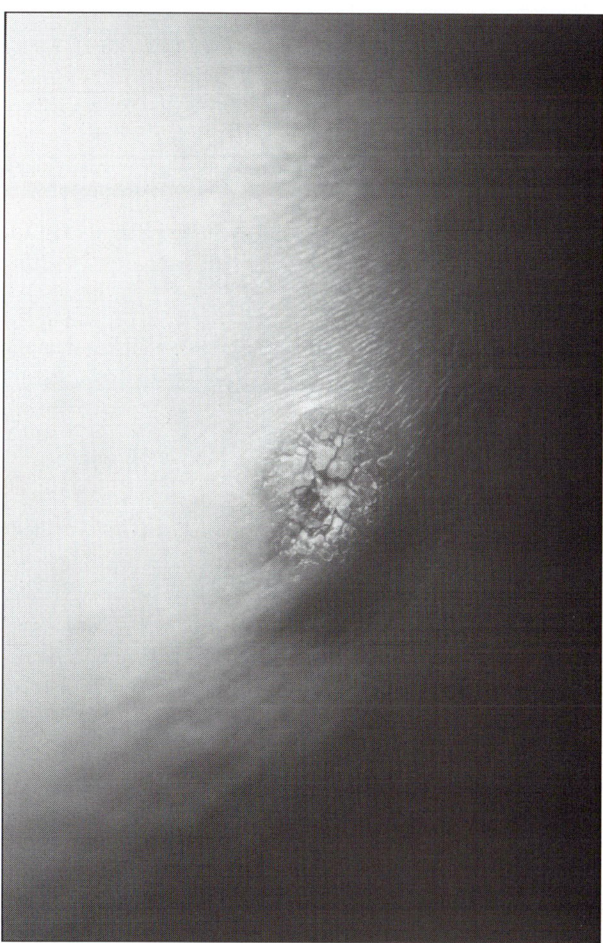

FIGURE 13.72 Paget's disease.

Other Imaging Modalities

Mammography is currently the only imaging modality with the proven capability of detecting early breast cancer. However it has limitations in both sensitivity and specificity, with only 80% to 90% of breast cancers being detected in reported studies. These limitations have stimulated interest in other breast imaging techniques that can be used as adjuncts to mammography in the detection or diagnosis of breast cancer. Some have proven inadequate and been discarded; others are in varying stages of development and evaluation.

COMPUTED TOMOGRAPHY

During the 1970s, CT scanning, based on tumor uptake of iodinated contrast, was investigated as a means of breast cancer detection. Scans were taken before and after the IV injection of contrast and differentiation between benign and malignant lesions was assessed on changes in CT density. Although one study reported some success, it could not be corroborated in a further study, and the overriding disadvantages of CT breast scanning (higher radiation dose than mammography, the time factor involved in the procedure, and the cost) have precluded its use as a screening tool.

Consequently CT is currently used as an adjunct to mammography:

- To guide preoperative needle localization of lesions that cannot be successfully identified on two mammographic views
- To ascertain whether the breast cancer has invaded the chest wall (Figure 13.73)
- To better image and evaluate breast prostheses, especially rupture (Figure 13.74)
- To assist in assessing the number and size of axillary lymph nodes before breast cancer surgery

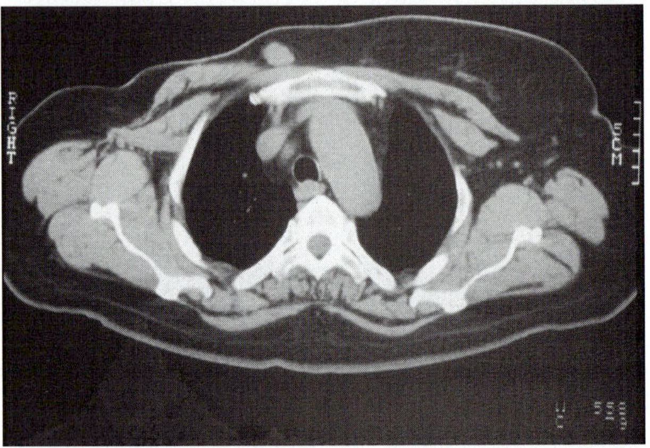

FIGURE 13.73 **CT demonstrating metastases.**

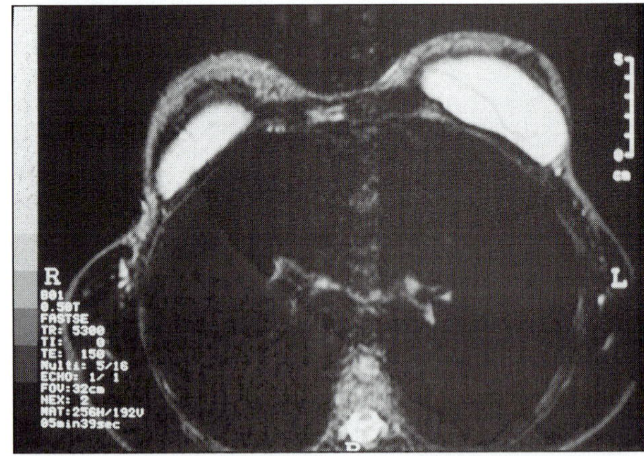

FIGURE 13.74 **CT demonstrating implant rupture.**

MAGNETIC RESONANCE IMAGING

The advantage of MRI of the breast is the possibility of achieving better image contrast than mammography without the use of ionizing radiation. Studies have been conducted to assess its ability to detect occult breast cancer. Limitations of early studies included relatively low resolution, large slice thickness, long acquisition times, and limited ability to characterize tissues. Recent advances in MRI technology have allowed improvements in its ability to characterize breast lesions. These improvements include:

- The replacement of body coils with surface coils to improve the signal-to-noise ratio (Figure 13.75)
- Better gradient-echo sequences to allow thinner slice imaging
- The introduction of three-dimensional, gadolinium-enhanced fat suppression techniques to improve tissue differentiation (Figure 13.76).

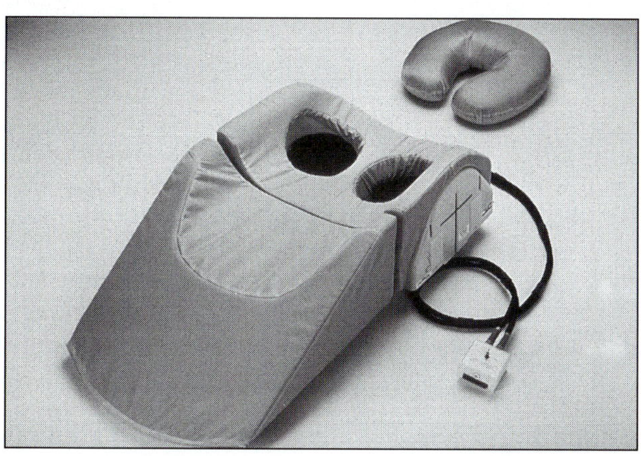

FIGURE 13.75 MRI breast coil.

Lengthy examination time, the availability of equipment, and the cost of the procedure are still limiting factors to the use of MRI for breast cancer screening. However, its potential role in breast cancer diagnosis and management cannot be discounted, and further research is being undertaken. It is currently considered the most accurate method of assessing breast prosthesis rupture.

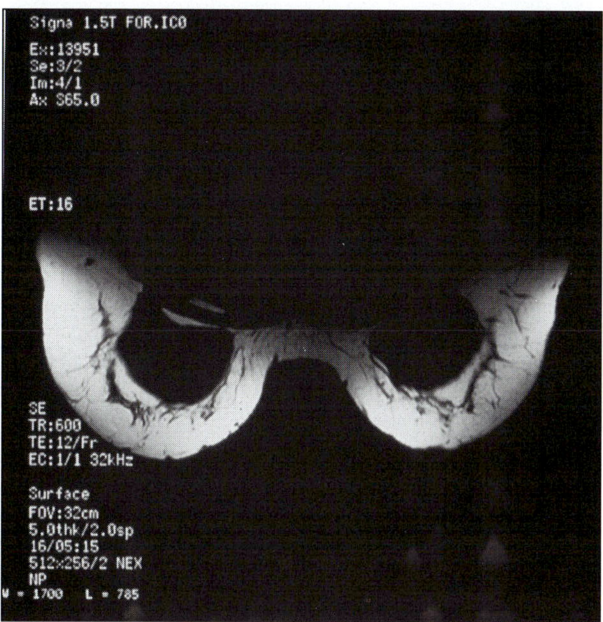

FIGURE 13.76 Breast MRI.

ULTRASOUND

Ultrasound is well established as a useful adjunct to mammography.

Its indisputable role is the differentiation of a cyst (Figure 13.77) from a solid mass (Figure 13.78) when a nonpalpable mass is seen mammographically. If the sonographic "mass" displays the strict criteria for a cyst (smooth sharp borders, posterior acoustic enhancement and the absence of internal echoes), then the need for further workup, including biopsy, is eliminated. The cyst may be drained under ultrasound control if necessary. Any suggestion that the sonographic lesion is solid should encourage aspiration biopsy, taking into account the clinical and mammographic findings.

Ultrasound may also be useful in the evaluation of a clinically palpable mass that cannot be seen mammographically. Cyst/solid differentiation will be helpful, but it should be noted that some solid masses will not be visible on ultrasound.

Ultrasound can be used to guide interventional procedures such as cyst aspiration and fine needle aspiration or core biopsy of solid lesions. These are simpler and quicker than similar x-ray guided procedures.

Ultrasound is often preferred as the initial imaging modality for the young patient with clinical symptoms, on the basis that it provides better imaging of dense breast tissue. Studies investigating ultrasound as an alternative method of breast cancer screening,

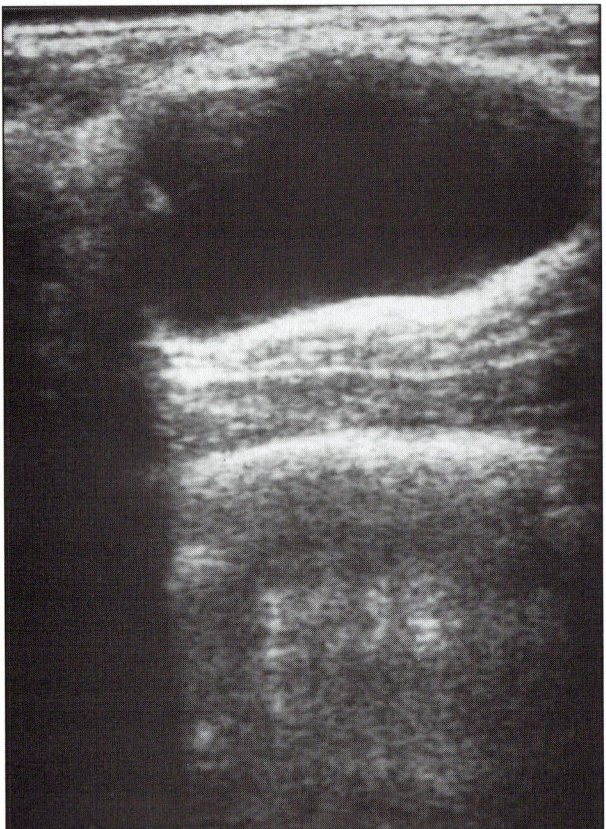

FIGURE 13.77 Ultrasound demonstrating cyst.

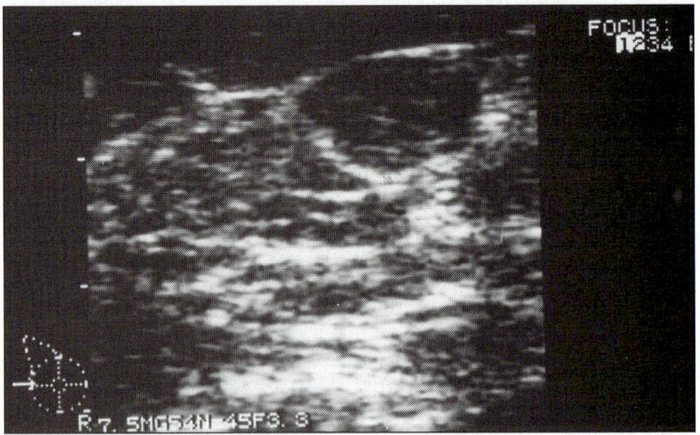

FIGURE 13.78 Fibroadenoma.

especially for the mammographically dense breast, have suggested that it is of limited value in detecting nonpalpable cancers. Also the fine microcalcifications, which are important for identifying cancer in younger women, are not imaged as well on ultrasound as on mammography.

Ultrasound cannot currently differentiate with certainty benign from malignant lesions. Some sonographic imaging criteria have been reported for the identification of malignant lesions (Figure 13.79), but a definitive answer still relies on pathologic assessment. Doppler ultrasound and color Doppler are being investigated as possible aids in differential diagnosis. Cancer detection may be improved by the use of color Doppler to demonstrate the increased blood flow through malignant lesions.

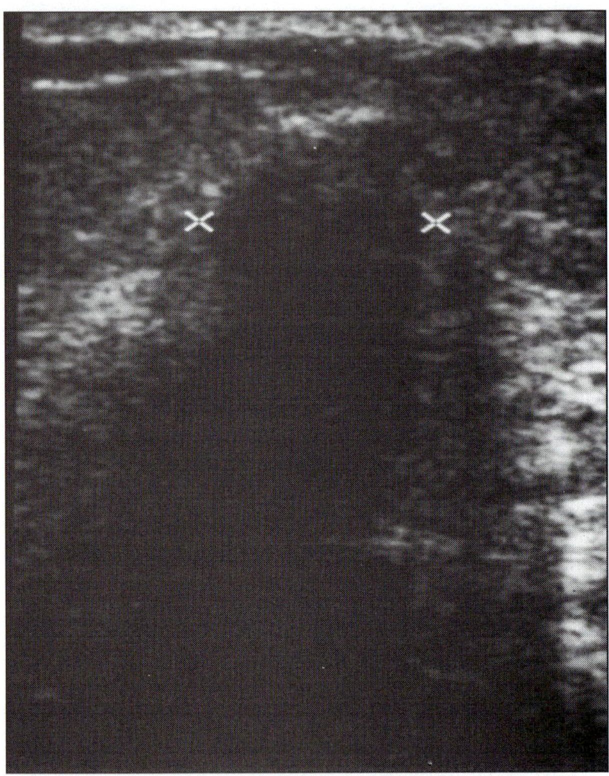

FIGURE 13.79 Ultrasound demonstrating adenocarcinoma.

THERMOGRAPHY

Thermography was aimed at detecting changes in skin temperature, which indicated an underlying breast cancer. The technique was based on the premise that the cancer would generate more heat than normal breast tissue. From studies conducted in the 1970s, the role of thermography in the detection of breast cancer looked promising. However, the Breast Cancer Detection Demonstration Project showed a high false-positive rate for the detection of clinically occult cancers by thermography, and no subsequent studies have supported the effectiveness of thermography in either cancer detection or as a cancer risk indicator.

TRANSILLUMINATION

Transillumination, light scanning or diaphanography, is a technique that uses the transmission effects of red and near-infrared light through breast tissue to detect tumors. It is founded on the basis that the hypervascularity of breast cancers will result in their higher absorption of light and distinguish them from the surrounding tissue. Initial studies were promising with sensitivity and specificity comparable to those of mammography. However, later studies have demonstrated that mammography is more accurate than transillumination in detecting small cancers that have a good prognosis. The limited sensitivity of the technique is due to light scattering in the breast. Today the interest in transillumination has been revived with the availability of computer-assisted technology to electronically enhance the light pattern emerging from the breast. Some success has been reported in imaging the dense glandular breast and the augmented breast, both of which are difficult areas for mammography. A future role for transillumination cannot be discounted, but currently no conclusive clinical data support the use of this technique as a screening or diagnostic tool.

POSITRON EMISSION TOMOGRAPHY (PET) SCANNING

Recently, PET scanning has assumed a role in the imaging of breast tumors although it was primarily used to image the brain and heart. Evaluation of both primary and metastatic tumors is achieved by the use of two compounds, 2-[F-18]-fluoro-2-deoxy-D-glucose (FDG) and 16-[F-18]-fluoroestradiol-17 (F-18-ES). Some success has been reported with FDG imaging of relatively large breast cancers (> 3 cm) that are clinically palpable but mammographically occult. Further scanning to record the results of FDG uptake after chemotherapy has suggested that it is possible to monitor tumor response to treatment before a change in tumor size can be identified. PET imaging with F-18-ES fluoroestradiol has been used as a method of providing in vivo information on the **estrogen** receptor status of breast tumors. This information can assist in assessing treatment and management options, especially the potential use of antiestrogens. The major limitation of PET is the necessity of an on-site or nearby cyclotron.

DIGITAL MAMMOGRAPHY

Digital mammography is emerging as the technology of the future for breast cancer detection and diagnosis. Advantages over screen/film mammography include:

- Lesser amount of radiation for image acquisition resulting in reduced patient dose
- Increased contrast resolution
- Wider gray-scale latitude
- Ability for electronic postprocessing to improve image information
- Rapid acquisition of information for needle guidance during interventional procedures
- Use of teleradiology for off-site radiologic consultation

One of the main limitations of currently available digital imaging systems is the relatively low spatial resolution that is achievable (6 line pairs/mm). At present levels of technology, pixel size needs to be decreased considerably for digital imaging to match the spatial resolution of screen/film mammography (16–20 line pairs/mm). Research continues to develop improvements in image processing technology, which may negate the necessity for such stringent spatial resolution requirements.

The potential of digital imaging to achieve greater sensitivity and specificity in mammography is enormous. Although the prospects for digital mammography are promising, further technologic improvement and further clinical evaluation are needed before it can replace screen/film mammography.

Interventional Procedures

DUCTOGRAPHY

Ductography, or **galactography** (gă-lăk-tŏg´ră-fē), is a procedure involving the introduction of a radiopaque contrast medium into the lactiferous ducts. Discharges from the nipple in the nonlactating breast are not uncommon, but most are of a typically benign origin associated with **fibrocystic changes**. The indication for the performance of ductography is the presentation of an abnormal unilateral blood-stained or serous **nipple discharge**. Outlining of the **ducts** with contrast medium aims to determine the site and cause of the discharge. The procedure can often detect papillomas or carcinomas that are not imaged on routine mammography and provide guidance to the area requiring open surgical biopsy. The main purpose of ductography is to demonstrate the location of a **lesion**.

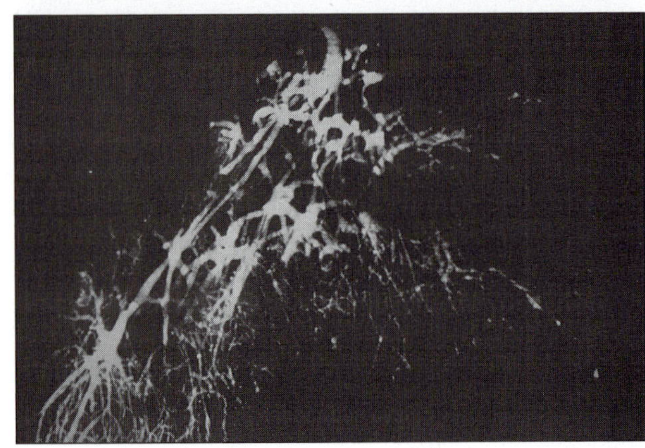

FIGURE 13.80 Ductogram.

It is important that the discharge be spontaneous or expressible on the day of the examination so that the correct duct opening can be cannulated. A small gauge (22–30) sialographic cannula is inserted into the identified duct opening and up to 3 mL of an iodinated contrast, such as Conray 60 or Optiray 320, is injected. Injection should be stopped when the patient indicates a feeling of discomfort in the breast. With the cannula still in position, mild compression is applied to the breast as images are obtained in the CC (Figure 13.80) and 90° lateral projections. Stereo and magnified views of the contrast-filled ducts may be useful to separate and better visualize overlapping structures. Lesions are demonstrated on the images as filling defects.

FINE NEEDLE ASPIRATION AND PNEUMOCYSTOGRAPHY

Fine needle aspiration (FNA) is performed to aspirate fluid from a cyst. The procedure involves the use of a 23-gauge needle and syringe, and may be performed for the following reasons:

- To drain a large "tension" cyst that is causing the patient discomfort or limiting accurate physical examination. Fluid may be aspirated by needling the cyst under clinical or sonographic guidance.
- When the sonographic appearances suggest a lesion is cystic but there is some internal echogenicity. The fluid should be aspirated and analyzed for the presence of blood or cellular material, which may alter the differential diagnosis.

Pneumocystography is a procedure that may be used as an adjunct to FNA and involves the introduction of air into the cyst after the aspiration of fluid. CC and 90° lateral mammographic projections are obtained to demonstrate the cystic cavity filled with air. It is performed when there is a suspicion of an intracystic tumor (Figure 13.81) or as a prophylactic measure if a cyst continues to fill with fluid after repeated drainage.

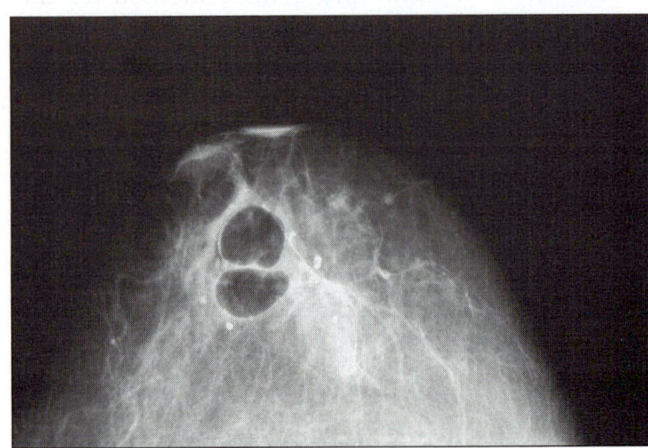

FIGURE 13.81 Pneumocystogram.

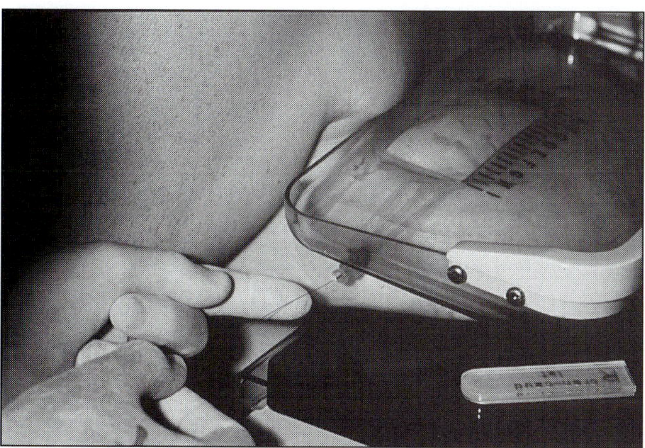

FIGURE 13.82 Compression for breast lesion localization.

Preoperative Localization The introduction of high-quality screen/film mammography has resulted in an increase in the discovery of small, nonpalpable lesions that require assessment. The management of these lesions has necessitated overcoming the problems of "blind" surgical biopsy and the associated difficulty in correct histologic sampling of the specimen. Techniques for preoperative localization of nonpalpable lesions have been developed. The procedures involve the placement of a hookwire or carbon track in the breast to guide the surgeon to the area for excision. The mammographic projection chosen for the localization procedure depends on achieving the shortest possible track from the skin surface to the lesion. The advantage of carbon track localization is that it can be performed at the time of fine needle biopsy, thus eliminating the necessity for a further procedure just before surgery.

Localization can be performed under ultrasound guidance if the lesion is clearly visible sonographically. This is the easier and quicker method for the patient. Localization under x-ray guidance requires compression of the breast with a perforated or fenestrated plate (Figure 13.82) throughout the procedure and is more uncomfortable for the patient. The needle/wire or needle is placed in the lesion (or just beyond) with the aid of a stereotactic device or by manual adjustment using two orthogonal views. Stereotactic devices use a computer for calculation of lesion depth and may be "add-on" units (Figure 13.83) to routine mammography equipment or part of a prone table used for core biopsy (Figure 13.84). Digital imaging, incorporated into more recently manufactured core biopsy units, has assisted in lessening procedure time.

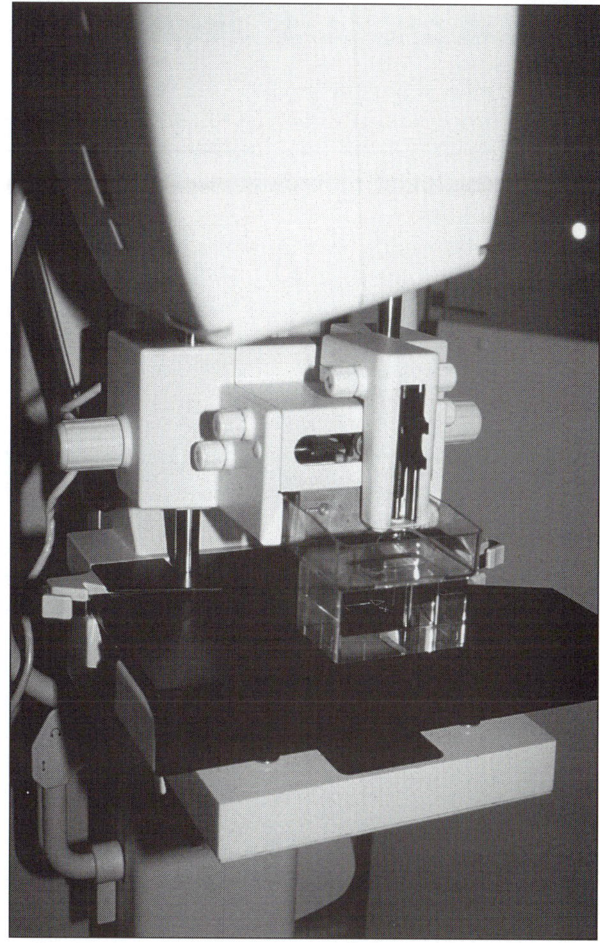

FIGURE 13.83 Stereotactic "add-on" unit.

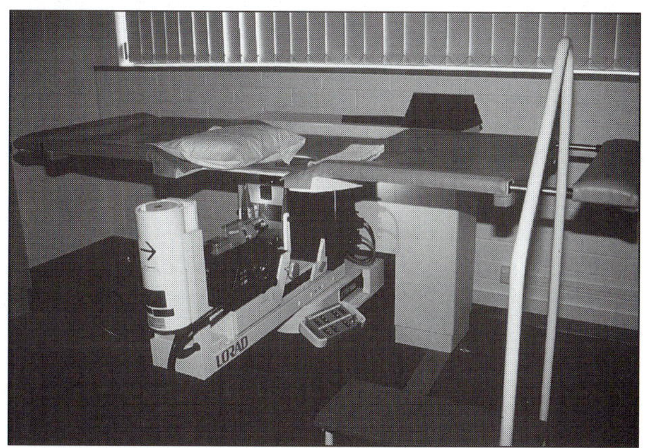

FIGURE 13.84 Prone table for core biopsy.

FINE NEEDLE ASPIRATION BIOPSY

A **fine needle aspiration biopsy (FNAB)** of a breast lesion involves the aspiration of a small amount of cellular material for cytologic assessment, using a 23-gauge needle. The procedure may be performed under clinical, sonographic, or x-ray guidance depending on whether the lesion is palpable or not. Sampling of a nonpalpable lesion under x-ray guidance involves the use of a perforated compression plate or stereotactic unit as described for preoperative localization procedures.

The FNAB **cytology** can add useful information to the clinical, mammographic, and sonographic findings and assist in clarifying treatment and management options. By confirming malignancy or benignity the necessity for open surgical biopsy can be eliminated, and the patient can proceed straight to surgical excision of the lesion or return to routine follow-up.

CORE BIOPSY

Core biopsy is a recent development that assists in the diagnosis of breast cancer. It involves biopsying the breast with a 14-gauge needle in a long-throw gun, and providing a "core" of tissue for histologic diagnosis. The procedure usually includes the acquisition of at least five specimens and may be performed under clinical, sonographic, or stereotactic guidance. The stereotactic procedure provides a better means of immobilizing the breast to cater for the "throw" of the biopsy gun and is currently the preferred option. The advantage of core biopsy is that it provides a simple, highly accurate method of confirming malignancy with surprisingly little discomfort or trauma to the patient and obviates the necessity for open surgical biopsy. In comparison, the evaluation of FNAB is very dependent on accurate sampling and a skilled pathologist experienced in breast cytology.

SPECIMEN RADIOGRAPHY

The surgical biopsy specimen should always be radiographed to ensure that the mammographic lesion has been excised. Mild compression will assist in spreading the tissue and better identifying a mass lesion. Magnification views may be useful for visualization of microcalcifications. The localizing wire or carbon marker, visible in the specimen, will serve as a point of reference to aid the pathologist in slicing for histopathology studies. The sliced specimen may also be radiographed after the surgery for better clarification of the area to be analyzed.

To ensure that a core biopsy for microcalcifications has been successful, the core specimens may be radiographed immediately after the procedure (Figure 13.85).

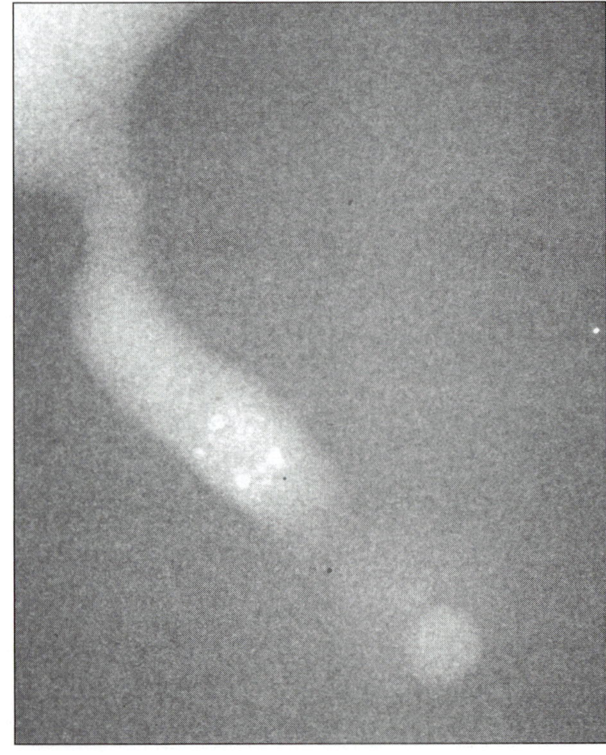

FIGURE 13.85 Radiograph of postsurgical core specimens.

Review Questions

1. Describe the essential components of a dedicated mammographic x-ray unit. Explain the purpose of these components.

2. Radiation dose and image quality may be perceived as having conflicting requirements. Discuss mammographic imaging with respect to this statement.

3. A comprehensive quality assurance program is essential to maintain a high standard of mammographic imaging. Discuss the role and responsibility of the radiographer with regard to quality assurance.

4. Good spatial and contrast resolution are important in mammographic images because:
   a. breast tissue is primarily fat
   b. breast calcifications are large
   c. there are subtle density differences between normal and pathological structures in the breast
   d. "extended" processing is used for mammographic images

5. Discuss the benefits and risks for women undergoing mammographic screening for breast cancer.

6. The most common radiation dose measurement for mammography is
   a. skin dose
   b. mean glandular dose
   c. half-value layer dose
   d. mid-breast dose

7. Discuss the role of ultrasound in breast imaging.

CASE STUDY

A 55-year-old woman received a letter of invitation to attend a screening mammogram. An asymmetrical density identified in her left breast resulted in her being recalled for assessment of the lesion. Available expertise at the assessment clinic includes a radiographer, radiologist, surgeon, pathologist, and nurse counselor. Describe the critical pathway that would be followed to further categorize the abnormality and determine a diagnosis. Include specialized views, other imaging modalities, and interventional techniques that might be appropriate. Comment on the necessity for continuous counseling and information sharing as the diagnosis is revealed.

References and Recommended Reading

Andolina, V. F., Lille, S., & Willison, K. M. (1992). *Mammographic imaging: A practical guide.* Philadelphia: Lippincott .

Azzopardi, J. G. (1979). *Problems in breast pathology.* London: Saunders.

Baker, L. H. (1982). Breast cancer detection demonstration project: Five year summary report. *CA, 32,* 194–226.

Bassett, L. W., & Kimme-Smith, C. (1991). Breast sonography. *AJR American Journal of Roentgenology, 156,* 449–455.

Bohm-Velez, M., & Mendelson, E. B. (1989). Computed tomography, duplex Doppler ultrasound, and magnetic resonance imaging in evaluating the breast. *Seminars in Ultrasound, CT and MRI, 10,* 171–176.

Cole-Beuglet, C., Golberg, B. B., Kurtz, A.B., et al. (1981). Ultrasound mammography: Comparison with radiographic mammography. *Radiology, 139*(3), 693–698.

Dodd, G. (1977). Present status of thermography, ultrasound, and mammography in breast cancer detection. *Cancer, 39,* 2796–2805.

Eklund, G. W., Busby, R.C., Miller, S. H., & Job, J.S. (1988). Improved imaging of the augmented breast. *AJR, American Journal of Roentgenology, 151* 469–473.

Feig, S. A. (1989). The role of ultrasound in a breast imaging center. *Seminars in Ultrasound, CT and MR, 10,* 90–105.

Geslien, G. E., Fisher, J. R., & Delaney, C. (1985). Transillumination in breast cancer detection: Screening failures and potential. *AJR, American Journal of Roentgenology, 144,* 619–622.

Gisvold, J. J., Brown, L. R., & Swee, R. G. (1986). Comparison of mammography and transillumination light scanning in the detection of breast lesions. *AJR, American Journal of Roentgenology, 147,* 191–194.

Gisvold, J. J., Reese, D. F., & Carsell, P. R. (1979). Computed tomographic mammography (CTM). *AJR, American Journal of Roentgenology, 133,* 1143.

Kimme-Smith, C., Bassett, L. W., & Gold, R. H. (1992). *Workbook for quality mammography.* Philadelphia: Williams & Wilkins.

Kopans, D. B. (1989). *Breast imaging.* Philadelphia: Lippincott.

Lanyi, M. (1986). *Diagnosis and differential diagnosis of breast calcifications.* New York: Springer-Verlag.

Logan-Young W., & Hoffman, N. Y. (1994). *Breast cancer: A practical guide to diagnosis, Volume 1—procedures.* Rochester, NY: Mt. Hope Publishing.

Shaw-de Parades, E. (1989). *Atlas of film-screen mammography.* Baltimore: Urban & Schwarzenberg.

Sickles, E. A. (1988). Practical solutions to common mammographic problems: Tailoring the mammographic examination. *AJR, American Journal of Roentgenology, 151,* 31–39.

Sickles, E. A., Filly, R. A., & Callen, P. W. (1983). Breast cancer detection with sonography and mammography: Comparison using state-of-the-art equipment *AJR, American Journal of Roentgenology, 140,* 843–845.

Tabar, L., & Dean, P. B. (1985). *Teaching atlas of mammography* (2nd ed.). New York: Thieme.

Wahl, R. L., Cody, R. L., Hutchins, G. D., et al. (1991). Primary and metastatic breast carcinoma: Initial clinical evaluation with PET with the radiolabeled glucose analogue 2-[F-18]- Fluoro-2-deoxy-D-glucose. *Radiology, 179*(3), 765–770.

Wentz, G., Parsons, W. C. (1992). *Mammography for radiologic technologists.* Scarborough: McGraw-Hill.

SECTION VII

NERVOUS SYSTEM

CHAPTER 14

Brain

CYNTHIA COWLING, BSc, MEd, MRT(R), ACR

OBJECTIVES

At the completion of this chapter, the student should be able to:

1. List the procedures used in the diagnostic studies of the brain.
2. Identify the major features of the anatomy of the brain.
3. Describe the four usual plain radiographs used to visualize the skull and state their use in the demonstration of neurologic conditions.
4. List the pathologies visualized in tomography that may indicate a neurologic condition.
5. Identify relevant equipment for each study and procedure.
6. Identify radiation protection methods used.
7. Describe the relevant procedure sequences.
8. List common pathologies visualized for each examination and procedure.
9. Describe the basic concepts of alternative imaging routines.

Introduction and Historical Overview

The brain, which together with the heart was often shrouded in mystery and mystique, was one of the first areas of human anatomy that the general public wanted to see through the miracle new medium of x-rays. As early as 1896, Randolph Hearst asked Thomas Edison to take a cathodograph of the human brain for the *New York Journal.* Edison failed at this time, placing blame on the insuperable obstacles imposed by the skull itself. Initially, head x-rays were performed for fractures and foreign bodies. The father of neuroradiology was considered to be Arthur Schuller, who published his first textbook on radiology in 1912, but the very first localization of a brain tumor was reported by Church in 1899 (on the basis of the calcification of the tumor).

The introduction of air into the brain as a contrast agent created the primary form of brain imaging for the next 30 years. Dandy first experimented with ventriculography (vĕn-trĭk´´ū-lŏg´ră-fē) in 1918 at Johns Hopkins Hospital in Baltimore when he bubbled air directly into the ventricles. Studies of the blood supply to the brain (cerebral angiography) were begun in the 1920s and radionuclide brain scanning was born in 1948, when George Moore, a surgeon from Minneapolis, used a Geiger counter to measure the amount of radiation being emitted from the brain after an injection of diiofluorescin 131. Since that time, nuclear medicine has played an increasingly important role in the demonstration of the function of the brain. Modern advances such as PET and SPECT have added to the variety of functions nuclear medicine can perform.

Major changes to brain imaging occurred with the advent of CT and then MRI. These two modalities have become the primary methods of brain imaging. However, the need for plain films should not be discounted. Conventional tomography can still occasionally be used to demonstrate certain bony pathologies that have implications neurologically. Encephalography and ventriculography were examinations of the brain by the insertion of air as a contrast medium either by direct injection or via the spinal cord. These procedures have virtually ceased. CT and MRI are able to image the ventricles well, without the prolonged pain and discomfort that frequently accompanied air-contrast examinations. These procedures will therefore not be covered in this text.

Anatomy

The chief functions of the nervous system are the transmission of nerve impulses, the interpretation of nerve stimuli, and the storage of nerve stimuli. The principle divisions of the nervous system include the:

1. Central nervous system (CNS) consisting of the brain and spinal cord (Figure 14.1).
2. Peripheral nervous system consisting of the cranial nerves, spinal nerves and the autonomic nervous system (Figure 14.2).

CENTRAL NERVOUS SYSTEM

Brain

On the basis of its development, the brain consists of three divisions

1. Forebrain
2. Midbrain
3. Hindbrain

The forebrain includes the cerebrum, thalamus, hypothalamus, pineal gland, and the neural part of the pituitary gland. The largest part of the forebrain,

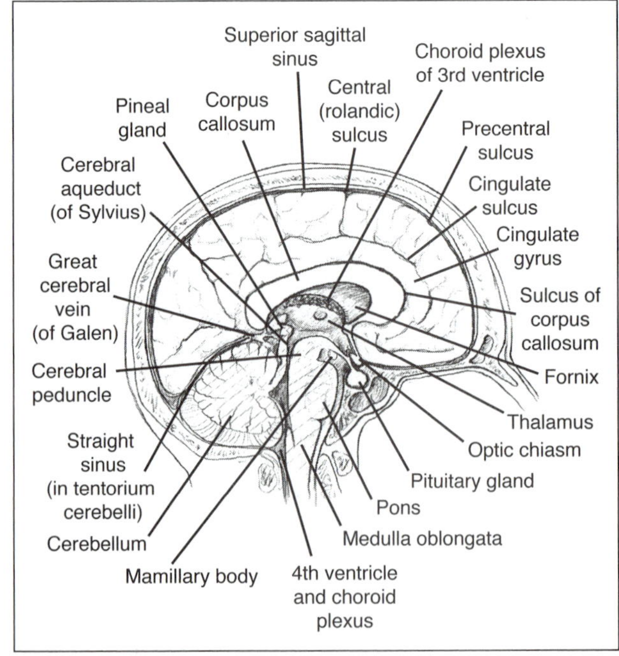

FIGURE 14.1 The nervous system.

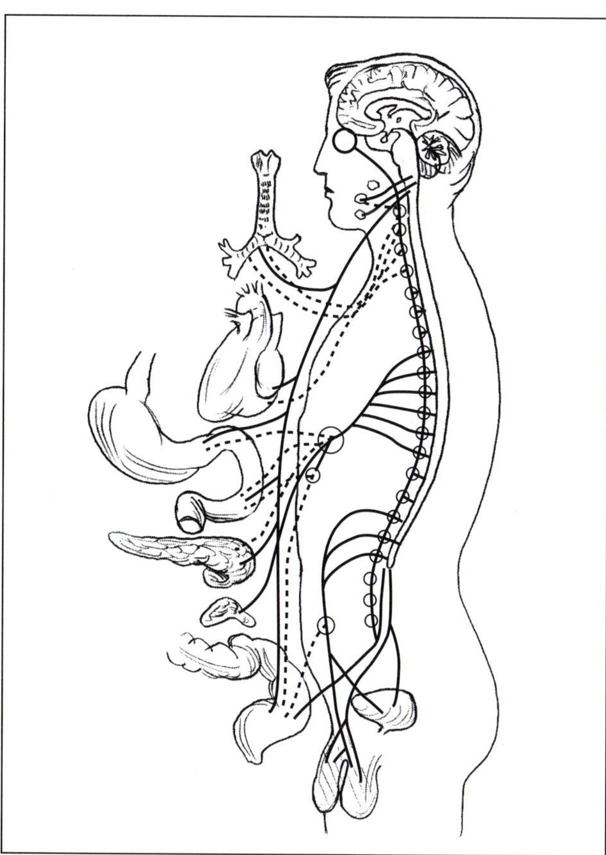

FIGURE 14.2 The autonomic system.

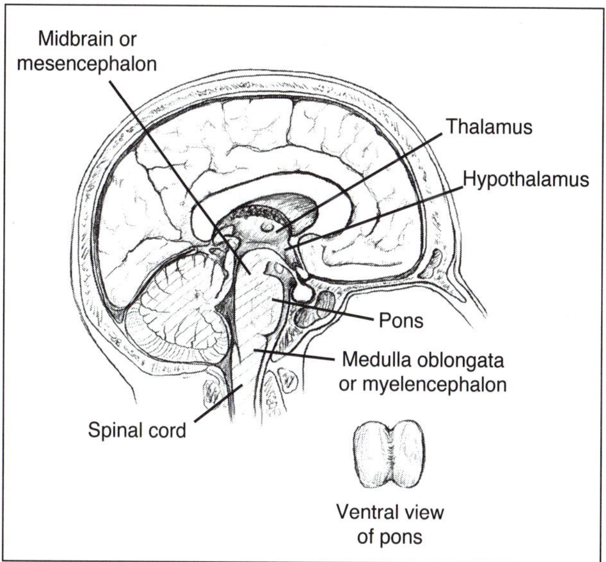

FIGURE 14.3 Main sections of the brain.

the cerebrum, consists of two hemispheres connected by a mass of white matter, the corpus callosum. Each hemisphere will occupy the anterior cranial fossa and the superior half of the posterior cranial fossa. The thalamus and hypothalamus occupy the central part of the middle cranial fossa (Figure 14.3).

As the cerebrum develops, a number of grooves or sulci and twisted folds or gyri appear on its surface. Two of these, the central sulcus and lateral fissure, define the lobes of the cerebrum. The frontal lobe lies anterior to the central sulcus and superior to the lateral fissure, the parietal lobe lies posterior to the central sulcus and superior to the lateral fissure; the temporal lobe lies inferior to the lateral fissure, and the occipital lobe is located posterior to the termination point of the lateral fissure.

The midbrain, the smallest part of the brain, is positioned in the upper central part of the posterior cranial fossa. On its dorsal aspect are a superior pair of superior caliculi and an inferior pair of inferior caliculi. Together, the caliculi are known as the corpora quadrigemina (kwŏd′′rĕ-jĕm′ĭn-ă). Ventrally, two bundles of nerve fibers known as the cerebral peduncles, convey impulses to and from the cerebral hemispheres.

The hindbrain is located in the inferior part of the posterior cranial fossa. On the dorsal aspect of the upper end of the hindbrain lies the cerebellum. The pons forms the ventral aspect. The lower half of the hindbrain is comprised of the medulla, a cone-shaped structure, which continues as the spinal cord at the level of the foramen magnum of the skull.

Ventricles

The ventricular apparatus consists of four cavities and their associated foramina and ducts. Three ventricles are located in the forebrain; the fourth is found in the hindbrain, anterior to the cerebellum (Figure 14.4).

Located one in each cerebral hemisphere, the lateral ventricles consist of an anterior, posterior and inferior horn, extending into the frontal, occipital and temporal lobes respectively. A small aperture, the interventricular foramen, allows each lateral ventricle to communicate with the third ventricle, a midline slit lying between the two halves of the thalamus. The cerebral aqueduct passes through the midbrain to connect the third and fourth ventricles. Three foramina open from the fourth ventricle, a median foramen of Magendie and two lateral recesses, the foramina of Luschka.

Coverings of the Brain

In addition to protection of the brain offered by the skull, the brain is further covered by three membranes, the meninges. The dura mater, the outer layer is a

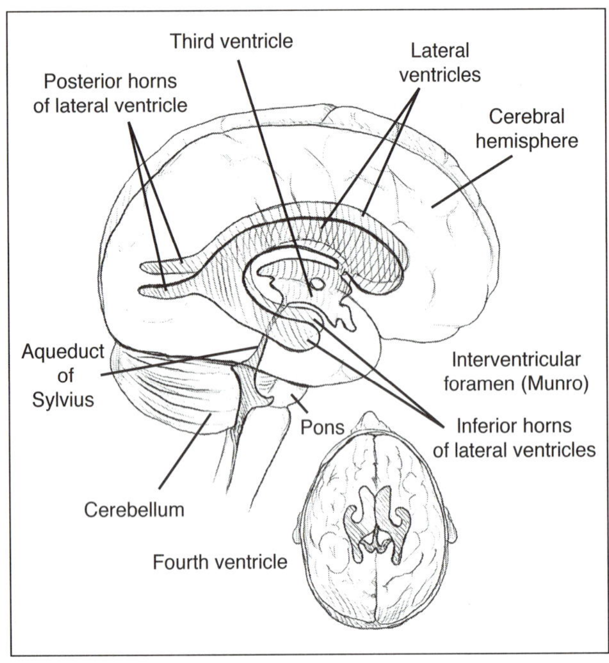

FIGURE 14.4 Ventricles of the brain.

tough avascular membrane. Its outer part is adherent to the periosteum of the anterior part of the skull, its inner component lies adjacent to the arachnoid mater. Where the two cerebral hemispheres come together on their medial aspects, the dura covering them unite to form the falx cerebri. Between the cerebellum and the cerebral hemisphere, the dura forms an extension called the tentorium cerebelli.

In certain areas of the brain, the two layers of dura separate to form the dural sinuses, channels that convey venous blood from the brain and head in general. A significant dural sinus is the superior sagittal sinus, located on the superior aspect of the falx cerebri. Into this sinus will project the arachnoid villi, through which passes cerebrospinal fluid (CSF) from the subarachnoid space.

The arachnoid mater is a delicate membrane that lines the mater and forms the outer limit of the subarachnoid space, which contains the CSF. The pia mater is a delicate vascular membrane that closely covers the brain. It passes into the depths of all the sulci and surrounds the cranial nerves emerging from the brain and the blood vessels entering the substance of the brain.

PERIPHERAL NERVOUS SYSTEM

Cranial Nerves

A total of twelve cranial nerves emerge from the base of the brain. Except for the first pair, the olfactory nerves, all the nerves extend from the brain stem. They are numbered 1 to 12, based on their origin from the anterior to the posterior brain stem. Some of the cranial nerves have primary sensory or motor fibers and are classed as sensory or motor nerves, respectively. Often nerves include both sensory and motor nerve fibers and are termed mixed nerves. In general the cranial nerves are involved with voluntary activities, although four, the oculomotor, facial, glossopharyngeal, and vagus nerves, are involved in regulating parasympathetic functions of the autonomic nervous system.

Cranial Nerves	Exit from Skull	Function
Olfactory I	Cribiform plate	Sensory, smell
Optic II	Optic foramen	Sensory, vision
Oculomotor III	Superior orbital fissure	Mixed; eye muscles
Trochlea IV	Superior orbital fissure	Mixed; superior oblique muscles of the eye
Trigeminal V	Superior orbital fissure	Sensory, face
	Foramen rotundum	Sensory, maxilla
	Foramen ovale	Mixed, mandible
Abducens VI	Superior orbital fissure	Mixed, lateral muscles of the eye
Facial VII	Stylomastoid foramen	Mixed, facial muscles
Vestibulocochlear VIII	Internal auditory meatus	Sensory, hearing and equilibrium
Glossopharyngeal IX	Jugular foramen	Mixed, taste, pharynx
Vagus X	Jugular foramen	Mixed, thoracic and abdominal viscera
Accessory XI	Jugular foramen	Motor, trapezius muscle
Hypoglossal XII	Hypoglossal canal	Motor, tongue

Procedures

PLAIN RADIOGRAPHS

Plain radiographs can demonstrate normal variants or pathologic processes that give rise to neurologic symptoms not necessarily caused by brain lesions.

Applied Anatomy (Figure 14.5)

Indications

- Vault fractures
- Early enlargement of pituitary fossa
- Raised intracranial pressure
- Bone erosion, **sclerosis**

Contraindications

- Plain radiography is noninvasive and therefore does not have the potential risks due to reaction or disease.
- Most soft tissue pathology and the blood supply to the brain require specialized procedures.

Equipment General radiographic equipment can provide good radiographs of the skull.

Contrast Media None

Radiation Protection

- To the gonadal area and thyroid where possible
- Greatest collimation possible

Preliminary Radiographs None because plain radiographs of the head are usually initial studies

Patient Preparation Removal of all radiopaque materials from the head area

Procedure Sequence See Chapter 12, Basic Skull Positions, in Volume I for positioning technique.

Procedure Radiographs Deformities of the bony skull are well demonstrated on plain radiographs and these can sometimes lead to neurologic conditions and symptoms.

Position	Demonstrates
Lateral view of the skull	Calcifications of the pineal gland
PA 20° caudad (Figure 14.6)	
AP 30° caudad fronto-occipital	(If greater than 1 cm a pineal tumor should be suspected.) Metastatic deposits usually from primary tumors of prostate or breast
Optic foramen view	Enlarged optic foramen can indicate presence of optic nerve glioma.
Pediatric skull	
Lateral view	
AP 30° caudad fronto-occipital (Figure 14.7)	Raised intracranial pressure by evidence of separation of lambdoid and sagittal sutures.

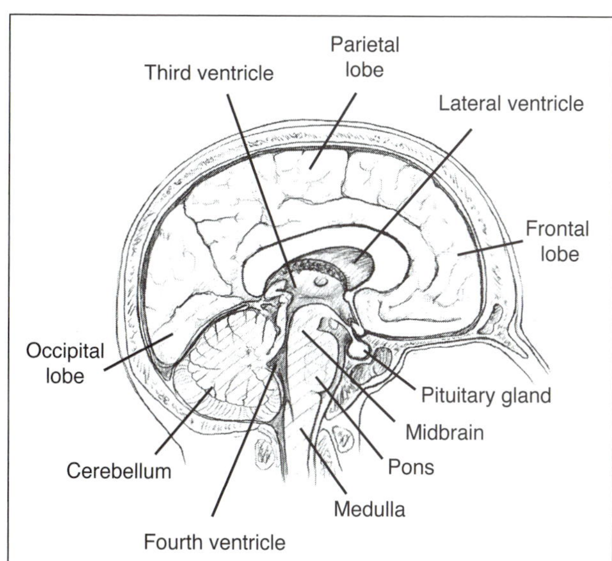

FIGURE 14.5 Cross section of the brain.

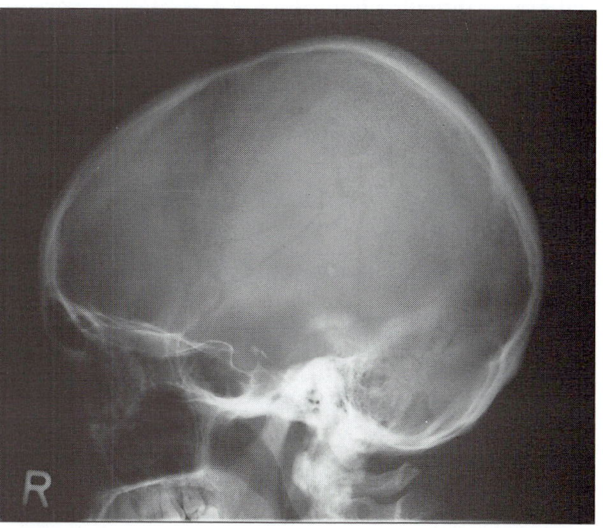

FIGURE 14.6 Lateral view of skull to demonstrate possible calcification.

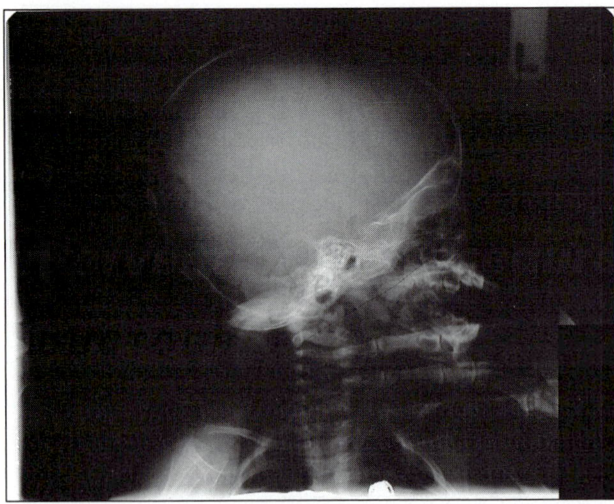

FIGURE 14.7 Lateral view of pediatric skull to demonstrate sutures.

Alternative Radiographs/Indications Conventional tomography has been mainly superseded by CT and MRI but can still be useful as an initial and inexpensive screening of suspected pathologies such as fractures of the skull base, petrous bones, and cribiform plate.

Postprocedure Care None specific to procedure

Common Pathologies

- Fractures
- Calcifications
- Metastases
- Raised intracranial pressure
- Bony erosion, sclerosis

ANGIOGRAPHY

Prior to the introduction of CT and MRI, angiography was the primary method of imaging cerebral vessels. It is used less now, but still useful in the demonstration of aneurysms, arteriovenous malformations, and certain vascular lesions. It is also used as part of detailed studies required during interventional procedures. The description of cerebral angiography and associated interventional procedures is covered in Chapter 9, Head and Neck Vessels, Arterial and Venous.

Other Imaging Modalities

COMPUTED TOMOGRAPHY

The introduction of CT revolutionized the imaging of the brain. Initially plain film CT was used to demonstrate the full range of densities between bone and air. Subsequently, brain scans were sometimes enhanced by iodinated contrast media or air that is introduced into the subarachnoid spaces or ventricles to visualize certain structures or pathologies.

Indications

- Suspected head injury
- Tumor
- Stroke
- Intracranial infection
- Subarachnoid hemorrhage
- Bone destruction

Contraindications

- No special considerations apart from discomfort and difficulty in imaging a severely injured patient.
- Allergy to contrast, if being used
- Imaging of vascular intracranial bleeds is contraindicated if contrast is being used.

Equipment CT scanner

Contrast Media Iodinated contrast media is administered as a bolus or as an IV infusion technique. Occasionally, air is administered (rare).

Radiation Protection

- A complete study of the brain using 10-mm slices will provide about 2 to 3 rads (0.2–0.3 Gy) to the skin in the immediate vicinity of the head. Although this is a higher dose than conventional radiographic study, it is very localized.
- Shield gonadal area and thyroid if possible.

Patient Preparation

- It is advisable to have the patient fast for 4 hours before a brain study in case contrast is to be administered.
- Very restless or uncooperative patients may require some sedation.

Procedure Sequence

- The physician will advise as to the protocol for each patient. There are some basic principles that apply, whatever the pathology being investigated.
- The patient is placed in the AP position.
- Sections are usually coronal, occasionally sagittal. Some CT scanners will reconstruct through any desired plane (Figure14.8).
- For the orbits, the anterior portion of the temporal lobe, and the sella turcica, there is no angulation of the gantry, which is placed parallel to the infraorbital meatal line.
- For supratentorial cranial contents, the gantry is angled 20° to 30° caudad to the infraorbital meatal baseline.
- A standard scan will consist of 8 to 10 slices, 8 to 10 mm thick, from the posterior fossa to the vertex.

Procedure Radiographs Slices demonstrate the anatomy of the brain (Figure 14.9).

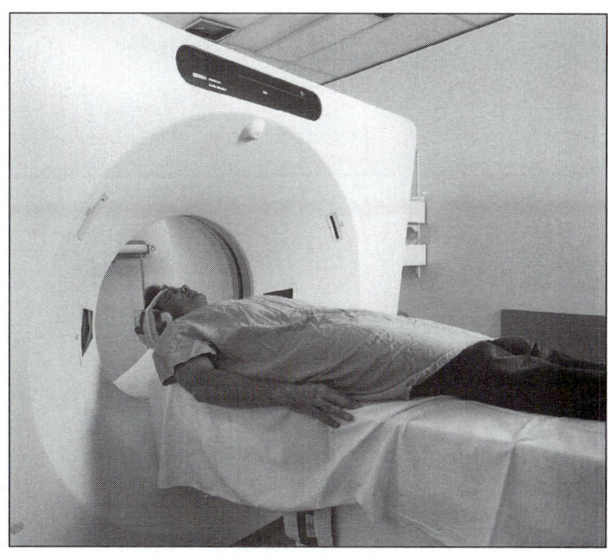

FIGURE 14.8 Patient positioned for CT of brain.

Brain structures are visualized according to their **Hounsfield number** (Figure 14.10).

Bone	>500
Gray matter	35–40
White matter	28–35
CSF	0–10
Fat	<–90– –100
Air	–500– –1000

Postprocedure Care Usually none

Common Pathologies

- Subarachnoid hemorrhage
- Astrocytoma
- Old infarctions
- Tumor (Figure 14.11)

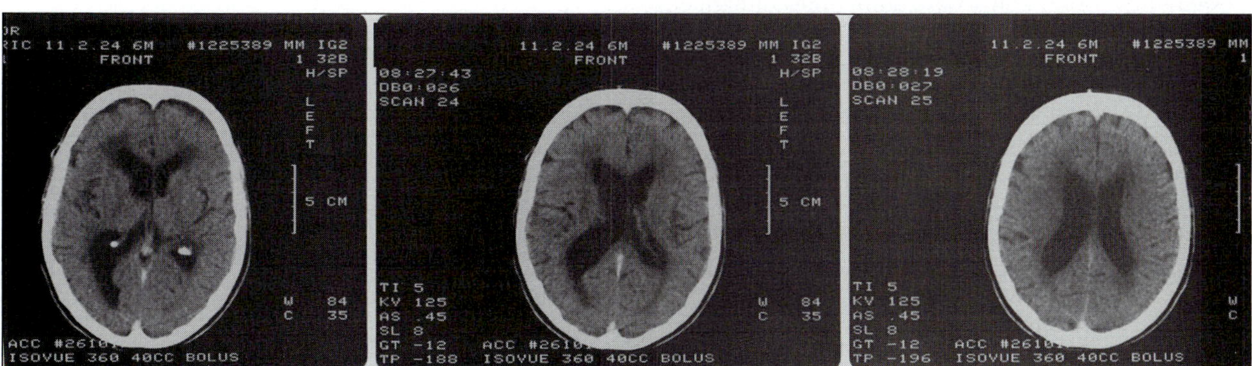

FIGURE 14.9 Examples of CT sections of brain.

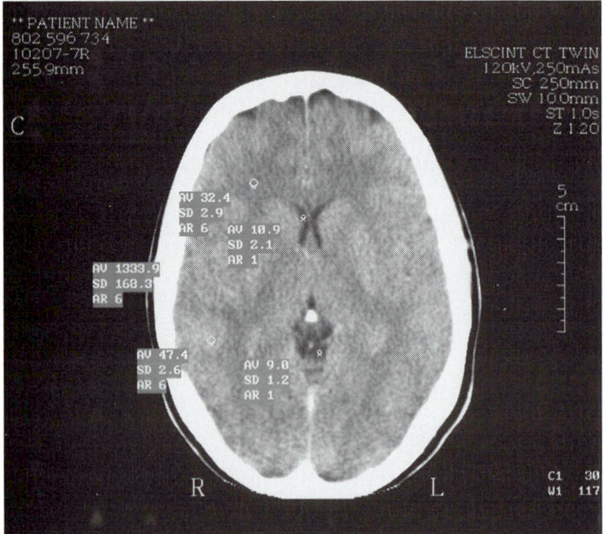

FIGURE 14.10 CT brain labelled with Hounsfield numbers.

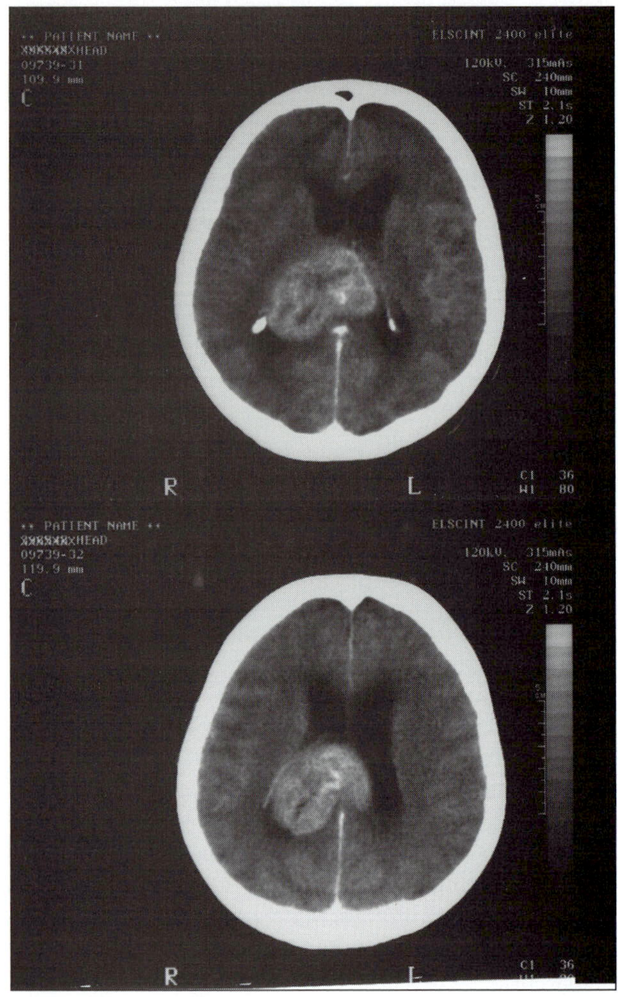

FIGURE 14.11 CT section with tumor.

MAGNETIC RESONANCE IMAGING

Magnetic resonance imaging has now become the most sensitive imaging modality for the detection of brain pathology. If availability and expense permit, it is the initial imaging procedure for any suspected pathology with the exception of subarachnoid hemorrhage and bone lesions.

Applied Anatomy (Figure 14.12)

Indications

- Cerebral infarction
- Study of white matter disease (i.e., multiple sclerosis)
- Lesions at the base of the skull, including pituitary lesions
- Lesions of the posterior fossa
- Acoustic neuroma

Contraindications

- Patient on life support systems
- Pacemaker insertion
- Metallic implants (e.g., cochlear implants)
- Uncontrollable seizures

Equipment MRI unit

Contrast Media Contrast agents in MRI are not imaged directly by their detection in tissues, but by the effect they have on relaxation time (known as a **paramagnetic agent**). Gadolinium, **chelated** to DTPA

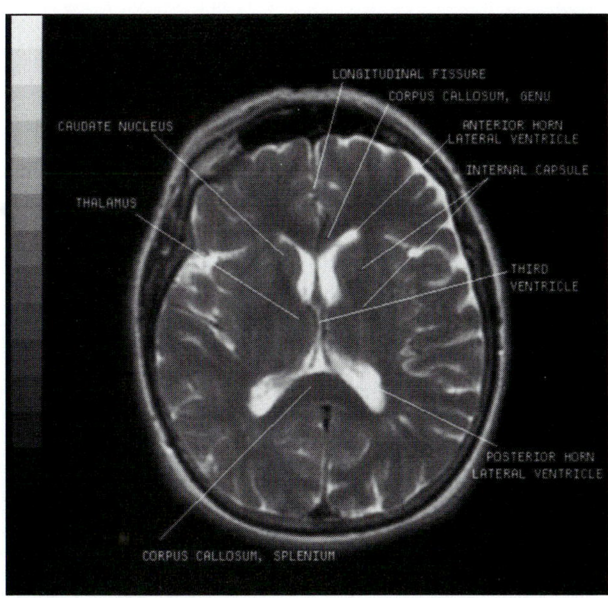

FIGURE 14.12 MR of head.

(Gd-DTPA), decreases the T1 relaxation time of that tissue in which it is deposited. It tends to be deposited in areas where there is a breakdown of the blood–brain barrier. It also increases the sensitivity of MRI to certain disease processes. As a general rule, enhancement is used in MRI and CT to detect the same pathologies.

Indications for Nonenhancement

- Hydrocephalus
- Congenital malformation
- Shunt malformation
- Acute head trauma
- Dementia
- Nonspecific headaches

Indications for Enhancement

- Tumors
- Acoustic neuromas
- Brain abscess
- Aneurysm
- Multiple sclerosis
- Vertigo
- Ataxia
- To improve poorly defined lesions in nonenhanced studies

Radiation Protection Not required

Preliminary Radiographs Screening radiographs of orbital area to detect presence of metals (see below)

Patient Preparation Every patient undergoing MRI must be screened for the presence of metals, including an eye examination for those from high-risk occupations, such as welding. Other high-risk patients include military veterans who may present with shrapnel.

Procedure Sequence

- T1 and T2 images are acquired.
- Protocol for each patient depends on their condition and presenting pathology.

Procedure Images The tissue densities vary from CT because of the different physical and physiologic principles applied to acquire these images. The densities also differ depending on the type of MRI used, T1 or T2. (Figures 14.13 and 14.14.)

Densities

	T1	T2
Bone	Very low	Very low
Marrow	High	Moderately low
CSF	Low	High
Lesions	Low	Moderately high
White matter	Moderately high	Moderately low
Gray matter	Moderately low	Moderately high
Edema	Moderately low	Very high

Postprocedure Care None specific

Common Pathologies

- Cerebral **infarction**
- Multiple sclerosis
- Tumor (Figure 14.15)

> MRI is now being used to map the brain, by following oxygen-enriched hemoglobin in the brain. Increased activity in the brain is identified by increased oxygen supply.

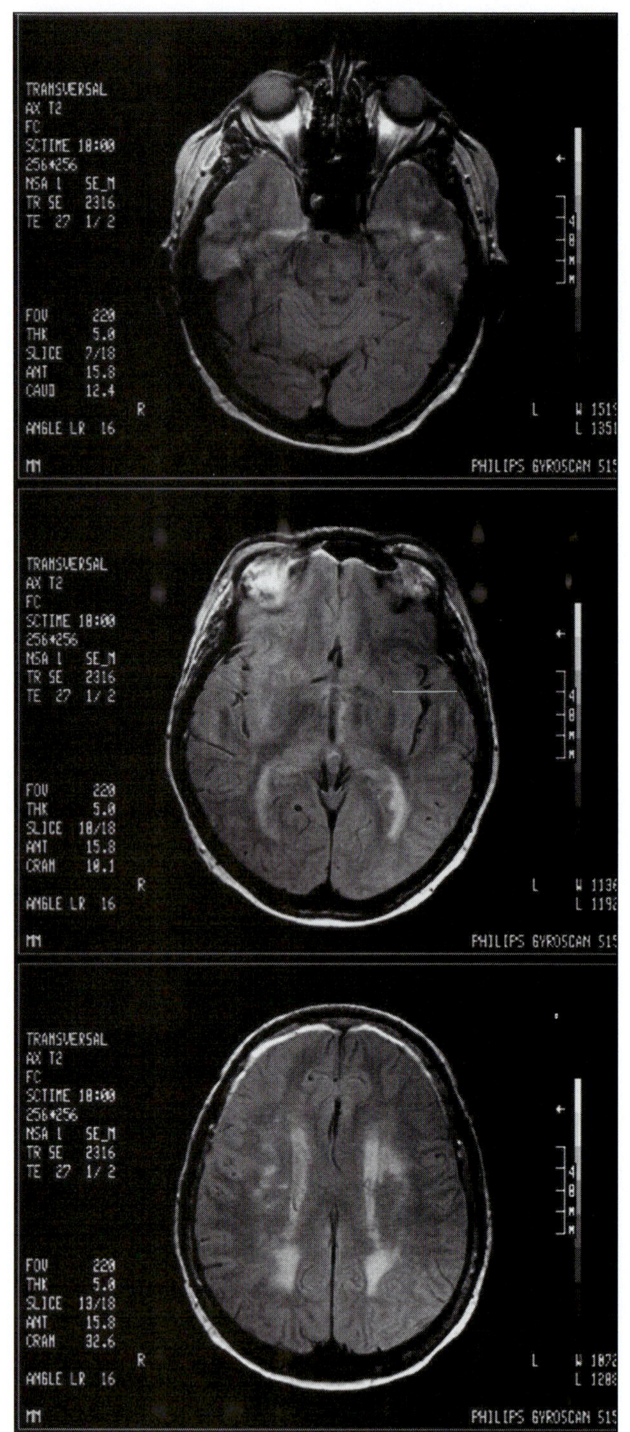

FIGURE 14.13 Examples of coronal sections—MRI.

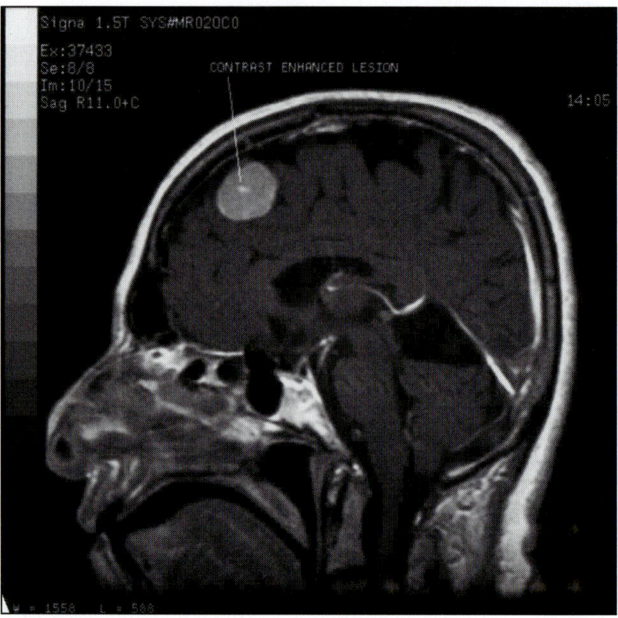

FIGURE 14.14 Tumor visualized on MRI.

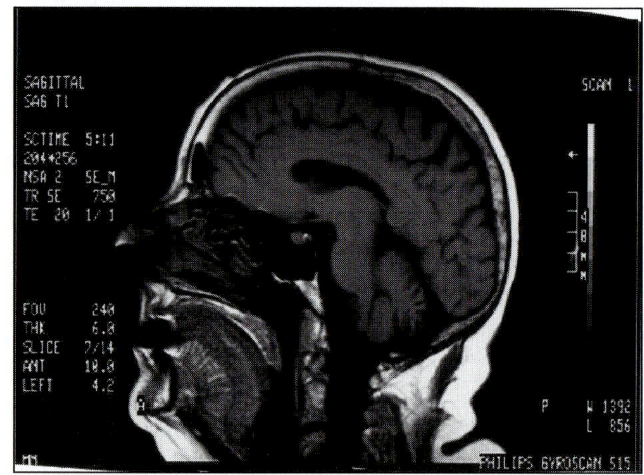

FIGURE 14.15 Lateral view of brain—MRI.

ULTRASOUND

Structures of the cranium can be achieved in infants by scanning through an unclosed fontanelle. Pathologies that can be visualized using this method include intraventricular hemorrhage and congenital abnormalities.

Duplex-scanning, a combination of B-mode imaging and pulsed Doppler flow detection, can identify disease of the carotid bifurcation, primarily atherosclerosis, and transcranial Doppler is being increasingly used to visualize intracranial vascularity.

RADIONUCLIDE IMAGING

The use of the conventional brain scan has decreased since the introduction of MRI. Studies using technetium 99m-labelled glucoheptonate (a radiopharmaceutical) are still performed to demonstrate blood flow by crossing a damaged blood–brain barrier (Figure 14.16).

SPECT imaging is also used, but although its spatial resolution is better than conventional radionuclide scanning, it is not as well defined as CT or MRI (Figure 14.17).

PET scanning can also be used to demonstrate physiologic information of the brain, but it is very expensive equipment and requires a cyclotron nearby to produce positron-emitting radionuclides (Figure 14.18).

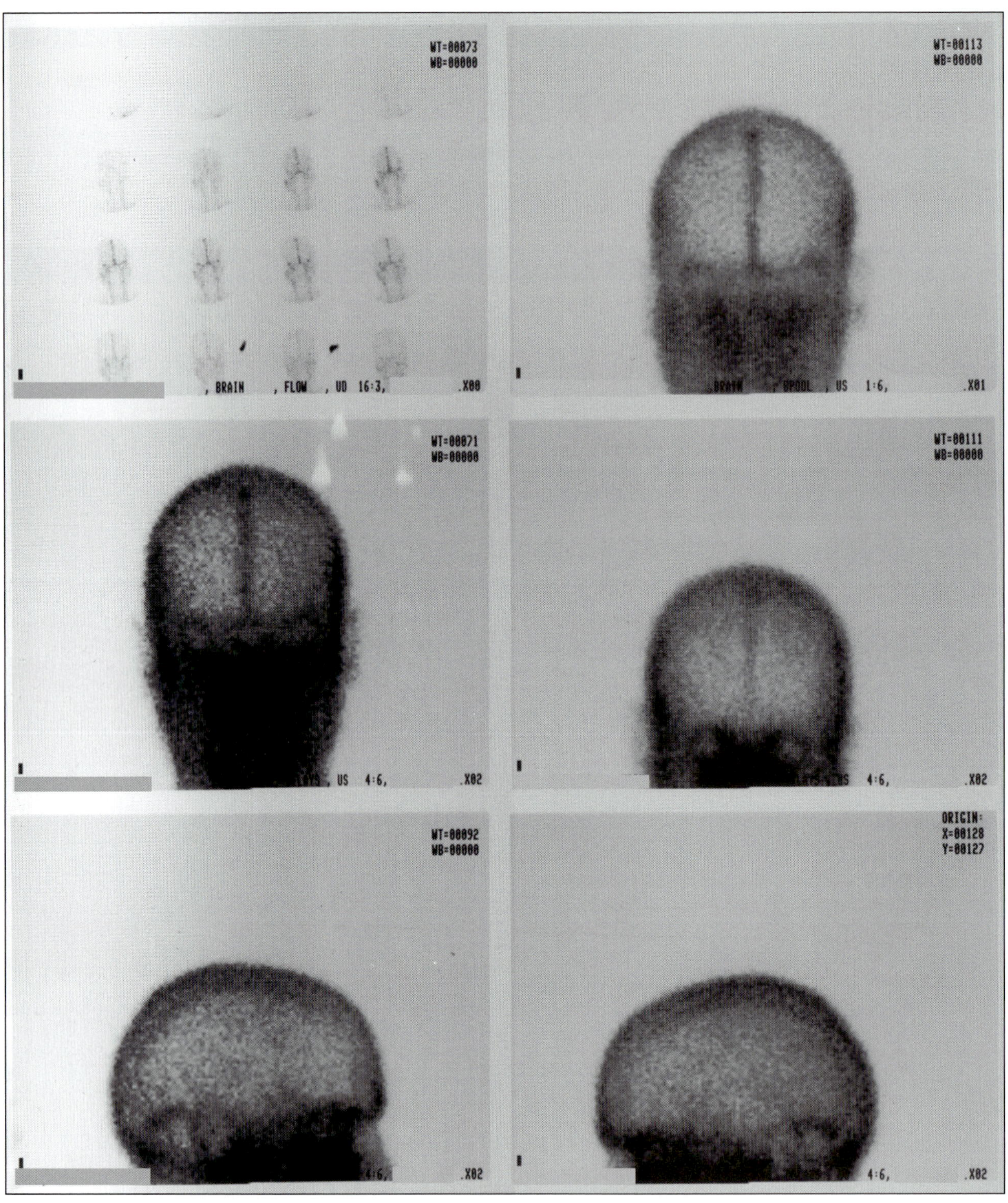

FIGURE 14.16 Normal brain scan.

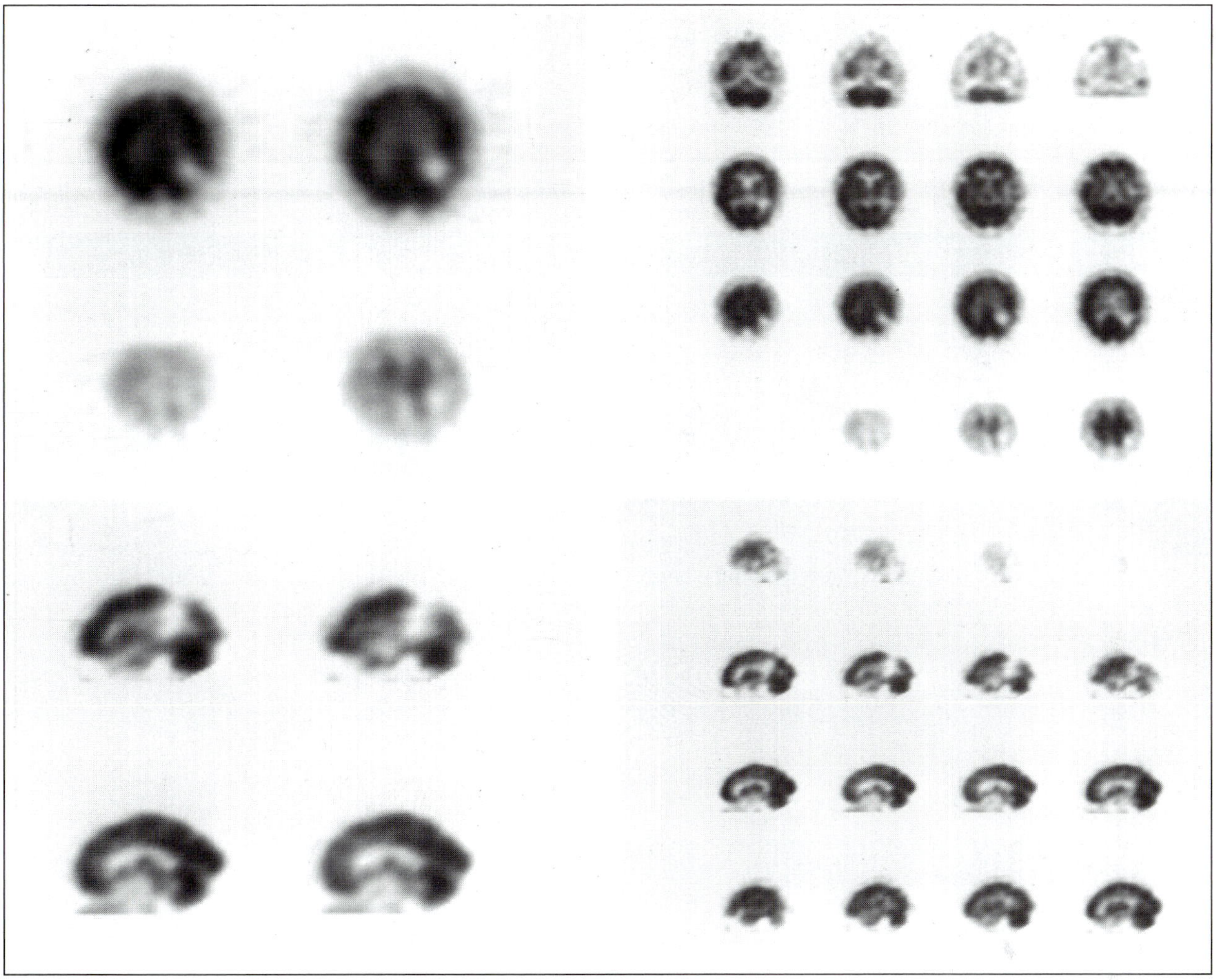

FIGURE 14.17 Example of SPECT imaging examination.

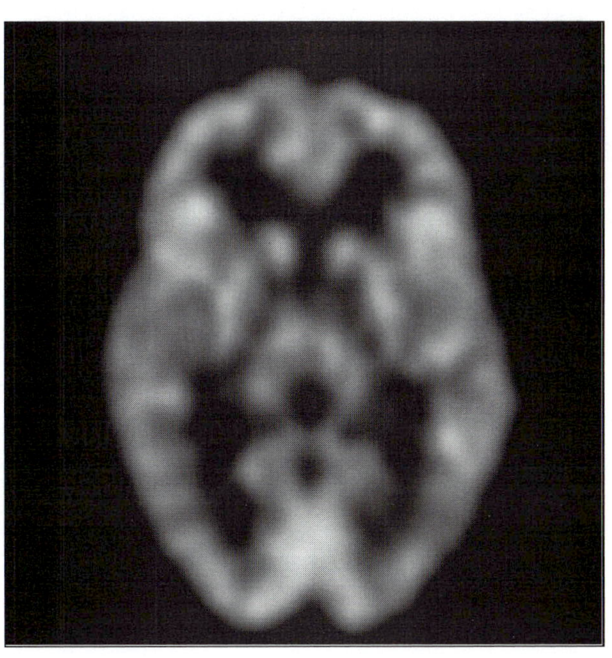

FIGURE 14.18
A transaxial slice from a normal 18FDG (fluoro-deoxy-glucose) PET (positron emission tomgraphy) brain scan, demonstrating areas of glucose metabolism.

Interventional Procedures

Many interventional procedures are used. They all involve the vascular system in some way and are described in Chapter 9, Head and Neck Vessels, Arterial and Venous. However, it is useful to be aware of the variety of methods, approaches, and techniques. The two main types of studies are defined as follows:

EMBOLIZATION

Embolization is the percutaneous treatment of arterial hemorrhage. Within the brain it is most often used to contain an arteriovenous malformation (see Chapter 1 and Chapter 6).

ANGIOPLASTY OR PERCUTANEOUS TRANSLUMINAL ANGIOPLASTY

This method increases the lumen diameter of a blood vessel by means of a balloon catheter. It has been used on carotid and vertebral arteries (see Chapter 9, Head and Neck Vessels, Arterial and Venous, for further discussion).

Review Questions

1. Discuss the advantages and disadvantages of using CT and MRI as methods of imaging the brain.

2. For the following pathologies, identify the best initial imaging examination:

   a. raised intracranial pressure in an infant
   b. astrocytoma
   c. multiple sclerosis
   d. neonate intraventricular hemorrhage

3. Discuss the role of contrast media in brain imaging.

4. Identify the different methods used to image the infant brain. Which pathologies are best seen in which imaging modality?

5. Which of the following is the imaging of choice for a patient with an acoustic neuroma?

   a. plain radiograph
   b. SPECT
   c. PET
   d. MRI
   e. CT

CASE STUDY

A young man is brought into the radiology department with acute head injuries due to a motor vehicle accident. Raised intracranial pressure is indicated. Describe the radiographs you might take, which ones would be of particular interest and why, and which other imaging modalities might be used to image this patient.

References and Recommended Readings

Ballinger, P. W. (1995). *Merrill's atlas of radiographic positioning and radiologic procedures* (8th ed.). St. Louis: Mosby-Year Book.

Bradshaw, J. (1989). *Brain imaging. An introduction.* London: Wright.

Brant, M., & Zawardski, M.D. (1988). MR imaging of the brain. *Radiology, 166*(1), 1–10.

Bryan, R. N. (1990). Imaging of acute stroke. *Radiology, 177*(3), 615–616.

Bryan, R. N., Levy, L. M., Whitlow W. D., et al. (1991). Diagnosis of acute cerebral infarction: Comparison of CT and MR imaging. *AJNR, American Journal of Neuroradiology, 12*(4), 611–620.

Chapman, S., & Nakielny, R. (1993). *A guide to radiological procedures* (3rd ed.). London: Bailliere and Tindall.

Church, A. (1899). *Cerebellar tumour. Recognised clinically, demonstrated by X-ray, proved by autopsy. American Journal of Medical Science, 117.*

Cope, C., Burke, D., & Meranze, S. (1990). *Atlas of interventional radiology.* Philadelphia: Lippincott.

Doyle, T., Hare, W., Thomson, K., & Tress, B. B. (1989). *Procedures in diagnostic radiology.* London: Churchill Livingstone.

Eisenberg, R., & Dennis, C. (1990). *Comprehensive radiographic pathology.* St. Louis: Mosby.

Eisenberg, R. L. (1992). *Radiology, an illustrated history.* St. Louis: Mosby-Year Book.

Keen, W. W., & Sweet, W. M. (1903). A case of gunshot wound of the brain in which the roentgen rays showed the presence of eight fragments of the bullet. *American Journal of Medical Science, 126.*

Kirkwood, J. R. (1988). *Essentials of neuroimaging*. New York: Churchill Livingstone.

Kreel, L., & Thornton, A. (1992). *Outline of medical imaging.* Oxford: Butterworth Heinemann.

Magnetic resonance imaging of the brain Part 1. (1991). *Canadian Association of Radiologists Journal, 42*(1).

Meyer, C. A., Minis, S. E., Wolf, A. L., Thompson, R. K., & Gutierrez, M. A. (1991). Acute Traumatic Midbrain Hemorrhage. *Radiology, 179.*

Osborn, A. (1991). *Handbook of neuroradiology.* St. Louis: Mosby-Year Book.

Shoji, H., Hirai, S., Ishiwaki K., et al. (1991). CT and MR imaging of acute cerebellar ataxia. *Neuroradiology, 33.*

Snopek, A. M. (1992). *Fundamentals of special radiographic procedures* (3rd ed.). Philadelphia: Saunders.

Sutton, D. A. (1993). *Textbook of radiology and imaging.* Edinburgh: Churchill Livingstone.

Wojtowycz, M. (1990). *Interventional radiology and angiography.* Chicago: Year Book Medical Publishers.

CHAPTER 15

Specialized Studies of the Spinal Cord and Spine

CYNTHIA COWLING, BSc, MEd, MRT(R), ACR

OBJECTIVES

At the completion of this chapter, the student should be able to:

1. Describe the main features of the spinal cord.
2. Identify the shape of the vertebral canal for each vertebral type.
3. List the main examinations used to demonstrate the spinal canal and cord.
4. List the indications and contraindications for these procedures.
5. Describe the equipment used during these procedures.
6. Describe the procedure sequence for each examination.
7. Identify the usual contrast media used.
8. Apply safe practice to each procedure.
9. List the main pathologies demonstrated.
10. Compare the different modalities and the resultant information obtained.
11. Describe interventional procedures used in the treatment of nervous and bony pathology.
12. Apply good patient care principles during all examinations.

Introduction and Historical Overview

In the early 1900s, it was realized that problems associated with the spinal cord could not be demonstrated on plain radiographs and the first contrast agent used was air, which was bubbled in via a lumbar puncture. The first use of a positive contrast agent, lipiodil, was actually an accident. In 1922, Dr. Forestier was attempting to inject lipiodil (an iodized poppy seed oil) into the epidural space. He pushed too hard and ended up with a drop in the subarachnoid space. There appeared to be no meningeal reaction and it flowed with gravity when viewed under the fluoroscope. From the 1930s onward, the method of visualization remained remarkably similar, but there was an ongoing search to find a nonoily substance that did not have to be removed from the subarachnoid space at the completion of the examination (for reasons of risk). Eventually, nonionic, water-soluble compounds were introduced that demonstrated an extremely low neurotoxicity making myelography a much safer procedure. Ironically it was at that time that CT and MRI were being developed to become the primary mode for imaging the spine.

The other spinal examination used in the past was the diskogram, which enabled the radiologist to examine the actual morphology of the disk by injecting contrast media directly into it, while at the same time attempting to mimic the pain the patient had been experiencing. For a while in the 1970s this procedure became a therapeutic, interventional procedure when a special substance was injected into the disk, which gradually dissolved parts of it. Risk factors together with poor long-term prognosis all but ended this procedure. MRI has largely supplanted the diskogram in the examination of the nucleus pulposus and **annulus** fibrosis of the disk. However, some in the profession still believe that the diskogram can provide the most accurate picture of the disk's condition before surgery.

Many comparative studies have been done assessing the success and usefulness of the different imaging modalities used for studying the spine and its contents. One study comparing radiologic diagnosis with surgical findings, found that MRI had a 96% accuracy rate, myelogram 81%, and CT 57%. When CT and myelography were combined, the accuracy increased to 84%.

Anatomy

SPINAL CORD

The spinal cord is considered part of the central nervous system (CNS), the spinal nerves being part of the peripheral nervous system.The spinal cord is a rod of nervous tissue that forms the portion of the nervous system that occupies the upper two-thirds of the vertebral canal. It extends from the lower border of the foramen magnum to the lower border of the first lumbar vertebra. It is approximately 45 cm long in the male and 42 cm long in the female. It is cylindrical in form with a slight fusiform enlargement in the lower cervical, lower thoracic, and lower lumbar regions (Figure 15.1).

Attached to the posterolateral aspect of the spinal cord are the sensory roots of the spinal nerves; the motor roots are found on the anterolateral aspect of the cord.

The sensory and motor nerve roots pass toward the intervertebral foramina, where they join to become the spinal nerve, which thus contains both sensory and motor fibers.

The coverings of the cord from the spinal cord outward are the pia, arachnoid, and dura mater, meninges also found encasing the brain. The pia mater, a delicate membrane adjacent to the cord, contains no superficial blood vessels. The cerebrospinal fluid (CSF) circulates in the subarachnoid space between the pia mater and the spinal cord. This space ends at the second sacral level. The arachnoid mater is a thin membrane that forms the outer boundary of the subarachnoid space and lines the inner aspect of the dura mater. The dura mater is a thick fibrous avascular membrane that ends at the second sacral segment (Figures 15.2 and 15.3).

The CSF bathes the spinal cord and is found in the subarachnoid space. A spinal needle punctures the dura and arachnoid mater to retrieve CSF and to inject contrast into the subarachnoid space.

The cord ends at the level of the L1 or L2, at the conus medullaris, but the subarachnoid space extends to the second sacral segment and is filled with CSF. The lower portion of the lumbar vertebral canal encases the cauda equina, a collection of nerve roots.

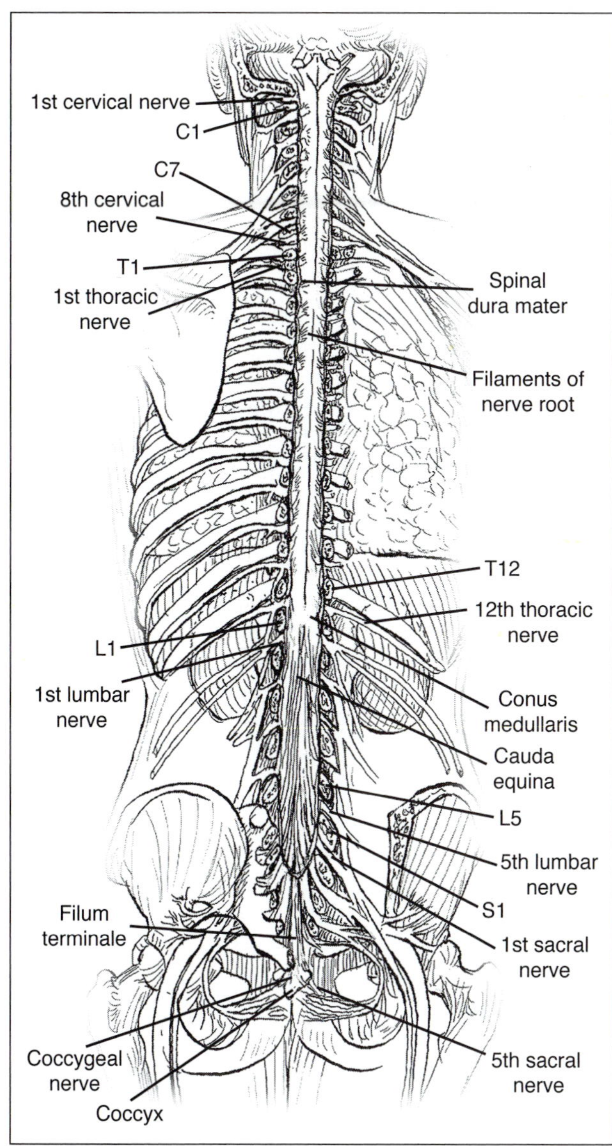

FIGURE 15.1 The spinal cord.

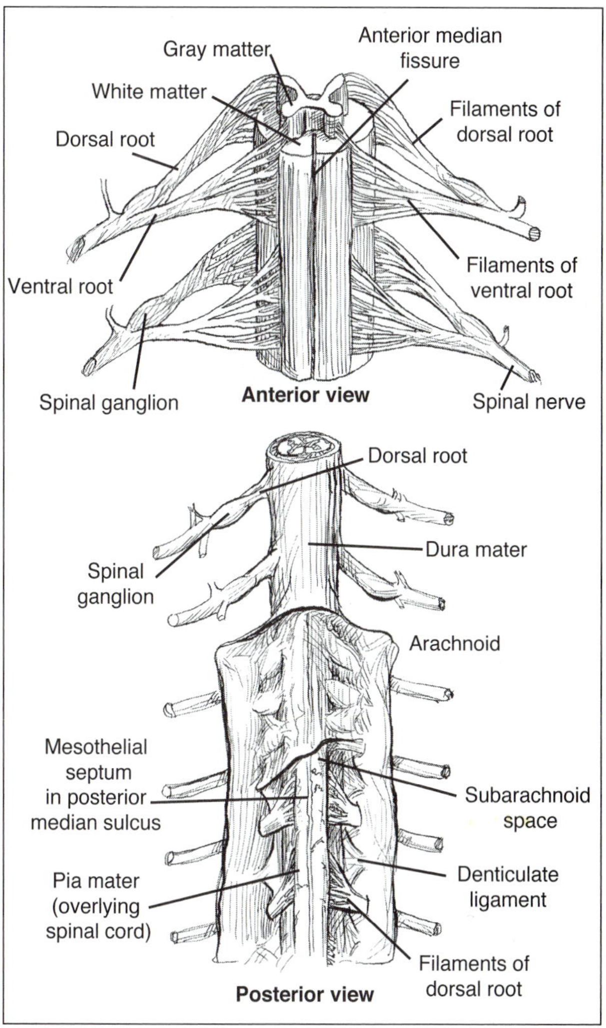

FIGURE 15.2 Spinal membranes and nerve roots.

The shape of the vertebral canal varies according to the type of vertebra (Figure 15.4).

Spinal Nerves. Thirty-one pairs of spinal nerves primarily emerge from the lateral aspects of the spinal cord to exit the vertebral canal via the intervertebral foramina. They are, by cord segment: 8 cervical, 12 thoracic, 5 lumbar, 5 sacral, and 1 coccygeal pair of spinal nerves.

On exiting the intervertebral foramina, each nerve, mixed in nature, will divide primarily into anterior and posterior rami. The anterior ramus provides sensory and motor fibers associated with the upper extremities, abdominal and pelvic regions, and the lower extremities. The posterior ramus is associated with the anterior and posterior thoracic area.

Associated with the anterior ramus is the white ramus, the preganglionic component of the sympathetic division of the autonomic nervous system.

AUTONOMIC SYSTEM

In comparison to the somatic nervous system, which is involved in voluntary actions, the autonomic system is that part of the nervous system that involves the innervation of tissues not under conscious control. In conjunction with the cerebral cortex, hypothalamus, and medulla, the autonomic nervous system consists of two divisions that regulate the heart, smooth muscle, and glandular tissues.

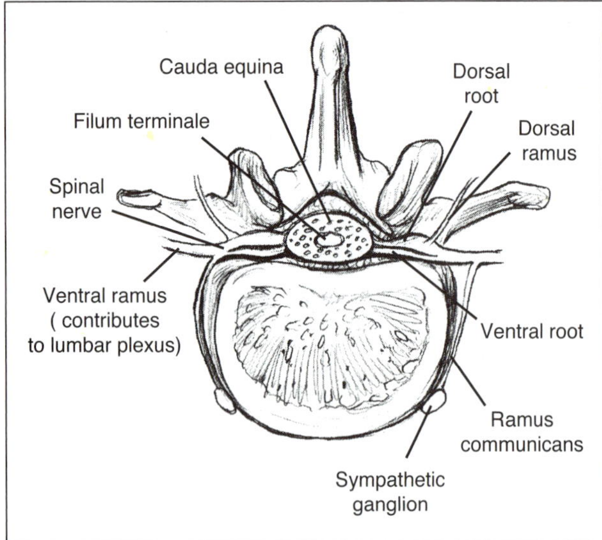

FIGURE 15.3 Section through lumbar vertebra.

The sympathetic division arises with spinal nerves thoracic one to lumbar two, to elicit a response to stress, such as increased heart rate, dilation of the pupils, and increased diameter of the bronchi. The parasympathetic division arising from ganglia in the medulla and sacral region elicits an action opposite by slowing the heart rate and restoring the size of pupils and bronchi.

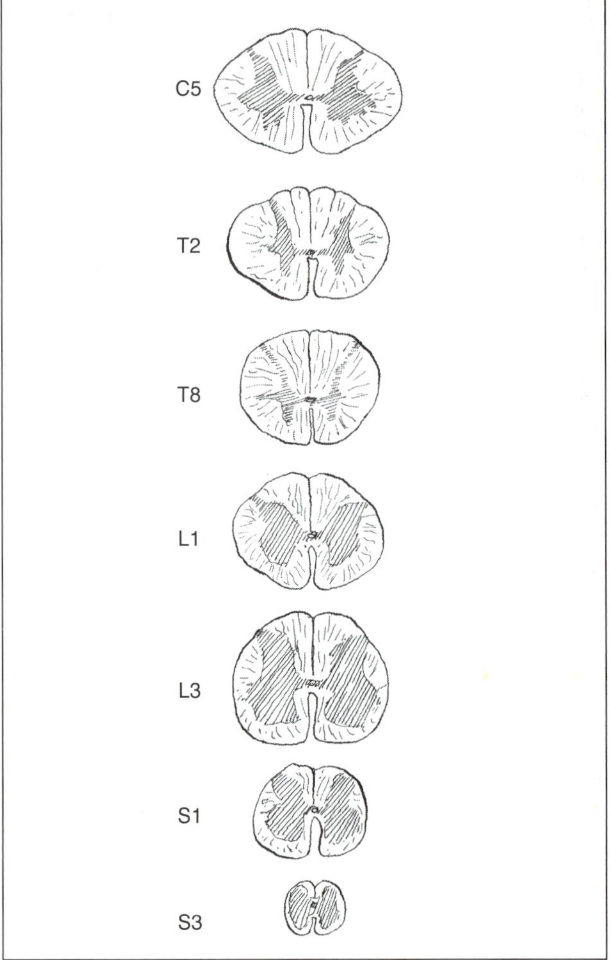

FIGURE 15.4 Sections through spinal cord at various levels.

Procedures

MYELOGRAPHY

Myelography (mī-ĕ-lŏg´ră-fē) is the radiographic examination of the spinal cord by the use of a radiopaque medium injected into the intrathecal space. Depending on the region of the spine to be imaged, these injections can be given at the cisternal, cervical, thoracic, or lumbar regions, the most common area being the lumbar region. Injection of the contrast medium, which is now generally a nonionic water-soluble agent, is usually into the subarachnoid space. Occasionally, epidural myelography is performed for specific pathologies. Distortions of the spinal canal demonstrated in a myelogram indicate the presence of extradural disease impinging on the cord, rather than the disease process itself, which is the case with CT and MRI, in which the pathology or structure is imaged directly.

LUMBAR MYELOGRAPHY

This is the most common type of myelography performed, not only because pathologies occur more often in this area, but because contrast media, injected via a lumbar puncture can be moved via gravity to examine all three areas of the spine—cervical, thoracic, and lumbar. The myelogram defines and details the subarachnoid space. Distortions of the spinal canal indicate evidence of extradural disease.

Applied Anatomy The following should be visualized on a myelogram:

- Spinal cord
- Conus medullaris
- Nerve roots and sheaths
- Spinal vessels
- Denticulate ligaments
- Arachnoidal septa (see Figure 15.1)

Indications

- Intraspinal abnormalities
- Any nerve root abnormalities
- Disk prolapse, herniation
- Spondylosis, **spondylolisthesis** (spŏn´´dĭ-lō-lis´´thē´sĭs)
- Spinal stenosis (dynamic studies)
- Tumors; most common in lumbar region are:
  —**Ependymoma** (ĕp-ĕn´´dĭ-mō´mă) of conus medullaris
  —**Lipoma**
  —Dermoid
  —Lymphoma
- Metastases

Contraindications

- Cerebral aneurysms, arteriovenous malformations, **papilledema** (păp´´ĭl-ĕ-dē´mă). Myelography can cause a raised intracranial pressure, which would adversely affect these conditions.
- Recent lumbar puncture. Myelography should not be performed within a week of a previous puncture. Sometimes CSF leaks into the subdural space and this can mistakenly be tapped, thus causing an injection into the subdural rather than subarachnoid space.
- Previous reaction to same contrast. Reaction to an IV contrast medium would not contraindicate use of contrast for a lumbar myelogram. In the case of necessity, steroid cover can be given.

Equipment

- Fluoroscopy unit with spot film device (100-mm cine film sometimes used)
- Digital fluoroscopic unit allows for postprocessing edge enhancement
- Tilting table top, able to tilt to 90° in both directions
- Spinal lumbar puncture tray (sterile) containing:
  —Luer-lok syringes
  —Spinal manometer (optional)
  —Needles (18 and 22 gauge)
  —Spinal needle (20 or 22 gauge with removable stilette)
  —Three-way stopcock
  —Towels, gauze
  —Medicine glass
  —Specimen tube

Contrast Media

- **Iohexol** (Omnipaque)—a nonionic, water-soluble contrast that is less neurotoxic than previous contrast media used in myelography. It does not cause epileptic seizures or psychological changes. It can also be used without having to withdraw other drugs patients may be taking.
- **Iopanodol**—similar to iohexol.
- **Iotrolan** (Isovist)—a more recent nonionic, water-soluble contrast agent that tests have shown to be less toxic even than iohexol.

NOTE: In the past, numerous agents were used but have since been discarded.

- Gas—CO_2 or air: provided poor contrast
- Lipiodil—very oily and toxic, produced arachnoiditis
- Myodil, Pantopaque—less toxic than lipiodil, but still sometimes caused arachnoiditis. Sometimes these oily contrasts occluded the root sleeves and masked other conditions.
- Amipaque (metrizamide)—first nonionic, low-osmolar, water-soluble contrast medium. It was safer but still produced neurotoxic effects such as hallucinations and transient confusion. It was also expensive because it came as a freeze-dried solute and had to be dissolved with dilute sodium bicarbonate.

Radiation Protection

- Minimize fluoroscopy time as much as possible
- Not possible to protect the gonadal area

Preliminary Radiographs

- It is usually essential that plain radiographs are taken of the lumbar region, although it is recognized that it does not always provide useful clinical information for individuals suffering from low back pain.
- The list below summarizes their use:
  —To determine accurate bony anatomy
  —To exclude such pathologies as ankylosing spondylitis and bone tumors that may not need further examination
  —To distinguish any congenital lumbosacral anomalies
  —To correlate with myelography, MRI and CT images during reporting. The plain radiographs provide good contrast between bone and tissue and thus help in the interpretation of subsequent imaging.
- Radiographs taken before a myelogram are:
  —AP projection
  —Lateral view
  —Both anterior oblique views to demonstrate the pars interarticularis
  —Lateral view of L5–S1

Patient Preparation

- Improved contrast agents have meant that this examination can be an outpatient procedure, performed without premedication or special preparation except for children who might require sedation.
- High fluid intake should be encouraged. A light meal may be eaten before the procedure.
- Patients must be informed of the procedure and its potential hazards, and a history should be taken identifying any previous myelograms, lumbar punctures, or adverse allergic reactions.
- Vital signs are taken before the procedure to give a baseline reading.
- The patient should be dressed only in a back-opening gown and when placed on the table should have the injection site shaved if necessary.

Procedure Sequence

- The patient is placed in the lateral decubitus position or prone. Although a lumbar puncture is easier to perform with the patient sitting, leaning forward, it is easier to determine needle placement with fluoroscopy with the patient lying down.
- The table is tilted slightly feet-down to ensure pooling of CSF in the subarachnoid space of the lumbar region.
- The area to be punctured is cleaned and injected with a local anesthetic.
- Using aseptic technique, a lumbar puncture needle (usually 22 gauge) is inserted at the level of L3–L4 or L2–L3. Because pathologies in the lumbar spine are more often found in the lower regions, the higher injection point is usually preferred.
- The needle is slowly advanced until fluid appears from the lumen of the needle once the stilette has been withdrawn. The stilette is returned and the needle advanced another 2 mm to ensure that the entire bevel of the needle is within the subarachnoid space.
- At this time CSF may be taken, as well as cranial pressures measured by attaching a spinal manometer to the needle via a three-way stopcock. Once appropriately opened the CSF can move up the core of the manometer.
- Contrast media is injected after a small amount of CSF has been withdrawn. This will help maintain stasis. Approximately 10 to 15 mL is injected under fluoroscopy. The amount depends on the pathologies to be observed and the iodine content of the contrast (the higher the concentration, the lower the amount required).
- The flow of the contrast is monitored under fluoroscopy. If the thoracolumbar region or higher is required the table is tilted slowly head-down, to allow gravity to move the contrast.
- Before radiographs are taken of the lumbar region, the patient is tilted slightly to the feet to allow for pooling of the contrast in the subarachnoid space below L1.
- Radiographs are taken, usually with the patient in the semierect position. It depends again, on body type and pathologic conditions.

Procedure Radiographs The following radiographs are usually taken with the spot film device:

- AP projection (using under table tube)
- PA projection (using over table tube)
- Both oblique views with the patient positioned under fluoroscopy to demonstrate the origin of the nerve roots. This is usually a 15° to 30° oblique.
- Lateral view to include L5–S1.
  (Figures 15.5, 15.6, and 15.7)

Alternative Radiographs

- Lateral views with flexion and extension will demonstrate any dynamic stenosis, spinal instability, and degree of movement of a disk protrusion.
- Lateral and AP views of the thoracolumbar region, taken when the contrast has been moved to this

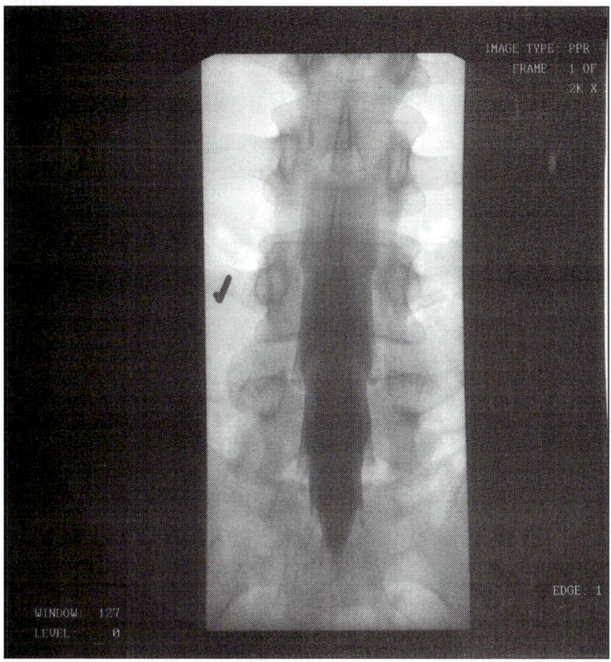

FIGURE 15.5 PA lumbar myelogram.

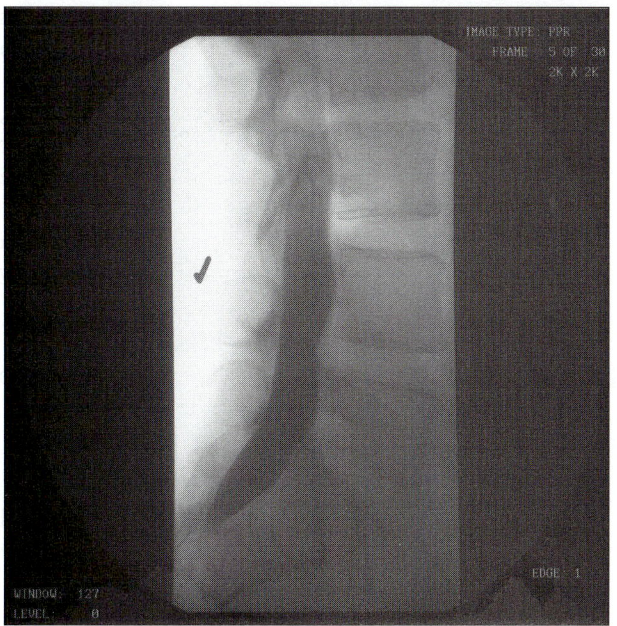

FIGURE 15.6 Lateral lumbar myelogram.

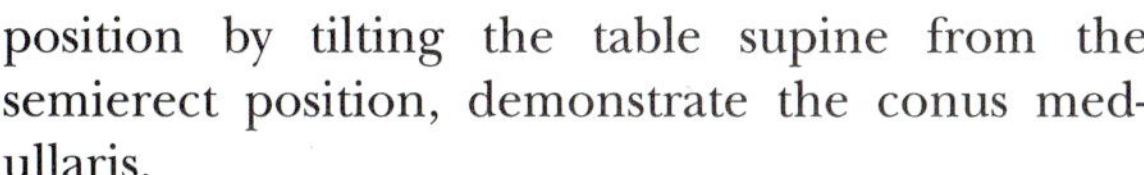

position by tilting the table supine from the semierect position, demonstrate the conus medullaris.

- An overcouch decubitus (shoot-through) lateral view with the patient prone (Figure 15.8)

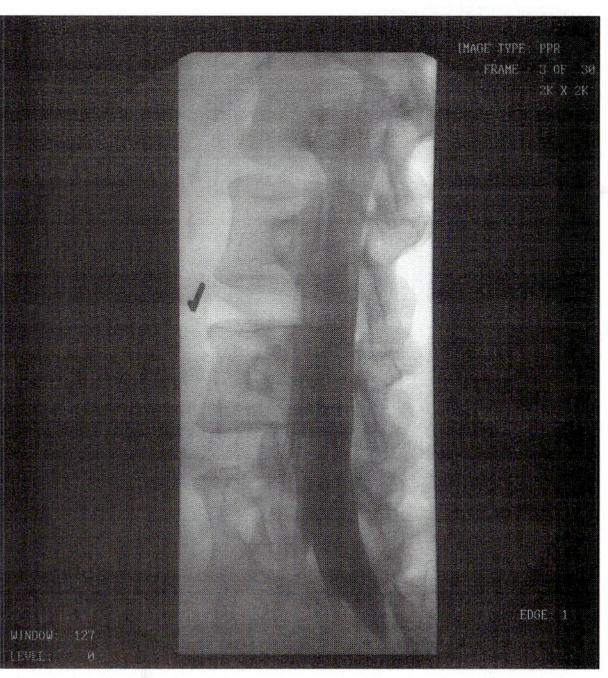

FIGURE 15.7 Oblique lumbar myelogram.

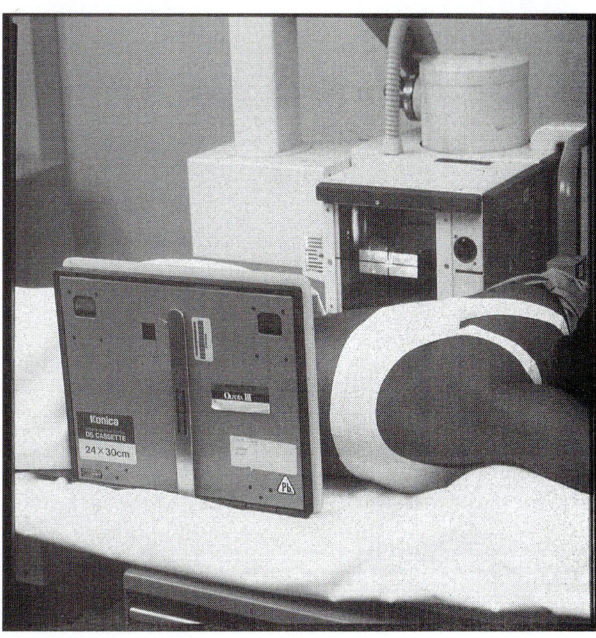

FIGURE 15.8 Decubitus view positioning.

- An overcouch decubitus (shoot-through) PA with the patient lateral
- An overcouch decubitus with the patient obliqued 15° to 30° from the prone position
- An erect lateral view

Common Pathologies

- Herniated or prolapsed intervertebral disk (Figure 15.9)
- Spinal stenosis
- Spondylolisthesis
- Tumors, causing blockage to the spinal cord (Figure 15.10)

Postprocedure Care

- Several complications can result from a myelogram, but they have been minimized with the introduction of low neurotoxic contrast media.
  —Headache—more frequent with females and dependent on dose administered
  —Nausea
  —Slight, temporary increase in lumbar or sciatic pain
  —Convulsions (rare)—treatment is to use diazepam
  —Confusion/hallucinations (very rare with new contrast)
- There are also complications that can arise as a result of the lumbar puncture itself.
  —Hypotension
  —Headache, nausea, vomiting

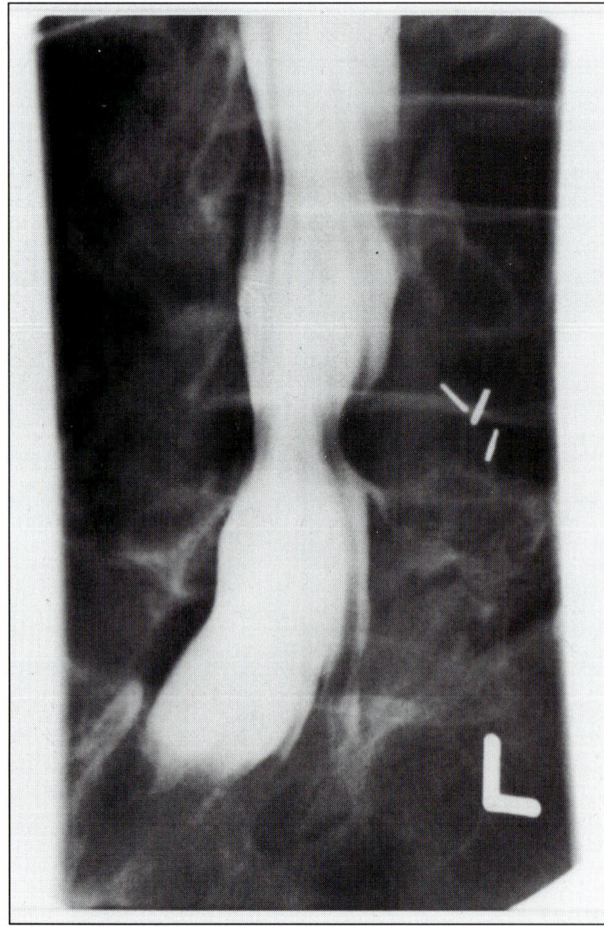

FIGURE 15.9 Herniated disk.

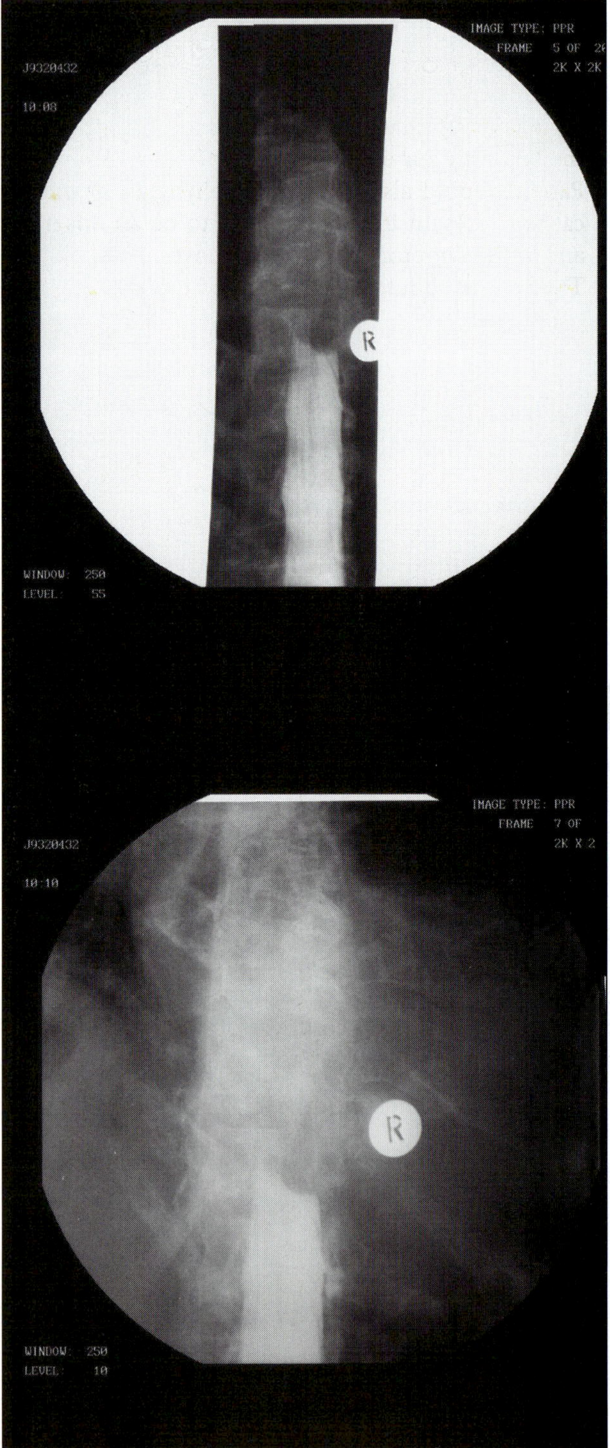

FIGURE 15.10 Blockage due to tumor.

—Incorrect injection of contrast material:
  —Subdural
  —Extradural
  —Intramedullary
- These do not necessarily result in pain to the patient, but in a nondiagnostic procedure.
  —Hemorrhage into the subarachnoid space, resulting in bloody CSF (very rare, a small amount is not significant)
  —Stiff neck, numbness of limbs (extremely rare)
- Patient should have bed rest for 8 to 24 hours, with the head slightly elevated.
- Patient should also inform the physician or medical staff present if there appears to be an onset of any of the symptoms described above.
- The patient should be encouraged to drink.

Arachnoiditis (ă-răk′noyd-ī′tĭs)
This is an inflammatory disease of the pia-arachnoid membrane, which is chronic and progressive. It has been called a major cause of the "failed back surgery syndrome." It is diagnosed by myelography, demonstrating clubbing of nerve roots and their adherence to the margins of the dura. Ironically, the use of certain contrast media was thought to be one cause of this very painful and unrelenting disease. Some oily contrasts and some ionic contrasts such as meglumine iothalamate have been linked to arachnoiditis. Although these have not been used for several years and although the nonionic contrasts do not cause arachnoiditis, the chronic and progressive nature of the disease means that some patients can still present with signs and symptoms that could have partially been caused by a myelogram many years previous. The British Society of Neuroradiology and the Council of Royal College of Radiologists issued a joint statement in 1991, saying that studies have indicated that only 1% of myodil (oily contrast) myelogram patients experienced arachnoiditis after the procedure.

THORACIC MYELOGRAPHY

The contrast medium for this myelogram is generally injected via the lumbar region unless there is known pathology to prohibit this. All factors are the same as for the lumbar spine except that the patient is positioned slightly headdown to allow the contrast to move throughout the thoracic region. The patient's head must always remain slightly elevated to prevent contrast from entering the head. As soon as the thoracic area is filled with contrast, the patient must be replaced in the horizontal position.

Procedure Radiographs AP projection and lateral views with the table horizontal (Figures 15.11 and 15.12)

Common Pathologies Disk herniations are rare and occur mainly at T11 and T12.

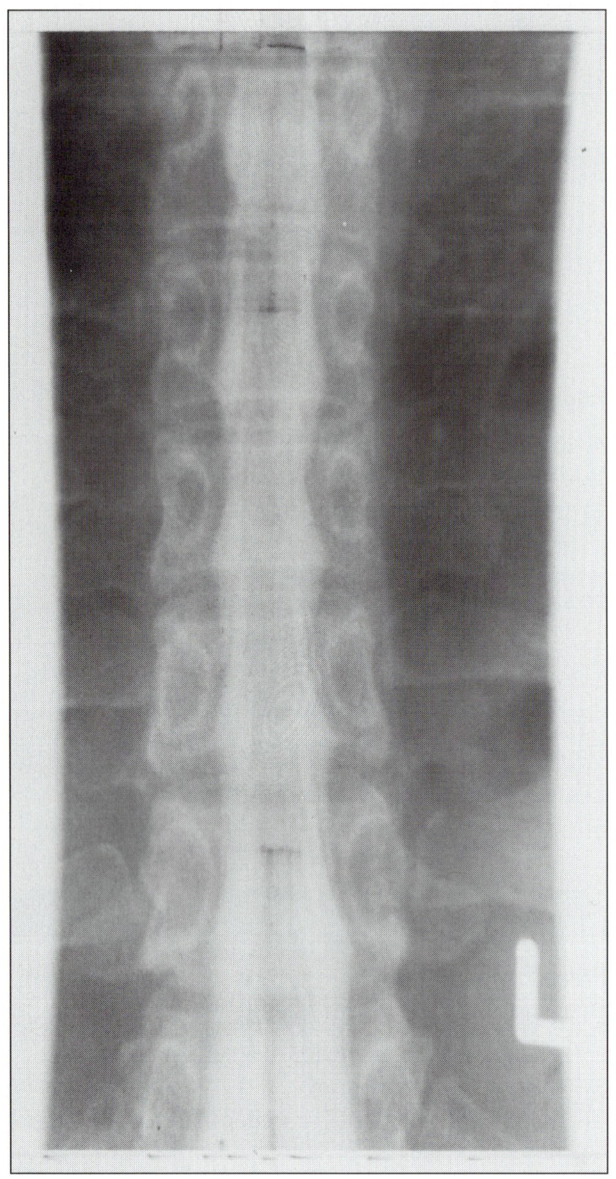

FIGURE 15.11 PA projection thoracic myelogram.

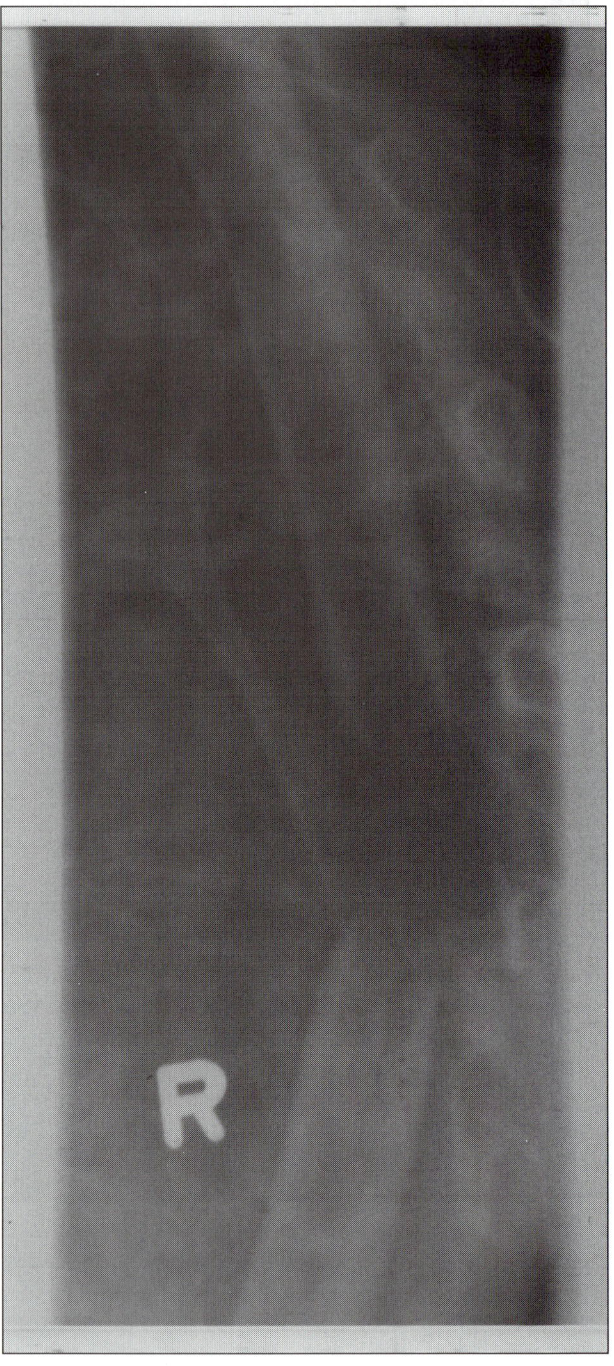

FIGURE 15.12 Lateral view demonstrating blockage.

CERVICAL MYELOGRAPHY

This examination can be carried out via two methods of approach:

- Via a lumbar puncture (the most common approach)
- Via an injection at the level of C1–C2 or through the cisterna magna (in the case of suspected spinal blockage)

Applied Anatomy (Figure 15.13)

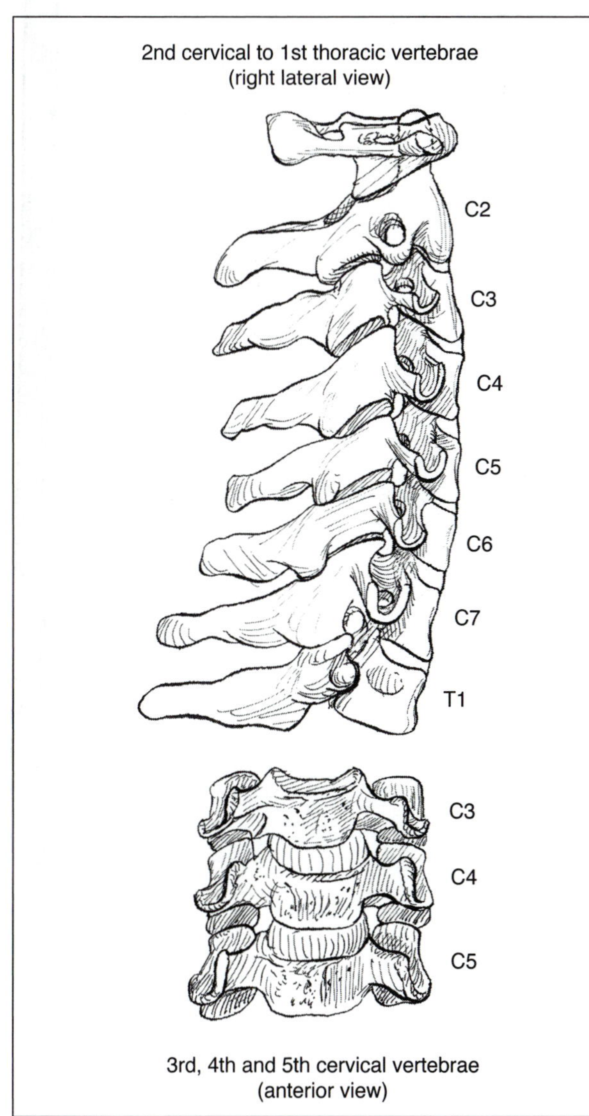

FIGURE 15.13 Cervical anatomy.

Indications

- Cervical disk herniation
- Presence of a spinal block
- Tumors—neurofibroma, astrocytoma
- Degenerative changes
- Inflammatory disease

Contraindications Same as lumbar myelography

Equipment

- Fluoroscopy unit with tilting mechanism
- Biplane facility, useful for needle placement

Contrast Media

- For lumbar approach—7 to 10 mL higher concentration of iodine content
- For the cisternal or C1–C2 approach—5 mL at a slightly lower concentration

Radiation Protection Minimize field size and fluoroscopy time.

Preliminary Radiographs AP projection and lateral views of the cervical spine

Patient Preparation

- Same as for the lumbar myelogram
- In the case of a cervical or cisternal puncture, phenobarbitone sodium or diazepam can be administered 30 minutes before and 4 hours after. This reduces any likelihood of epileptic seizures.

Procedure Sequence

For C1–C2

- Patient lies prone on the fluoroscopy table
- The neck is slightly extended and supported. Hyperextension is not advised because it causes discomfort and increases the difficulty of inserting the needle.
- The chin should rest on a soft radiolucent pad.
- Hair should be restrained with a cap and the area lateral to and posterior to the level of C1–C2 may need to be shaved.
- Injection area is anesthetized locally.
- A 22-gauge spinal needle is directed at right angles to the neck and parallel to the table.

- The needle is advanced until it passes the dura, at which time CSF should drop from the needle, following removal of the stilette.
- The patient's head must be gently held at this time to minimize movement and to provide comfort for the patient. This is not a painful procedure but it can be a distressing one.
- A small amount of contrast is introduced (about 3 mL) to confirm correct placement and then the remainder is introduced.

Procedure Radiographs AP projection and lateral views. The lateral view is a cross-table lateral and the arms are pulled down to clear the shoulder girdle from C7–T1 (Figure 15.14).

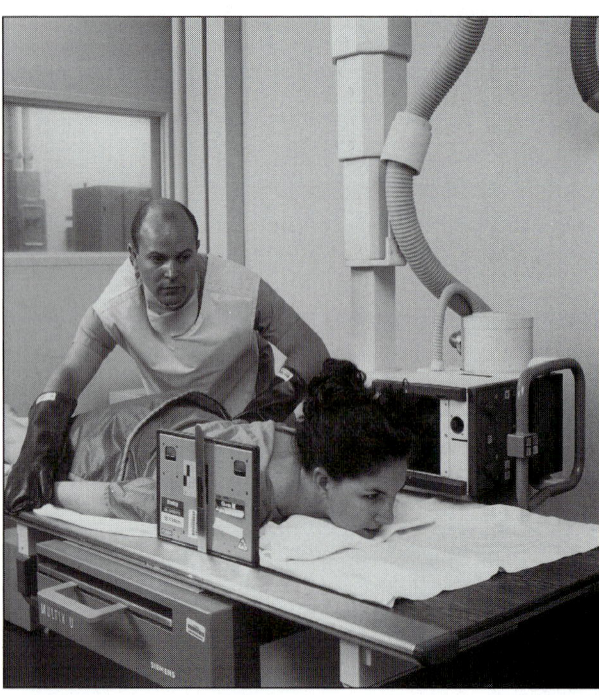

FIGURE 15.14 Lateral cervical myelography.

Alternative Radiographs

- Swimmer's view to visualize C7–T1
- AP with angulation to bring that section of the neck required to be imaged at right angles to the central ray

Procedure Sequence

Cisternal Puncture

- Patient lies in the lateral decubitus position.
- The neck is held horizontal on its side by radiolucent pads.
- The area around the occipital protuberance may need to be shaved.
- Hair must be contained within a cap.
- Area around C2 is anesthetized locally.
- A 20-gauge spinal needle is introduced at this level, parallel to the table at the midpoint of the neck and directed toward the nasion.
- The needle is pushed through the atlanto-occipital membrane and then advanced slowly until CSF appears from the needle, following removal of the stilette. The needle is then advanced about 0.5 cm to ensure correct positioning within the cisterna magna.
- Contrast is then injected under fluoroscopic control.

Procedure Radiographs AP and lateral. A cross-table lateral is usually performed (Figure 15.15).

Postprocedural Care It is suggested that the patient remain semirecumbent for about 6 hours to avoid headache and the possibility of contrast moving into the head.

Common Pathologies

- Degeneration of the disk
- Cervical disk herniation (Figure 15.16)

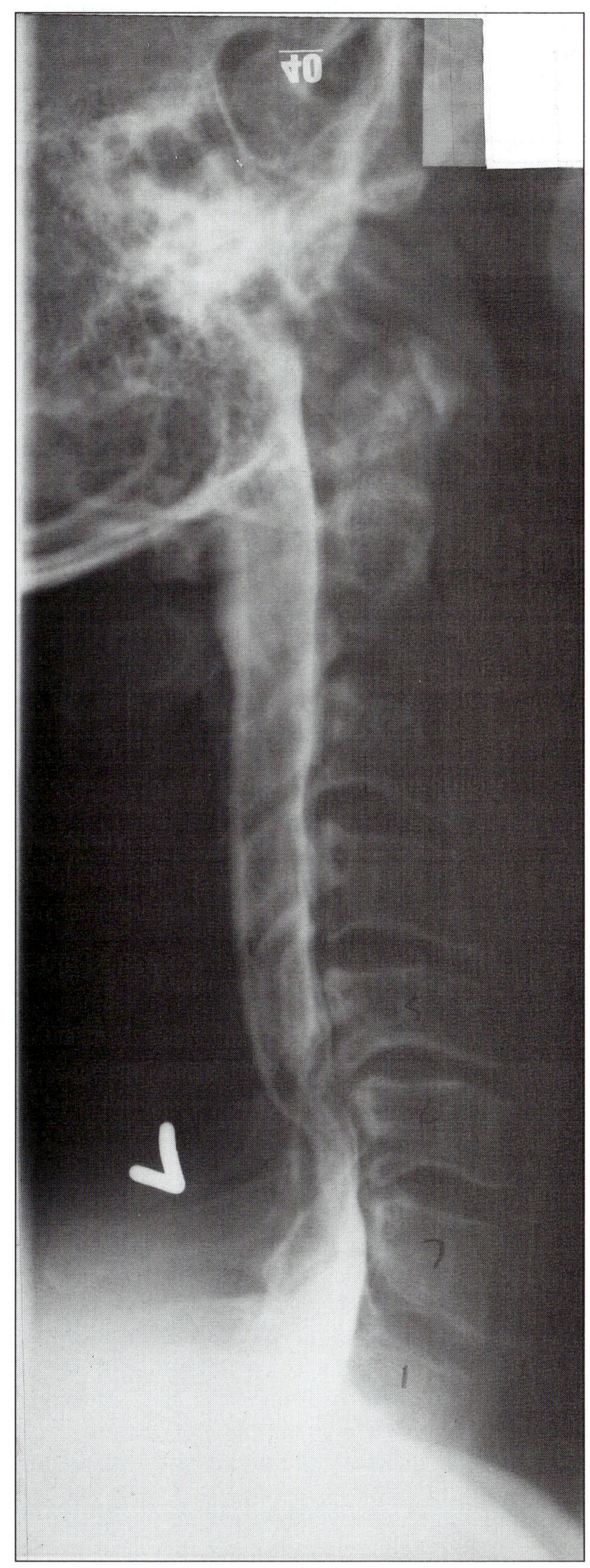

FIGURE 15.15 Cross table lateral view.

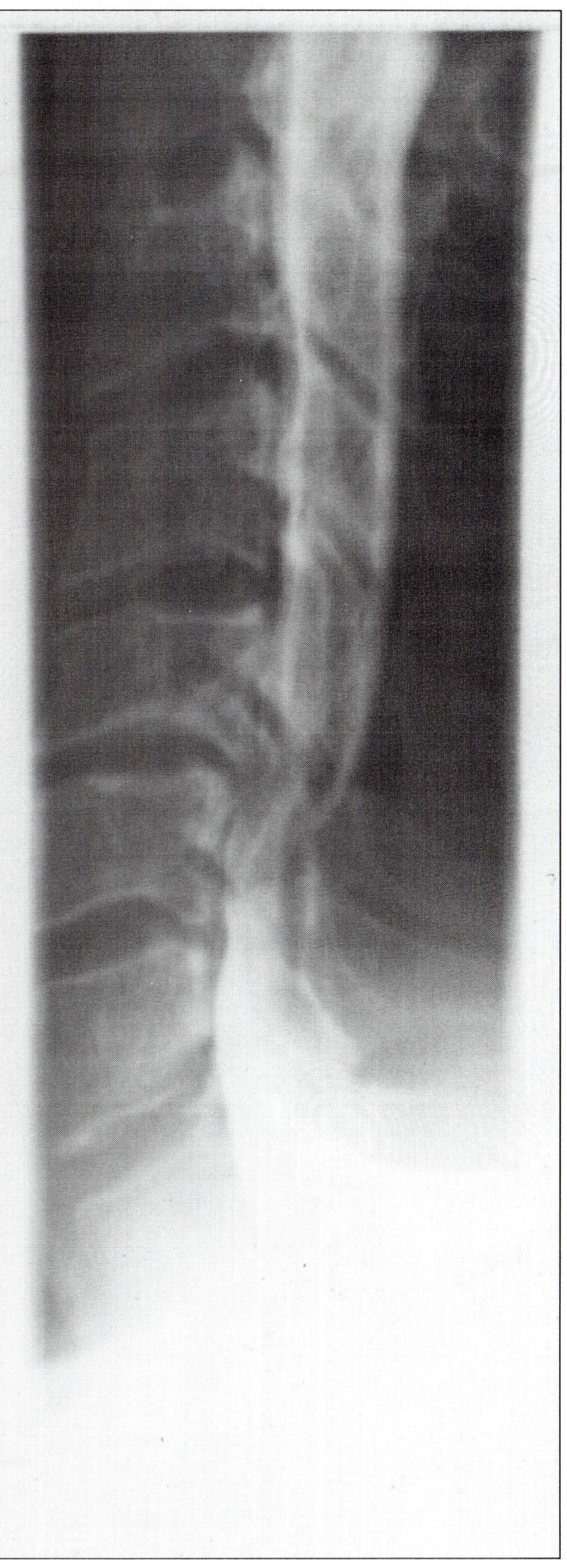

FIGURE 15.16 Cervical disk herniation.

DISKOGRAPHY

This is an examination of the intervertebral disks by means of a direct injection of contrast media. This has been a controversial examination and many in the field believe that it should be considered obsolete with the advent of CT and MRI. However, some believe that diskography can still play a significant role in dealing with patients experiencing pain, prior to a surgical fusion.

When a diskogram is performed, it has two main functions: to determine the **morphology** of the disk, including the nucleus pulposus and annulus, and to reproduce the pain caused by the disk disease, thus determining which disk is causing the problem and which are healthy.

Applied Anatomy The main features of a lumbar intervertebral disk (Figure 15.17)

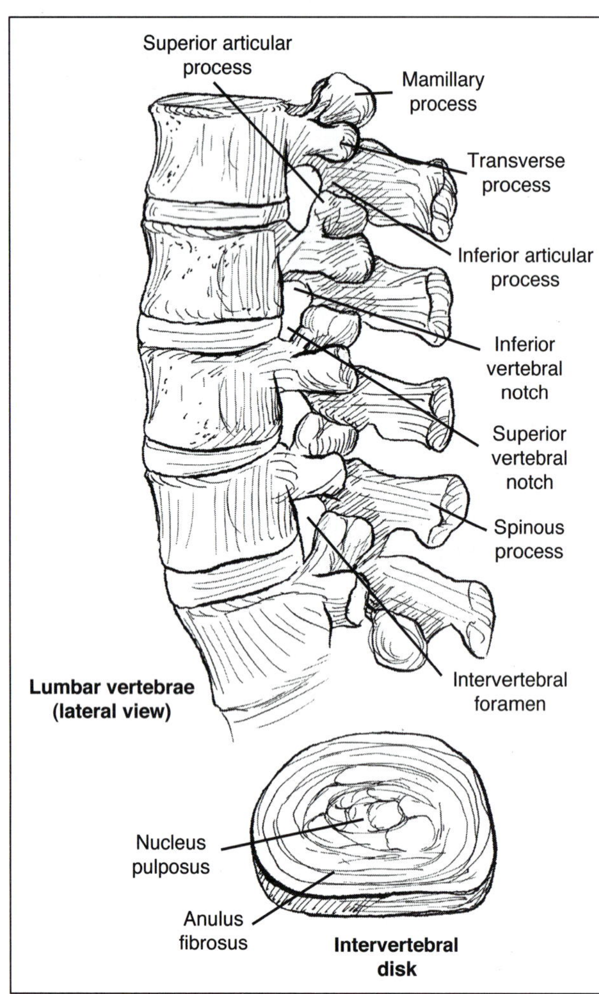

FIGURE 15.17 Intervertebral disk in lumbar area.

Indications

- Suspected prolapse on a negative myelogram patient
- Acute traumatic interosseous disk herniation
- Assessment of normal disks above and below proposed surgical fusion (very rarely performed now)
- Postdiskectomy syndromes or fusion complications
- Delineation of annular disease

Contraindications

- No major contraindications
- Sometimes painful for the patient

Equipment

- Fluoroscopy with spot film device
- Use of an overcouch tube for use with Bucky mechanism to produce a more accurate radiograph
- A second image intensifier (C-arm) may be used for biplane localization of the needle.
- Sterile tray containing diskography needles.
  —Outer needle is 21 gauge and 12.5 cm.
  —Inner needle is 26 gauge and 15.8 cm.

Contrast Media Nonionic compounds such as iohexol should be used. Damaged disks sometimes allows communication into the spinal canal. Use of iohexol abolishes risks associated with contrast in this area (see lumbar myelography).

Radiation Protection Reduce field size to disk area only and minimize fluoroscopy time.

Preliminary Radiographs

- AP projection and lateral views of lumbar spine
- Myelogram—diskograms are sometimes done after a myelogram has demonstrated no abnormalities.

Patient Preparation

- It is very important that patients are aware that the physician be told of any pain experienced during the procedure. Avoid telling them that it may be their symptomatic pain because this sometimes results in a programmed response.
- No strong analgesics are given so that pain is not completely masked.
- Anxious patients may receive a sedative.
- Broad-spectrum antibiotics can be given to reduce the likelihood of infection.

Procedure Sequence

- Patient is placed in the left lateral decubitus position on the fluoroscopy table.
- Needles are inserted under fluoroscopic guidance either posteriorly through the dura or laterally, avoiding puncturing the dura.
- Contrast is injected (up to 1 mL) into each disk as required.
- Patient is asked to describe any pain felt.

Procedure Radiographs

- Spot lateral views and PA projection with needles in situ (Figures 15.18 and 15.19)
- After needle removal, AP projection and lateral views

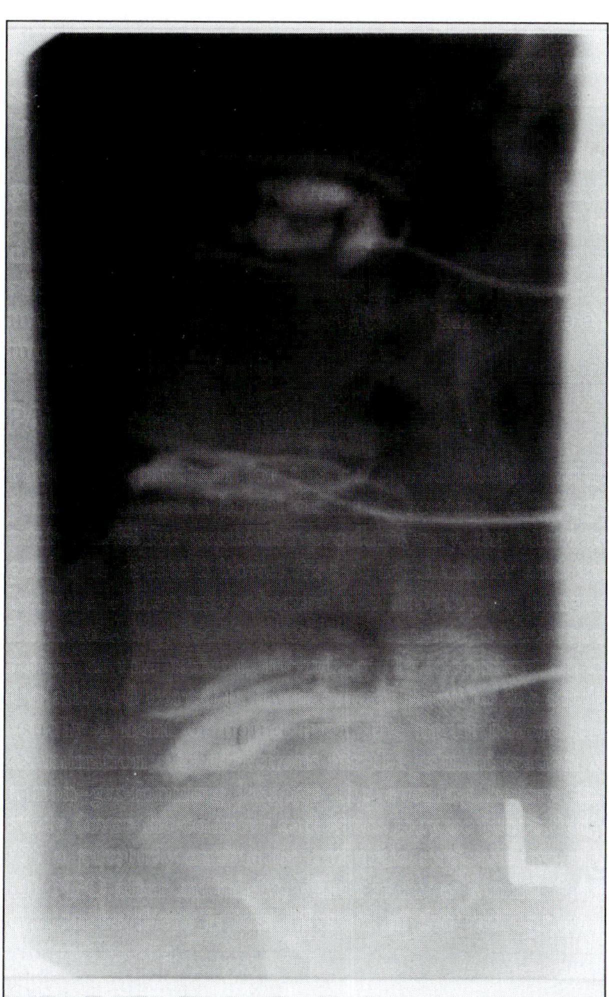

FIGURE 15.18 Lateral view diskogram.

Alternative Radiographs

- Erect lateral view
- Flexion/extension views

Postprocedure Care Depending on the degree of discomfort, the patient may require bed rest.

Common Pathologies

- Prolapsed disk
- Annular disease

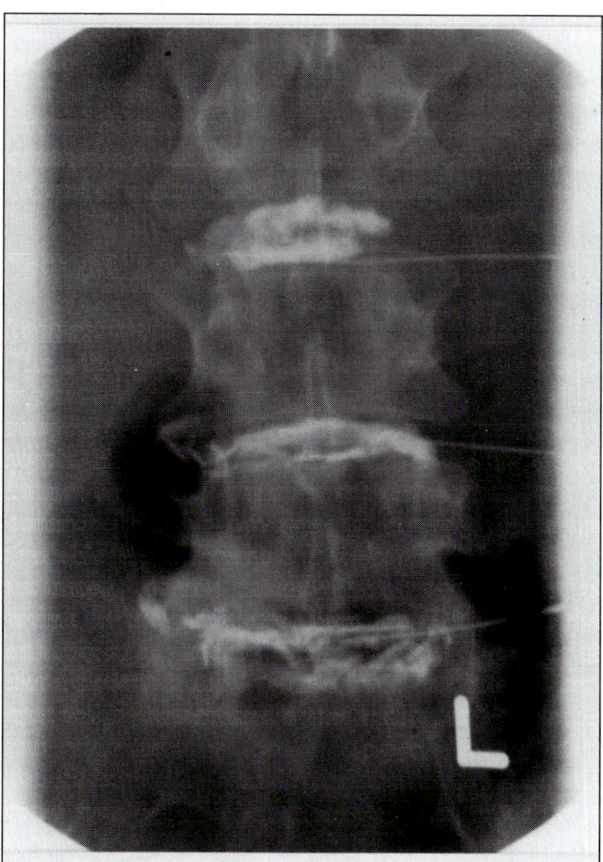

FIGURE 15.19 PA projection diskogram.

Other Imaging Modalities

COMPUTED TOMOGRAPHY

Initially, it was CT and CT myelography that supplanted myelography as the primary imaging method. MRI has now taken that position. However, CT is still used extensively for spinal imaging, often in combination with an injection of contrast media, creating the CT myelogram. Advantages of using CT include the fact that it is faster, less expensive, and often more accessible than MRI. It is an important imaging method for any spinal trauma and demonstrates degenerative disk disease and spinal stenosis well. Visualization of nerve roots is good in the lumbar region where the epidural fat is thick and more visible on the CT scan.

Disadvantages of CT are that the varying bone densities of the vertebra, interspersed with foramina and a relatively narrow canal make intrathecal imaging quite exacting. Sections can only be transverse axial. (This can be resolved in part if the CT scanner has reformatting and three-dimensional reconstruction capabilities.) The need for high resolution and many thin slices results in high radiation doses.

Applied Anatomy (Figure 15.20)

Indications for Plain CT

- Spinal stenosis
- Congenital abnormalities
- Spondylolisthesis

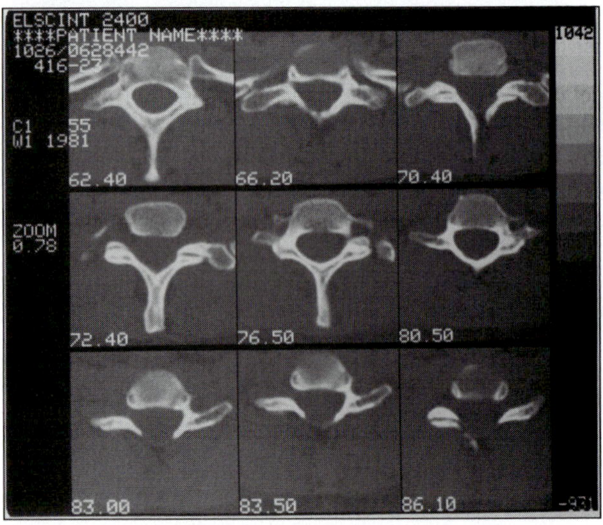

FIGURE 15.20 Labelled section CT.

- Disk degeneration
- Some tumors (e.g., hemangioma)

Indications for CT Myelography

- Intradural, extramedullary lesions
- Disk herniations
- Arachnoiditis
- Spina bifida
- Postoperative conditions of nerve roots

Contraindications As for myelography, otherwise none

Radiation Protection

- This procedure necessitates high doses.
- Every effort must be made to reduce field size and avoid repeats.

Equipment CT scanner with tilting gantry, variable section width capabilities and the ability to reformat in any plane, especially sagittal

Patient Preparation

- If a CT myelogram is required, it can be done after a conventional myelogram using the contrast in place. A delay of 2 to 4 hours is suggested to reduce the density of the contrast.
- The higher sensitivity of CT requires a lower concentration of contrast.
- If there has been no previous myelogram, a lumbar puncture is performed (as per lumbar myelogram) but with only 3 to 5mL dilute contrast administered.

Procedure Radiographs

- Thin, contiguous sections (2 mm) are taken through the area of interest, using the highest resolution possible. This is so that reformatting can be successfully accomplished.
- Larger sections (8–10 mm) can be used for general scanning of the area of interest for stenosis (Figure 15.21).

Postprocedure Care None, unless as for myelogram

Common Pathologies Cord stenosis

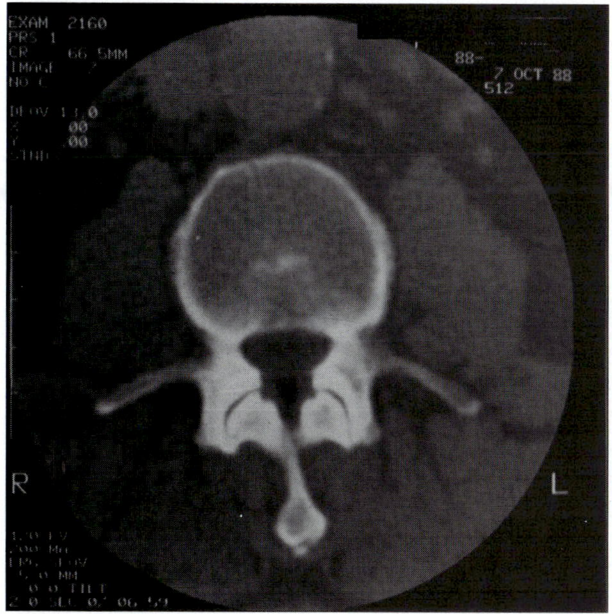

A

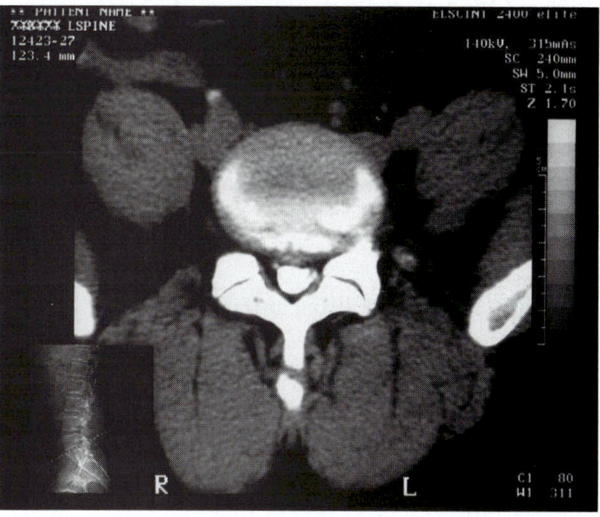

B

FIGURE 15.21 CT sections (A) without contrast (B) with contrast.

MAGNETIC RESONANCE IMAGING

Magnetic resonance has become the imaging method of choice for the majority of spinal conditions. In comparison to CT, it allows for visualization along any plane, including sagittal, there are no bone-produced artifacts, all intrathecal structures are well visualized, as are the intramedullary lesions, tumors, and cystic spaces. Finally, there is no ionizing radiation.

There are some disadvantages. Artifacts do occur due to patient motion. MRI is expensive and not always accessible.

Applied Anatomy (Figure 15.22)

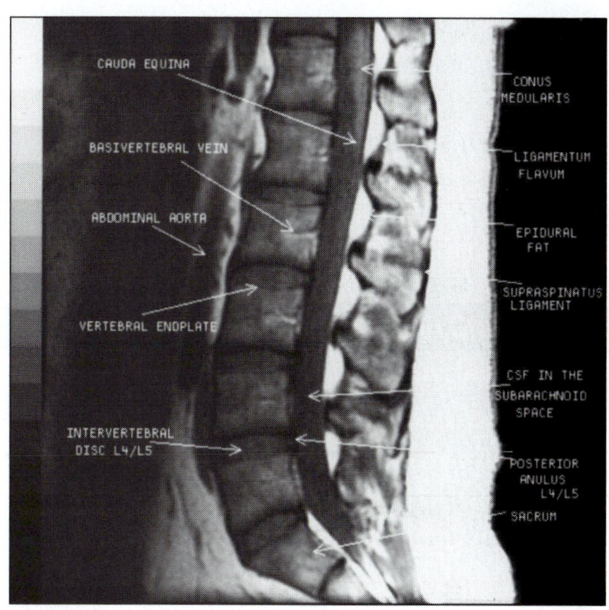

FIGURE 15.22 Labelled MRI of spine.

Indications

- Disk herniation
- Any intrathecal abnormalities
- Tumors
- Postsurgical examination

Contraindications

- Presence of pacemakers, surgical clips
- Acute anxiety, claustrophobia (open-sided equipment will help eliminate this problem)

Equipment MRI unit

Contrast Media Occasionally, gadolinium (gd-DTPA) is used for enhancement. Pathologies better visualized using gadolinium include:

- Differentiation of post-operative scar from disk herniation
- Metastatic and cord tumors
- Arachnoiditis
- Multiple sclerosis

Radiation Protection Not applicable

Procedure Sequence

- T1- and T2-weighted images both provide information although T2 is more useful. It provides a "myelogram-like" appearance, as well as differentiating white and gray matter well.
- Edema in the cord produces a high signal intensity.
- Bones and ligaments are well defined as a low signal density (Figure 15.23).

Postprocedure Care None related to examination

Common Pathologies Tumor

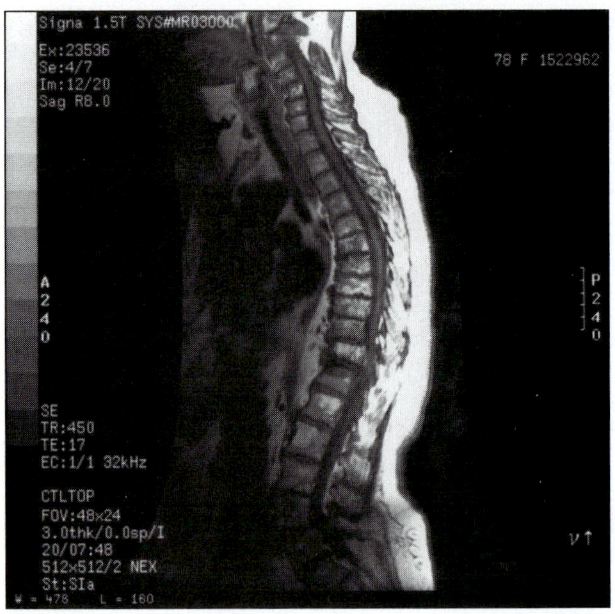

FIGURE 15.23 **MRI of spine.**

ULTRASOUND

Applications for this technology in this area are growing. Currently, ultrasound is useful to:

- Verify the contents of meningoceles
- Detect intramedullary cysts
- Measure spinal diameters

Ultrasound can be used as an intraoperative tool after the surgical removal of the laminae to assess the spinal cord.

The complex bony composition tends to obscure the image but in the case of neonates with unossified elements in the spine, ultrasound is an excellent, noninvasive method of demonstrating spinal anomalies.

RADIONUCLIDE IMAGING

Injected radiopharmaceuticals can determine:

- Spinal metastases
- Presence of bone tumors
- Presence of inflammatory process
- Localization of lower back pain

These scans are highly sensitive, but nonspecific (Figure 15.24).

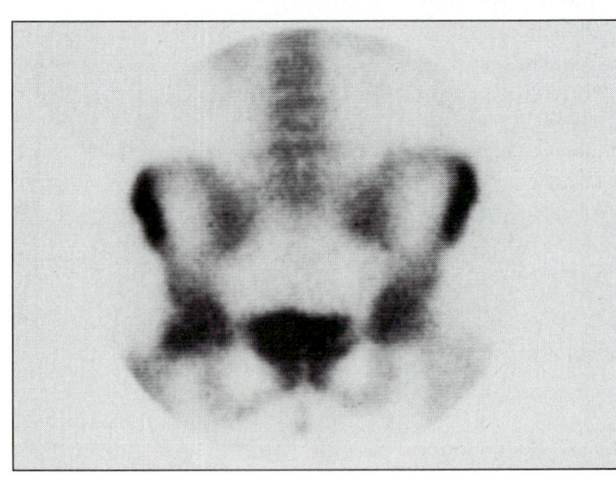

FIGURE 15.24 **Radionuclide scan of lower lumbar spine and pelvis.**

SPINAL ANGIOGRAPHY

This has a limited role and is used mainly in collaboration with interventional procedures such as the embolization of arteriovenous malformations. Digital subtraction angiography should be used where possible (see Chapter 7, Heart and Arterial System). Spinal venography, a relatively simple procedure was an excellent tool for determining any encroachment of the epidural space. However, CT has replaced this, being a more reliable and safer procedure.

Interventional Procedures

A number of interventional procedures are related to the spine, which can be divided into vascular and bone. Vascular interventions are covered in Chapter 8, Venous System.

BONE BIOPSY

(See also Chapter 3, Specialized Studies of the Skeletal System.)

The percutaneous spinal biopsy is a relatively safe and simple method of obtaining samples of tumors before therapy or surgery. It avoids the trauma of unnecessary open surgery and, if needed, allows the immediate commencement of therapy. Its primary use has been to define metastatic lesions. Opinions differ whether the samples obtained are large enough to definitively diagnose a primary tumor.

Applied Anatomy Labeled lateral view of lumbar spine with needle in situ

Indications

- To determine state and type of metastatic disease, which can assist in determining the primary site if it is currently unknown
- As follow-up to a positive but inconclusive nuclear scan
- To acquire tissue samples for analysis of tumor cell markers
- To demonstrate condition of cells within a treated tumor

Contraindications

- Abnormal, excessive bleeding, with a low platelet count
- Highly vascular tumor
- If a similar lesion is available within an extremity, it is advisable to biopsy that rather than the slightly higher risk vertebra.

Equipment

- Fluoroscopic unit
- Sterile tray containing biopsy needles, which are usually thin-walled, 18 to 23 gauge, with a central stilette. Larger bore needles (12 gauge) do provide clearer histologic samples.

Radiation Protection Minimize fluoroscopic imaging.

Preliminary Radiographs AP and lateral views of tumor site

Patient Preparation Patient should be sedated, and in certain conditions a general anesthetic is preferred.

Procedure Sequence

- Patient is placed in the lateral decubitus position on the fluoroscopy table or under C-arm fluoroscopy unit.
- The injection area is cleansed and a local anesthetic is administered.
- The spinal needle is advanced at the midline, along the sagittal plane under fluoroscopic control so that the tip of the needle is in the posterior third of the vertebral body.
- The position should be checked in both planes and then the needle advanced into the identified lesion.
- With the stilette removed the remaining cannula is advanced slightly and twisted to obtain a core of tissue.

- Suction is applied by means of a syringe as the cannula is removed.
- The specimen is retrieved to be analyzed by histology, possibly cytologic, cytogenetic, or bacterial analysis.

Procedure Radiographs Radiographs are generally not taken.

Postprocedure Care

- It is generally recommended that overnight care be given, with analgesics administered if necessary.
- Care should be taken to observe for bleeding or nerve root damage, both very rare.

Common Pathologies Metastatic lesion of lumbar spine

INTRADISKAL THERAPY

A number of methods have been devised to relieve the problems and conditions associated with disk disease, primarily disk herniation, while avoiding surgery. There is some controversy regarding their efficacy and new microsurgical procedures have reduced their use. They are still used where conservative treatment has been unsuccessful and surgery is contraindicated at that time.

Intradiskal Steroids

Injection of steroids can reduce the inflammation associated with disk herniation. Results using this have never been dramatically successful.

Chemonucleolysis

Chemical compounds have been used to reduce the pressure exerted by a bulging disk by destroying the water-binding properties of the nucleus pulposus. This would then reduce nerve compression and pain. Unfortunately, evidence appeared of some serious neurologic complications and in many countries this procedure has been banned.

Percutaneous Diskectomy

The disk is cut, sliced, and aspirated under fluoroscopic control.

Percutaneous Laser Disk Decompression

This is still in the developmental stage, but it appears to have potential. A laser beam is emitted percutaneously, which vaporizes a portion of the nucleus pulposus, which in turn reduces nerve compression.

Review Questions

1. Discuss the role of MRI in the imaging of the spine. Identify advantages and disadvantages of MRI compared to conventional myelography.

2. Conventional diskography has supporters and detractors. Discuss.

3. Define arachnoiditis and explain its significance in the development of myelography.

4. Which statement is incorrect?
   a. Cervical myelography can be performed using a lumbar puncture.
   b. Contrast medium is injected into the subarachnoid space.
   c. Trauma to a vertebral body is best demonstrated by myelography.
   d. Nerve roots can be visualized on a lumbar myelogram.

5. Which is the safest contrast media to use for a myelogram.
   a. Iotrolan
   b. Myodil
   c. Iohexol
   d. Omnipaque

6. Postprocedural conditions can include
   a. Hypertension
   b. Hives
   c. Hypotension
   d. Elevated blood sugar levels

CASE STUDY

Design a critical pathway in the imaging department for a patient who is admitted with acute back pain. The patient has a previous history of carcinoma and is 50 years old.

References and Recommended Reading

An, H. S., & Haughton, V. M. (1993). Nondiscogenic lumbar radiculography; imaging considerations. *Seminars in Ultrasound, CT and MR 14*(6), 414–424.

Ballinger, P. W. (1995). *Merrill's atlas of radiographic positions and radiologic procedures* (8th ed.). St. Louis: Mosby-Year Book.

Berland, L. L. (1987). *Practical CT technology and techniques.* New York: Raven Press.

Bischoff, R. J., et al. (1993). A comparison of computed tomography-myelography, magnetic resonance imaging and myelography in the diagnosis of herniated nucleus pulposus and spinal stenosis. *Journal of Spinal Disorders, 6*(4).

Blaser, S., & Harwood-Nash, D. (1993, summer). Pediatric spinal neoplasms. *Topics in Magnetic Resonance Imaging.*

Castaneda-Zuniga, W. R., & Tadavarthy S. M. (1992). *Interventional Radiology* (2nd ed.). Baltimore: Williams and Wilkins.

Chapman, S., & Nakielny, R. (1993). *A guide to radiological procedures* (3rd ed.). London: Bailliere and Tindall.

Coleman, L. T., & Zimmerman, R. A. (1994). Pediatric craniospinal spiral CT: Current applications and future potential. *Seminars in Ultrasound, CT and MR. 15*(2), 148–155.

Grossman, Z., Ellis, D. A., & Brigham, S. (1983). *The clinician's guide to diagnostic imaging.* New York: Raven.

Hasuo, K. et al. (1993). MR imaging compared with CT, angiography and myelography supplemented with CT in the diagnosis of spinal tumors. *Radiation Medicine, 11*(5).

Janssen, M. E., Bertrand, S. J., & Levine, M. I. (1994). Lumbar herniated disk disease: Comparison of MRI, myelography and post-myelographic CT scan with surgical findings. *Orthopedics, 17* (2).

Kawakami, N., et al. (1994). Intra-operative ultrasonographic evaluation of the spinal cord in cervical myelography. *Spine, 19* (1).

Kido, D. K., Wippold, F. J. 2nd, & Wood, R. C., Jr. (1993). The role of nonionic myelography in the diagnosis of lumbar disk herniation. *Investigative Radiology, 28* (Suppl. 5P).

Kirkwood, J. R. (1990). *Essentials of Neuroimaging.* New York: Churchill Livingstone.

Kliewer, M. A., et al. (1993). Acute spinal ligament disruption: MR imaging with anatomic correlation. *Journal of Magnetic Resonance Imaging, 3*(6).

Osborn, A. (1991). *Handbook of neuroradiology.* St. Louis: Mosby-Year Book.

Shapiro, R. (1984). *Myelography.* Chicago: Year Book Medical Publishers.

Snopek, A. M. (1992). *Fundamentals of special radiographic procedures,* (3rd ed.). Philadelphia: Saunders.

Sutton, D. A. (1993). *Textbook of radiology and imaging.* Edinburgh: Churchill Livingstone.

Thornbury, J. R., et al. (1993). Disk-caused nerve compression in patients with acute low back pain. Diagnosis with MR, CT myelography and plain CT. *Radiology, 186* (3).

Zuleger, S., & Staubesand, J. (1977). *Atlas of the central nervous system in sectional planes.* Baltimore: Urban and Schwarzenberg.

SECTION VIII

RESPIRATORY SYSTEM

CHAPTER 16

Respiratory System

CYNTHIA COWLING, BSc, MEd, MRT(R), ACR

OBJECTIVES

At the completion of this chapter, the student should be able to:

1. List the procedures used in the diagnostic studies of the respiratory system.
2. Identify the major features of the anatomy of the respiratory system.
3. Describe the tomographic procedures used to demonstrate certain pathologies and anatomy.
4. Identify relevant equipment for each study or procedure.
5. Describe the types of contrast media used for each procedure.
6. Identify radiation protection methods used.
7. Describe the relevant procedure sequences.
8. List common pathologies visualized for each examination and procedure.
9. Describe the basic concepts of alternative imaging routines.
10. Discuss the benefits of and problems with the various imaging modalities in the visualization of the respiratory system.
11. Describe the main radiologic interventions used to assist in the treatment of respiratory pathologies.

Introduction and Historical Overview

The radiography of the chest has a long history and continues to be one of the primary diagnostic tools used in respiratory disease. Chest x-rays were discussed as early as 1897 and by 1900, fluoroscopy was being used to determine various chest conditions such as pleurisy and **pneumothorax** (nū-mō-thō´răks). This method evolved to become a screening process for tuberculosis for many years.

In 1906, Karl Springer first attempted to outline the bronchial tree by catheterizing dogs through the trachea and blowing in a powder consisting of bismuth and iodoform. After the discovery of lipiodol in 1924, human bronchography became routine. A disadvantage to this contrast was the fact that it took a long time to dissipate away from the lungs. Water-soluble contrast proved too irritating and it was not until Dionosil (an oily and aqueous solution) was discovered in the 1950s that bronchograms became anything less than suffocating (literally!) for the patient. In 1968, powdered tantalum was first used, which coated the mucosa without clogging the bronchial tree. It was at about this time, however, that conventional tomography, then CT imaging and the effective and extensive use of the **bronchoscope**, dramatically reduced the use of bronchography as a diagnostic tool. It still remains the definitive method for imaging **bronchiectasis** (brŏng´´kē-ĕk´tă-sĭs).

Anatomy

Structurally, the respiratory tract consists of a series of passages that convey air from outside the body to a large expanse of respiratory membrane, the lungs, which lie on close proximity to blood capillaries. Here, oxygen is released to the vascular system and carbon dioxide is released by the blood in a process called external respiration.

Beginning at the external nares, inspired air passes through the nasal cavity and, in sequence, to the nasopharynx and oropharynx to the larynx. The air passes through the **glottis** (glŏt´ĭs) (the vocal apparatus) of the larynx to enter the trachea.

The trachea extends from the larynx, anterior to the esophagus, to its bifurcation point into the right and left mainstem (primary) bronchi. Each of these enters their respective lung through the hilum, with the right bronchus shorter and more vertical than the left.

On entering the lung each bronchus divides into secondary and tertiary bronchi and then continues, resulting in the bronchial tree. The fine bronchial tubes at the periphery of the tree are the bronchioles. The terminal branches of these are called the respiratory bronchioles and each of these in turn gives rise to several branches known as the alveolar ducts. The alveoli open directly into the ducts or pass through an intervening structure, the alveolar sac (Figures 16.1 and 16.2).

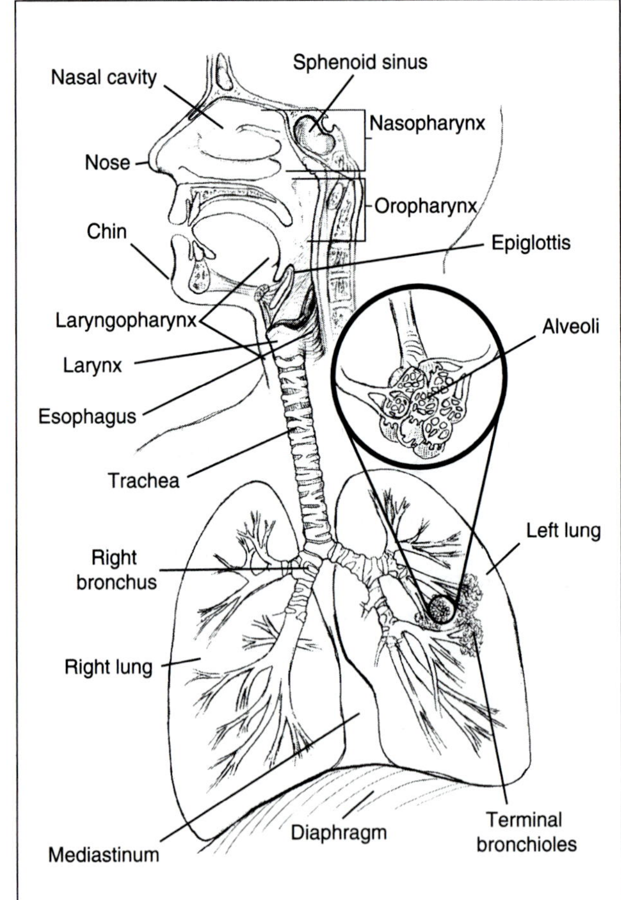

FIGURE 16.1 The respiratory system.

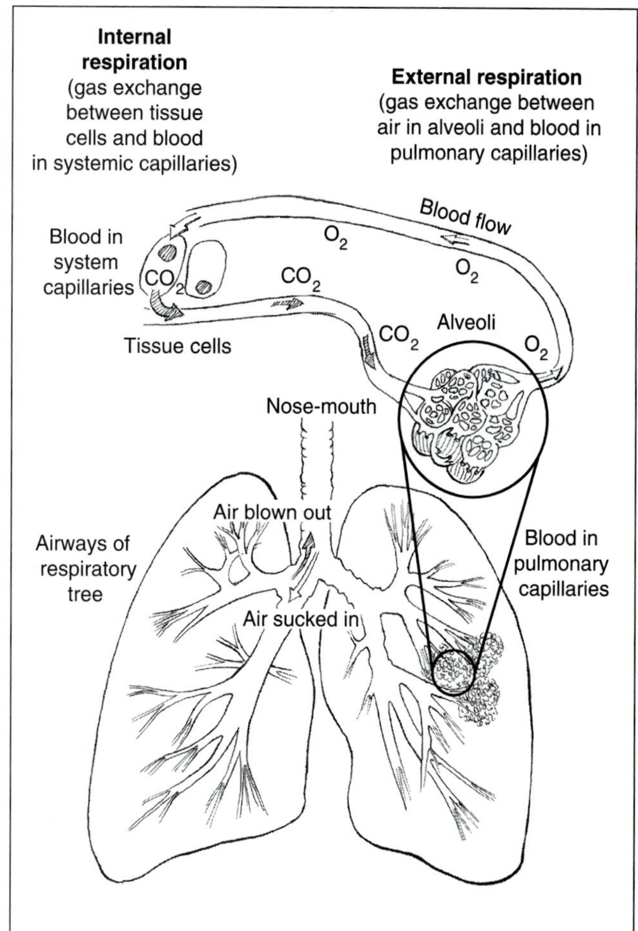

FIGURE 16.2
The respiratory mechanism.

Procedures

CONVENTIONAL TOMOGRAPHY

This technique has been superseded by CT in most instances, but tomography is still performed as a mechanism for localizing single known lesions quickly and inexpensively. Tomography should be performed on low-risk patients with a high likelihood of a benign lesion. The technique for tomographic examinations is covered in Volume I.

Indications

- To assess position of a single lesion (e.g., intrapulmonary, **hilar**)
- To improve visualization of a single lesion
- To demonstrate benign calcifications
- To evaluate the chest wall and **mediastinum** (mē′′dē-ăs-tī′nŭm)

Contraindications

- Any high-risk patient (i.e., high likelihood of malignant condition)
- Presence of multiple lesions

Equipment

- In most instances a linear tomographic unit is sufficient.
- Trispiral movements are occasionally used.

Contrast Media None

Radiation Protection

- Gonadal shielding
- Thyroid shielding may be problematic if the suspected lesion is high in the chest.
- Exposures are kept to a minimum with suitable collimation.

Preliminary Radiographs

- A recent plain chest radiograph is essential.
- PA and lateral views and occasionally an oblique view will provide an initial assessment of the presence of a lesion.
- Sometimes nipple markers are required to exclude false-positive interpretation.

Patient Preparation None specific. The patient may be required to lie at a particular angle for some time.

Procedure Sequence

- Linear tomography is performed using 1-cm cuts.
- Patient is placed in the AP position for peripheral lesions.
- Patient is placed in the 55° APO position to demonstrate hilar lesions. The side obliqued dependents on the position of the lesion. In an APO projection of the chest, the side down and closest to the film or image detector will be best demonstrated. Therefore, a right oblique will demonstrate the right side.
- The fulcrum level of the tomographic cut is estimated by evaluating the chest radiographs.
- All radiographs should be taken at the same degree of suspended respiration.

Procedure Radiographs

- AP and oblique cuts are taken through the lesion to extend beyond either side of the lesion (Figure 16.3).
- Occasionally lateral views are taken.
- If the lesion is deep within the hilum, at the **carina** (kă-rī′nă), overpenetrated views may be needed.

Alternative Radiographs CT examinations are usually required with any lesion not well visualized or with any risk of malignancy.

Postprocedure care None

Common Pathologies Single calcified, benign lesions

> Fluoroscopy is a conventional imaging modality that is still useful when determining the movement of a lesion or the degree of movement of the chest wall or the diaphragm. It is interesting to note that it is sometimes possible to determine whether a lesion is of pleural or vascular origin by asking the patient to perform the **Valsalva** maneuver. The vascular lesion will tend to change size, but the pleural lesion will not.

BRONCHOGRAPHY

Bronchography is the examination of the lower respiratory tract. It is performed infrequently because it is an uncomfortable procedure for the patient. It does, however, give an excellent demonstration of the outline of the bronchial tree and is still considered the best way to demonstrate bronchiectasis.

Applied Anatomy (Figure 16.3)

Indications

- Bronchiectasis
- Other obstructions of the lower bronchial tree
- Recurrent **hemoptysis**

Contraindications

- Impairment of pulmonary function
- Recent pneumonia
- Active tuberculosis
- Known allergies

Equipment

- Conventional image intensification unit with overhead source for radiographs
- Prepared sterile tray for introduction of contrast medium, dependent on route administered (see procedure sequence)
- Emergency tray equipment

Contrast Media

- A low **osmolaric** water-based contrast medium such as iotrolan 300 or iohexol is used. These are rapidly absorbed from the bronchi but are considered more irritable on the mucosal lining.
- Oil-based compounds, such as Dionosil have been frequently used, but their viscosity and inability to mix with bronchial secretions sometimes prohibits good coverage; residual oily contrast can sometimes cause fever.

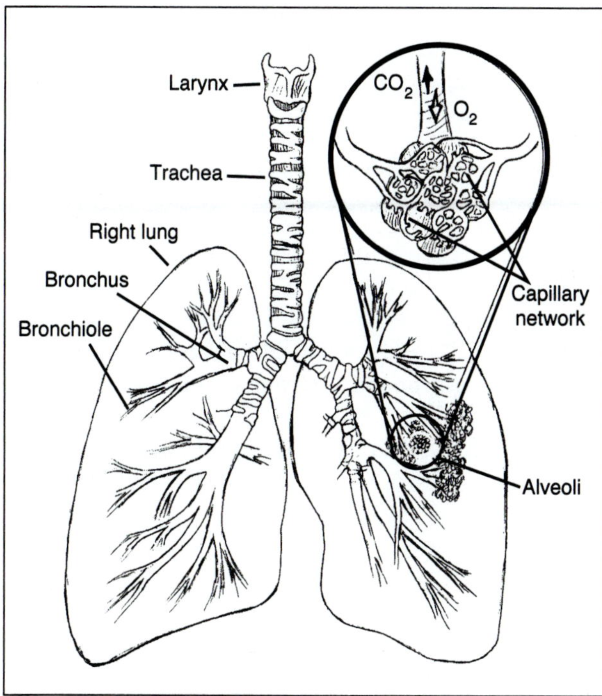

FIGURE 16.3 The bronchial tree.

Radiation Protection

- Gonadal protection
- Minimize fluoroscopic time.

Preliminary Radiographs

- Recent chest radiographs, PA and lateral
- Oblique views may be required.

Patient Preparation

- Nothing by mouth at least 2 hours before examination; there have been instances of mild headache, nausea, and vomiting during the procedure.
- Mild sedation is advised for adults, but patient must be alert to respond to instructions.
- Chest physiotherapy before the examination will clear mucosa.
- In the presence of infection, antibiotic therapy is recommended.
- Asthmatics should have appropriate **prophylactic therapy** before examination.
- Patients must be advised that the examination is uncomfortable giving them a choking sensation and that it will be important to refrain from coughing when asked.
- Administration of a topical anesthetic immediately before the procedure is advised to suppress the cough reflex.

Procedure Sequence In any method, if a bilateral study is performed, the right side is examined and imaged before the left because of the anatomic situation of the bronchi and because it is the larger lung.

Via Bronchoscope

- This is the preferred method because it allows for accurate placement of the contrast medium, which can be directed to a specific segment of the lung.
- A bronchoscope is introduced via the nose or mouth into the trachea. This can be performed in the fluoroscopy room or before the patient coming to the imaging department.
- The bronchoscope is advanced using visual sighting of the bronchial tree by means of fiberoptics.
- When the tip of the bronchoscope is appropriately positioned, contrast medium is administered under fluoroscopic control.
- Radiographs are taken with the spot film device when needed. The water-based contrast agent disperses quickly so these images must be taken as quickly as possible.
- The patient can be rotated during injection to ensure complete filling.

Other Methods of Contrast Administration

- Catheter—A catheter is inserted via fluoroscopic control either through the mouth or the nose.
- It is advanced to the general area required and contrast is introduced and distributed by moving the patient and by gravity.
- Transtracheal puncture—The cricothyroid membrane is punctured and the contrast is injected via a special 17-gauge needle. This method requires hospitalization for the patient.
- Aspiration method—The patient is seated and the contrast is introduced via a cannula placed either above the glottis (supraglottis) or into the glottis (intraglottis) and the contrast is introduced into the bronchial system.

Procedure Radiographs

- In addition to spot radiographs taken during the examination, conventional chest radiographs may be required. PA, lateral, and oblique views should be taken erect at 200- or 180-cm distance (Figures 16.4 and 16.5).
- A delay PA projection chest radiograph at 4 hours is recommended to determine continued presence of contrast medium and any respiratory complications.

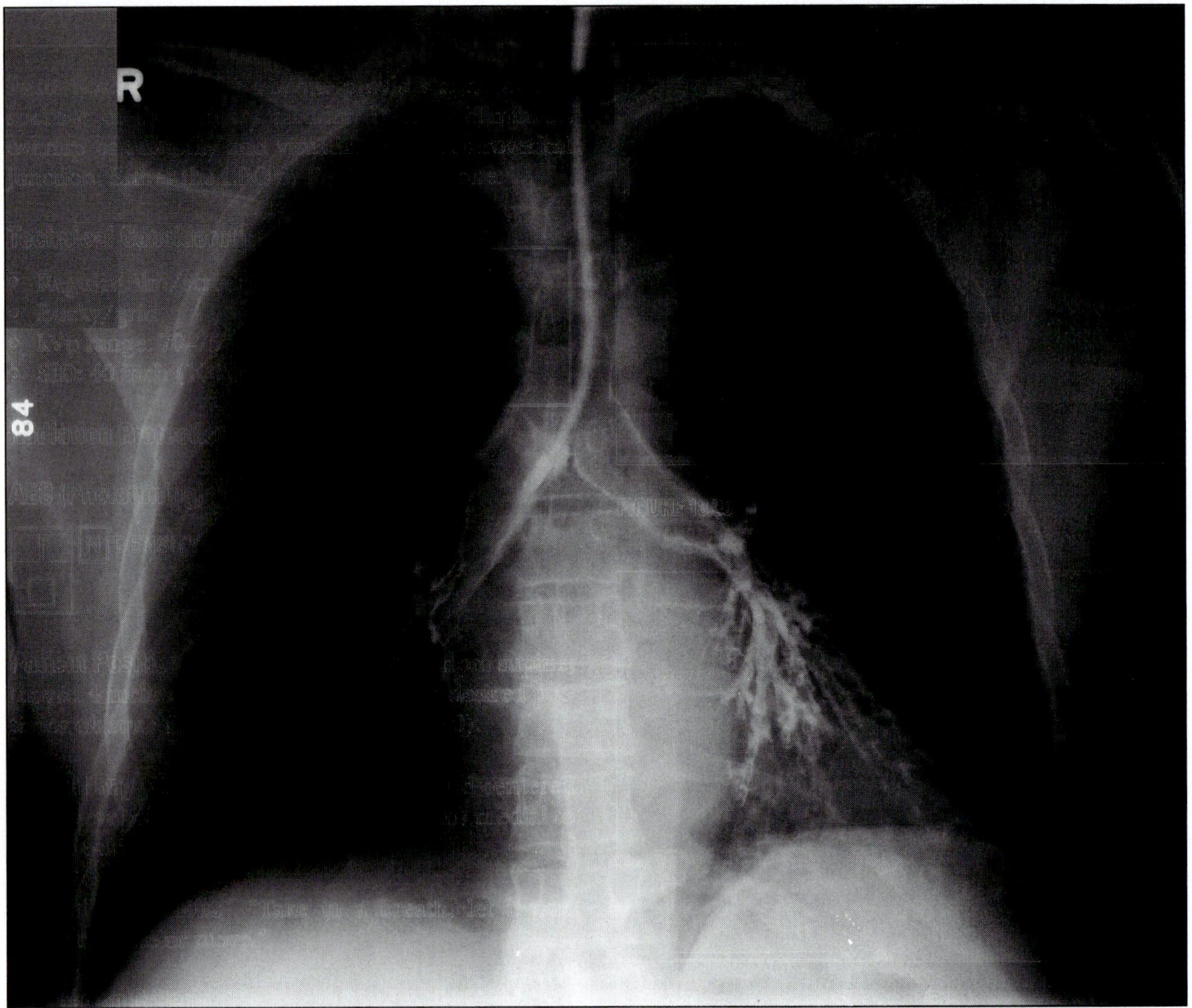

FIGURE 16.4 PA projection of bronchial tree.

Postprocedure Care

- Bronchospasm and impaired respiratory function should be checked by observation up to 4 hours postexamination.
- Postural drainage may be required in extreme conditions.

Common Pathologies

- Bronchiectasis
- **Adenoma** due to carcinoma

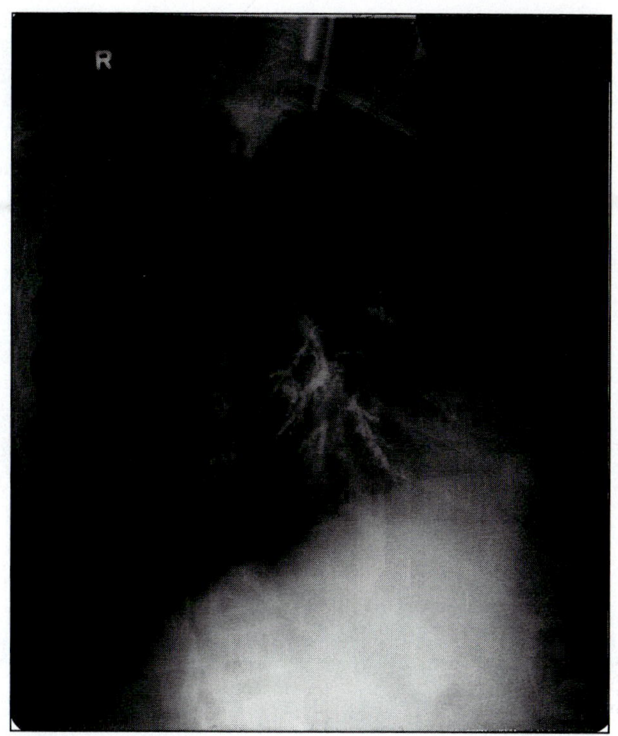

FIGURE 16.5
Right anterior oblique view demonstrating left lung.

Other Imaging Modalities

COMPUTED TOMOGRAPHY

Scanning with CT has been proven to be extremely useful as a follow-up to any chest radiograph indicating **lobar** or **segmental disease**. Contiguous slices passing through the area are required and a short scanning time is recommended because each slice should be taken with the same degree of inspiration and with the minimum of mediastinal movement. Inspiration generally improves the visualization of structures and pathologies, particularly mediastinal structures. The phase of inspiration will also affect the density visualized on the image.

Several mechanisms are used to improve the quality of CT images, including:

1. Enhancement with IV contrast medium (Figure 16.6).
2. The use of high-resolution, thin-section CT

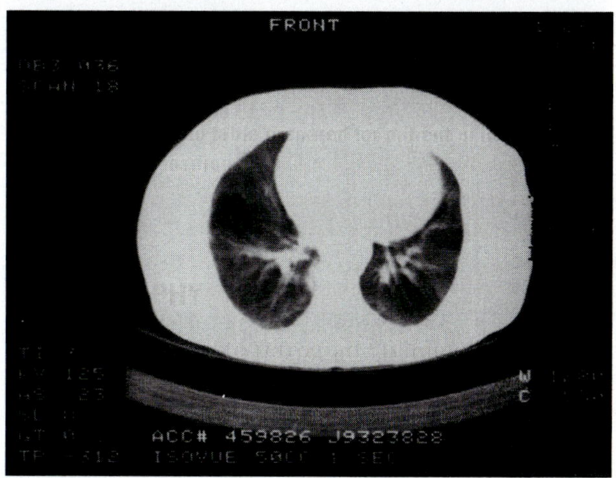

FIGURE 16.6 CT of lungs.

CT can be used for treatment planning in radiotherapy and for monitoring of nodules before and after treatment (Figure 16.7). It also provides an accurate method for the placement of biopsy needles and drainage tubes (see below).

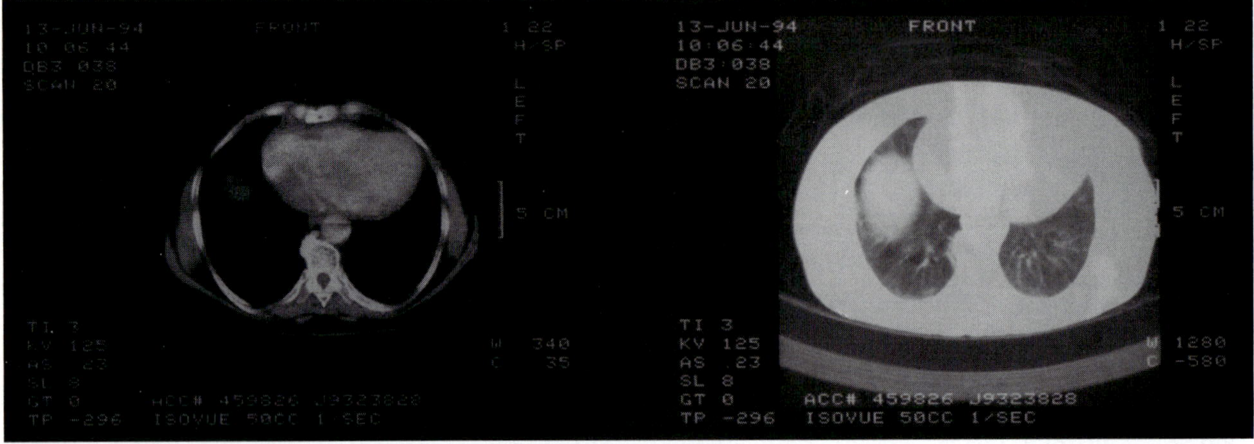

FIGURE 16.7 Enhanced CT images to demonstrate a lesion.

MAGNETIC RESONANCE IMAGING

Tissue differentiation is extremely high using MRI without any contrast enhancement, but the problems related to mediastinal movement prevents it from replacing CT as the imaging modality of choice for the respiratory system. It is able to discriminate mediastinal masses from normal or abnormal vessels but is unable to produce the same anatomic detail as high-resolution CT. Advances in the technology such as faster MRI scan times and a good signal-to-noise ratio may improve the quality of images (Figure 16.8).

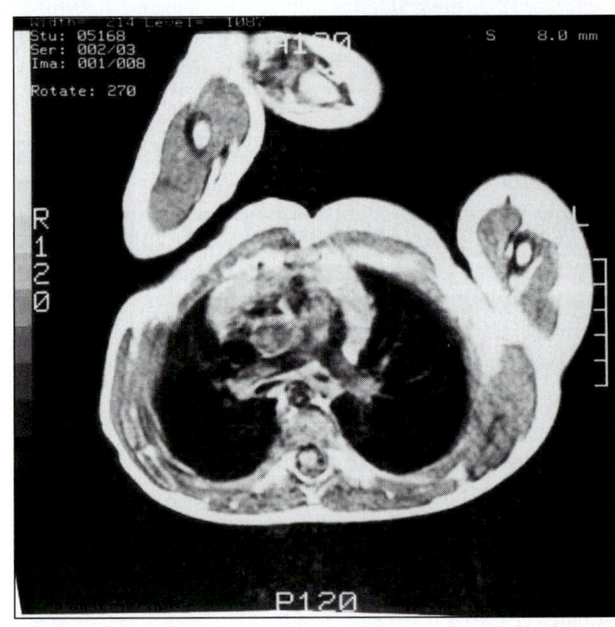

FIGURE 16.8 MRI of lungs.

ULTRASOUND

The acoustic shadows thrown by the chest wall and the lung fields limit the use of ultrasound in the respiratory system and it is generally used only to localize pleural **effusions** (ĕ-fū´zhŭn) and other homogenous-like fluid-filled collections such as a **subphrenic abscess**. It can also be used to position a biopsy needle if there is a well defined lesion. Scanning of the diaphragmatic area can be aided by passing the signals via the liver on the right side or through a water-filled stomach on the left.

RADIONUCLIDE IMAGING

Nuclear medicine is used extensively in the diagnosis of certain conditions within the chest. The most common examination is the ventilation/perfusion scan, which excludes the presence of pulmonary embolism. When this condition is indicated, nuclear medicine will be the first imaging modality of choice. For a definitive diagnosis, pulmonary angiography will be performed (see Chapter 7, Heart and Arterial System).

Lung ventilation and perfusion scans complement each other and depending on the type of gas (**xenon** [zē´nŏn] or **krypton** radionuclide) or other radionuclide a **technetium** (tĕk-nē´shē-ŭm) compound are performed sequentially. The basic principle is that the patient is asked to breathe through a special dispensing equipment (Figure 16.10), which will diffuse the radionuclide throughout the lungs while images are taken in the anterior, posterior, and oblique views. These images will demonstrate areas of obstruction, low activity, or increased uptake. There is a certain lack of specificity to the studies, but they are relatively simple and inexpensive to perform and provide essential initial information, principally on the diagnosis of pulmonary emboli and chronic obstructive disease such as **emphysema**. They are useful in the detection of malignancies associated with AIDS and in monitoring the effects of therapy (Figure 16.10).

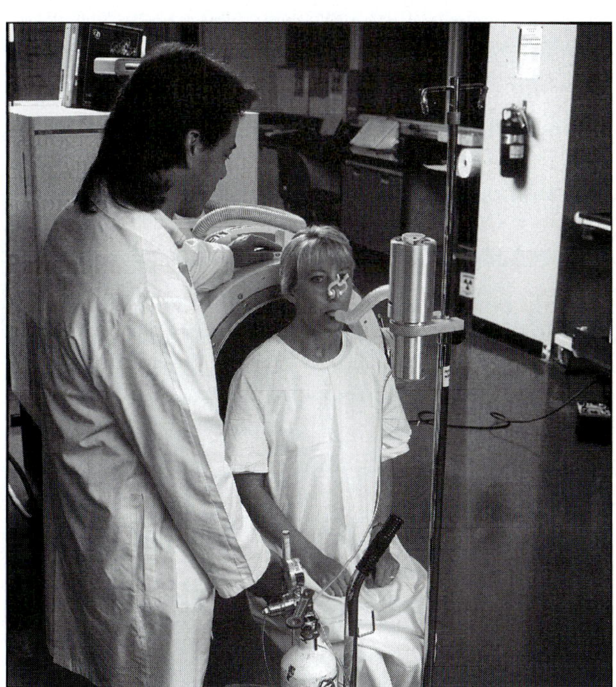

FIGURE 16.9 Patient undergoing NM ventilation.

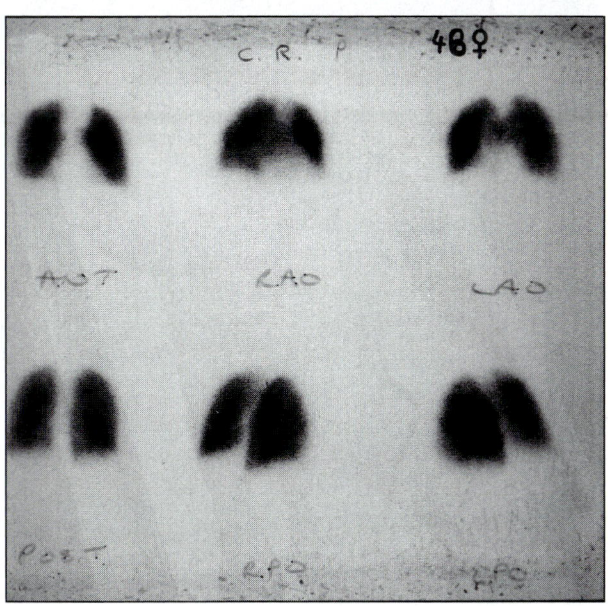

A

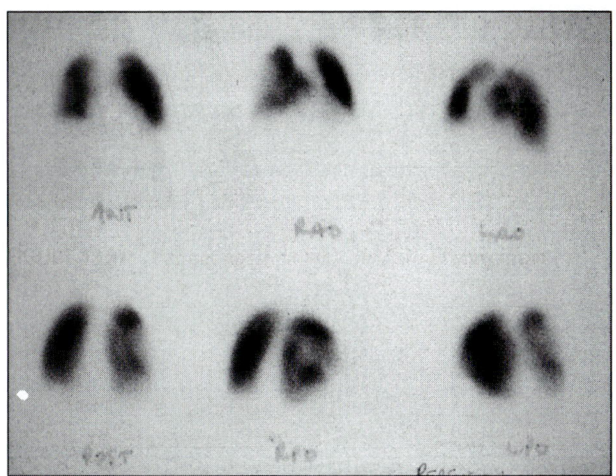

B

FIGURE 16.10 (A) Normal perfusion lung scan (B) perfusion scan demonstrating pneumonia.

Interventional Procedures

LUNG BIOPSY

Indications

- Bronchogenic carcinoma
- Solitary pulmonary nodule
- Multiple pulmonary nodules
- **Immunocompromised** patient with nodule

Contraindications

- Severe chest infections
- Suspected vascular lesion
- Seriously impaired respiratory function. There is a possibility of a pneumothorax being incurred during this procedure. The patient must be able to tolerate this condition.

Equipment

- Conventional fluoroscopy

or

- C-arm fluoroscopy unit
- CT equipment. CT is generally used only when the lesion cannot be visualized with fluoroscopy.
- Ultrasound can be used if the lesion is well defined or fluid filled.
- Biopsy needle, usually **Chiba** type. The gauge and length depend on the position of the lesion. Gauges range from 18 to 23 and length from 15 to 20 cm.
- Resuscitation equipment

Contrast Media

None used

Radiation Protection

- Minimize exposure time.
- Minimize fluoroscopy time.
- Protect gonadal area.

Preliminary Radiographs

- PA and lateral chest radiographs
- CT of relevant area

Patient Preparation

- As with all procedures, the patient is made aware of risks and benefits of the procedure.
- Clotting time test (**prothrombin**)
- Pulmonary function test
- Mild sedation is advisable, but the patient must remain reasonably alert to ensure a consistent breathing pattern.

Procedure Sequence

- The patient is positioned on the fluoroscopy table, prone for posterior lesions and supine for anterior lesions.
- The lesion is localized by using the biplane fluoroscopy and chest radiographs.
- The skin directly above the lesion is marked as the entry point and local anesthetic administered to the area and as far as the pleura.
- It is important to determine position of ribs and diaphragm during respiration. The needle is inserted during rested, suspended respiration and under fluoroscopic control.
- The needle is inserted so that the end is placed in the periphery of the lesion to avoid possible necrotic tissue.
- Suction is applied to the needle as it is moved around to obtain a sample, but the suction is stopped when the needle is being withdrawn to prevent contamination of the sample.
- If a fine needle is used (22 gauge) it is considered safe to have three passes into the lesion to obtain a sample.
- The sample is immediately placed in a sterile container and given to a cytologist for examination.

Procedure Radiographs

- None usually taken during the procedure
- A follow-up chest radiograph is taken to check for pneumothorax or other complications (see below).

Postprocedure Care

- A pneumothorax occurs in about 15% of cases, but they are usually small, resolving without need of a suction pump. However, such patients should be closely monitored until the pneumothorax is resolved. Patients with any doubtful conditions or difficulty breathing should be hospitalized overnight.
- There is also a 5% incidence of hemoptysis, which is usually very temporary.
- **Empyema** (ĕm´´pī-ē´mă) can occur.
- In extremely rare cases, malignant cells can be seeded along the needle track.

PERCUTANEOUS ASPIRATION OF LUNG NODULES AND DRAINAGE OF FLUID

The use of CT has allowed significantly clearer display of chest lesions, which permits extremely accurate placement of needles and tubes. The use of drainage in the abdomen has led to the development of small drainage techniques for abscesses and empyemas in the chest with very positive results. The procedure is the same as for a biopsy, but with a larger gauge needle, enabling the physician to remove fluid in adequate quantities. Because fluid is demonstrated as a homogenous ultrasound image, the positioning of the needle for the drainage of empyemas and pleural effusions is sometimes performed using ultrasound control.

PERCUTANEOUS PLACEMENT OF CHEST TUBES

Small tubes can be placed under fluoroscopy, CT, or ultrasound control for the alleviation of pneumothoraces. Under fluoroscopic control and in an aseptic environment small drainage kits are inserted into the pleural cavity, usually between the third and fourth costal interspace. The kits contain a **heimlich** valve, which is a one-way air device, allowing the **aspiration** of air from the lung space without air entering. As with biopsies and large conventional drainage tubes, there is the risk of **hemothorax** or a **hematoma** or infection. This method is generally only used for small pneumothoraces. Larger ones require a standard thoracostomy (thō´´răk-ŏs´tō-mē) tube.

Review Questions

1. Devise a chart that demonstrates which imaging modality best demonstrates which respiratory pathology.

2. Describe the role of the technologist during a lung biopsy.

3. Which of the following statements about bronchiectesis is untrue?

a. it is best demonstrated on a bronchogram
b. air is trapped in the lower lobes of the lungs
c. it is well demonstrated on a plain chest radiograph
d. a low osmolaric contrast will provide a better defined image of bronchiectasis

4. CT images of the lung can be improved by:

a. using a thicker section
b. having the patient perform the Valsalva maneuver
c. using IV contrast medium
d. using a longer scanning time

5. Ultrasound is not the ideal imaging modality for the lungs because:

a. respiration causes too much movement
b. the heartbeat produces abnormal acoustic shadows
c. the variation of the chest wall and lung tissue produce abnormal acoustic shadows
d. there are no lung pathologies that produce a homogenous shadow

6. For a lung biopsy:

a. the patient is placed on the side
b. only one puncture is permitted
c. the needle must be as close to the periphery of the lesion as possible
d. pneumothorax occurs in 50% of lung biopsies

CASE STUDY

A patient with a chronic history of breathing difficulties goes to the doctor. Bronchiectasis or emphysema is suspected. Suggest the imaging modalities that may be used and discuss variations in procedures that may be required depending on the pathology.

References and Recommended Reading

Ballinger, P. W. (1995). *Merrill's atlas of radiographic positioning and radiologic procedures* (8th ed.). St. Louis: Mosby-Year Book.

Berland, L. (1987). *Practical CT technology and techniques.* New York: Raven.

Castenada-Zuniga, W., & Tadavarthy, S. (1992). *Interventional radiology* (Vol 2, 2nd ed.). Baltimore: Williams & Wilkins.

Eisenberg, R. L. (1993). *Radiology, an illustrated history.* St. Louis: Mosby-Year Book.

Goddard, P. (1986). *Diagnostic imaging of the chest.* Edinburgh: Churchill Livingstone.

Grossman, Z., Ellis, D., & Brigham, S. (1983). *The clinician's guide to diagnostic imaging.* New York: Raven.

Kang, E. Y. (1995). Bronchiectasis: Comparison of pre-operative thin section CT and pathologic findings in resected specimens. *Radiology, 195*(3), 121–122.

Lamers, R. J., et al. (1994). Chronic obstructive pulmonary disease: Evaluation with spirometrically controlled CT lung densitometry. *Radiology, 193*(1), 109–113.

Ontario Association of Radiologist. (1994, June). *Magnetic resonance position paper.*

Reed, J. G., et al. (1991). Interventional procedures used for diagnosing and treating lung cancer. *Journal of thoracic imaging* 7(1), 48–56.

Sharp, P. F., Gemmell, H. G., & Smith, F. W. (Eds.). (1989). *Practical nuclear medicine.* Oxford: Oxford University Press.

Snopek, A. (1992). Fundamentals of special radiographic procedures (3rd ed.). Philadelphia: Saunders.

Sutton, D. A. (1993). *Textbook of radiology and imaging.* Edinburgh: Churchill Livingstone.

Swensen, S. J., et al. (1995). Pulmonary nodules: CT evaluation of enhancement with iodinated contrast material. *Radiology, 194*(2), 393–398.

Glossary

abscess infection process that has formed a pocket of pus; seen in the breasts of lactating women.

absorptiometry measurement of absorption rates of radiation by bone to determine chemical composition. (Densitometry measures the amount of calcium in the bone).

absorption values numerical value given to the amount of radiation each tissue type absorbs.

acinus small sac-like dilatation found in glands.

acoustic impedance mismatch difference in stiffness and density between adjacent tissues.

acoustic shadowing black area produced posterior to a highly attenuating structure.

ACR-NEMA conjoint committee of the American College of Radiologists and the National Electrical Manufacturers Association that includes medical imaging equipment manufacturers and is responsible for the definition and maintenance of industrial standards for digital image transfer in medicine.

ADC (analog to digital conversion) device that converts analog representations of a measured property to a digital form. This conversion process is integral to digital image processing instruments.

adenocarcinoma malignant neoplasm of epithelial cells in glandular tissue.

adenoma neoplasm of glandular epithelium; benign tumor with gland-like structures and intervening supporting stroma, usually well circumscribed tending to compress rather than "invade" adjacent tissue.

adenosis benign breast change marked by an increase in proportion of glandular (adeno) tissue to the other kinds of tissue in the breast. This change is not associated with an increased risk of breast cancer.

adipose tissue fatty tissue.

adnexal adjacent to.

ALARA principle as low as reasonably achievable.

albumin (of blood) a plasma protein.

algorithm unambiguous series of steps by which a problem may be solved.

align in MRI, this term refers to spins in the low energy state that "align" or point in the direction of the static magnetic field.

alpha particle particle that is identical to the helium nucleus, consisting of two protons and two neutrons. It carries a positive charge of 2.

amenorrhea failure to menstruate.

amniotic fluid the albuminous fluid that fills the amniotic cavity and surrounds the fetus.

ampulla local dilation of the excretory duct that functions as a reservoir of milk.

analgesia the absence of sensibility to pain.

analog quantity or signal that varies in a continuous unbroken fashion.

anastomosis communication between two vessels. It can occur naturally or by surgical connection.

angiography the general term used to describe the study of vessels using contrast media introduced through a lymphatic, venous, or arterial route by needle puncture.

angioplasty following angiography, a procedure used to repair blood vessels, which results in improved blood flow without the use of invasive surgery.

anion an ion carrying a negative charge.

annular ring shaped; pertaining to the annulus of the intervertebral disc.

anorexia lack or loss of appetite.

antegrade (anterograde) extending or moving forward; going forwards as, for example, the contrast agent introduced in the direction of normal urine flow.

aplasia failure of an organ to develop normally.

apocrine metaplasia benign breast change in which the cells lining the breast ducts, normally shaped like cubes, become longer and shaped like columns. This change is not associated with an increased risk of breast cancer.

arachnoiditis inflammation of the arachnoid membrane.

areola pigmented ring of tissue that surrounds the nipple.

arteriography term used to describe the study of arteries using contrast media introduced by needle puncture.

arthrography study of the articulations of the body (from the Greek "arthro", meaning articulation).

arthroscopy examination of the interior of a joint with an arthroscope; a type of endoscope.

artifacts artifact is any false feature in the MRI caused by the imaging process.

ascites collection of fluid in the abdominal peritoneal cavity due to obstruction of the lymph or venous system.

aspiration removal of fluid or cells from a mass or thickening by means of a hypodermic syringe; withdrawal of fluid for therapeutic reasons or for testing.

atherosclerosis common form of arteriosclerosis in which deposits of plaques are formed within the lumen of arteries.

attenuation decrease in the intensity of an x-ray beam caused by absorption upon interaction with matter.

atypia the condition of having abnormal cells. This can be demonstrated only by diagnosis of tissue obtained by biopsy. It carries an increased risk of subsequent breast cancer.

atypical hyperplasia cells that are abnormal in appearance and increased in number.

augmentation insertion of silicone or saline-filled pouches in the breast to enhance the breast size.

axial tomography conventional tomography since the plane of the image is parallel to the long axis of the body used interchangably with transaxial tomography.

axilla underarm area that contains lymph nodes and channels, blood vessels, muscles and fat.

B_0 B_0 is the scientific notation that is generally used to represent the main, or primary, magnetic field (that field within the magnet itself).

becquerel (Bq) measure of radioactive decay stated as the decay rate of 1 disintegration per second.

benign non-cancerous growth that does not spread to other parts of the body.

beta decay radioactive disintegration of a nucleus resulting in the emission of an electron (beta particle).

beta particle electron, either positive or negative. Positive beta particles are called positrons (B+). Negative beta particles are sometimes called negatrons (B-). The terms "beta particle" and the symbol "B" are reserved for electrons originating in a nucleus.

bi-plane two x-ray sources and receptor devices (film or image intensifier) positioned at right angles to each other. Usually the two systems can be energized simultaneously.

bile thick, viscous, dark green fluid that is secreted by the liver. Bile is an alkaline liquid that is composed of mainly water, bile salts, cholesterol, bilirubin, and mucin. Bile's primary function is to aid in digestion by emulsifyng dietary fat. This is essential for the absorption of fat and fat-soluble vitamins.

bilirubin bile pigment casued by the breakdown of blood products in the liver.

biophysical profile number of measurements and tests that provide the fetal age and condition.

biopsy surgical removal and microscopic examination of a piece of tissue to diagnose a problem.

bit smallest numeral in the binary scale of notation. This digit may be zero (0) or one (1). It may be equivalent to an on or off condition, a yes, or a no statement, or black and white depending on context.

bit depth term used to describe the number of quantization levels available at digitization. It is generally expressed in the unit bit. For example, where 8 bits is a depth of digitization 256 discrete levels are available to quantize the analog waveform.

bolus single concentration of material; in contrast injection a single injection of contrast media.

breech delivery the buttocks rather than fetal head are presented first for delivery through the birth canal.

bronchiectasis chronic dilatation of the bronchus or bronchi, with associated infection in the lower lobes of the lung.

bronchoscope endoscope which allows visual inspection of the trachea and bronchial tree.

bronchospasm narrowing of the bronchus due to the spasm of the smooth muscle.

byte group of binary characters operated on as a unit. A byte is a sequence of 8 adjacent bits. It is also used as the standard unit to describe memory storage capacity.

C-, U-arm mount term used to describe the shape of the mounting system in radiologic imaging. A C-arm has the x-ray tube and imaging device mounted on the end of the arc that forms the letter. These forms of mounts are capable of rotations in three planes allowing precise angles to be achieved for imaging procedures.

calcifications tiny white specks of calcium salt that can sometimes be seen on mammograms. In clusters they can be the only sign of ductal carcinoma in situ.

calculus from the latin for pebble, this can mean any pathologic concretion in the body. In the kidney, they are usually composed of cyrstalline urinary salts, held together by an organic compound.

cannula tub or sheath; in angiography, a blunt portion of the needle.

cardiac pacemakers cardiac pacemaker is used to regulate the heartbeat of patients, and is incompatible for MRI. Pacemaker patients are contraindicated for MRI.

cardiomyopathy general diagnostic term identifying primary disease pertaining to the muscle tissue of the heart.

carina ridge separating the two bronchi at the base of the trachea.

casting calcifications reliable sign for the presence of ductal carcinoma, representing the cast of a segment of the ductal lumen. Sometimes extends into the branches of the duct as well. These calcifications are always fragmented, irregular in contour, and their width is determined by the ductal lumen.

catheter tubular, flexible instrument passed through body channels for withdrawal or the introduction of fluids.

catheter sheath tubular case or envelope used to prevent the leakage of blood when catheters are exchanged or removed.

cathode ray tube (CRT) image display device used to record an event by exciting its phosphor.

cation ion carrying a positive charge.

cephalically toward the head.

chelate molecule combined with a metal.

chelation bonding of an ion and an organic molecule to create a complex molecule.

chemonuclolysis injection of chymopapain into the nucleus pulposus of the intervertebral disc in order to dissolve it.

chemotoxic function of a substance to affect the chemical balance of the body.

Chiba needle a fine needle with a stylet used to obtain samples during a biopsy.

cholangiocarcinoma primary biliary neoplasm affecting the biliary tree. Often associated with ulcerative colitis; 33% are associated with gallstones.

cholangitis inflammation of the biliary ducts. Symptoms include right upper quadrant pain, fever, chills, nausea, jaundice, and an elevated white blood count.

cholecystitis imflammation of the gallbladder and biliary system.

choledocholithiasis presence of gallstones within the bile ducts.

cholelithiasis formation or presence of gallstones within the gallbladder. The etiology of gallstones includes abnormal bile composition, stasis, and infection.

cirrhosis chronic disease of the liver that often causes a reduction in blood flow and increased blood pressure (portal hypertension).

clot accumulation of aggregates of blood also termed thrombus.

collateral circulation secondary circulation that often becomes established as a result of an accidental, pathologic, therapeutic, or surgical intervention.

collimator apparatus, often consisting of a pair of slits, used to confine radiation to a narrow beam.

colloid solution in which dissolved particles remain uniformly distributed.

colostomy the formation of a permanent colonic fistula.

compression compressed portion of a sound wave.

constant potential used in relation to radiologic high-tension generators to indicate the rectified high tension is ideally ripple free.

contiguous in contact; in CT, slices that are immediately adjacent.

contrast enhancement operation that seeks to increase or decrease contrast existing within an image to enable improved perception of a target object, feature, or region.

contrast manipulation process that changes the contrast range of an image.

contrast resolution term used to describe the contrast range of the image. For a digital image it can be expressed in the number of quantization levels (by the number of bits) available for assignment at digitization.

coronary bridging anatomic status of the overlaying of muscle tissue over a blood vessel surrounding the heart.

coupling device conventional radiologic imaging, it generally refers to the optical coupling system between the image intensifier and the photofluorographic and television camera. Complex coupling systems contain a semitransparent mirror that is able to rotate and direct the light image to several outputs (ports). Single port systems using only a television camera may use fiberoptics instead of optical lenses.

curie (Ci) measure of radioactive decay equaling 3.7×10^{10} disintegrations per second.

cyclotron device used to produce neutron-poor radionuclides; apparatus that accelerates atomic particles, allowing for the production of certain radionuclides.

cyst sac or capsule containing a liquid or semisolid material; usually harmless and can be removed by aspiration.

cytology study of cells for the presence of cancer.

cytosarcoma unusually large fibroadenoma-like lesion of the Phyllodes mammary gland with a cellular, sarcoma-like stroma. There are benign and malignant types.

DAC (digital to analog conversion) device that serves to convert each digital quantity at each sample point into an equivalent analog level such as a voltage. Such a conversion allows display of a digital image on a video display unit.

DAT tape permanent storage mechanism for digital information.

data collection of quantities or representations used as an information resource for a particular application.

daughter decay product produced by a radioactive nuclide. When the parent nuclide undergoes decay, a daughter nuclide is produced.

decay radioactive disintegration of a nucleus.

deep vein thrombosis (DVT) collection of blood clots in the deep vein system of the legs.

detector single receptor device used to measure the intensity of the X- radiation passing through the patient.

detector array entire assembly of detectors.

diagnostic procedure any procedure that is performed to identify or recognize a disease.

DICOM (digital image and communication in medicine) DICOM 3.0 is the successor of ACR-NEMA 2.0 standard for the transfer and exchange of digital images and associated data in medicine.

digital representation of data or physical quantities in the form of discrete measurements, rather than in a continuous stream.

digital computer electronic device that processes information represented by sequences and combinations of discrete signals. Specifically it is a specialized collection of electronic circuits (hardware) that performs logic and arithmetic functions under the direction of a program (software) to obtain specific outcomes.

digital image image composed of discrete sample points. In medical imaging applications each sample point correlates typically to a fixed volume (voxel) or area within the object being imaged, which then is translated to discrete picture elements (pixels or pels) to form the image on the display monitor.

digitization general term used to describe the process used to obtain a digital representation of the magnitude of a physical quantity from an analog representation of that magnitude. Is also known as A/D conversion.

dilatation and curettage surgical procedure where expansion of the cervix allows for the scraping of the uterine wall.

dissection surgical division or separation of tissues. In treating breast cancer, this usually refers to removal of the axillary lymph nodes and lymph vessels.

doppler recording of the velocity of blood flow.

dose calibrator specially designed gas-filled ionization chamber used to measure the amount of radioactivity in a sample such as a syringe, vial, or test tube.

double contrast use of a combination of positive and negative contrast agents.

duct channel for transporting milk from the lobules out to the nipple.

ductal carcinoma form of breast carcinoma confined to the breast in situ (DCIS) ducts, which often reveals itself as microcalcification on mammography. Noninvasive duct carcinoma.

duct ectasia benign breast change in which large or small ducts in the breast become dilated and retain secretions, often leading to nipple discharge, and sometimes a lump in the nipple/areolar areas or nipple retraction. This change is not associated with increased risk of breast cancer.

ductography injection of an opaque contrast medium into the lactiferous ducts and subsequent imaging of the structures.

dynamic image nuclear medicine image representing the distribution of a radiopharmaceutical over a specific time period. Also called a "flow study" which refers to the blood flow being imaged in a particular area. This is a sequential or time-lapse sequence in which images are collected every few seconds for a preset time.

dysphagia diffiuculty in swallowing.

dysplasia abnormality of development. Alteration of size, shape and organization of mature cells.

echo time (TE) time from the first RF pulse to the echo. This parameter is set in MR to control the T2 effect on image contrast.

ectopic pregnancy implantation of the embryo outside the uterine cavity, usually in the fallopian tubes.

edema presence of abnormally large amounts of fluids in the intercellular tissue spaces of the body.

edematous swelling caused by abnormal collection of fluid in the tissues.

edge enhancement spatial imaging operation that generally accentuates edge details within an image by increasing the relative contrast of the boundary.

effusion fluid in the pleural cavity.

ejection fraction assessment of cardiac output that determines the percentage of blood flow that passes through the ventricles of the heart.

EKG electrocardiograph.

electrolytes chemical substances which dissolve into charged particles when mixed with water and which are associated with vital metabolic activities in the body.

electromagnet magnet generally made up of turns of wire, through which current is passed. In an electromagnet, the magnetic field is generated by the current passing through the wires.

electron elementary particle of nature having a charge of 1 and a mass of 9.1×10^{-28} grams.

embolization obstruction of a blood vessel by means of an introduced, artificial substance.

embolus collection of obstructive material in a blood vessel, caused by natural products within the body or by artificial means.

emphysema distention of the lung tissues often with associated destruction of bronchiole tissue.

empyema pus within the lumen of the gallbladder. The microorganisms involved are the enteric bacteria and staph cocci. Symptoms include right upper quadrant pain, fever, jaundice, and an elevated white blood cell count.

encapsulated enclosed in a capsule or sheath. Breast implants may become encapsulated in fibrotic tissue.

endometrium lining of the uterus, composed of mucus membrane tissue.

endorectal scanning the prostate and seminal vesicles by inserting the transducer into the rectum.

endoscopy visual inspection of a body cavity using a fiber optic instrument (endoscope).

endovaginal scanning the uterus and adnexa by inserting a transducer into the vagina.

engaged in obsteric terms, point where the fetal head moves into the pelvic inlet, during delivery.

enhancement any digital imaging process that seeks to selectively increase the perception of a select parameter of an image.

enteral within the intestine.

ependynoma tumor arising from an inclusion of fetal tissue.

epistaxis bleeding from the nose.

epithelium cellular covering of skin and mucous membrane. Milk ducts are lined with epithelium. It consists of cells joined by "cementing" substances.

esophageal varices twisted, enlarged veins found around the base of the esophagus and often caused by portal hypertension.

estrogen female hormone, produced by the ovaries and adrenal glands.

excitation in MRI, excitation comes as the result of adding RF energy to a spin system in thermal equilibrium.

excitation pulse short intense burst of RF energy used to transfer the magnetization from a position along the longitudinal (Z) axis to a position in the transverse (XY) plane.

extrahepatic outside the liver capsule.

extravasation discharge or escape. In this context the escape of contrast from a vessel or organ; abnormal flow of fluid into tissue; in the case of an IV injection, an escape of blood or injected material into the tissues surrounding the vein.

extrinsic of exterior origin.

fat necrosis a benign breast change in which the breast responds to trauma of the fatty tissue of the breast (including surgical biopsy sometimes) with a firm, irregular mass, often years after the event.

feature prominent or conspicuous part, object, or characteristic within an image that can be individually identified as having properties related to pattern recognition, texture, size, shape, gray scale.

fenestrated a surgical drape with a round or slit like opening in the center.

fibroadenolipoma a benign tumor made up of fatty and glandular tissue.

fibroadenoma a benign breast condition common in young adult women in which the breast develops a solid lump, either firm or soft, but usually moveable. The lump is named according to the amount of glandular (adeno-) and fibrous (fibro-) tissue present.

fibrocystic changes a term used to describe changes in the fibrous tissue in the breast with the formation of cysts or more broadly, for any benign breast change. Common symptoms are general lumpiness in the breasts, cystic lumps, and cyclic tenderness. This condition does not indicate increased risk of breast cancer.

fibroma tumor composed mainly of fibrous tissue.

fibrosis the formation of fibrous tissue.

film badge piece of photographic film contained in a light proof holder and worn by an individual to measure the amount of radiation to which he or she is exposed.

filter in spatial domain local image operations refers to the small matrix of. This matrix, which contains weighting factors, is used in local operations to determine the new output value in the enhanced image. Filters are used to produce spatial enhancements like edge sharpening.

fine needle aspiration biopsy (FNAB) diagnostic technique utilised to diagnose "lumps". Cells from the lumps are aspirated and smeared on a glass slide. The slides are stained and a pathologist reviews them to make a diagnosis.

flocculation dispersal of material into discrete particles.

foramen ovale septal opening in the fetal heart, which normally closes after birth; failing to close after birth is referred to as a patent (open) foramen ovale.

fourier domain also known as frequency domain or Fourier or frequency space. A region where quantities are expressed in terms of their component complex frequencies.

Fowler's position semierect position, with the head raised and the body at 45° to the vertical.

free induction decay (FID) signal voltage induced within the receiver coil after the RF pulse.

french system used to describe the outer diameter of a catheter. It is usually written as [F]. Each unit is approximately 0.33 mm and therefore 6F would be approximately 1.9 mm in diameter.

frequency of precession rate at which protons wobble in a magnetic field.

galactocele cystic enlargement containing milk, usually occurring during nursing or weaning.

galactography injection of a milk duct with contrast medium, to delineate the size, type, and extent of a pathologic lesion causing nipple discharge.

gamma rays electromagnetic radiation having its origin in an atomic nucleus.

gantry houses the x-ray tube and detectors.

gas detector device using a gas plus a high-voltage power supply for detection of radiation.

gating attachment and synchronizing of two pieces of measuring equipment.

gauss (g) measure of magnetic field strength whereby 10,000 g = 1 tesla.

Geiger-Mueller Survey Meter small ionization chamber operated by gas amplification and used to detect small quantities of radioactivity.

generations term used to differentiate the various tube detector geometric designs.

gestation time between conception and birth, in humans the average time being 40 weeks.

global operator in spatial domain processing, where all the values of a pixel in the input digital image are treated as a single set and the new output image calculated by a global mathematical manipulation. An example of a global operation is rotation or size reduction.

glottis vocal apparatus of the larynx.

granular calcifications. Ductal calcifications resembling granulated sugar are often a sign of malignancy. They are characteristically localized in a small cluster.

granulocytes white blood cells that contain large granules in their cytoplasm.

gravid pregnant.

gray scale the luminance's/brightness available as valid gray levels for pixels in an image processing system. A gray scale is used to map the individual quantization levels of an image into a visible form. An 8 bit gray scale can display accurately 256 levels.

guidewires generally made of stainless steel used to give support to a catheter and prevent injury to the vessel wall during catheter placement.

gynaecomastia excessive development of the male mammary glands, even to the functional state.

gynecological study of diseases pertaining to women.

gyromagnetic ratio (g) measure of the spin angular momentum and the magnetic moment. This factor is constant for each atom. For example, the gyromagnetic ratio for hydrogen is approximately 42.6 MHz/T.

half-life time required for one-half of a given number of radioactive atoms to undergo decay; symbol $T^1/_2$.

hamartoma mass containing multiple areas of fatty and fibroglandular densities surrounded by a fibrotic pseudocapsule.

heimlich mechanism whereby increased pressure forces movement of an obstruction.

helix coil or spiral.

hemangioma benign tumor of blood vessels.

hematoma localized mass of extravasated blood in the tissues. May occur in the breast after trauma or surgery; collection of blood in tissue; a bruise.

hematuria blood in the urine.

hemiplagia one-sided paralysis.

hemodynamic monitoring continuous monitoring of the blood pressures and flow in veins, arteries, and chambers of the heart. Common measurements include intra-arterial blood pressure, pulmonary artery pressure, left atrial pressure, and central venous pressure.

hemoptysis coughing of blood from the respiratory system.

hemostasis stoppage of blood by clot formation or vessel spasm. Artificial blood flow stoppage can be produced by providing pressure or ligation (suturing).

hemothorax blood in the pleural cavity; can be caused by trauma or by repeated puncture of a biopsy needle.

hertz unit for frequency; cycles per second.

heterogeneous composed of many different elements. Many different types of breast cancer cells within one tumor.

high energy state spins in the magnetic field whose magnetic moments oppose the magnetic field are in the high energy state.

hilar region the root of the lungs at the level of the 5th and 6th thoracic vertebrae.

Hodgkin's disease malignant tumor of the lymph system, usually beginning in the lymph nodes. Considered curable in 70% of cases.

homogeneous having a similarity of structure, uniform tissue throughout a structure.

Hounsdfield number numeric applied to each pixel of information of a CT scan, related to the degree of density demonstrated. Water is considered zero.

Houndsfield unit (CT number) generally accepted unit for attenuation values within the pixels.

hydration addition of water to the body. In angiographic care, the patient is encouraged to hydrate, that is, drink additional water after the examination.

hydronephrosis distention of the pelvis and calices of a kidney with urine, due to ureteric obstruction.

hyperplasia abnormal but benign increase in number of normally arranged cells.

hypertrophy morbid enlargement of an organ or part, due to increase in size of the constituent cells.

hypotonic possessing less than the normal muscular tone or tension in response to stimuli.

image acquisition general term relating to the method in which the imaging energy is produced, controlled, applied to the patient, and detected in an imaging mode. All image acquisition processes involve analog transitions.

imaging mode (modality) generic term in medical imaging to refer to differing forms of medical image acquisition, such as x-ray imaging, ultrasound imaging, nuclear imaging, magnetic resonance imaging.

imaging planes views that are used to acquire an MRI. Imaging planes are sagittal, axial, coronal, and oblique.

immunocompromised having an immune system incapable of reacting to pathogens or tissue damage.

implants metallic devices that are placed in the body during surgery. Some metallic implants are adversely effected by the magnetic field and are contraindicated for MRI.

infarct tissue necrosis or death caused by an interruption of the blood supply to that area.

infarction a localized area of necrosis caused usually by an interruption of blood supply.

infiltrating carcinoma a cancer that can grow beyond its original origin into neighboring tissues. Infiltrating does not imply that the cancer has spread beyond the breast. It has the same meaning as invasive.

inflammation condition into which tissues enter as a reaction to various conditions, resulting in pain, heat or redness.

in situ confined to site of origin, not having invaded adjoining tissue or metastasized to other parts of the body.

inspissated being thickened, dried or rendered less fluid. Usually refers to the hardened secretions that form intraductal calcifications.

interventional radiologic examinations that can be extended to provide remedied measures.

intrauterine device (IUD) mechanical method of contraception which when placed in the uterus causes the uterus to reject an ovum.

intrahepatic within the liver capsule.

intra-arterial within an artery.

intracardiac within the heart.

intracranial vascular clips metallic clips that are placed in the brain during surgery to repair aneurysms. Some vascular clips are adversely effected by the magnetic field and are contraindicated for MRI.

intradermal calcifications calcifications that are tiny, rounded homogenous, or ring-shaped in their appearance. They are radiolucent in density and usually the same size as skin pores. These calcifications are usually benign.

intraocular foreign bodies metallic objects located within the eye. Metallic objects in the eye are adversely effected by the magnetic field and are contraindicated for MRI.

intrathecal within the spinal canal.

intubation insertion of a tube.

in vitro within a glass; observable in a test tube; or in an artificial environment. This term is used to describe the nonimaging laboratory studies performed in nuclear medicine.

in vivo within the living body. The term is used to describe many of the routine nuclear medicine imaging studies.

involution regressive change in vital processes or in an organ after fulfilling its function. In the breast this occurs over a long period of time, beginning as early as the third or fourth decade of life.

iohexol type of contrast media that is less neurotoxic because of its non-ionic nature. Also Iopanodol and Iotrolan.

ischemia decreased blood supply to an area marked by pain or organ dysfunction; usually due to partially blocked circulation.

isotope one of a group of nuclides of the same element (same Z) having the same number of protons in the nucleus but differing in number of neutrons, resulting in different values of A.

jaundice yellowish discoloration of tissues and bodily fluids with bile pigment caused by any of several pathological conditions in which the normal processing of bile is interrupted.

klatskin tumor neoplasm of the bile ducts at the level of the right and left hepatic duct bifurcation.

krypton gas used to demonstrate the functioning of the lungs in radionuclide imaging.

lactation secretion of milk.

lactiferous producing or conveying milk.

larmor equation $w_0 = b_0 g$ equation used to calculate the processional frequency (w_0) by multiplying the magnetic field strength (b_0) with the gyromagnetic ratio (g).

left heart refers to procedures involving placement of a catheter in the left side chambers of the heart and coronary arteries for the purpose of pressure measurement and contrast injection.

lesion general term for a change in tissue structure or function due to injury or other processes. Most lesions in the breast are benign.

leukocytes white blood cells.

ligand molecule that binds to another molecule; this term is used especially to refer to a small molecule that binds specifically to a larger molecule (e.g., an antigen binding to an antibody, a hormone binding to a receptor).

lipofibroadenoma mass containing multiple areas of fatty and fibroglandular densities surrounded by a fibrotic pseudocapsule.

lipofibroma fibroma (benign) containing fatty elements.

lipoma benign tumor made up of fat cells.

lithotomy position patient position commonly used for some urinary procedures. The patient lies supine, legs raised, flexed, and open and supported on stirrups.

lithotripsy the disintegration of renal calculi using high frequency shock waves.

liver function tests tests performed that help correlate clinical history and presenting symptoms with radiographic evaluation. These routinely include alanine aminotransferase(ALT), asparate aminotransferase(AST), bilirubib, lactic dehydrogenase(LDH), alkaline phosphatase(ALP), Y-glutamyl transpeptidase(GGT), albumin and prothrombin time(PT).

lobar disease disease found in a lobe of the lung.

lobe portion of the breast that contains a complete unit for producing, transporting and delivering milk.

lobular carcinoma in situ form of breast carcinoma in-situ characterized by multiple areas of highly atypical cells, often in both breasts. Occurs in the terminal ducts of the breast lobules. It is considered a marker for increased future risk of development of breast cancer.

lobule branching ducts terminate in lobules, the functional unit of the breast.

local operator in spatial domain processing, where the value of a new pixel in the processed digital image is calculated by the weighted magnitudes of a local group of pixels in the original digital image. Edge sharpening and smoothing are local operations.

localizer first image or series of images acquired during the MRI examination. This is generally a relatively fast, T1-weighted image acquired in the plane that best demonstrates the anatomy.

logarithmic conversion mathematical conversion of data using a logarithmic expression. Such conversions compress large differences between data values seen in linear systems into a smaller scale for improved data manipulation and final image production.

long film cassette changer an angiographic serial changer with oversized cassettes designed to visualize the entire limb on one film.

longitudinal relaxation time constant by which spins recover along the Z (longitudinal) axis, also known as T1 recovery or spin-lattice.

Look Up Table (LUT) system where a mathematical conversion factor between two data sets is precalculated and stored as a conversion table.

low energy state in MRI, this term refers to spins that “align” or point in the direction of the static magnetic field.

lumen opening through the length of a tube-like structure, such as a needle, vessel, or catheter.

lumpectomy surgical procedure in which a cancerous tumor or “lesion” or “lump” is removed, leaving intact most of the remaining breast tissue.

lymph nodes bean-shaped structures scattered along vessels of the lymphatic system. The nodes act as filters, collecting bacteria or cancer cells that may travel through the lymph system.

lymphedema abnormal swelling due to an obstruction in the lymph system.

lymphoma tumor of lymphoid tissue; general term applied to any neoplastic disorder of the lymphoid tissue.

macroangiography use of magnification radiographic technique to produce an enlarged image of a vessel or area.

macrocyst cyst large enough to feel with the fingers.

magnetic field gradient magnetic field that is high in one location and low in another that is superimposed over the main magnetic field.

magnetic moment small magnetic field associated with the spinning charged proton.

magnetic susceptibility ability for something to be magnetized.

magnetic tape permanent storage mechanism for digital information.

mammary dysplasia literally, poorly structured tissue in the breast.

mammoplasty plastic reconstruction of the breast(s).

manometer apparatus used to measure pressure, such as spinal fluid.

mask in subtraction of an image, a reverse tone image of the area required, without contrast.

mastalgia pain in the breast.

mastectomy surgical removal of all the breast and sometimes adjoining structures, usually done for breast cancer.

mastitis inflammation of the mammary gland.

matrix display collection of rows and columns of pixels displayed across the image.

mediastinum the organs which separate the two lungs; namely, the heart, great vessels and esophagus, lymph vessels, connective tissue.

medullary carcinoma circumscribed carcinoma named because of its fleshy appearance. The consistency is soft and it can attain a relatively large size.

megahertz (mhz) measurement of radiofrequency whereby 1 hertz is 1 cycle per second and 1 megahertz is one million cycles per second.

meningoceles protrusion of the meninges into the spial column; it is of congenital origin.

menisectomy operation to remove a meniscus of the knee.

metastases (in bone) secondary malignant neoplasms transferred from other primary sites, usually breast, bronchus or prostate.

metastasis the spread of cancer from the primary tumor to another part of the body.

microcalcifications tiny white specks of calcium salts that can sometimes be seen on the mammogram. In clusters, they can be the only sign of ductal carcinoma in situ or early invasive cancer; they can be associated with benign breast changes.

microcurie (uCi) one millionth of a curie.

microcyst a cyst too small to feel with the fingers.

millicurie (mCi) one thousandth of a curie.

modified radical mastectomy surgical procedure in which the breast and the lymph nodes are removed, while underlying chest muscles are largely left intact.

montgomery's tubercles visible pores or tiny lumps on the areola. Openings for the oil glands that lubricate the nipple and areola during breast feeding.

morbidity condition of being diseased.

morphology structure and form in anatomy, not function.

mortality frequency of death; death rate.

myoblastoma rare benign tumor of striated muscle made up of groups of cells that resemble primitive myoblasts. Otherwise known as granular cell tumor.

necrosis pathologic death of one or more cells, or of a portion of tissue or organ, resulting from irreversible damage.

necrosis death of tissue; dead tissue, sometimes found in the center of a lesion and often caused by insufficient blood supply.

neoplasm new or abnormal growth, such as a tumor.

nephrostomy surgical incision into the pelvis of a kidney.

nephrotoxic function of a substance to damage kidney tissue.

net magnetization vector sum of the magnetic moments of the leftover spins in line with the magnetic field expressed as a vector quantity.

net magnetization sum of the magnetic moments of the leftover spins in line with the magnetic field.

network computer network refers to an established group of linked computers capable of data exchange and communication via common protocols.

neurolept sedation a state of quiescence. Altered awareness or sedation caused by the use of a neuropharmacologic agent.

neurotoxic substance having a poisoning effect upon the nervous system.

neutron neutral elementary particle having a mass number of 1. In the free state (outside the nucleus), it is unstable, having a half-life of about 12 minutes. It decays by the process n = p + e + v.

nevus circumscribed new growth of skin of congenital origin. Commonly called a mole.

nipple discharge secretion of fluid that comes out of the nipple, either spontaneously or elicited when the nipple area is squeezed. It often results from benign breast changes or minor hormonal irregularities. A history of spontaneous discharge is more worrisome than an expressible discharge, which is often normal.

nodularity general "lumpiness" or normal textured tissue consistency, often bilateral.

nodule discrete lump, as opposed to normal nodularity.

noise products undesired variations in the magnitude of an imaging signal which are unrelated to the information contained within that signal.

non-proliferative benign breast changes in which there is no cell multiplication beyond the limits of normal. These changes, such as fibroadenomas and cysts, are not associated with increased risk of breast cancer.

notochord embryonic axial skeleton.

nuclear magnetic resonance (NMR) study of the reactions of nuclei in a magnetic field with RF interaction (now referred to as MRI).

nuclear reactor device for supporting a self-sustained nuclear chain reaction under controlled conditions.

nuclei center of the atom is a nucleus; nuclei is the plural.

nucleus positively charged core of an atom in which almost all the mass of the atom is concentrated.

nuclide any one of the more than 1000 species of atoms characterized by the number of protons and number of neutrons in the nucleus.

nyquist limit refers to the spatial frequency at which a digital image will contain no useful information. Practically it refers to the smallest features that can be accurately imaged.

obstetrics management of women during pregnancy.

obstruction blockage of a duct or passage.

occlusion obstruction or a clotting off.

oncology study of malignant tumors.

optical disk permanent storage mechanism for digital information.

orifice entrance to any bodily cavity.

osmolaric pertaining to the osmotic characteristic of a solution.

osmolarity concentration of a solution.

osteoblast germ cell that assists in the formation of bone.

osteophytes abnormal bony outgrowth.

ostium refers to an opening into or a mouth of a tubular organ or cavity. In angiography, the origin or opening of the coronary artery.

paget's disease inflammatory cancerous process affecting the areola and nipple, usually associated with an underlying ductal carcinoma.

pan to move the radiographic table during angiography.

pantomograph single radiographic examination of the teeth, jaw and temporomandibular joints by using a moving source and an equal and opposite movement of the film.

papilledema swelling of the optic nerve, often caused by a brain tumor.

papilloma small, cauliflower-like growth inside a mammary duct usually near the nipple, which can produce a clear or bloody discharge from the nipple.

papillomatosis development of a group of papillomas.

paramagnetic agent contrast medium used in MRI which affects the speed of the relaxation time.

parenchyma supporting elements of an organ.

patent open, accessible.

PCWP pulmonary-capillary wedge pressure.

percutaneous performed through the skin.

peritonitis inflammation of the peritoneum.

permanent magnet magnet made up of ferrous materials that have been exposed to a magnetic field and have retained magnetization.

phase coherence spins that precess together maintain phase coherence. When they no longer precess together they become out of phase.

photocathode photosensitive layer (cathode) of a photomultiplier tube.

photomultiplier tube (PMT) phototube of exceptionally high sensitivity; the electron or electrons released at the photocathode initiate a cascade from one dynode to another with resultant electron amplification as high as 10 times.

phyllodes term applied to tumors that on section show a lobulated, leaf-like, cauliflower appearance.

piezoelectric effect ability of a structure to change one form of energy into another.

pitch combination of table speed, slice thickness and tube rotation.

pixel (PEL) abbreviation for picture element. The smallest discrete representation of a digital image on the display screen. An alternative term is pel.

pixel size field of view divided by matrix size.

pneumobilia air within the biliary tree. It is often a complication of sphincterectomy of the hepatopancreatic ampulla.

pneumoperitonenum air in the abdominal cavity.

pneumothorax air in the pleural cavity usually caused by a perforation of the pleura. This can be as a result of trauma, rupture of an abscess or repeated puncture by biopsy needle. It is often associated with a collapsed lung.

point operator in spatial domain processing, where the value of a pixel in the processed digital image is directly calculated from the corresponding pixel in the original image.

polymastia a condition in which more than two breasts are present.

portosystemic joining of the portal and systemic venous system, usually by some type of intervention.

positron positive electron.

positron emission tomography (PET) scanning method used to determine physiological information of the brain, utilizing the administration of positron-emitting radionuclides.

postprocessing image processing routines applied to data after information is processed by the computer. Postprocessing routines allow the operator to manipulate the image data for analysis. Contrast and spatial manipulations are possible.

precess when the net magnetization is precessing, it is wobbling in the transverse plane, after RF interaction.

preprocessing image processing routines applied to data before they are processed by the computer. Preprocessing routines are applied to correct flaws in the image data that have occurred as a result of the analog processes in image acquisition or nonlinearity of the transducer or an excessive magnitude of results. These routines in many modes cannot be altered by the operator.

progesterone female hormone, produced by the ovary's corpus luteum, only during a specific time of a woman's menstrual cycle. This antiestrogenic hormone is needed for the egg to mature and prepare the uterus for a possible pregnancy. Menstruation occurs after the secretion of progesterone stops.

prolactin female hormone that stimulates the development of the breast and later is essential for starting and continuing milk production.

prophylactic therapy preventive therapy.

prosthesis artificial substitute for a missing body part.

prothrombin coagulating agent found in the blood that interacts with calcium salts to produce thrombin. The amount of prothrombin found in the blood will determine whether a patient is likely to experience clotting problems.

protocol recipe of parameters that are used to complete the MRI examination; an operating convention that exists to ensure that data are communicated correctly and error free between computers in a network.

proton density number of leftover spins in the low-energy state during thermal equilibrium. Also known as the spin excess.

proton positively charged elementary particle having a mass number of 1; the nucleus of a hydrogen atom of mass 1.

pulse height analysis electronic circuitry used to select some pulses and reject others that are not within a desired preset range.

purulent containing pus.

quantization process in which discrete image samples (produced from scanning and sensing in a digitization process) are awarded a discrete level from a discrete range of values (Quantization range) according to their relative analog value.

quantization error potential and actual error that occurs in digitization when at quantization a discrete level must be awarded to a continuously variable function. To diminish these errors a large quantization range must be used. Theoretically an infinite quantization range would produce zero error.

quantization range range of values possible to be assigned to the analog data in the A/D conversion process. Typically it is expressed in terms of bits. Typical ranges are 10 bit (1024 levels) to 12 bit (4096 levels) in medical imaging applications.

radioactive giving off radiant energy in the form of alpha, beta, or gamma rays by the breaking up of atoms.

radioimmunoassay (RIA) highly sensitive and specific assay method that uses the competition between radiolabeled and unlabeled substances in an antigen-antibody reaction to determine the concentration of the unlabeled substance.

radioisotope any isotope that is unstable, thus undergoing decay with emission of a characteristic radiation. Synonym for radioactive isotope.

radiolucent transparent to the x-ray.

radionuclide generator method of producing radioactivity in a nuclear medicine department.

radionuclide chemical compound that disintegrates causing the emission of electromagnetic radiation and/or particulate radiation.

radiopaque opaque to the x-ray.

radiopharmaceutical radioactive substance used especially for diagnostic purposes or treatment of disease.

radiowaves electromagnetic energy that is used to excite proton spins.

RAM (Random Access Memory) refers to computer memory that allows direct and fast access to all its memory locations and stores and retrieves data in relation to its location only. When such memory is switched off it retains no information.

rarefaction relaxed portion of a sound wave.

real time image that can be visualized as it is being produced.

rectilinear scanner device that generates an image of an organ by detecting radioactivity within that organ and recording it on film.

renin enzyme produced in the kidney. Elevated levels can indicate renal hypertension.

repetition time (TR) time from the first RF pulse to the next. This parameter is set in MRI to control the T1 effect on image contrast.

resolution relates to range of accurate measurements made by a measuring instrument. Is generally characterized by a statement of this range or by the magnitude of the smallest measurement possible.

resonance when the RF pulse is applied at the appropriate frequency, spins precess in the transverse plane, at this time resonance has been achieved.

retraction (skin) a visual change in either breast contour or the nipple, often caused by an alteration in the tension of a Cooper's ligament on the skin or nipple. The skin develops a dip, dimple, or hollow.

retrograde going backwards as, for example, the contrast agent introduced in the opposite direction to the normal flow of urine; moving against the normal flow or, in angiography, blood flow toward the origin of the vessel.

rf coil hardware designed to either transmit or receive the MRI signal.

rf pulse short intense blast of energy used to excite proton spins.

right heart referring to procedures involving placement of a catheter in the right side chambers of the heart, usually for pressure measurement.

sampling part of the digitization process. Is the process that divides the analog waveform into small samples generally in relation to time.

sanguineous abounding in blood.

sarcoma tumor made of closely packed stromal or mesenchymal cells as opposed to epithelial cells; usually highly malignant.

scanogram single AP film taken by the CT Scanner to determine anatomical levels before CT scans are calculated; localizing image obtained by the continuos movement of the patient through the gantry with no tube rotation.

scintillation flash of light produced in a phosphor by radiation.

scintillation camera imaging device using all of the components of a scintillation counter.

scintillation counter counter using a phosphor, photomultiplier tube, and associated circuits for the detection of radiation.

scirrhous a hard cancer with marked predominance of connective tissue.

sclerosing adenosis a common form of adenosis which occurs in two phases

1. A solid, benign breast lump develops.
2. Sclerosis (hardening) replaces the cells of the breast lump.

If the areas of sclerosis calcify, they may be seen on the mammogram and can sometimes appear similar to the microcalcifications found with malignancy.

sclerosis a hardening of tissues from a variety of sources.

scout another term for a scanogram.

sebaceous secretions of an oily, cheesy material by the skin glands.

sector field of view pie-shaped image.

segmental disease disease found in a segment of the lung.

Seldinger technique percutaneous method of introducing a catheter into a vessel or organ by first inserting a needle, followed by a guidewire through the needle. The needle is then removed. A catheter is threaded over the guidewire. Finally the guidewire is removed leaving the catheter in place.

sepsis generalized poisoning by microorganisms of tissues or blood, often termed blood poisoning.

Single Photon Emission Computed Tomography (SPECT) imaging technique in which the gamma camera rotates around the patient to collect and reconstruct data in various planes including transaxial, sagittal, and coronal orientations.

sinus cavity or hollow space.

slice thickness depth of the voxel.

slip ring technology arrangement of cables within the gantry as to allow continuous circular rotation of the tube and detectors in the same direction.

sludge composed mainly of calcium bilirubinate, cholesterol, and pigment crystals. Often seen as an indicator of abnormal biliary dynamics.

spatial resolution relates to the size of the smallest spatial feature imaged. In a digital image it is critically influenced by the sampling process at digitization, which ultimately determines the number of pixels that can be displayed to form the image.

spin echo signal produced as the result of two RF pulses.

spin excess number of leftover spins in the low energy state during thermal equilibrium. Also known as the proton density.

spin states possible locations for proton spins, for hydrogen there are two spin states allowed including high- and low-energy states.

spin-lattice time constant by which spins recover along the Z (longitudinal) axis, also known as T1 recovery or longitudinal recovery.

spondylolithesis the forward slipping of one vertebral body on top of the other. Usually occurs at L5/S1.

staging process used to classify tumors so that management of them can be organized.

static image single stationary nuclear medicine image of a particular structure.

stellate star-shaped, referring to an unusual arrangement of breast fibers sometimes seen on mammography, suspicious of breast cancer, although it occurs with benign conditions also.

stenosis narrowing or constriction of a passage or opening.

stent device or mold to provide support to a graft or tubular structure that has been anastamosed. Can also be used to maintain patency of a stricture.

stepping table an angiographic table used for lower limb arteriography. It moves as films are taken over the entire length of the legs.

stilette solid, sharp-pointed part of a needle used in the introduction of a catheter into the body. It sits within the cannula, is also spelled stylet, and is sometimes called a trocar.

stoma small opening; the opening established in the abdominal wall by a colostomy.

streptokinase enzyme used in therapeutic interventions to reduce thrombi.

stricture abnormal narrowing of a duct or passage.

stroma tissue forming the ground substance, frame-work, or matrix of an organ.

subarachnoid hemorrhage escape of blood into the space between the arachnoid and pia mater of the brain.

subphrenic abscess collection of pus beneath the diaphragm.

subareolar beneath the nipple-areolar complex.

subcutaneous situated or occurring immediately beneath the skin.

subcutaneous mastectomy surgical removal of most of the breast tissue that usually is replaced with an implant. This procedure is sometimes done for a woman at high risk of developing breast cancer as a prophylactic (preventive) measure.

superselection catheterization of a vessel from another vessel that has already been selected. It often involves the changing of the angiographic catheters.

Swan-Ganz pulmonary catheter that permits measurement of pulmonary artery diastolic and systolic pressures, pulmonary-capillary wedge pressure (PCWP), left atrial filling pressure, central venous pressure, and cardiac output.

synovitis inflammation of the synovial membrane.

syringe shield a device used to house syringes containing radioactive material. These shields are made of lead and include leaded glass, with the primary purpose of decreasing radiation exposure from the radioactive material within the syringe.

system clock term used in computing to describe the rate of control pulses generated within a particular computer to coordinate the flow of internal digital data and associated processing routines. Measured in the unit Hertz, the higher this specification the faster the system will process information (>100 MHz is now typical).

T1 relaxation time constant by which spins recover along the Z (longitudinal) axis, also known as spin-lattice or longitudinal recovery.

T2 decay time constant by which spins lose transverse magnetization, also known as transverse decay or spin-spin relaxation.

tamponade (cardiac) pathological compression of the heart due to the collection of blood or fluid in the pericardium.

tangential position assumed to demonstrate the periphery of a curve. In radiography, the degree of head movement needed to demonstrate a curved structure in profile.

"tea-cup" calcifications lobular type calcification that is usually associated with an extensive fibrosis throughout the breast. There may be stagnation of fluid in the cystically dilated lobules, which contains many calcium particles (milk of calcium). In larger cystic dilatations, milk of calcium settles to the dependent portion of the cavity, giving rise to the so called "tea-cup" calcification. Lobular type calcifications can be distributed throughout the breast and are often bilateral.

technetium synthetic element, an isotope of technetium is used in many radionuclide studies.

tesla (T) measure of magnetic field strength whereby 10,000 gauss = 1 tesla.

thermal equilibrium point at which there is no thermal exchange between proton spins that have either aligned or opposed the magnetic field.

thermoluminescent dosimetry (TLD) method of measuring radiation exposure.

thoracotomy resection of the chest wall in order to allow drainage of the chest cavity.

three-phase an efficient method of supplying electric operating voltage at high current to a radiologic generator. Consists of three alternating currents carried on a three- or four-wire system, with a phase relationship of 120¡ in relation to each other.

thrombophlebitis inflammation in the venous system caused by the presence of a thrombus.

thrombus a blood clot that causes an obstruction to a blood vessel.

through transmission increase in brightness (reflection amplitude) of reflections that lie behind a weakly attenuating structure.

torque force producing a rotary motion; pulling force exerted on metallic objects in a magnetic field.

tortuosity object or part, such as a blood vessel, that turns and twists.

tortuous having many twists and turns.

tourniquet instrument that exerts pressure on and constricts blood vessels; usually a stretchable band.

transaxial tomography image is perpendicular to the long axis of the body.

transducer any device that converts one energy form to another. Most medical imaging transducers are analog devices (such as CT detectors, film/screens, gamma camera scintillation crystals, radiofrequency coils, ultrasound peizo electric crystals etc.).

transient ischemic attacks (TIA) intermittent blood flow, interrupting the blood supply to the brain.

translate to move the aligned x-ray tube and detectors in a linear fashion across the area to be scanned.

transluminal through the lumen of a vessel.

trimester 3-month period. Pregnancies are divided into three trimesters.

trocar sharp-pointed instrument used with a cannula for tapping.

tumor abnormal growth of tissue.

vaginal speculum instrument that opens the vaginal canal and allows for the examination of the uterus.

valgus bending outward.

Valsalva's maneuver during exhalation the mouth remains closed, trapping air in the respiratory and nasal passages. It is used in radiography to provide a negative contrast image, using air as the medium. This maneuver compresses the vena cava by constricting of the diaphragm, which in turn tends to keep blood (and contrast) longer in the lower body and limbs.

valvular regurgitation retrograde flow of blood through a valve in the heart.

varicose ulcer ulcer that forms on the skin; usually the leg, as a result of the presence of a varicose vein.

varicose vein superficial veins that have become enlarged and deformed, usually caused by dysfunctioning venous valves.

varus bending inward.

video signal electronic representation of an optical scene produced by an orderly scanning pattern across a photosensitive element in a television camera. A video signal conforms to a particular standard and contains a series of synchronization pulses to allow display.

viscus any large interior organ in any part of the four great body cavities, especially those in the abdomen.

vocedure interference designed to accomplish a goal. Commonly used to refer to angiographic procedures that repair a pre-existing condition.

voxel represents a volume of tissue being scanned; consists of a pixel and has an extension of depth.

window level operator-selected raw digital image sample value mapped to the center gray scale value of the dynamic range of the display monitor; center of the range of Houndsfield unit displayed; range of the raw digital image sample values mapped to the dynamic range of the monitor.

window width range of the raw digital image sample values mapped to the dynamic range of the monitor; range of displayed Houndsfield units.

windowing the selection of range of digital image quantization values to be displayed within the dynamic range of the display monitor. Those digital image values outside this range are displayed as white or black.

xenon a gas; the isotope of xenon is used to demonstrate the functioning of the lungs in radionuclide imaging.

Index

Page numbers followed by *f* and *t* are for figures and tables respectively

F

G

M

P

Q

R

T

V

W

X

Z